Clinical Asthma

Enormous progress in asthma research has been made in the past 50 years, including a greater understanding of its complex pathogenesis and new and more effective therapies. Consequently, the scientific literature has grown vast and can be difficult to integrate. With contributions from a distinguished panel of world-renowned authors, the Second Edition of ***Clinical Asthma: Theory and Practice*** presents a comprehensive study of both the common and the more challenging problems faced by all healthcare personnel who treat patients with asthma.

The book is divided into seven sections, starting with the basics of asthma and ending with a discussion on the approach to asthma worldwide and in the primary care setting. Reflecting a strong clinical emphasis, each chapter begins with a patient case study supported by essential background information on the basic science and clinical decision-making process. This is followed by a discussion of clinical evaluation and management.

The multidisciplinary coverage explores a range of topics including genetics, inflammation, immunology, and the identification of different endotypes. Using a bench-to-bedside approach, the book links basic science to the clinical management of asthma and explores options for improvement. The carefully selected authorship from experts worldwide presents a truly global outlook.

Jonathan A. Bernstein, MD, FAAAAI, FACAAI, FACP, FACCP
Professor of Medicine, University of Cincinnati, Department of Internal Medicine, Division of Rheumatology, Allergy and Immunology; Partner Advanced Allergy Services, LLC; Partner Bernstein Clinical Research Center, Cincinnati, Ohio

Mark L. Levy, MBChB (Pret), FRCGP
Semi-Retired General Practitioner in London, United Kingdom, with a special interest in asthma. Currently a General Practice Appraiser, London; Member of the Board of Directors and Chair of the Dissemination Working Group of the Global Initiative for Asthma (GINA)

CLINICAL ASTHMA

THEORY AND PRACTICE

Second Edition

Edited by

Jonathan A. Bernstein, MD, FAAAAI, FACAAI, FACP, FACCP

Professor of Medicine, University of Cincinnati, Department of Internal Medicine, Division of Rheumatology, Allergy and Immunology; Partner Advanced Allergy Services, LLC; Partner Bernstein Clinical Research Center, Cincinnati, Ohio

Mark L. Levy, MBChB (Pret), FRCGP

Semi-Retired General Practitioner in London, United Kingdom, with a special interest in asthma. Currently a General Practice Appraiser, London; Member of the Board of Directors and Chair of the Dissemination Working Group of the Global Initiative for Asthma (GINA)

CRC Press
Taylor & Francis Group
Boca Raton London New York

CRC Press is an imprint of the
Taylor & Francis Group, an **informa** business

Second edition published 2026
by CRC Press
2385 NW Executive Center Drive, Suite 320, Boca Raton FL 33431

and by CRC Press
4 Park Square, Milton Park, Abingdon, Oxon, OX14 4RN

CRC Press is an imprint of Taylor & Francis Group, LLC

First edition published by CRC Press 2014

ISBN: 978-1-032-26225-3 (hbk)
ISBN: 978-1-032-26230-7 (pbk)
ISBN: 978-1-003-28720-9 (ebk)

DOI: 10.1201/9781003287209

Typeset in Times
by Apex CoVantage, LLC

This book is dedicated to my wife Lisa of 42 years, our 4 children and their spouses (Alison and Danny; Joshua and Kayla; Rebecca and Ronnie; and Caren and Robb and our 7 grandchildren (Micah, Miri, Ezra, Ruby, Leo, Shai, Maya) + 1 (Liv) who passed away at 2 months of age. I am grateful for their love and support.
Jonathan A. Bernstein

This book is for Celia with thanks for the last 51 years.
Mark L. Levy

Contents

SECTION VI Asthma and Special Populations

SECTION VII Approach to Asthma Worldwide and in the Primary Care Setting

About the Editors

Jonathan A. Bernstein, MD, is Professor of Clinical Medicine in the Department of Internal Medicine, Division of Rheumatology, Allergy and Immunology at the University of Cincinnati Medical Center and a partner of Advanced Allergy Services and Bernstein Clinical Research Center. He received his MD from the University of Cincinnati College of Medicine (1981–1985), completed his residency in Internal Medicine at the Cleveland Clinic Hospital (1985–1988) and Allergy/Clinical Immunology training at Northwestern University (1988–1990). He has been a faculty member of UC since 1990. He is the immediate past president of the AAAAI (2022–2023). He is also a member of the Joint Task Force Guideline committee, the WAO board of directors, President of Interasma, GINA advocacy council, HAEA organization medical advisory board, and WE CU patient advocacy organization. He is a member of the Cincinnati Alpha Lambda Omega society. Dr. Bernstein is a DIA-certified clinical trial investigator and conducting multicenter and physician-initiated clinical therapeutic trials for a number of clinical conditions including asthma, chronic urticaria, hereditary angioedema, atopic dermatitis, and systemic mastocytosis and is considered a key opinion leader in these areas. He was the editor-in-chief of the *Journal of Asthma* from 2009 to 2022 and is currently on the editorial board for the *Journal of Allergy Clinical Immunology*; *Journal of Allergy in Practice*; *Annals of Allergy, Asthma & Immunology;* and *Allergy Proceedings*. Dr. Bernstein is the recipient of many awards, including the Distinguished Clinician Awards from the AAAAI and World Allergy Organization (2019). He is currently an author or coauthor of over 510 scientific articles and five books pertaining to asthma, rhinitis, and immunodeficiency. Dr. Bernstein is actively involved with the University of Cincinnati Allergy Fellowship Training Program in the education of fellows and also teaches residents and medical students. Dr. Bernstein has been voted "Best Doctor" in Cincinnati from 1999 to 2025 by *Cincinnati* magazine and has been ranked by *US News & World Report* as being in the top 1% of doctors in his specialty. He is director or codirector for several centers of excellence in Cincinnati, including the WAO center of excellence, the American Initiative for Mast Cell Diseases (AIM), Urticaria Centers of Excellence and Reference (UCARE), Angioedema Centers of Excellence and Reference Care (ACARE), Atopic Dermatitis Centers of Excellence and Reference Care (ADCARE), and Anaphylaxis Centers of Excellence and Reference Care (ANACARE).

Mark L. Levy, FRCGP, did his medical training in South Africa where he lived until 1977. He has been a United Kingdom (UK) General Practitioner for over 45 years, was a GP trainer for 13 years, and was an expert assessor for the National Clinical Assessment service in England for 6 years. He was a voluntary first line responder for the London Ambulance service for six years. His interest in respiratory disease started in medical school, followed by six months working in a respiratory intensive care unit in Johannesburg, and has since developed a special interest in asthma. He has authored and coauthored over 180 papers and six books on asthma. He was one of the six founder members, first chairman and past editor of the Primary Care Respiratory Society UK (formerly the GPIAG), and is currently Editor Emeritus for the *NPJ Primary Care Respiratory Medicine journal.* He was Clinical Lead for the UK National Review of Asthma Deaths (NRAD) (2011–2014) and has since been expert witness for coroners in preventable asthma deaths. He was a member of the UK acute asthma guidelines (BTS/SIGN) from 1992 to 2017 and is currently an Executive Board member and Chair of the Dissemination Working Group of the annually updated, evidence-based Global Initiative on Asthma (GINA, www.ginasthma.org). He was Clinical Lead for the NHS England Data and Digital Transformation program workstream for children and young people and currently is an adviser for the UK All Party Parliamentary Respiratory Group on asthma, COPD, and allergy.

X: @bigcatdoc, BlueSky: markllevy.bsky.social, Ln: https://www.linkedin.com/nhome/?trk=

Asthma Spotlight Podcast: https://bigcatdoc.com/prevent-asthma-attacks-and-asthma-deaths/; also on Spotify and Apple podcasts

Webs and Full CV: www.bigcatdoc.com

Contributors

Engi Ahmed
PhyMedExp
University of Montpellier
Montpellier, France

Neil E. Alexis
Department of Pediatrics
UNC Chapel Hill
Chapel Hill, North Carolina, USA

Leonard B. Bacharier
Department of Pediatrics
Division of Allergy, Immunology and Pulmonary Medicine
Monroe Carell Jr Children's Hospital
Vanderbilt University Medical Center
Nashville, Tennessee, USA

Alan P. Baptist
Division of Allergy and Clinical Immunology
University of Michigan School of Medicine
Ann Arbor, Michigan, USA

Sachin Baxi
Harvard Medical School, Division of Immunology
Boston Children's Hospital
Boston, Massachusetts, USA

Joshua S. Bernstein
University of Cincinnati
College of Medicine
Cincinnati, Ohio, USA

Clément Boissin
PhyMedExp
University of Montpellier
Montpellier, France

Louis-Philippe Boulet
Department of Medicine
Laval University
and
Québec Heart and Lung Institute
Québec, Canada

Arnaud Bourdin
PhyMedExp
University of Montpellier
Montpellier, France

Jean-Marie Bruzzese
Columbia University School of Nursing
New York, New York, USA

Andrew Bush
Professor of Paediatrics and Paediatric Respirology
Imperial College
and
Director of Imperial Centre for Paediatrics and Child Health
and
Consultant Paediatric Chest Physician
Royal Brompton Hospital
London, UK

Chris Carlsten
Respiratory Medicine Division
The University of British Columbia
Vancouver, Canada

Thomas B. Casale
Morsani College of Medicine
University of South Florida
Division of Allergy and Immunology
Tampa, Florida, USA

Jérémy Charriot
PhyMedExp
University of Montpellier
Montpellier, France

Laura Chen
Yale School of Medicine
New Haven, Connecticut, USA

Chris J. Corrigan
King's College London
School of Medicine
London, UK

Álvaro Augusto Cruz
Faculdade de Medicina da Universidade Federal da Bahia
Salvador, Brazil

Sarah Diver
Department of Respiratory Sciences
University of Leicester
Leicester, UK

Liesbeth Duijts
Erasmus University Rotterdam
Rotterdam, The Netherlands

Tolly E.G. Epstein
Division of Immunology, Allergy, and Rheumatology
University of Cincinnati School of Medicine
Cincinnati, Ohio, USA
and
Allergy Partners of Central Indiana
Indianapolis, Indiana, USA

Louise Fleming
Professor of Practice, Paediatric Respiratory Medicine
Imperial College London
and
Consultant Respiratory Paediatrician
Imperial College Healthcare NHS Trust and Royal Brompton Hospital
London, UK

Peter G. Gibson
School of Medicine and Public Health
The University of Newcastle
Newcastle, Australia

Krystelle Godbout
University Institute of Cardiology and Pulmonology
Laval University
Quebec, Canada

Justin Greiwe
Bernstein Allergy Group, Inc.
and
Division of Immunology/Allergy Section
Department of Internal Medicine
The University of Cincinnati College of Medicine
Cincinnati, Ohio, USA

Pranabashis Haldar
Department of Respiratory Sciences
University of Leicester
Leicester, UK

Bart Hilvering
Amsterdam University Medical Center
Respiratory Medicine and Experimental Immunology
Academic Medical Center
University of Amsterdam
Amsterdam, The Netherlands

Chi Yan Hui
The University of Edinburgh
Edinburgh, UK

Laureen Hurault
PhyMedExp
University of Montpellier
Montpellier, France

Alan G. Kaplan
Department of Family and Community Medicine
University of Toronto
Toronto, Canada

Tarik Karramass
Erasmus University Rotterdam
Rotterdam, The Netherlands

Federico Lavorini
Department of Experimental and Clinical Medicine
University of Florence
Florence, Italy

Adam Lawton
Great Ormond Street Hospital
London, UK

Deborah Lee
Division of Allergy and Clinical Immunology
University of Michigan School of Medicine
Ann Arbor, Michigan, USA

Jenny J. Lee
Division of Allergy and Clinical Immunology
University of Michigan School of Medicine
Ann Arbor, Michigan, USA

René Lutter
Amsterdam University Medical Center
Respiratory Medicine and Experimental Immunology
Academic Medical Center
University of Amsterdam
Amsterdam, The Netherlands

Luane Marques de Mello
Ribeirão Preto Medical School
University of São Paulo
São Paulo, Brazil

Vanessa M. McDonald
NHMRC Centre of Research Excellence in Severe Asthma
The Centre of Research Excellence in Asthma Treatable Traits
The Priority Research Centre for Healthy Lungs
The University of Newcastle
Newcastle, Australia

Alison C. McLeish
Department of Psychological and Brain Sciences
University of Louisville
Louisville, Kentucky, USA

Kirsten R. Murray
The University of Newcastle
Newcastle, Australia

S. Shahzad Mustafa
Rochester Regional Health
Rochester, New York, USA

Anil Nanda
Asthma and Allergy Center
Lewisville and Flower Mound
and
Division of Allergy and Immunology
University of Texas Southwestern Medical Center
Dallas, Texas, USA

Sharmilee M. Nyenhuis
Division of Pulmonary, Critical Care, Sleep and Allergy
Department of Medicine
University of Illinois at Chicago
and
Center for Dissemination and Implementation Science
Department of Medicine
University of Illinois at Chicago
Chicago, Illinois, USA

Andrew Nyman
Consultant Paediatric Intensivist
Evelina London Children's Hospital
Guy's and St Thomas's NHS Foundation Trust
London, UK

Paul M. O'Byrne
Firestone Institute for Respiratory Health
St. Joseph's Hospital
and
Department of Medicine
McMaster University
Hamilton, Ontario, Canada

Sara Patrawala
Department of Medicine, Allergy/Immunology and Rheumatology
University of Rochester Medical Center
Rochester, New York, USA

Wanda Phipatanakul
Harvard Medical School, Division of Immunology
Boston Children's Hospital
Boston, Massachusetts, USA

Hilary Pinnock
Usher Institute
College of Medicine and Veterinary Medicine
The University of Edinburgh
Edinburgh, UK

Meghan E. Rebuli
University of North Carolina
School of Medicine
Chapel Hill, North Carolina, USA

Richard Russell
Lymington New Forest Hospital
and
Hampshire Community Integrated Respiratory Service
and
Respiratory Medicine Department
University of Oxford
Oxford, UK

Glenis K. Scadding
University College London
Division of Infection and Immunity
London, UK

Guy Scadding
National Heart and Lung Institute
Imperial College London
London, UK

Anchalee Senavonge
BNH Allergy and Asthma Center
Bangkok Nursing Home Hospital
and
Department of Pediatrics, Faculty of Medicine
Chulalongkorn University
Bangkok, Thailand

Syed Ahmar Shah
Usher Institute
College of Medicine and Veterinary Medicine
The University of Edinburgh
Edinburgh, UK

Beverley J. Sheares
Yale School of Medicine
New Haven, Connecticut, USA

Aziz Sheikh
Usher Institute
College of Medicine and Veterinary Medicine
The University of Edinburgh
Edinburgh, UK

Colin Simpson
Wellington Faculty of Health
Te Herenga Waka–Victoria University of Wellington
Willington, New Zealand

Andrew M. Smith
Allergy Associates of Utah
Murray, Utah, USA

Alessandra Sorano
Department of Experimental and Clinical Medicine
University of Florence
Florence, Italy

Jeffrey R. Stokes
Department of Pediatrics
Division of Allergy, Immunology, and Pulmonary Medicine
Washington University School of Medicine
and
St. Louis Children's Hospital
St. Louis, Missouri, USA

Isabelle Vachier
PhyMedExp
University of Montpellier
Montpellier, France

Job F.M. van Boven
Faculty of Medical Sciences
University of Groningen
Groningen, The Netherlands

Barbara P. Yawn
University of South Dakota
School of Medicine
Vermillion, South Dakota, USA
and
University of Minnesota
School of Medicine
Minneapolis, Minnesota, USA

Arzu Yorgancioglu
Celal Bayar University
Department of Chest Diseases
Manisa, Turkey

Anna Zhang
Tufts Children's Hospital
and
Boston Children's Hospital
Boston, Massachusetts, USA

Preface

Asthma is an enigma. Despite its formal recognition in medical texts for more than a millennium, we still lack a single, unequivocal test or biomarker to confirm the diagnosis. Instead, we rely on clinical history, physiological testing, and a handful of biomarkers—many of which provide limited insight into the underlying disease process. This diagnostic ambiguity is especially striking when juxtaposed against the sheer prevalence of the condition: Asthma affects nearly 1 in 30 individuals globally. Most people, even those outside the medical field, know someone who experiences asthma symptoms—whether or not they carry the formal label of "asthma."

While our understanding of asthma's pathobiology continues to evolve, it remains incomplete. Nonetheless, the clinical imperative to recognize and manage asthma is undeniable. Asthma does not manifest uniformly. Instead, it presents in diverse forms that may mimic other respiratory illnesses or appear subtly in ways that only a physician's experience and clinical insight can decipher. For healthcare professionals—particularly those in general practice, pediatrics, allergy, pulmonology, and emergency care—having a nuanced, practical approach to asthma is not optional; it is essential.

This is why the second edition of *Clinical Asthma: Theory and Practice* by Jonathan Bernstein and Mark Levy is such a valuable contribution. More than a didactic text, this book is grounded in the clinical realities of asthma care. Most of its 27 chapters are anchored by a case vignette, bringing the patient's experience into focus and setting the stage for a discussion that integrates current biological understanding with real-world therapeutic guidance.

The case-based format not only enhances engagement but also reinforces the variability of asthma and the necessity of individualized treatment. This book serves both as a reference and as a guide for practitioners who seek to move beyond textbook definitions and treat the person—not just the disease. It belongs in the library of every clinician who encounters asthma in their practice.

Jeffrey M. Drazen, MD

Section I

Basics of Asthma

1 Understanding Asthma
A Global Epidemiological Perspective

Syed Ahmar Shah, Aziz Sheikh, and Colin Simpson

1.1 INTRODUCTION

Epidemiology focuses on understanding the causes, distribution, occurrence, and patterns of diseases within populations. Epidemiologists are particularly concerned with defining diseases and their subtypes, as well as identifying data sources to calculate both numerators and denominators for determining disease frequency, patterns, and outcomes (1).

Asthma is now recognised as one of the most prevalent chronic conditions globally, causing considerable morbidity and, in some cases, mortality. Its prevalence has increased over recent decades (2), particularly in countries adopting westernised lifestyles, with recent studies indicating that asthma affects approximately 262 million individuals globally (3).

This chapter represents a comprehensive update to the original publication in 2014 (4). It incorporates the latest epidemiological data, research findings, and evolving understanding of asthma's global impact over the past decade. This revision reflects significant advancements in our knowledge of asthma prevalence, risk factors, and outcomes, providing an up-to-date perspective on this complex and widespread condition.

The economic impact of asthma is substantial. In the United States, the total cost of asthma—including direct medical costs and indirect costs due to lost productivity—was estimated at $81.9 billion in 2013 (5). Furthermore, uncontrolled asthma is projected to cost the US economy approximately $300.6 billion in direct medical costs over the next 20 years (2019–2038) (6). When considering indirect costs, the overall economic burden of uncontrolled asthma in the US is expected to reach a staggering $963.5 billion during this same period (6).

Health-wise, a recent study based on the Global Burden of Disease (GBD) estimated that asthma caused an annual loss of 21.55 million disability-adjusted life years (DALYs) in 2019 (7). In the US, it is projected that uncontrolled asthma will result in a loss of 15.46 million quality-adjusted life years (QALYs) over the next two decades (6). Asthma remains the most common chronic childhood disorder and significantly impacts children's lives by leading to school absences, regular medication use, and hospital admissions (6).

1.2 DEFINITIONS OF ASTHMA

Asthma is a complex, heterogeneous disorder characterised by chronic airway inflammation, variable airflow obstruction, and bronchial hyperresponsiveness (8). While our understanding of asthma has evolved significantly since the 19th century, a comprehensive definition remains elusive due to the condition's multifaceted nature and diverse clinical presentations (9).

The Global Initiative for Asthma (GINA) defines asthma as "a heterogeneous disease, usually characterised by chronic airway inflammation. It is defined by the history of respiratory symptoms such as wheeze, shortness of breath, chest tightness and cough that vary over time and in intensity, together with variable expiratory airflow limitation" (8).

Diagnosing asthma remains challenging due to its variable and intermittent nature (8). In preschool-age children, differentiating between viral-associated wheeze and other causes of wheezing is crucial (10). For adults, conditions such as vocal cord dysfunction, chronic obstructive pulmonary disease (COPD), and occupational asthma must be considered (11).

Recent research has highlighted the importance of biomarkers in asthma diagnosis and management (12). Type 2 inflammation, characterised by elevated levels of interleukin-4, interleukin-5, and interleukin-13, is now recognised as a key feature in many asthma phenotypes (13). Fractional exhaled nitric oxide (FeNO) testing has emerged as a valuable tool for assessing airway inflammation and guiding treatment decisions (14).

Clinicians typically diagnose asthma based on a combination of (8, 9, 15):

1. Patient history of characteristic symptoms (e.g. cough, wheeze, breathlessness);
2. Objective evidence of variable airflow limitation, measured through spirometry or peak expiratory flow rates;
3. Bronchial provocation tests using agents such as methacholine, mannitol, or exercise; and
4. Response to asthma medications, particularly inhaled corticosteroids and bronchodilators.

In primary care settings, symptom assessment and response to bronchodilators often guide initial diagnosis (8, 9). However, there's growing emphasis on confirming the diagnosis with objective tests to avoid misdiagnosis and the potential for unnecessary treatment (16).

The concept of treatable traits in asthma has gained traction, focusing on identifying specific characteristics that can guide targeted therapies (17). Recent guidelines stress the importance of assessing both symptom control and

DOI: 10.1201/9781003287209-2

future risk when managing asthma (8, 18). This includes evaluating factors such as exacerbation history, lung function, and comorbidities to guide treatment decisions (8, 18).

These updates reflect the evolving understanding of asthma as a complex, heterogeneous condition requiring a nuanced approach to diagnosis and management.

1.3 ASTHMA PHENOTYPES AND ENDOTYPES

Our understanding of asthma has evolved significantly in recent years, moving beyond a one-size-fits-all approach to recognising distinct phenotypes and endotypes. Asthma phenotypes are observable characteristics of the disease, such as symptom patterns and response to treatment, while endotypes refer to the underlying biological mechanisms or pathways driving these observable traits. Modern asthma research has shifted focus from a binary classification (intrinsic vs. extrinsic) to recognising multiple phenotypes and endotypes, each with distinct pathophysiological mechanisms (19). This complexity underscores the need for personalised approaches to diagnosis and treatment (15).

Current research recognises several key phenotypes:

- **Early-Onset Allergic Asthma:** This phenotype typically begins in childhood and is associated with allergies and elevated IgE levels. It is often characterised by type 2 inflammation, driven by T-helper type 2 (Th2) cells and involving cytokines such as IL-4, IL-5, and IL–13 (19, 20).
- **Late-Onset Eosinophilic Asthma:** More common in adults, particularly women, this phenotype is characterised by persistent eosinophilic inflammation despite high-dose corticosteroid treatment. It often involves thickening of the airway basement membrane and can be associated with nasal polyps and aspirin sensitivity (20, 21).
- **Exercise-Induced Bronchoconstriction (EIB):** While not exclusively an asthma phenotype, EIB can occur in individuals with or without underlying asthma. It involves airway narrowing triggered by sustained exercise, likely due to airway cooling and dehydration (22).
- **Obesity-Associated Asthma:** This phenotype is characterised by less eosinophilic inflammation and a poor response to standard asthma treatments. It may involve mechanical factors and systemic inflammation related to adipose tissue (23).
- **Neutrophilic Asthma:** Associated with more severe disease and relative corticosteroid resistance, this phenotype involves neutrophilic airway inflammation. It may be linked to environmental factors such as air pollution or bacterial endotoxins (24).
- **Aspirin-Exacerbated Respiratory Disease (AERD):** This distinct phenotype involves asthma, chronic rhinosinusitis with nasal polyps, and respiratory reactions to aspirin and other nonsteroidal anti-inflammatory drugs (NSAIDs). It's associated with increased production of pro-inflammatory leukotrienes (21).
- **Infection-Associated Asthma:** Respiratory infections, particularly viral infections, can trigger asthma exacerbations and may play a role in asthma development. This phenotype may involve altered immune responses to pathogens (25).
- **Severe Asthma:** This heterogeneous group includes patients with persistent symptoms and exacerbations despite high-dose treatment. It may encompass several underlying endotypes and requires careful evaluation for targeted therapies (18).

Recent advances in molecular and genetic studies have further refined our understanding of asthma endotypes. Genetic variations in the IL-33 pathway have been strongly associated with eosinophilic inflammation in asthma. For instance, a loss-of-function mutation in the IL-33 gene was identified in patients and associated with reduced blood eosinophils and protection from asthma (26).

Polymorphisms in human IL-33 and ST2 genes have been shown to be associated with increased numbers of eosinophils (27). Furthermore, IL-33 has been found to significantly promote eosinophil survival and upregulate the expression of adhesion molecules like ICAM-1 on eosinophils (27). While the association between IL-1β pathway variations and neutrophilic inflammation is less direct, research has shown that neutrophilic asthma is characterised by distinct genetic and molecular features. For example, α-defensins, neutrophil cathepsin G, and neutrophil elastase genes are significantly increased in neutrophilic asthma (28). Additionally, S100A9, a calcium-binding protein, is associated with neutrophilic asthma (29).

Understanding these diverse phenotypes and endotypes is crucial for implementing precision medicine approaches in asthma management. It allows for more targeted use of biologicals and other advanced therapies such as CRISPR gene editing (30), potentially improving outcomes for patients with severe or difficult-to-treat asthma (15, 18).

1.4 KEY MEASURES, STUDY DESIGNS EMPLOYED, AND DATA SOURCES AVAILABLE

Epidemiologists employ various study designs and data sources to estimate the frequency and patterns of asthma, understand its aetiology, and assess outcomes. Recent advancements have expanded our toolkit for studying asthma epidemiology, allowing for more comprehensive and nuanced investigations (1, 31–33).

1.4.1 Key Measures of Disease Frequency

Several measures are used to quantify the frequency and impact of asthma in populations:

1. **Incidence:** The rate of occurrence of new asthma cases in a period of time

2. **Cumulative Incidence:** The number of new asthma cases divided by the population at risk
3. **Person-Time Incidence:** The number of new asthma cases divided by the person-time at risk
4. **Point Prevalence:** The proportion of a population with asthma at one point in time
5. **Period Prevalence:** The proportion of people with asthma presenting during a period of time, usually one year
6. **Lifetime (Ever) Prevalence:** The proportion of people in a population who have ever been diagnosed with asthma
7. **Case Fatality Ratio:** The proportion of people diagnosed with asthma who die from it, within a specific time period after diagnosis
8. **Disability-Adjusted Life Years (DALYs):** A measure that combines years of life lost due to premature mortality and years lived with disability due to asthma

These measures help researchers and policymakers understand the burden of asthma, track changes over time, and evaluate the effectiveness of interventions and treatments.

1.4.2 Study Designs Commonly Employed

Study designs commonly used in asthma epidemiology include cohort studies, cross-sectional surveys, case-control studies, ecological studies, and interrupted time series analysis (31, 34–43). Each design has its strengths and limitations for investigating asthma incidence, prevalence, risk factors, and outcomes.

Cohort Studies: Cohort studies remain crucial for identifying host and environmental influences on asthma development, incidence, and progression. These studies follow groups of individuals over time, allowing for the assessment of exposure effects on asthma incidence and outcomes (34). While traditionally expensive and time-consuming, advancements in data collection methods have made cohort studies more feasible.

Genome-Wide Association Studies (GWAS): GWAS have become increasingly important in asthma research, elucidating novel genes and markers associated with asthma susceptibility (44). These studies have opened new avenues for understanding asthma's genetic underpinnings and potential therapeutic targets.

Cross-Sectional Studies: Cross-sectional surveys continue to be valuable for assessing asthma prevalence and associated factors at a specific point in time (41). These studies are often cost-effective and can provide rapid insights into population-level asthma burden.

Case-Control Studies: Case-control studies remain useful for exploring risk factors, particularly for less common exposures or in resource-limited settings (42). These studies compare individuals with asthma to those without, examining past exposures to identify potential causal factors.

Ecological Studies: Ecological studies have gained prominence in asthma research, allowing for the investigation of environmental and socio-economic factors at the population level (45). These approaches help in understanding geographical variations in asthma prevalence and identifying area-level risk factors.

Interrupted Time Series Analysis: Interrupted time series (ITS) analysis is an effective method for assessing the impact of large-scale events or policy changes on asthma outcomes over time. For example, ITS analysis has been used to evaluate the impact of COVID-19 lockdowns on asthma exacerbations and the imposition of a soft drinks levy on childhood asthma-related hospital admissions (39, 40). By examining trends before and after these interventions, ITS helps isolate their specific impact on asthma outcomes. This design is particularly valuable for understanding both immediate and long-term effects of population-level interventions in real-world settings.

1.4.3 Data Sources

Data sources for asthma epidemiology have expanded significantly beyond traditional survey-based methods, offering researchers a rich array of information to study asthma prevalence, risk factors, and outcomes. This expansion has enabled more comprehensive and nuanced investigations into the complex nature of asthma across diverse populations. The integration of these varied data sources, coupled with advanced analytical techniques, is enhancing our understanding of asthma's aetiology, progression, and management (36, 46).

Key data sources in modern asthma epidemiology include:

1. **Global Population Surveys:** Large-scale international studies like the International Study of Asthma and Allergies in Childhood (ISAAC) and the European Community Respiratory Health Survey (ECRHS) provide valuable cross-national data on asthma prevalence and risk factors (41, 47).
2. **National Health Surveys:** Many countries conduct regular health surveys that include asthma-related questions, offering insights into national trends and population health needs (48).
3. **Electronic Health Records and Administrative Databases:** The growing availability of electronic health records and healthcare utilisation databases has transformed asthma epidemiology, enabling large-scale, longitudinal studies of real-world asthma patterns, healthcare costs, treatment patterns, and outcomes at a population level (49, 50).
4. **Biobanks and Genetic Databases:** These resources have become invaluable for studying genetic and environmental interactions in asthma (51).
5. **Mobile Health Technologies:** Emerging data collection methods, such as smartphone apps and wearable devices, offer new opportunities for real-time monitoring of asthma symptoms and environmental exposures (52, 53).

6. **Environmental Monitoring Data:** Integration of air quality and other environmental data with health outcomes has enhanced our understanding of environmental influences on asthma (52).

1.5 FREQUENCY OF ASTHMA

Asthma is a significant global health concern, affecting millions of people worldwide. Recent estimates indicate that approximately 262 million people are living with asthma globally, with prevalence rates varying considerably across different regions, populations, and time periods (3). Understanding these variations in asthma frequency is crucial for developing targeted prevention strategies and improving asthma management on a global scale.

1.5.1 Frequency of Asthma by Place

Global comparisons of asthma prevalence have been primarily determined by large-scale international studies, particularly the ISAAC and the ECRHS, with more recent data coming from the Global Burden of Disease (GBD) studies. Figure 1.1 illustrates the age-standardised prevalence of asthma per 100,000 populations in 2019, highlighting significant regional variations in asthma burden globally.

The ISAAC Phase Three study, conducted between 2000 and 2003, provided comprehensive data on global asthma prevalence (54). This study involved approximately 1,200,000 children from 233 centres in 98 countries. The study revealed that, for adolescents aged 13–14 years, the global prevalence of current asthma symptoms (wheeze in

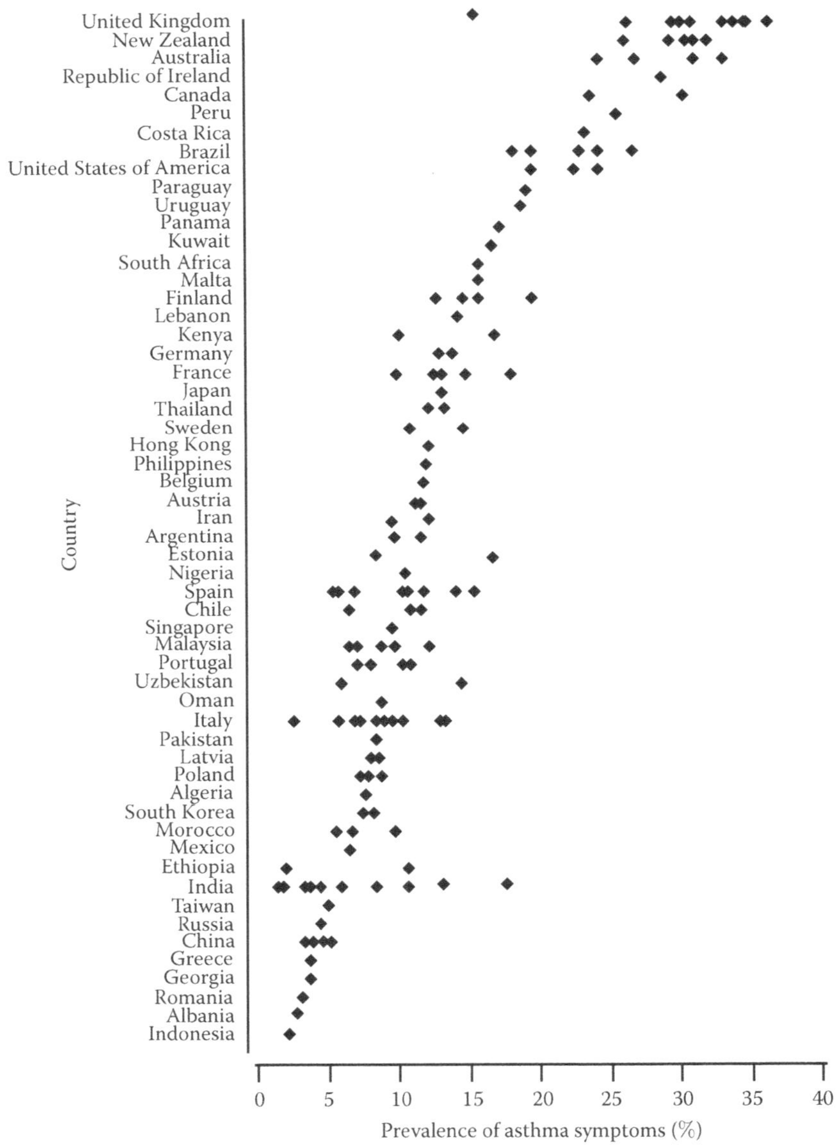

FIGURE 1.1 Age-standardized prevalence of asthma per 100,000 population in 2019. (This figure is reproduced from the study by Wang et al. [7] under the terms of the Creative Commons CC BY license, which allows for unrestricted use, distribution, and reproduction in any medium, as long as the original work is properly cited.)

the last 12 months) was 14.1%. Additionally, for children aged 6–7 years, the global prevalence of current asthma symptoms was 11.7%.

More recent estimates combine data from several population-based studies and modelling provides updated data (33). The global prevalence of current asthma in 2019 was estimated at 5.4% (95% CI: 3.2–9.0) for people aged 5–69 years. This translates to approximately 357.4 million (95% CI: 213.0–590.8) cases worldwide.

There are large regional variations in asthma prevalence across different parts of the world (33). The African Region showed the highest prevalence of current wheezing at 13.2% (95% CI: 10.5–16.5) among individuals aged 5–69 years. In contrast, the Americas Region had the lowest prevalence at 10.0% (95% CI: 8.0–12.5). Additionally, high-income countries (HICs) generally exhibited a slightly higher prevalence (12.1%, 95% CI: 9.7–15.2) compared to low- and middle-income countries (LMICs), where the prevalence was 11.0% (95% CI: 8.8–13.8).

Country-specific data from recent studies reveal significant variations in asthma prevalence (55). In countries such as India, Taiwan, Kosovo, Nigeria, and Russia, the prevalence rates range from 1.3% to 5.9% (55). Conversely, higher rates are observed in Costa Rica, Honduras, New Zealand, Kingdom of Saudi Arabia, Brazil, and Spain, where prevalence ranges from 11.6% to 29.0% (55). The ECRHS findings, focusing on young adults, remain relevant and show similar patterns of variation, with higher rates in English-speaking countries (56).

Moreover, studies indicate significant differences in asthma prevalence between urban and rural areas. A systematic review found that the risk of asthma is higher in urban environments, with a relative risk of 1.3 (95% CI, 1.1–1.4) (57). Additionally, research in Nigeria reported an age-adjusted prevalence of asthma at 3.4% in urban areas compared to just 0.5% in rural regions, highlighting the increased odds of asthma associated with urban living (58).

These international studies consistently highlight significant global variations in asthma prevalence, suggesting that environmental, genetic, and lifestyle factors play crucial roles in the development and expression of asthma. The persistence of these patterns across different studies and time periods underscores the complex, multifactorial nature of asthma aetiology and the need for targeted, region-specific approaches to asthma prevention and management.

1.5.2 Frequency of Asthma by People

The prevalence of asthma varies significantly across different demographic groups, with notable differences based on age, sex, race/ethnicity, and socio-economic factors.

Age and Sex Differences: Asthma prevalence exhibits a distinct pattern across age groups and between sexes. In children, asthma is more prevalent in boys than girls. Recent data from the American Lung Association shows that among children, current asthma rates are higher for males (7.0%) compared to females (5.4%) (59). However, this trend reverses in adulthood, with females (10.8%) more likely than males (6.5%) to have current asthma (59).

The shift in prevalence from male to female predominance occurs around puberty, suggesting a role for sex hormones in asthma pathogenesis (60–62). The Childhood Asthma Management Program (CAMP) study found that asthma symptoms in girls increased around age 10, coinciding with the onset of puberty, while symptoms in boys declined (63).

Race and Ethnicity: Significant disparities in asthma prevalence exist among different racial and ethnic groups. In, for example, the United States, Black individuals (10.3%) have higher current asthma rates compared to White individuals (8.4%) (59). Hispanic individuals generally have lower rates (6.7%), except for Puerto Rican individuals, who have the highest rate among all racial/ethnic groups at 14.0% (59).

Socio-Economic Factors: Asthma prevalence is inversely related to family income. In 2022, the highest rates (11.3%) were observed among those with a family income below the poverty threshold (59). Additionally, health insurance coverage plays a role, with higher rates among adults on Medicaid compared to those with private insurance or no insurance (59).

Severe Asthma: Severe asthma, which affects approximately 5–10% of all people with asthma, shows distinct demographic patterns. Females are more likely to have severe asthma, particularly in the premenopausal years (60). However, this trend may reverse after menopause, with some studies showing increased severity in older males (60).

These demographic patterns highlight the complex interplay of genetic, hormonal, environmental, and socio-economic factors in asthma prevalence and severity. Understanding these variations is crucial for developing targeted prevention strategies and improving asthma management across different population groups.

1.5.3 Frequency of Asthma Over Time

Tracking trends in asthma incidence and prevalence is crucial for understanding the disease's aetiology and developing effective prevention strategies. While the 20th century saw a well-documented increase in asthma prevalence, recent studies suggest a more complex picture of asthma trends globally.

The Global Asthma Network (GAN) Phase I cross-sectional study, conducted between 2015 and 2020, provides the most recent comprehensive data on global asthma trends amongst school-aged children (41). This study, which included 119,795 participants from 27 centres in 14 countries, revealed:

1. About 1 in 10 individuals in both childhood (6–7 years) and adolescent (13–14 years) age groups reported wheeze in the preceding year.
2. Over a 27-year period (1993–2020), adolescents showed a significant decrease in severe asthma

symptoms (−0.4 percentage points per decade, 95% CI −0.7 to −0.04).
3. An increase in lifetime asthma prevalence (1.3 percentage points per decade, 95% CI 0.7–1.8) and night cough (4.3 percentage points per decade, 95% CI 3.1–5.4) was observed in adolescents, with similar trends in children.

The study also found that trends varied by country income level, with low-income countries showing a decrease in current wheeze prevalence, lower-middle-income countries experiencing an increase, and upper-middle-income and high-income countries showing stable prevalence rates (41).

These findings contrast with earlier studies like ISAAC Phase Three (1999–2004), which reported increases in asthma symptom prevalence in many centres, particularly in the 6–7 year age group (64). The ISAAC study found that increases were twice as common as decreases, suggesting a continuing rise in global asthma burden.

These recent findings suggest that, while the global burden of asthma remains high, the trends are not uniform across regions and age groups. The apparent stabilisation or even decrease in some high-income countries may reflect improvements in asthma management and environmental interventions. However, the rising prevalence in some lower-middle-income countries is concerning and warrants further investigation.

It's important to note that interpreting these trends is challenging due to various factors, including changes in diagnostic criteria, healthcare access, and environmental conditions. Additionally, the COVID-19 pandemic may have impacted recent asthma trends, although its full effects are yet to be fully understood (50).

Future research should focus on understanding the drivers of these divergent trends, particularly in different socio-economic contexts, to inform targeted prevention and management strategies.

1.6 RISK FACTORS FOR ASTHMA

Asthma is a complex disease with multifactorial aetiology, involving interactions between genetic predisposition and environmental exposures. Recent research has further elucidated the role of various risk factors in asthma development and exacerbation.

Genetic Factors: GWAS have identified several genetic variants associated with asthma risk. A GWAS study, which analysed data from 376,358 British White individuals from the UK Biobank, identified 61 independent asthma loci (65). Of these, 23 were specific to childhood-onset asthma, one was specific to adult-onset asthma, and 37 were shared between both forms.

Environmental Factors:

1. **Air Pollution:** Recent studies have strengthened the evidence linking air pollution to asthma development and exacerbations. Long-term exposure to traffic-related air pollution, particularly fine particulate matter (PM2.5) and nitrogen dioxide (NO_2), is associated with increased asthma incidence in children (43).
2. **Allergens:** House dust mites, pet dander, and pollen remain significant risk factors (66). Climate change is altering pollen seasons, potentially increasing allergen exposure (67).
3. **Early-Life Exposures:** The hygiene hypothesis has evolved into the "microbiome hypothesis." Reduced microbial diversity in early life, influenced by factors such as caesarean delivery and antibiotic use, may increase asthma risk (68).
4. **Occupational Exposures:** Over 300 substances have been identified as occupational asthmagens (69). Recent research has focused on various occupational exposures, including those in healthcare settings, that may contribute to the development of occupational asthma (70).
5. **Tobacco Smoke:** Both active smoking and second-hand smoke exposure remain significant risk factors. E-cigarette use has emerged as a potential concern, with some studies suggesting increased asthma risk in adolescents (71).

Lifestyle Factors:

1. **Obesity:** The relationship between obesity and asthma has been further clarified. Obesity is now recognised as both a risk factor for asthma development and a modifier of asthma severity (72).
2. **Diet:** While the evidence for specific dietary interventions remains mixed, a Mediterranean diet rich in fruits, vegetables, and omega-3 fatty acids may have protective effects against asthma (73).
3. **Physical Activity:** Regular physical activity may reduce asthma risk and improve symptoms in those with existing asthma, possibly through anti-inflammatory effects (74, 75).

Emerging Risk Factors:

1. **Stress and Psychological Factors:** Chronic stress and adverse childhood experiences have been associated with increased asthma risk and worse outcomes in those with asthma (76).
2. **Vitamin D Deficiency:** Low vitamin D levels have been linked to increased asthma risk and severity, though the benefits of supplementation remain unclear (77).
3. **Maternal Factors:** Maternal obesity, gestational diabetes, and certain medications during pregnancy have been associated with increased asthma risk in offspring (78).

Understanding these risk factors is crucial for developing targeted prevention strategies and personalised treatment approaches. Future research should focus on elucidating the complex interactions between these factors and identifying modifiable targets for intervention.

1.7 OUTCOMES (MORBIDITY, HEALTHCARE UTILISATION, MORTALITY)

Monitoring asthma outcomes is crucial for assessing the effectiveness of management strategies and identifying areas for improvement in asthma care. Key outcomes at the population level include asthma exacerbations, healthcare utilisation, and mortality rates.

Global Mortality: Recent estimates indicate that asthma-related deaths remain significant despite some improvements. According to a comprehensive study on the global, regional, and national burden of asthma, there were an estimated 461,070 (95% UI 366.58–559.01) deaths due to asthma in 2019 (7).

Morbidity and Healthcare Utilisation: Asthma continues to be a major cause of morbidity worldwide. According to a comprehensive study on the global, regional, and national burden of asthma, the *Global Burden of Disease* (*GBD*) 2019 study estimated that asthma caused approximately 21.6 million disability-adjusted life years (DALYs) globally in 2019 (7). Figure 1.2 presents the number of DALYs globally and the DALY rate of asthma per 100,000 population, differentiated by age and sex in 2019, illustrating the disease's varied impact across different demographic groups.

Healthcare utilisation due to asthma remains high across various regions. In the United States, the American Lung Association reported that in 2020, there were approximately 94,560 hospitalisations with asthma listed as the primary cause, translating to a rate of 28.5 per 100,000 people (79). Additionally, the same year saw around 898,000 emergency room visits related to asthma, which corresponds to a rate of

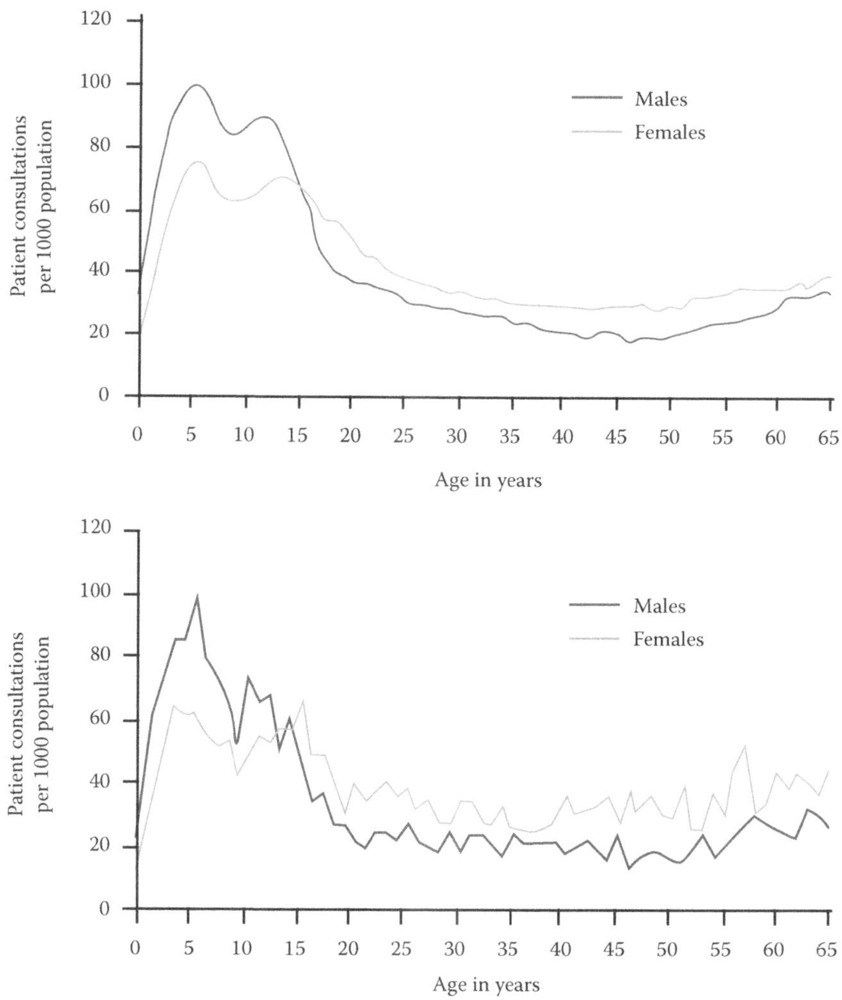

FIGURE 1.2 Number of DALY cases globally and DALY rate of asthma per 100,000 population, by age and sex in 2019. Boxes indicate DALY cases with 95% uncertainty intervals for men and women. DALY: disability adjusted life year. (This figure is reproduced from the study by Wang et al. [7] under the terms of the Creative Commons CC BY license, which allows for unrestricted use, distribution, and reproduction in any medium, as long as the original work is properly cited.)

271.0 per 100,000 people (79). In the United Kingdom, Asthma + Lung UK noted that asthma hospital admission rates have consistently exceeded 60,000 annually since the publication of the National Review of Asthma Deaths (NRAD), peaking at 67,015 in 2018/2019 (80). This highlights the significant burden asthma places on healthcare systems.

Disparities in Outcomes: Significant disparities in asthma outcomes persist across various demographic groups:

1. **Socio-Economic Factors:** Lower-income individuals consistently show poorer asthma outcomes. A study in the UK found that patients from the most deprived socio-economic status (SES) quintile were more likely to report uncontrolled disease (OR: 1.54, 95% CI: 1.16, 2.05) and to have an exacerbation during follow-up (OR: 1.27, 95% CI: 1.13, 1.42) than the least deprived quintile (81). A study across six countries found that lower household income during early childhood was associated with increased risk of ever asthma (RR 1.28, 95% CI: 1.15–1.43), wheezing/asthma attacks (RR 1.22, 95% CI: 1.03–1.44), and asthma with medication control (RR 1.25, 95% CI: 1.01–1.55) in children aged 9–12 years (82).
2. **Race and Ethnicity:** Disparities in asthma outcomes among racial and ethnic groups continue to be observed. In the United States, Black children bear a disproportionately high burden of severe and uncontrolled asthma (83). Moreover, asthma-related mortality rates are about four times higher in Puerto Rican and Black populations compared to White individuals (83). In the UK, socio-economic disparities in exacerbations were larger among those from ethnic minority groups (OR: 1.94, 95% CI: 1.40, 2.68) than White patients (OR: 1.24, 95% CI: 1.10, 1.39; p interaction = 0.012) (81).
3. **Age:** The effect of deprivation on asthma control was greater among those aged over 75 years (OR = 1.81, 95% CI: 1.20, 2.73) compared to those aged less than 35 years (OR: 1.22, 95% CI: 0.85, 1.74; p interaction = 0.019) (81). Asthma control was assessed using the Royal College of Physicians' three questions, which evaluate the presence or absence of symptoms through patient-reported answers (84).

1.8 IMPLICATIONS FOR POLICY, PRACTICE, AND FUTURE RESEARCH

The implications of the findings presented in this chapter extend across policy, clinical practice, and future research, particularly given the high prevalence of asthma worldwide. The global burden of asthma is expected to increase in the coming decades, with a disproportionate rise anticipated in LMICs, potentially linked to urbanisation (85). A systematic review by Rodriguez et al. (85) found that urban residence was consistently associated with a higher prevalence of asthma, with odds ratios ranging from 1.46 to 1.96 compared to rural areas.

As urbanisation accelerates in LMICs, healthcare systems in these regions may be ill-equipped to manage the increasing prevalence of asthma and other chronic conditions and their associated morbidity. Without improved access to effective treatments and targeted interventions, a rise in asthma-related hospitalisations and mortality rates is likely. This underscores the urgent necessity for comprehensive policy measures aimed at addressing the growing impact of this chronic condition.

From a policy perspective, there is a critical need for targeted interventions to address the global burden of asthma. Policymakers should prioritise improving healthcare access, particularly in LMICs where asthma prevalence is rising. This includes implementing environmental regulations aimed at reducing exposure to pollutants and other risk factors, such as tobacco smoke, which are known to exacerbate asthma symptoms. Public health education initiatives are essential to raise awareness about asthma management strategies and the importance of early diagnosis and treatment and the risks associated with smoking.

In terms of clinical practice, the evolving understanding of asthma phenotypes is shifting towards personalised medicine. Clinicians should consider individual characteristics when devising treatment plans, utilising biomarker testing to guide therapy decisions effectively. This personalised approach should extend to managing comorbidities that can complicate asthma control, such as obesity, gastroesophageal reflux disease, and asthma-COPD syndrome.

Looking ahead, several future research directions emerge from the current understanding of asthma. Investigating the interactions between genetic predispositions and environmental factors will be crucial in determining the underlying mechanisms of asthma development and progression. There is also a pressing need for research into novel therapeutics tailored to specific asthma endotypes, particularly those that do not respond well to standard treatments. Additionally, exploring primary prevention strategies for high-risk populations could significantly impact asthma incidence rates.

By focusing on these areas, stakeholders can significantly enhance our understanding of asthma, leading to improved prevention strategies, more effective treatments, and ultimately better health outcomes for individuals affected by this complex condition. The global nature of this challenge requires coordinated efforts across nations, with a particular focus on supporting LMICs in developing robust healthcare systems capable of managing the anticipated increase in asthma prevalence.

REFERENCES

1. Lash T, VanderWeele T, Haneuse S, Rothman KJ. *Modern Epidemiology*. 4th ed. Wolters Kluwer; 2021.

2. Anandan C, Nurmatov U, Van Schayck OCP, Sheikh A. Is the prevalence of asthma declining? Systematic review of epidemiological studies. *Allergy*. 2010;65(2):152–67.
3. Momtazmanesh S, Moghaddam SS, Ghamari SH, Rad EM, Rezaei N, Shobeiri P, et al. Global burden of chronic respiratory diseases and risk factors, 1990–2019: an update from the global burden of disease study 2019. *EClinicalMedicine*. 2023;59.
4. Simpson CR, Sheikh A. Epidemiology of asthma: a worldwide perspective. In: *Clinical Asthma*. CRC Press; 2014. p. 3–12.
5. Nurmagambetov T, Kuwahara R, Garbe P. The economic burden of asthma in the United States, 2008–2013. *Ann Am Thorac Soc*. 2018;15(3):348–56.
6. Yaghoubi M, Adibi A, Safari A, FitzGerald JM, Sadatsafavi M. The projected economic and health burden of uncontrolled asthma in the United States. *Am J Respir Crit Care Med*. 2019;200(9):1102–12.
7. Wang Z, Li Y, Gao Y, Fu Y, Lin J, Lei X, et al. Global, regional, and national burden of asthma and its attributable risk factors from 1990 to 2019: a systematic analysis for the global burden of disease study 2019. *Respir Res*. 2023;24(1):169.
8. Reddel HK, Bacharier LB, Bateman ED, Brightling CE, Brusselle GG, Buhl R, et al. Global initiative for Asthma strategy 2021: executive summary and rationale for key changes. *Am J Respir Crit Care Med*. 2022;205(1):17–35.
9. Asthma N. Diagnosis, Monitoring and Chronic Asthma Management. Guidance and Guidelines. Available from: https://www.nice.org.uk/guidance/ng80 (accessed on 3 July 2018). 2020.
10. Brand PLP, Baraldi E, Bisgaard H, Boner AL, Castro-Rodriguez JA, Custovic A, et al. Definition, assessment and treatment of wheezing disorders in preschool children: an evidence-based approach. *Eur Respir J*. 2008;32(4):1096–110.
11. Tarlo SM, Lemiere C. Occupational asthma. *N Engl J Med*. 2014;370(7):640–9.
12. Erzurum SC, Gaston BM. Biomarkers in asthma: a real hope to better manage asthma. *Clin Chest Med*. 2012;33(3):459–71.
13. Fahy J V. Type 2 inflammation in asthma—present in most, absent in many. *Nat Rev Immunol*. 2015;15(1):57–65.
14. Khatri SB, Iaccarino JM, Barochia A, Soghier I, Akuthota P, Brady A, et al. Use of fractional exhaled nitric oxide to guide the treatment of asthma: an official American Thoracic Society clinical practice guideline. *Am J Respir Crit Care Med*. 2021;204(10):e97–109.
15. Pavord ID, Beasley R, Agusti A, Anderson GP, Bel E, Brusselle G, et al. After asthma: redefining airways diseases. *Lancet*. 2018;391(10118):350–400.
16. Aaron SD, Vandemheen KL, FitzGerald JM, Ainslie M, Gupta S, Lemière C, et al. Reevaluation of diagnosis in adults with physician-diagnosed asthma. *JAMA*. 2017;317(3):269–79.
17. Agusti A, Bel E, Thomas M, Vogelmeier C, Brusselle G, Holgate S, et al. Treatable traits: toward precision medicine of chronic airway diseases. *Eur Respir J*. 2016;47(2):410–9.
18. Holguin F, Cardet JC, Chung KF, Diver S, Ferreira DS, Fitzpatrick A, et al. Management of severe asthma: a European respiratory society/American thoracic society guideline. *Eur Respir J*. 2020;55(1).
19. Wenzel SE. Asthma phenotypes: the evolution from clinical to molecular approaches. *Nat Med*. 2012;18(5):716–25.
20. Pavord ID. Eosinophilic phenotypes of airway disease. *Ann Am Thorac Soc*. 2013;10(Supplement):S143–9.
21. Laidlaw TM, Boyce JA. Aspirin-exacerbated respiratory disease—new prime suspects. *N Engl J Med*. 2016;374(5):484–8.
22. Parsons JP, Mastronarde JG. Exercise-induced bronchoconstriction in athletes. *Chest*. 2005;128(6):3966–74.
23. Scott HA, Wood LG, Gibson PG. Role of obesity in asthma: mechanisms and management strategies. *Curr Allergy Asthma Rep*. 2017;17:1–10.
24. Ray A, Kolls JK. Neutrophilic inflammation in asthma and association with disease severity. *Trends Immunol*. 2017;38(12):942–54.
25. Jackson DJ, Johnston SL. The role of viruses in acute exacerbations of asthma. *J Allergy Clin Immunol*. 2010;125(6):1178–87.
26. Smith D, Helgason H, Sulem P, Bjornsdottir US, Lim AC, Sveinbjornsson G, et al. A rare IL33 loss-of-function mutation reduces blood eosinophil counts and protects from asthma. *PLOS Genet*. 2017;13(3):e1006659.
27. Cayrol C, Girard JP. IL-33: an alarmin cytokine with crucial roles in innate immunity, inflammation and allergy. *Curr Opin Immunol*. 2014;31:31–7.
28. Simpson JL, Scott R, Boyle MJ, Gibson PG. Inflammatory subtypes in asthma: assessment and identification using induced sputum. *Respirology*. 2006;11(1):54–61.
29. Quoc QL, Choi Y, Thi Bich TC, Yang EM, Shin YS, Park HS. S100A9 in adult asthmatic patients: a biomarker for neutrophilic asthma. *Exp Mol Med*. 2021;53(7):1170–9.
30. Goodman MA, Moradi Manesh D, Malik P, Rothenberg ME. CRISPR/Cas9 in allergic and immunologic diseases. *Expert Rev Clin Immunol*. 2017;13(1):5–9.
31. Ndlovu V, Chimbari MJ, Sibanda E. Assessing the nature of asthma in African epidemiological studies: a scoping review protocol. *Syst Rev*. 2020;9:1–7.
32. Kallis C, Maslova E, Morgan AD, Sinha I, Roberts G, van der Valk RJP, et al. Recent trends in asthma diagnosis, preschool wheeze diagnosis and asthma exacerbations in English children and adolescents: a SABINA Jr study. *Thorax*. 2023;78(12):1175–80.
33. Song P, Adeloye D, Salim H, Dos Santos JP, Campbell H, Sheikh A, et al. Global, regional, and national prevalence of asthma in 2019: a systematic analysis and modelling study. *J Glob Health*. 2022;12.
34. Stern J, Pier J, Litonjua AA. Asthma epidemiology and risk factors. In: *Seminars in Immunopathology*. Springer; 2020. p. 5–15.
35. Anto JM, Bousquet J, Akdis M, Auffray C, Keil T, Momas I, et al. Mechanisms of the Development of Allergy (MeDALL): Introducing novel concepts in allergy phenotypes. *J Allergy Clin Immunol*. 2017;139(2):388–99.
36. Beasley R, Semprini A, Mitchell EA. Risk factors for asthma: is prevention possible? *Lancet*. 2015;386(9998):1075–85.
37. Dharmage SC, Perret JL, Custovic A. Epidemiology of asthma in children and adults. *Front Pediatr*. 2019;7:246.
38. Asher MI, Twiss J, Ellwood E. The epidemiology of asthma. In: Wilmott RW, Boat TF, Bush A, editors. *Kendig & Chernick's Disorders of the Respiratory Tract in Children*. Elsevier Saunders; 2012. p. 647–76.
39. Rogers NT, Cummins S, Jones CP, Mytton OT, Roberts CH, Shaheen SO, et al. The UK Soft drinks industry levy and childhood hospital admissions for asthma in England. *Nat Commun*. 2024;15(1):4934.
40. Shah SA, Quint JK, Nwaru BI, Sheikh A. Impact of COVID-19 national lockdown on asthma exacerbations: interrupted time-series analysis of English primary care data. *Thorax*. 2021;76(9):860–6.

41. Asher MI, Rutter CE, Bissell K, Chiang CY, El Sony A, Ellwood E, et al. Worldwide trends in the burden of asthma symptoms in school-aged children: Global Asthma Network Phase I cross-sectional study. *Lancet.* 2021;398(10311):1569–80.
42. Mpairwe H, Namutebi M, Nkurunungi G, Tumwesige P, Nambuya I, Mukasa M, et al. Risk factors for asthma among schoolchildren who participated in a case-control study in urban Uganda. *Elife.* 2019;8:e49496.
43. Khreis H, Kelly C, Tate J, Parslow R, Lucas K, Nieuwenhuijsen M. Exposure to traffic-related air pollution and risk of development of childhood asthma: a systematic review and meta-analysis. *Environ Int.* 2017;100:1–31.
44. Pividori M, Schoettler N, Nicolae DL, Ober C, Im HK. Shared and distinct genetic risk factors for childhood-onset and adult-onset asthma: genome-wide and transcriptome-wide studies. *Lancet Respir Med.* 2019;7(6):509–22.
45. Khreis H, Kelly C, Tate J, Parslow R, Lucas K, Nieuwenhuijsen M Exposure to traffic-related air pollution and risk of development of childhood asthma: a systematic review and meta-analysis. *Environ Int.* 2017;100:1–31.
46. Dharmage SC, Perret JL, Custovic A. Epidemiology of asthma in children and adults. *Front Pediatr.* 2019;7:246.
47. Janson C, Anto J, Burney Pobot, Chinn S, de Marco R, Heinrich J, et al. The European Community Respiratory Health Survey: what are the main results so far? *Eur Respir J.* 2001;18(3):598–611.
48. Zahran HS. Vital signs: asthma in children—United States, 2001–2016. *MMWR Morb Mortal Wkly Rep.* 2018;67.
49. Nissen F, Morales DR, Mullerova H, Smeeth L, Douglas IJ, Quint JK. Validation of asthma recording in the Clinical Practice Research Datalink (CPRD). *BMJ Open.* 2017;7(8):e017474.
50. Shah SA, Quint JK, Sheikh A. Impact of COVID-19 pandemic on asthma exacerbations: retrospective cohort study of over 500,000 patients in a national English primary care database. *Lancet Regional Health–Europe.* 2022;19.
51. Pividori M, Schoettler N, Nicolae DL, Ober C, Im HK. Shared and distinct genetic risk factors for childhood-onset and adult-onset asthma: genome-wide and transcriptome-wide studies. *Lancet Respir Med.* 2019;7(6):509–22.
52. Chan AHY, Stewart AW, Harrison J, Camargo CA, Black PN, Mitchell EA. The effect of an electronic monitoring device with audiovisual reminder function on adherence to inhaled corticosteroids and school attendance in children with asthma: a randomised controlled trial. *Lancet Respir Med.* 2015;3(3):210–9.
53. Tsang KCH, Pinnock H, Wilson AM, Salvi D, Shah SA. Home monitoring with connected mobile devices for asthma attack prediction with machine learning. *Sci Data.* 2023;10(1):370.
54. Mallol J, Crane J, von Mutius E, Odhiambo J, Keil U, Stewart A, et al. The International Study of Asthma and Allergies in Childhood (ISAAC) phase three: a global synthesis. *Allergol Immunopathol (Madr).* 2013;41(2):73–85.
55. Mortimer K, Lesosky M, García-Marcos L, Asher MI, Pearce N, Ellwood E, et al. The burden of asthma, hay fever and eczema in adults in 17 countries: GAN Phase I study. *Eur Respir J.* 2022;60(3).
56. Pearce N, Sunyer J, Cheng S, Chinn S, Björkstén B, Burr M, et al. Comparison of asthma prevalence in the ISAAC and the ECRHS. *Eur Respir J.* 2000;16(3):420–6.
57. Song M, Hwang S, Son E, Yeo HJ, Cho WH, Kim TW, et al. Geographical differences of risk of asthma and allergic rhinitis according to urban/rural area: a systematic review and meta-analysis of cohort studies. *J Urban Health.* 2023;100(3):478–92.
58. Desalu OO, Adeoti AO, Ojuawo OB, Aladesanmi AO, Oguntoye MS, Afolayan OJ, et al. Urban–rural differences in the epidemiology of asthma and allergies in Nigeria: A population-based study. *J Asthma Allergy.* 2021;1389–97.
59. American Lung Association. Current Asthma Demographics [Internet]. 2024 [cited 2024 Oct 21]. Available from: https://www.lung.org/research/trends-in-lung-disease/asthma-trends-brief/current-demographics
60. Zein JG, Erzurum SC. Asthma is different in women. *Curr Allergy Asthma Rep.* 2015;15:1–10.
61. Shah SA, Tibble H, Pillinger R, McLean S, Ryan D, Critchley H, et al. Hormone replacement therapy and asthma onset in menopausal women: national cohort study. *J Allergy Clin Immunol.* 2021;147(5):1662–70.
62. Nwaru BI, Pillinger R, Tibble H, Shah SA, Ryan D, Critchley H, et al. Hormonal contraceptives and onset of asthma in reproductive-age women: population-based cohort study. *J Allergy Clin Immunol.* 2020;146(2):438–46.
63. Fuhlbrigge AL, Jackson B, Wright RJ. Gender and asthma. *Immunol Allergy Clin.* 2002;22(4):753–89.
64. Pearce N, Aït-Khaled N, Beasley R, Mallol J, Keil U, Mitchell E, et al. Worldwide trends in the prevalence of asthma symptoms: phase III of the International Study of Asthma and Allergies in Childhood (ISAAC). *Thorax.* 2007;62(9):758–66.
65. Pividori M, Schoettler N, Nicolae DL, Ober C, Im HK. Shared and distinct genetic risk factors for childhood-onset and adult-onset asthma: genome-wide and transcriptome-wide studies. *Lancet Respir Med.* 2019;7(6):509–22.
66. Shin JW, Sue JH, Song TW, Kim KW, Kim ES, Sohn MH, et al. Atopy and house dust mite sensitization as risk factors for asthma in children. *Yonsei Med J.* 2005;46(5):629–34.
67. Ziska L, Knowlton K, Rogers C, Dalan D, Tierney N, Elder MA, et al. Recent warming by latitude associated with increased length of ragweed pollen season in central North America. *Proc Natl Acad Sci.* 2011;108(10):4248–51.
68. Fujimura KE, Lynch SV. Microbiota in allergy and asthma and the emerging relationship with the gut microbiome. *Cell Host Microbe.* 2015;17(5):592–602.
69. Crewe J, Carey R, Glass D, Peters S, Abramson MJ, Benke G, et al. A comprehensive list of asthmagens to inform health interventions in the Australian workplace. *Aust N Z J Public Health.* 2016;40(2):170–3.
70. Nicholson PJ, Cullinan P, Taylor AJN, Burge PS, Boyle C. Evidence based guidelines for the prevention, identification, and management of occupational asthma. *Occup Environ Med.* 2005;62(5):290–9.
71. McConnell R, Barrington-Trimis JL, Wang K, Urman R, Hong H, Unger J, et al. Electronic cigarette use and respiratory symptoms in adolescents. *Am J Respir Crit Care Med.* 2017;195(8):1043–9.
72. Peters U, Dixon AE, Forno E. Obesity and asthma. *J Allergy Clin Immunol.* 2018;141(4):1169–79.
73. Vassilopoulou E, Guibas G V, Papadopoulos NG. Mediterranean-type diets as a protective factor for asthma and atopy. *Nutrients.* 2022;14(9):1825.
74. Kuder MM, Clark M, Cooley C, Prieto-Centurion V, Danley A, Riley I, et al. A systematic review of the effect of physical activity on asthma outcomes. *J Allergy Clin Immunol Pract.* 2021;9(9):3407–21.

75. Francisco C de O, Bhatawadekar SA, Babineau J, Reid WD, Yadollahi A. Effects of physical exercise training on nocturnal symptoms in asthma: Systematic review. *PLOS ONE*. 2018;13(10):e0204953.
76. Rosenberg SL, Miller GE, Brehm JM, Celedón JC. Stress and asthma: novel insights on genetic, epigenetic, and immunologic mechanisms. *J Allergy Clin Immunol*. 2014;134(5):1009–15.
77. Jolliffe DA, Greenberg L, Hooper RL, Griffiths CJ, Camargo CA, Kerley CP, et al. Vitamin D supplementation to prevent asthma exacerbations: a systematic review and meta-analysis of individual participant data. *Lancet Respir Med*. 2017;5(11):881–90.
78. Forno E, Young OM, Kumar R, Simhan H, Celedon JC. Maternal obesity in pregnancy, gestational weight gain, and risk of childhood asthma. *Pediatrics*. 2014;134(2):e535–46.
79. American Lung Association. Asthma Trends and Burden [Internet]. 2024 [cited 2024 Oct 21]. Available from: https://www.lung.org/research/trends-in-lung-disease/asthma-trends-brief/trends-and-burden
80. Asthma+Lung UK. "Asthma care is in crisis" – charity sounds the siren as asthma death toll rises [Internet]. 2024 [cited 2024 Oct 21]. Available from: https://www.asthmaandlung.org.uk/media/press-releases/asthma-care-crisis-charity-sounds-siren-asthma-death-toll-rises
81. Busby J, Price D, Al-Lehebi R, Bosnic-Anticevich S, van Boven JFM, Emmanuel B, et al. Impact of socio-economic status on adult patients with asthma: a population-based cohort study from UK primary care. *J Asthma Allergy*. 2021;1375–88.
82. González Burchard E, Borrell LN. Need for racial and ethnic diversity in asthma precision medicine. *N Engl J Med*. 2021;385:2297–8.
83. Hoskins G, Williams B, Jackson C, Norman PD, Donnan PT. Assessing asthma control in UK primary care: use of routinely collected prospective observational consultation data to determine appropriateness of a variety of control assessment models. *BMC Fam Pract*. 2011;12:1–12.
84. Yang-Huang J, McGrath JJ, Gauvin L, Nikiéma B, Spencer NJ, Awad YA, Clifford S, Markham W, Mensah F, Andersson White P, Ludvigsson J, Faresjö T, Duijts L, van Grieken A, Raat H; EPOCH Collaborative Group. Early family socioeconomic status and asthma-related outcomes in school-aged children: Results from seven birth cohort studies. *J Epidemiol Community Health*. 2024 Dec 10;79(1):1–11. doi: 10.1136/jech-2023-220726. PMID: 38849153; PMCID: PMC11672016.
85. Rodriguez A, Brickley E, Rodrigues L, Normansell RA, Barreto M, Cooper PJ. Urbanisation and asthma in low-income and middle-income countries: a systematic review of the urban–rural differences in asthma prevalence. *Thorax*. 2019;74(11):1020–30.

2 Immunopathogenesis

Chris J. Corrigan

Anne is a 46-year-old patient who first developed breathlessness and chest tightness at the age of 32. She had no history of childhood asthma or atopic diseases. She had never smoked but did suffer from severe pneumonia as an infant caused by respiratory syncytial viral infection. For the past 10 years she was employed as a laboratory animal technician, with daily exposure to rats, mice, and other animals. Spirometry confirmed airways obstruction, which was significantly but not completely reversible with bronchodilators, consistent with a diagnosis of asthma associated with persistent airway obstruction. There was also a significant degree of gas trapping with elevated residual volume. Anne was treated routinely with inhaled corticosteroids and bronchodilators, which afforded some control of her symptoms, but she remained breathless nearly every day and suffered from 2–3 admissions to hospital almost every year with presumed infective exacerbations of her disease, which she consistently claimed showed little response to the courses of oral corticosteroid therapy that she was invariably prescribed in these situations. A formal trial of oral corticosteroid therapy for two weeks was not associated with a significant (<10%) improvement in her forced expiratory volume in one second (FEV_1). A computed tomography (CT) scan of her chest showed generally thickened bronchial walls, consistent with asthma, but no bronchiectasis or interstitial lung disease. Anne was reviewed for possible therapy of her asthma with biological agents.

2.1 INTRODUCTION

Asthma is a common and potentially fatal disease: there are currently 340 million sufferers worldwide, while nearly 1000 die of the disease annually in the United Kingdom alone. Symptoms (and death) are caused by obstruction of the airways. Although current mainstay therapies (inhaled glucocorticoids and bronchodilators) control symptoms tolerably well in most patients if used regularly and delivered reliably to the airways (which in turn requires excellent concordance with therapy and maintenance of exemplary inhaler technique), they are essentially palliative: they do not eliminate symptoms of breathlessness, wheeze, and the constant anxiety of possible acute breathlessness; neither do they eliminate the possibility of remodelling of the airways mucosa, which causes irreversible airways obstruction and may result in chronic, severe symptoms, frequent exacerbations, and increased mortality in a substantial minority of patients. Mortality is not by any means, however, limited to patients with irreversible airways obstruction: a substantial proportion of deaths from asthma occur in patients documented to suffer from mild or moderate disease (1). Thus bronchospasm alone is potentially life threatening. The relatively recent availability of "biological" agents, targeting IgE or particular inflammatory cytokines or their receptors has, in general, not yet proved the panacea that was hoped for: this partly reflects lack of understanding, by which patients will benefit most from each particular therapy, and also the fact that, at present, these therapies tend to be employed later on in the progress of the disease, rather than prophylactically to prevent irreversible airways obstruction and remodelling in susceptible individuals.

In this chapter is an account of the pathophysiology of the key components of airways obstruction in asthma (bronchial smooth muscle hyperresponsiveness, airways mucosal inflammation and remodelling, and excessive mucus production), and some recent, exciting avenues for advances in asthma therapy which have arisen from a deeper understanding of its immunopathogenesis.

2.2 BRONCHIAL SMOOTH MUSCLE HYPERRESPONSIVENESS: CAUSE OF ASTHMA

Non-specific hyperresponsiveness of the smooth muscle surrounding the larger airways, causing excessive contraction of the muscle in response to various non-specific stimuli such as smoke, cold air, exercise, and respiratory tract infection, as well as specific, pharmacological stimuli, is the essential pathognomonic feature of asthma that defines the disease and that may occur in the absence of inflammation of the airways mucosa (2). In patients with asthma, exposure to such stimuli may precipitate wheezing and breathlessness. Symptoms and lung function in asthmatic patients are typically diurnally variable according to the endogenous circadian plasma cortisol profile (worse when endogenous production is lowest in the early hours of the morning, or the opposite if the circadian rhythm is reversed). Demonstration of this phenomenon forms the basis of asthma diagnosis: in mild/moderate patients, it is typically diagnosed by documenting short-term variability in FEV_1, PEF, or airways resistance in children, either by diurnal, morning, and evening monitoring or, if low at baseline, in response to a pharmacological bronchodilator such as a β2-adrenoreceptor agonist ("reliever"). In patients with less marked airways obstruction at baseline, the diagnosis may be confirmed by a positive histamine or methacholine challenge test, which quantifies the fall in baseline FEV_1 in response to inhalation of serial, doubled concentrations

DOI: 10.1201/9781003287209-3

of these bronchoconstrictors: asthmatic airways constrict in response to these stimuli to a degree that reflects the degree of airways smooth muscle hyperresponsiveness, whereas non-asthmatic airways do not (3).

Breathlessness and impaired exercise tolerance in asthmatics arise from the increased ventilatory effort that is required to move air into and out of abnormally narrow airways and from the obstruction of the small airways, which causes "gas trapping" in the alveoli, which, if severe, results in hyperinflation of the chest and reduced tidal volume. Airways obstruction also results in a feeling of tightness in the chest, and turbulent airflow, which is perceived as wheeze.

Until recently, little was known about the pathogenesis of bronchial smooth muscle hyperresponsiveness in asthma. A key recent study (4) has, however, convincingly implicated over-expression of the Calcium Sensing Receptor (CaSR) on the airways smooth muscle cells of asthma patients as being responsible for this, since it results in non-specific, elevated contraction of the muscle in response to any contractile stimulus by releasing intracellular calcium from stores and promoting influx through ion channels in the plasma membrane. The CaSR is a G-protein-coupled receptor originally identified as the body's master controller for extracellular calcium homoeostasis. It is widely expressed and mediates many physiological functions other than calcium metabolism (5). It is also expressed widely by many cells, including in particular inflammatory cells involved in the genesis of asthmatic airways inflammation including T lymphocytes, eosinophils, dendritic cells, and structural cells of the airways mucosa, as well as bronchial smooth muscle cells. It is expressed in the cell membrane as a homodimer with large extracellular domains that enclose a ligand-binding cleft, which is also a binding site for positive allosteric modulators including polyamines such as spermine, spermidine, putrescine, and drugs, termed calcimimetics, which potentiate CaSR-mediated intracellular Ca^{2+} mobilization. Negative allosteric modulators of the receptor, termed calcilytics, have been developed by pharma (6), and it has recently been established that it should be possible to deliver these topically and safely to the airways of asthmatic patients, both children and adult (7). This in turn would be expected to abolish bronchial hyperresponsiveness and bronchospasm in asthmatic patients: an extremely exciting prospect for the future.

2.3 AIRWAYS MUCOSAL INFLAMMATION IN ASTHMA

Traditionally, asthma has been labelled as an "inflammatory disease of the airways," implying that inflammation of the airways is integral to its pathogenesis. Inflammation of the airways is not, however, integral to the pathophysiology of bronchial smooth muscle hyperresponsiveness, which is the defining feature of asthma. Some cases of bronchopulmonary dysplasia in premature infants are characterized by bronchial smooth muscle hyperresponsiveness to methacholine in the absence of any evidence of airways inflammation or clinical responsiveness to topical corticosteroid therapy, consistent with the hypothesis that it exists in the absence of such inflammation (8–10). Studies of adult asthmatics also support the view, albeit indirectly from clinical observation, that some patients who clearly have bronchial smooth muscle hyperresponsiveness show no evidence of inflammation or fixed obstruction of their airways (11). Conversely, bronchial mucosal inflammation may exist in the absence of asthma, as illustrated, for example, by the phenomenon of "eosinophilic bronchitis," in which patients with eosinophilic airways inflammation very similar to that observed in many patients with asthma nevertheless do not manifest the latter disease (12). This said, it is also true to say that many patients with asthma do also display evidence of inflammation of the airways mucosa, as first described by Dunnill and his colleagues (13) and many others since. These studies have revealed that the airways inflammation typically seen in patients with asthma is defined by local, elevated expression of Th2-type cytokines such as interleukin (IL)-5, IL-4, and IL-13, thought originally to be derived entirely from local, activated Th2-type, CD4+ T lymphocytes (6, 14, 15), although it was never clear at this time why and how such cells could be induced to differentiate at this site. Some of these T cells are specific for conventional aeroallergens, but their full potential repertoire of specificities has never been documented: other possible antigens include local environmental proteins, either inhaled (as with conventional aeroallergens) or derived from local, commensal organisms. It later became clear that differentiation of these Th2-type T cells was driven by the production of much larger quantities of Th2-type cytokines by innate immune cells within the epithelial mucosa of the airways, in particular innate, type 2 lymphocytes (ILC2s), which are in turn activated by the alarmin cytokines IL-33, thymic stromal lymphopoietin (TSLP) and IL-25, which are released from bronchial epithelial cells in response to environmental damage from a variety of agents including particulate pollution, inhaled proteins with intrinsic protease activity acting on protease-activated receptors (PARs) and viral and bacterial infections (6, 16, 17). The key molecular switch for Th2-type T cell development is interaction of the T cell accessory molecule OX40 with its ligand OX40L, the expression of which is induced on local antigen-presenting cells primed by IL-33 or TSLP (18, 19).

Thus in the bronchial mucosa of some individuals who are susceptible to damage of their airways epithelial cells by inhaled, environmental agents, epithelial damage results in the release of alarmin cytokines, which in turn promote the release of Th2-type cytokines by ILC2s, which in turn promote the local development of Th2-type, CD4+ T lymphocytes. Quantitatively, ILC2s contribute more to the local production of Th2-type cytokines than Th2-type T lymphocytes. In addition, both the release of epithelial alarmins, which follows cellular damage, and the release of Th2-type cytokines from ILC2s activated by the alarmins is resistant to inhibition by glucocorticoids, whereas Th2-type lymphocytes are variably sensitive to glucocorticoid inhibition (6). Local and systemic release of IL-5 from the inflamed airways promotes eosinophilopoiesis in the bone marrow and recruitment and development *in situ* of eosinophils within the bronchial mucosa, creating the bronchial mucosal, eosinophilic inflammation, which is typically (if not always) associated with the disease. As is the case with the natural history of bronchial hyperresponsiveness caused by over-expression of the CaSR, there is similarly relatively little known about what governs the susceptibility of individuals to respiratory epithelial damage by inhaled, environmental pollutants, proteases, and respiratory tract viral infections (20) (for a further discussion, see the section "Current Dilemmas"). In patients who develop progressive and severe airways inflammation despite treatment with topical and additional systemic glucocorticoid therapy, it seems reasonable to assume that these changes are driven principally by local alarmin production since, as noted previously, the production of Th2-type cytokines by ILC2 cells is resistant to inhibition by glucocorticoids (21). In patients with non-progressive, milder, or intermittent symptoms, it is on the other hand likely that these symptoms are driven predominantly by the local production of Th2-type cytokines by CD4+, Th2-type lymphocytes, since the clinical responsiveness of individual asthma patients with mild/moderate disease to systemically administered glucocorticoid therapy closely correlates, at least in the short term, with sensitivity of their lymphocytes to glucocorticoid inhibition (22, 23).

Although environmental stimuli acting on the respiratory tract mucosa commonly result in over-production of Th2-type cytokines by the mechanisms just described, some individuals react to such stimuli by manifesting predominantly neutrophilic inflammation of the airways mucosa, likely driven by cytokines such as IL-17A produced by local Th17 cells: cigarette smoking or passive exposure to smoke may be one trigger for this in susceptible individuals (24). There is also accumulating evidence that another trigger for neutrophilic airways inflammation in susceptible individuals is chronic bacterial infection of the airways, for example with non-encapsulated *Haemophilus influenzae* (see also the section headed "Current Dilemmas") (25). Often, both eosinophilic and neutrophilic infiltration may be apparent, again likely reflecting the susceptibility of different individuals to particular environmental insults.

As discussed previously, many subjects who develop bronchial smooth muscle hyperresponsiveness (asthma) also manifest airways mucosal inflammation. How may these phenomena interact to govern the severity of asthma symptoms? Firstly, inflammation of the airways mucosa causes swelling and oedema of the mucosa and thus reduces the internal diameter of the airways. According to Poiseuille's equation relating to fluid dynamics (discussed in [26]), the resistance to the flow of air through a cylindrical vessel such as a bronchus increases according to the fourth power of the reduction of its internal radius. Thus even a small reduction in the patency of the airways caused by mucosal inflammation and oedema exerts a very great influence on the resistance to airflow. This effect is independent of, but augments the effects of, excessive contraction of the surrounding smooth muscle. Secondly and critically, it is now clear (4) that many cationic products of inflammatory leukocytes, in particular the cationic proteins produced by eosinophils and the arginine metabolites spermine and spermidine produced by neutrophils, are direct or positive allosteric agonists of the CaSR: thus these products may directly trigger bronchospasm in asthmatic patients whose airways' smooth muscle cells over-express the CaSR. These interactions likely explain how glucocorticoid therapy ameliorates asthma: firstly, it reduces mucosal oedema and thus increases the internal diameter of the airways, and secondly, in the majority of patients it reduces the local accumulation of cells such as eosinophils, which release direct agonists of the CaSR. They also likely explain many previous studies linking the severity of asthma to the expression of CaSR agonists such as polyamines and eosinophil cationic proteins (27–29). Viral or bacterial respiratory tract infections are particularly liable to exacerbate asthma because they increase mucosal oedema in addition to inducing the influx of inflammatory granulocytes, which release basic proteins that activate the CaSR and thus induce bronchospasm.

Another possible contributor to the symptoms of asthma is the local release of the cysteinyl leukotrienes (leukotrienes C_4, D_4, and E_4), which are primarily products of activated eosinophils. These mediators, by acting on the cysteinyl leukotriene receptor 1 ($CysLT_1$), promote vascular leakage and therefore have the potential to increase airways mucosal oedema and blockage; in addition, they are also the most potent known natural constrictors of airways' smooth muscle. It is unclear what governs the susceptibility of individual patients with asthma to the possible effects of local leukotriene release in their airways: currently this is gauged empirically by their clinical responsiveness or lack of responsiveness to $CysLT_1$ receptor blockers such as montelukast and zafirlukast (30). For many patients, these drugs do not appreciably alter control of symptoms. Patients with aspirin-exacerbated asthma are in addition hyperresponsive to the bronchoconstrictor effects of leukotriene E_4, a phenomenon that also remains unexplained (31).

2.4 AIRWAYS REMODELLING IN ASTHMA

Features of remodelling of the airways mucosa in asthma include the laydown of structural proteins (including collagen, fibronectin, and tenascin) beneath the epithelial basement membrane and within the submucosa, hypertrophy of the mucus glands in the epithelial lining of the mucosa and neovascularization, resulting in proliferation of the vascular capillary beds within the submucosa (6). All of these features may contribute to irreversible obstruction of the airways, while excessive mucus production from hypertrophied mucus glands may acutely exacerbate this obstruction (and may indeed obliterate the airspace completely during disease exacerbations). It is likely that the majority of these changes are induced as a response to local release of the epithelial alarmins IL-33, TSLP, and IL-25, which cause partly overlapping and partly unique remodelling changes in the airways (32, 33) following environmental damage to the airways epithelial cells in susceptible individuals, some of whom may also exhibit bronchial smooth muscle hyperresponsiveness (asthma). These changes likely account for the accelerated decline in lung function, the irreversibility of airways obstruction, and the excessive mucus production observed in some patients with asthma.

2.5 ROLE OF IMMUNOGLOBULIN-E-(IGE)-MEDIATED MECHANISMS

It is salutary to reflect that, as late as the end of the 1980s, the pathophysiology of asthma was still viewed by many as periodic, histamine-induced spasm of the bronchial smooth muscle caused by allergen-induced degranulation of bronchial mucosal mast cells sensitized by the production of allergen-specific IgE. This view of asthma pathogenesis was curious in retrospect because it glossed over many obvious, implacable inconsistencies, for example that antihistamine therapy is of little or no clinical benefit in the management of chronic asthma or that not all atopic persons develop asthma, whereas some apparently non-atopic persons do. Because the local environment in the asthmatic bronchial mucosa is so conducive to Th2-type T cell activation and B lymphoblast switching to IgE synthesis (promoted by the high local release of the only two cytokines, which induce this switching, namely IL-4 and IL-13) (34), it seems reasonable to hypothesize that this is a site of the production of IgE against a wide variety of external antigens presented to the airways, including but not limited to conventional "aeroallergens" and likely also "self" antigens. This local IgE production may sometimes result in exacerbation of asthma symptoms and/or airways mucosal inflammation, for example by interference with innate immune mechanisms (discussed next) or, in the case of aeroallergens, sensitizing local mast cells by binding to their FcεRI receptors, cross-linking of which induces release of histamine on further exposure, exacerbating bronchospasm (hence the concept of "allergic" or "atopic" asthma). It is finally also conceivable that IgE produced in the airways mucosa to some local antigens plays no pathological role and is simply epiphenomenal. This hypothesis is well supported by consideration of the clinical benefits of monoclonal anti-IgE (omalizumab) therapy in severe asthma. This was originally conceived as an anti-asthma therapy which, in blocking the binding of IgE to its high- and low-affinity cellular receptors, would abolish the IgE-mediated "allergic" reactions (caused by cross-linking of allergen-specific IgE bound to its receptors on mast cells and basophils, resulting in histamine release) to environmental allergens thought then to drive asthma. It is now clear, however, from the excellent "inner-city" asthma studies (35) that this therapy actually reduces exacerbations of asthma by restoring impaired, innate immunity to respiratory viral infections: pretreatment of children and their parents for just a few months with omalizumab virtually wiped out the September epidemic of severe asthma exacerbations seen every year in North America and caused by asthmatic children returning to school, catching upper respiratory viral infections from their peers, and then passing them on to their asthmatic parents (36). This most likely reflects the fact that innate dendritic cells within the bronchial mucosa, which produce innate, immune interferons in response to respiratory viral infections which powerfully inhibit viral replication, are inhibited by cross-linking of IgE bound to their cell surface, high-affinity IgE receptors (FcεR1), an effect abrogated by anti-IgE (37, 38). It also underlines the fact that respiratory viral infections are a common exacerbator of asthma, increasing airways inflammation, reducing their internal diameter, and increasing the release of agonists of the CaSR, inducing bronchospasm. This effect of IgE on innate anti-viral immunity likely also accounts for the fact that asthmatic patients infected with rhinovirus in the laboratory develop a much greater viral load than non-asthmatics, with greatly elevated secretion of Th2-type cytokines, as well as alarmins such as IL-33, into their airways (20). The specificity of the IgE, which binds to and inhibits the dendritic cells, is unknown but might include IgE directed against conventional aeroallergens as well as respiratory viruses, which would account for some studies showing a synergistic effect of viral infection and allergen exposure in predisposing to acute exacerbation of asthma (39) or other local, non-allergen proteins: omalizumab therapy reduces bronchial mucosal IgE concomitantly with improving lung function in patients with non-atopic, as well as atopic asthma (40). Conversely, it is clear that inhaled aeroallergens, as with other environmental proteins and irritants, may induce the release of airways' epithelial alarmins in susceptible individuals quite independently of the presence of IgE (41), while approximately one-third of apparently eligible atopic asthmatics treated with omalizumab show no significant clinical response (42), supporting the hypothesis just referred to that IgE does not necessarily play a significant role in the pathophysiology of asthma in every patient, even if atopic.

2.6 EXCESSIVE AIRWAYS MUCUS PRODUCTION IN ASTHMA

As mentioned, severe and indeed fatal asthma attacks are often characterized by blockage of the airways with thick mucus. Mucus production throughout the respiratory tract is a physiological response to any noxious insult, but the problem may be greatly compounded by hypertrophy of the mucus glands in airways that may already be narrowed as a result of inflammation and remodelling changes, including mucous gland hypertrophy (43, 44). Again, given the clinical importance of this phenomenon, it is perhaps surprising that more research has not been directed at effective inhibition of mucus production in patients with asthma (45). In the light of our understanding that remodelling changes in the airways of susceptible individuals with asthma is likely driven by alarmin release following epithelial damage, it is possible that the problem of mucus hypersecretion may be pre-empted in the future by prophylactic environmental manipulation to minimize such damage and/or blockading the effects of these alarmins in susceptible individuals, either with monoclonal antibodies or with other inhibitors.

2.7 CURRENT DILEMMAS

The picture painted in this narrative so far (summarized graphically in Figure 2.1) is that the symptoms and clinical features of human asthma are governed by two independent, but interacting phenomena: bronchial smooth muscle hyperresponsiveness and inflammation and remodelling of the airways mucosa. They interact because inflammation results in the accumulation of inflammatory granulocytes, eosinophils, and neutrophils in the bronchial mucosa, which release cationic proteins that directly activate the calcium-sensing receptor (CaSR) on the smooth muscle, causing bronchoconstriction, the effects of which are amplified by narrowing of the lumen of the airways by the inflammatory infiltrate and, in some patients, also by remodelling. Because, in clinical practice, bronchial smooth muscle hyperresponsiveness, which defines asthma, is frequently accompanied by evidence of inflammation of the airways, it also seems very plausible that the natural histories of these two phenomena are linked, at least one possibility being that airways inflammation, causing elevated local concentrations of polycation agonists of the CaSR, induces over-expression of the CaSR *de novo* on bronchial smooth muscle cells in susceptible individuals, thus initiating asthma. Clearly there is still much to be learned about the aetiology and natural history of these phenomena that will allow us to explain, for example, why asthma typically develops in childhood but then often resolves or may appear for the first time later in life, sometimes after occupational exposure of the airways to potential agonists of the CaSR or to inhaled, environmental pollutants, which may initiate bronchial mucosal inflammation.

In susceptible individuals, environmental agents damage the bronchial mucosal epithelial cells, releasing the alarmin cytokines IL-33, IL-25, and thymic stromal lymphopoietin (TSLP), which activate local, innate, type 2 lymphoid cells (ILC2s), which release Th2-type cytokines (principally interleukins 5 [IL-5] and 13) and induce expression of CD40 ligand (CD40L) on local dendritic cells, thus priming the development of Th2-type T lymphocytes, which further

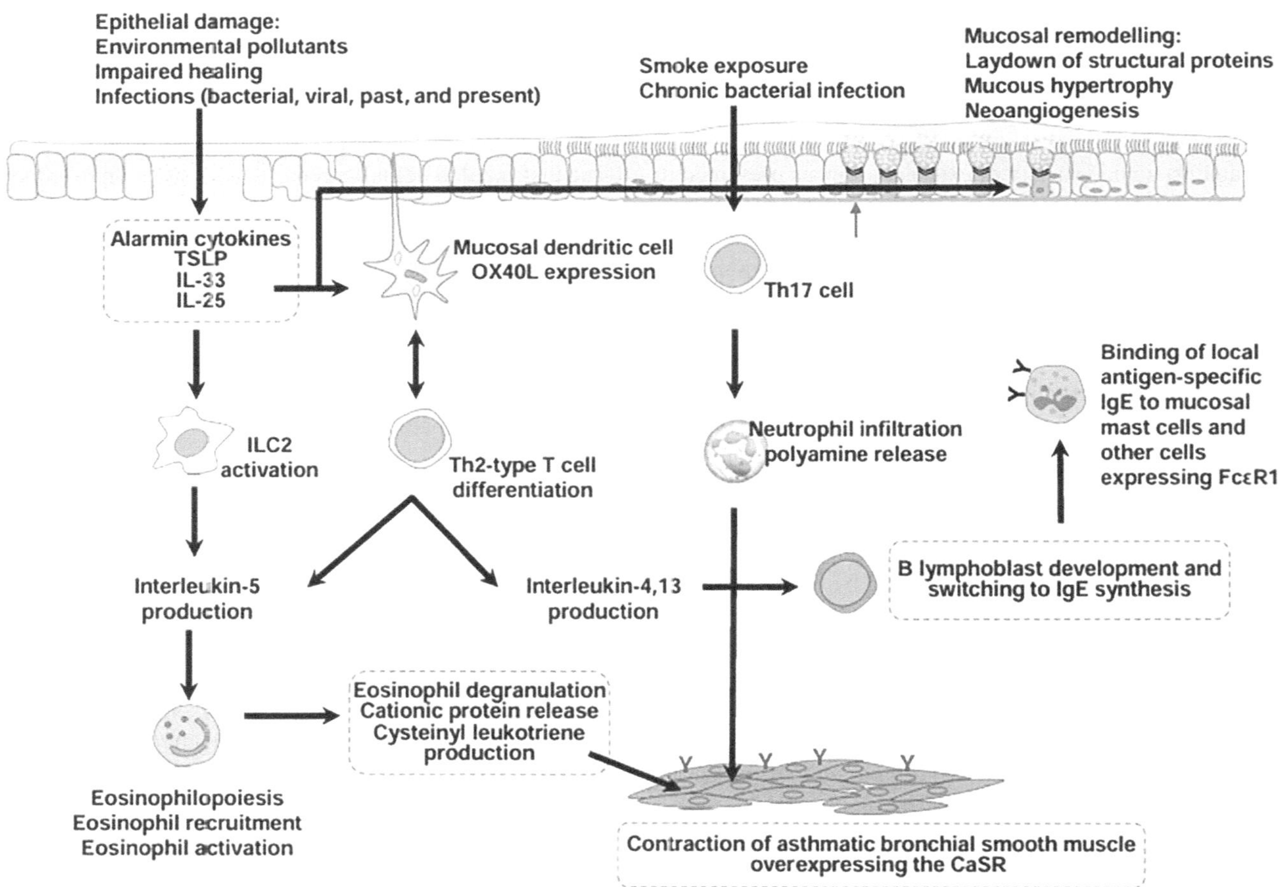

FIGURE 2.1 Diagrammatic portrayal of asthma pathogenesis and the interaction between mucosal inflammation and bronchial smooth muscle contraction.

contribute to local Th2-type cytokine production. Release of IL-5 into the systemic circulation promotes eosinophilopoiesis in the bone marrow and local eosinophil accumulation and activation in the bronchial mucosa. Production of other Th2-type cytokines (IL-4 and IL-13) by local Th2-type T lymphocytes also promotes local B lymphoblast proliferation and switching to IgE synthesis, thereby inducing IgE production against local antigens, including allergens. Th17 cellular activation in the respiratory mucosal epithelium of susceptible individuals, particularly from smoke exposure and bacterial infections, may in addition promote neutrophil influx into the mucosa. Cationic proteins (eosinophil basic proteins and neutrophil-derived polyamines) directly drive the excessive construction of the airways smooth muscle cells in patients with asthma, which overexpress the calcium-sensing receptor (CaSR). Cysteinyl leukotrienes released from activated eosinophils and histamine released from IgE-sensitized mast cells may also contribute to bronchoconstriction in some patients with asthma and bronchial smooth muscle hyperresponsiveness. Alarmin cytokines may also induce chronic structural changes in the airways epithelium and submucosa (remodelling), which may in turn result in irreversible airways obstruction. Susceptibility to airways smooth muscle hyperresponsiveness, caused by over-expression of the CaSR, and airways inflammation induced by a range of environmental exposures are independent phenomena but functionally linked in the sense that bronchial mucosal inflammation causes local, excessive production of eosinophil- and neutrophil-derived cationic proteins, which are direct agonists of the CaSR, and also narrows the internal diameter of the airways, greatly exacerbating the airways obstruction caused by bronchial smooth muscle contraction.

In addition to occupational exposure, many other environmental influences affecting asthma risk have now been identified: for example, children who grow up exposed to "farm-like" microbes are protected (46), whereas infection and/or colonization of the neonatal respiratory tract with potential respiratory tract pathogens, including bacteria (*Streptococcus pneumoniae*, *Haemophilus influenzae*, and *Moraxella catarrhalis*) (47) and viruses such as respiratory syncytial virus or rhinovirus, increases this risk (48–50). Experiments using animal surrogates of asthma suggest that early life infection of the respiratory tract with organisms such as *Streptococcus pneumoniae* may augment the airways inflammatory and remodelling changes induced by later exposure to environmental insults such as house dust mite, an environmental allergen that is also capable of activating protease-activated receptors on the airways' epithelial cells, inducing alarmin release (51). These observations are consistent with the hypothesis that early-life exposure to environmental factors such as respiratory pathogens or commensal organisms may somehow imprint, in the long term in susceptible individuals, the threshold, intensity, and character (52) of subsequent responses to environmental insults on the epithelial lining of the bronchial mucosa, which may result in immunity from or susceptibility to subsequent damage and the initiation of chronic inflammation. Little is known about the mechanistic basis of this phenomenon, although isolated studies have suggested, for example, that neonatal pneumonia may impair, in the long term, the integrity of the tight junctions between respiratory epithelial cells (53) which may permanently enhance vulnerability of the airways epithelium to environmental insults, inflammation, and remodelling. In the future it is to be hoped that such susceptible individuals and the environmental stimuli likely to trigger further damage can be identified *a priori*, so that the problem can be managed prophylactically, and irreversible airways obstruction caused by airways remodelling is eliminated (54, 55). Although these changes may be progressive throughout life in vulnerable individuals, there are also studies suggesting that some changes in the structure and function of the airways epithelium may result from a single insult in the past, the effects of which have persisted (56). Finally, in addition to environmental microorganisms, there is accumulating evidence that exposure of infants to a wealth of environmental "pollutants" in the household, such as tobacco smoke, gases from heating and cooking, moulds from dampness, and household cleaning products influences normal lung development and the risk of asthma in susceptible individuals, sometimes in a manner that is transmissible across generations (57).

Individual susceptibility to the development of all these phenomena described in the present chapter (bronchial smooth muscle hyperresponsiveness and airways inflammation and remodelling in response to past and ongoing environmental insults) is likely also partly inherited: the risk of developing asthma tends to run in families, and twin studies estimate the proportion of the asthma risk to be 50–60% genetically determined. Genome screens have linked the inheritance of various chromosomal regions with an increased risk of asthma (58). These genes may putatively regulate the expression, potency, and downstream effects of individual proteins key to the pathogenesis of bronchial smooth muscle hyperresponsiveness and inflammation and remodelling of the airways in asthma, as well as the susceptibility of individuals to initiation of this inflammation in the airways by particular environmental insults, both past and present, which may in turn reflect the development of the airways during embryogenesis. In addition to the properties of the airways epithelial cells themselves, epithelial function and permeability may also be regulated by structural proteins such as filaggrin (59). Impaired repair and "healing" of the airways epithelium is another well-described feature of asthma histopathology that may have a role in generating remodelling changes. Indeed, the observation (60) that simple repetitive distortion of the airway wall through bronchoconstriction can cause epithelial growth factor release and remodelling changes raises the possibility that these changes may arise independently of the asthma process as a "wound healing" response to repetitive epithelial distortion, although they may later become relevant to asthma pathophysiology if, for example, they eventually result in irreversible airways obstruction.

2.8 TOWARD THE FUTURE

The promise of treating asthma with topical calcilytic therapy, which is predicted to abolish bronchial smooth muscle hyperresponsiveness and may indeed also exert significant anti-inflammatory effects in the airways' epithelium (6, 26), is an exciting prospect for the future. It is also to be hoped that it will eventually be possible to identify, from their genetic background, family history and relevant past, and present environmental and occupational exposure, individual patients at increased risk of developing bronchial smooth muscle hyperresponsiveness and/or inflammation and remodelling of their bronchial mucosa and institute appropriate prophylactic measures wherever possible. At present, for those patients who do develop asthma that is poorly controlled despite receiving properly administered, full dosages of conventional anti-asthma therapy (bronchodilators and topical and systemic glucocorticoids), there is the further opportunity, at the time of writing, to offer treatment with monoclonal antibodies ("biological" therapies or "biologics"), which block the binding of IgE to its receptors (omalizumab, referred to previously), or block the activity of IL-5 (mepolizumab, reslizumab) or its receptor (benralizumab), or block the binding of IL-4 and IL-13 to their common alpha chain receptor (dupilumab), or block the alarmin cytokines IL-33 (tezepelumab) and TSLP (through blockade of its receptor ST2) (astegolimab) (61–64). All of these therapies have been reported to reduce the mean frequency of disease exacerbations in cohorts of severe asthmatics, while some modestly improve mean lung function. Since they all, with the possible exception of anti-IgE and anti-IL-4/13, likely reduce eosinophilopoiesis and the accumulation of eosinophils in the inflamed bronchial mucosa induced by IL-5 released from both glucocorticoid-sensitive, Th2-type T cells and glucocorticoid-resistant ILC2s, thus reducing the local concentrations of agonists of the CaSR and swelling and obstruction of the inflamed airways mucosa, this is perhaps not surprising. It seems reasonable to hypothesize, however, that a subgroup of these patients whose airways inflammation is predominantly neutrophilic and not driven by IL-5 will not respond. While many studies and meta-analyses are currently underway to identify clinical variables, such as the blood eosinophil count, which may earmark particular patients who are likely to derive maximal clinical benefit, at least in the short to medium term, or no benefit at all from any particular agent at the time of initiation of treatment (61), the real challenge for the future will surely be to identify patients at risk of glucocorticoid-resistant airways inflammation and remodelling *a priori* and use these agents, especially those targeting alarmins or their receptors, along with environmental manipulation wherever possible, to prevent, rather than manage, severe symptoms. With regard to remodelling of the airways mucosa causing long-term, irreversible obstruction, this problem is further complicated by the fact that all three alarmin cytokines (IL-33, TSLP, and IL-25) may induce both unique and shared remodelling changes in the airways mucosa (32, 33), thus reducing the potential impact of blockade of any single one of them. Again, early data, albeit from animal surrogates, provide great promise that topical calcilytic therapy of asthma, in addition to abolishing bronchial smooth muscle hyperresponsivess, will also inhibit the release of some alarmin cytokines, such as TSLP, from respiratory epithelial cells following damage from environmental insults (65) and, as a consequence of this and perhaps through additional mechanisms, will antagonize remodelling changes in the airways, potentially retarding or obviating irreversible obstruction (66).

REFERENCES

(1) The Royal Colleges of Physicians of the United Kingdom. Why asthma still kills. The National Review of Asthma Deaths (NRAD) Confidential Enquiry Report, May 2014. Available at: https://www.rcplondon.ac.uk/projects/outputs/why-asthma-still-kills

(2) Chan KN, Silverman M. Increased airway responsiveness in children of low birth weight at school age: effect of topical corticosteroids. *Arch Dis Child* 1993; 69(1):120–124.

(3) O'Byrne PM, Inman MD. Airway hyperresponsiveness. *Chest* 2003; 123 (Suppl 3): 411S–416S.

(4) Yarova PL, Stewart AL, Sathish V et al. Calcium-sensing receptor antagonists abrogate airway hyperresponsiveness and inflammation in allergic asthma. *Sci Transl Med* 2015; 7(284): 284ra260.

(5) Leach K, Fadil M Hannan FM, Josephs TM et al. International union of basic and clinical pharmacology. CVIII. Calcium-sensing receptor nomenclature, pharmacology, and function. *Pharmacol Rev* 2020 Jul; 72(3): 558–604. https://doi.org/10.1124/pr.119.018531.

(6) Riccardi D, Ward JPT, Yarova PL et al. Topical therapy with negative allosteric modulators of the calcium-sensing receptor (calcilytics) for the management of asthma: the beginning of a new era? *Eur Respir J* 2022; 10;60(2): 2102103. https://doi.org/10.1183/13993003.02103-2021.

(7) Yarova PL, Huang P, Schepelmann MW et al. Characterization of negative allosteric modulators of the calcium-sensing receptor for repurposing as a treatment of asthma. *J Pharmacol Exp Ther* 2021; 376(1): 51–63. https://doi.org/10.1124/jpet.120.000281.

(8) Baraldi E, Bonetto G, Zacchello F et al. Low exhaled nitric oxide in school-age children with bronchopulmonary dysplasia and airflow limitation. *Am J Respir Crit Care Med* 2005; 171(1): 68–72.

(9) Carraro S, Piacentini G, Lusiani M et al. Exhaled air temperature in children with bronchopulmonary dysplasia. *Pediatr Pulmonol* 2010; 45: 1240–1245.

(10) Chan KN, Silverman M. Increased airway responsiveness in children of low birth weight at school age: effect of topical corticosteroids. *Arch Dis Child* 1993; 69(1): 120–124.

(11) Haldar P, Pavord ID, Shaw DE et al. Cluster analysis and clinical asthma phenotypes. *Am J Respir Crit Care Med* 2008; 178(3): 218–224.

(12) Côté A, Russell RJ, Boulet LP et al. CHEST expert cough panel. Managing chronic cough due to Asthma and NAEB in adults and adolescents: CHEST Guideline and expert panel report. *Chest* 2020 Jul; 158(1): 68–96. https://doi.org/10.1016/j.chest.2019.12.021.

(13) Dunnill MS, Massarella GR, Anderson JA. A comparison of the quantitative anatomy of the bronchi in normal subjects, in status asthmaticus, in chronic bronchitis, and in emphysema. *Thorax* 1969; 24(2): 176–179.
(14) Corrigan CJ, Kay AB. CD4 T-lymphocyte activation in acute severe asthma: relationship to disease severity and atopic status. *Am Rev Respir Dis* 1990; 141: 970–977.
(15) Robinson DS, Hamid Q, Ying S et al. Predominant Th2-type bronchoalveolar lavage T-lymphocyte population in atopic asthma. *N Engl J Med* 1992; 326: 298–304.
(16) Mitchell PD, O'Byrne PM. Biologics and the lung: TSLP and other epithelial cell-derived cytokines in asthma. *Pharmacol Ther* 2017; 169: 104–112.
(17) Gavala ML, Bashir H, Gern JE. Virus/allergen interactions in asthma. *Curr Allergy Asthma Rep* 2013; 13: 298–307.
(18) Su Z, Lin J, Lu F et al. Potential autocrine regulation of interleukin-33/ST2 signaling of dendritic cells in allergic inflammation. *Mucosal Immunol* 2013; 6(5): 921–930.
(19) Baatjes AJ, Smith SG, Dua B et al. Treatment with anti-OX40L or anti-TSLP does not alter the frequency of T regulatory cells in allergic asthmatics. *Allergy* 2015; 70: 1505–1508.
(20) Jackson DJ, Makrinioti H, Rana BM et al. IL-33-dependent type 2 inflammation during rhinovirus-induced asthma exacerbations in vivo. *Am J Respir Crit Care Med* 2014; 190(12): 1373–1382.
(21) Li Y, Wang W, Lv Z et al. Elevated expression of IL-33 and TSLP in the airways of human asthmatics in vivo: a potential biomarker of severe refractory disease. *J Immunol* 2018; 200: 2253–2262.
(22) Corrigan CJ, Brown PH, Barnes NC et al. Glucocorticoid resistance in chronic asthma: glucocorticoid pharmacokinetics, glucocorticoid receptor characteristics and inhibition of peripheral blood T cell proliferation by glucocorticoids in vitro. *Am Rev Respir Dis* 1991; 144: 1016–1025.
(23) Corrigan CJ, Brown PH, Barnes NC et al. Glucocorticoid resistance in chronic asthma: peripheral blood T-lymphocyte activation and a comparison of the T-lymphocyte inhibitory effects of glucocorticoids and cyclosporin A. *Am Rev Respir Dis* 1991; 144: 1026–1032.
(24) Siew LQ, Wu SY, Ying S, Corrigan CJ. Cigarette smoking increases bronchial mucosal IL-17A expression in asthmatics, which acts in concert with environmental aeroallergens to engender neutrophilic inflammation. *Clin Exp Allergy* 2017; 47: 774–750.
(25) Brown MA, Jabeen M, Bharj G, Hinks TSC. Non-typeable Haemophilus influenzae airways infection: the next treatable trait in asthma? *Eur Respir Rev* 2022; 31: 220008. https://doi.org/10.1183/16000617.0008-2022.
(26) Corrigan CJ. Calcilytics: a non-steroidal replacement for inhaled steroid and SABA/LABA therapy of human asthma? *Expert Rev Respir Med* 2020 Aug; 14(8): 807–816. https://doi.org/10.1080/17476348.2020.1756779.
(27) Coyle AJ, Ackerman SJ, Irvin CG. Cationic proteins induce airway hyperresponsiveness dependent on charge interactions. *Am Rev Respir Dis* 1993; 147: 896–900.
(28) Koller DY, Halmerbauer G, Frischer T, Roithner B. Assessment of eosinophil granule proteins in various body fluids: is there a relation to clinical variables in childhood asthma? *Clin Exp Allergy* 1999; 29: 786–793.
(29) Kurosawa M, Shimizu Y, Tsukagoshi H, Ueki M. Elevated levels of peripheral blood, naturally occurring aliphatic polyamines in bronchial asthmatic patients with active symptoms. *Allergy* 1992; 47: 638–643.
(30) Ogawa Y, Calhoun WJ. The role of leukotrienes in airway inflammation. *J Allergy Clin Immunol* 2007; 118: 789–798.
(31) Arm JP, O'Hickey SP, Spur BW, Lee TH. Airway responsiveness to histamine and leukotriene E4 in subjects with aspirin induced asthma. *Am Rev Respir Dis* 1989; 140: 148–153.
(32) An G, Wang W, Zhang X et al. Combined blockade of IL-25, IL-33 and TSLP mediates amplified inhibition of airway inflammation and remodelling in a murine model of asthma. *Respirology* 2020 Jun; 25(6): 603–612. https://doi.org/10.1111/resp.13711.
(33) Li Y, Wang W, Lv Z et al. Elevated expression of IL-33 and TSLP in the airways of human asthmatics *in vivo*: A potential biomarker of severe refractory disease. *J Immunol* 2018; 200(7): 2253–2262.
(34) Takhar P, Corrigan CJ, Smurthwaite L et al. Class switch recombination to IgE in the bronchial mucosa of atopic and non-atopic asthmatics. *J Allergy Clin Immunol* 2007; 119: 213–218.
(35) Busse WW, Morgan WJ, Gergen PJ et al. Randomized trial of omalizumab (anti-IgE) for asthma in inner-city children. *N Engl J Med* 2011; 364: 1005–1015.
(36) Larsen K, Zhu J, Feldman LY et al. The annual September peak in asthma exacerbation rates. Still a reality? *Ann Am Thorac Soc* 2016; 13: 231–239.
(37) Gill MA, Bajwa G, George TA et al. Counterregulation between the FcepsilonRI pathway and antiviral responses in human plasmacytoid dendritic cells. *J Immunol* 2010; 184(11): 5999–6006.
(38) Teach SJ, Gill MA, Togias A et al. Preseasonal treatment with either omalizumab or an inhaled corticosteroid boost to prevent fall asthma exacerbations. *J Allergy Clin Immunol* 2015; 136(6): 1476–1485.
(39) Murray CS, Poletti G, Kebadze T et al. Study of modifiable risk factors for asthma exacerbations: virus infection and allergen exposure increase the risk of asthma hospital admissions in children. *Thorax* 2006; 61(5): 376–382.
(40) Pillai P, Chan YC, Wu SY et al. Omalizumab reduces bronchial mucosal IgE and improves lung function in non-atopic asthma. *Eur Respir J* 2016; 48: 1593–1601.
(41) Wang W, Li Y, Lv Z et al. Bronchial allergen challenge of patients with atopic asthma triggers an alarmin (IL-33, TSLP, and IL-25) response in the airways epithelium and submucosa. *J Immunol* 2018; 201: 2221–2231.
(42) Di Domenico M, Bisogno A, Polverino M et al. Xolair in asthma therapy: an overview. *Inflamm Allergy Drug Targets* 2011; 10: 2–12.
(43) Dunican EM, Watchorn DC, Fahy JV. Autopsy and imaging studies of mucus in asthma. Lessons learned about disease mechanisms and the role of mucus in airflow obstruction. *Ann Am Thorac Soc* 2018; 15 (Suppl 3): S184–S191.
(44) Martínez-Rivera C, Crespo A, Pinedo-Sierra C et al. Mucus hypersecretion in asthma is associated with rhinosinusitis, polyps and exacerbations. *Respir Med* 2018; 135: 22–28.
(45) Ha EV, Rogers DF. Novel therapies to inhibit mucus synthesis and secretion in airway hypersecretory diseases. *Pharmacology* 2016; 97(1–2): 84–100.
(46) Kirjavainen PV, Karvonen AM, Adams RI et al. Farm-like indoor microbiota in non-farm homes protects children from asthma development. *Nat Med* 2019; 25: 1089–1095.
(47) Bisgaard H, Hermansen MN, Buchvald F et al. Childhood asthma after bacterial colonization of the airway in neonates. *N Engl J Med* 2007; 357: 487–495.
(48) Rubner FJ, Jackson DJ, Evans MD et al. Early life rhinovirus wheezing, allergic sensitization and asthma risk at adolescence. *J Allergy Clin Immunol* 2017; 139: 501–507.

(49) Shi T, Ooi Y, Zaw EN et al. Association between respiratory syncytial virus-associated acute lower respiratory infection in early life and recurrent wheeze and asthma in later childhood. *J Infect Dis* 2020; 222: S628–S633.

(50) von Mutius E, Smits HH. Primary prevention of asthma: from risk and protective factors to targeted strategies for prevention. *Lancet* 2020; 396: 854–866.

(51) Peng D, Shi Y, Pang J et al. Early-life infection of the airways with Streptococcus pneumoniae exacerbates HDM-induced asthma in a murine model. *Cell Immunol* 2022; 376: 104536. https://doi.org/0.1016/j.cellimm.2022.104536.

(52) Thysen AH, Waage J, Larsen JM et al. Distinct immune phenotypes in infants developing asthma during childhood. *Sci Transl Med* 2020 May; 12(529): eaaw0258.

(53) Sugita K, Kabashima K. Tight junctions in the development of asthma, chronic rhinosinusitis, atopic dermatitis, eosinophilic esophagitis, and inflammatory bowel diseases. *J Leukoc Biol* 2020; 107: 749–762.

(54) James AL, Wenzel S. Clinical relevance of airway remodelling in airway diseases. *Eur Respir J* 2007; 30: 134–155.

(55) Banno A, Reddy AT, Lakshmi SP, Reddy RC. Bidirectional interaction of airway epithelial remodelling and inflammation in asthma. *Clin Sci* 2020; 134: 1063–1079.

(56) Jupelli M, Murthy AK, Chaganty BK et al. Neonatal chlamydial pneumonia induces altered respiratory structure and function lasting into adult life. *Lab Invest* 2011; 91: 1530–1539.

(57) Dai X, Dharmage SC, Lodge CJ. The relationship of early-life household air pollution with childhood asthma and lung function. *Eur Respir Rev* 2022; 31: 220020; https://doi.org/10.1183/16000617.0020-2022.

(58) Wills-Karp M, Ewart SL. Time to draw breath: asthma susceptibility genes are identified. *Nat Rev Genet* 2004; 5: 376–387.

(59) Scharschmidt TC, Man MQ, Hatano Y et al. Filaggrin deficiency confers a paracellular barrier abnormality that reduces inflammatory thresholds to irritants and haptens. *J Allergy Clin Immunol* 2009; 124: 496–506.

(60) Grainge CL, Lau LCK, Ward JA et al. Effect of bronchoconstriction on airway remodelling in asthma. *N Engl J Med* 2011; 364: 2006–2015.

(61) Lee T, Nair P, Corrigan CJ. Review of monoclonal antibody therapies in asthma and allergic diseases—a new paradigm for precision medicine. *Asian Pac J Allergy Immunol* 2020; 38(2): 78–90.

(62) Menzies-Gow A, Corren J, Bourdin A et al. Tezepelumab in adults and adolescents with severe, uncontrolled asthma. *N Engl J Med* 2021; 384: 1800–1809.

(63) Kelsen SG, Agache IO, Soong W et al. Astegolimab (anti-ST2) efficacy and safety in adults with severe asthma: a randomized clinical trial. *J Allergy Clin Immunol* 2021; 148: 790–798.

(64) Castro M, Corren J, Pavord ID et al. Dupilumab efficacy and safety in moderate-to-severe uncontrolled asthma. *N Engl J Med* 2018; 378: 2486–2496.

(65) Mansfield B, Ho T-R, Mudway I et al. Calcium-sensing receptor antagonists, calcilytics, prevent activation of human dendritic and epithelial cells by urban particulate matter. *Eur Respir J* 2020; 56 (Suppl 64): 1970.

(66) Bruce R, Huang P, Yarova P et al. Calcium-sensing receptor (CaSR) drives lung ECM remodelling and fibrosis in murine asthma models and in ageing mice. *Eur Respir J* 2019; 54 (Suppl. 63): PA4213.

3 Smartinhalers, Telemedicine, and Artificial Intelligence, and the Future of Asthma Care Worldwide

Job F.M. van Boven, Chi Yan Hui, and Hilary Pinnock

CASE STUDY

Charlotte is a 14-year-old girl, first diagnosed with asthma when she was seven years old. Initially she did well on low-dose inhaled corticosteroids (ICS), but in the last two years she has been in hospital twice with several other attacks, needing oral glucocorticoids. She takes a short-acting beta-agonist (SABA) inhaler frequently. Her family doctor has already stepped up treatment to a combined ICS and long-acting beta-agonist (LABA) inhaler and wonders whether a referral to be assessed for additional treatment options (e.g. biologics) is required. To rule out poor response to ICS due to nonadherence, he asked her whether she was able to take her inhaler daily. She responded that when she turned 12, she herself became responsible for her inhaler use instead of her parents and admits now and then missing some doses, but not too many in her opinion. One of her friends was recently prescribed a Smartinhaler that automatically gave feedback on the timing and quality of inhaler use via her smartphone. Charlotte loves her smartphone, and she asks her doctor whether this could be something for her as well. Will it suit my type of inhaler? She also wonders about the effectiveness of the Smartinhaler (will it improve my asthma control?) and whether it is affordable (are there any co-payments [for my parents]?). Her doctor makes a note of her question and decides to further look into these issues. What are the advantages and disadvantages of a Smartinhaler he wonders? Are there other digital asthma management opportunities he can provide to his patients? Could Charlotte monitor her control with smart devices—and maybe arrange remote follow-up appointments? Are digital self-management plans available? Will "physical doctors" still be needed in the future?

LIST OF ABBREVIATIONS

AI:	artificial intelligence
AGI:	artificial general intelligence
ANI:	artificial narrow intelligence
ASI:	artificial super-intelligence
AUROC:	area under the receiver operating characteristic curve
CDSS:	clinical decision support system
CE/UKCA:	Conformité Européenne/UK Conformity Assessed
EHR:	electronic health records
GINA:	Global Initiative for Asthma
ICS:	inhaled corticosteroids
ML:	machine learning
SABA:	short-acting beta-agonist
SMS:	short message service
WHO:	World Health Organization

3.1 INTRODUCTION

Asthma care is continuously evolving, fuelled by new discoveries and insights. Over the past decades, we have seen substantial improvements in asthma care thanks to, amongst others, inhaled corticosteroids (ICS) (1), innovative inhalers and regimens (2), supported self-management (3), identification of novel phenotypes (4), and the advent of targeted biologic therapies (5). Many of these new insights are incorporated in annually updated evidence-based guidelines such as those generated by the Global Initiative for Asthma (GINA) (6). Still, 20–70% of asthma remains undiagnosed and 30–35% is misdiagnosed (7). Moreover, even in those with an adequate diagnosis, suboptimal treatment, poor management, and nonadherence are common (8). As a result, an estimated 45% of asthma patients have poorly controlled asthma, which is associated with both poor clinical and economic outcomes (9).

DOI: 10.1201/9781003287209-4

While management could certainly be improved, this would require more resources to be allocated to asthma care. Whether this can be realized remains a matter of debate. On the one hand, we live in an era with an ageing population, increased pressure on the economic sustainability of healthcare systems, and a workforce of overburdened healthcare professionals. On the other hand, the last decade has been characterized by an accelerated development of novel digital technologies, offering opportunities for the improvement of asthma care, whilst reducing the burden on professionals. Digital technologies can support diagnostic algorithms, suggest management strategies, monitor the impact of treatment, and support the day-to-day decisions made by people living with asthma (10). Examples include digital spirometers, electronic air quality monitoring devices, and Smartinhalers. Not only can these devices offer data-informed and person-tailored feedback to individual patients and clinicians, their combined data may also allow population-wide analysis of large databases using machine learning and artificial intelligence (AI) (11, 12). While digital technologies seem promising in shaping the future of asthma care worldwide (13), there are many challenges to overcome before they are integrated into healthcare systems (10).

In this chapter, we provide an overview of digital technologies within asthma care, focusing primarily on their effectiveness but also on implementation barriers and facilitators. The chapter ends with a vision of future digitally supported asthma care.

3.2 WHAT IS DIGITAL ASTHMA CARE?

We define "digital asthma care" as a broad range of care and support tools that have an electronic component. Notably, this care could involve computers and smartphones but also stand-alone digital technologies developed to monitor a specific parameter such as quality of inhalation or lung function. Acknowledging that this is a very broad area to be covered in a single chapter, we will focus on three digital technologies that are expected to be used increasingly in asthma care: (1) Smartinhalers, (2) telemedicine, and (3) artificial intelligence.

3.3 SMARTINHALERS

Smartinhalers, also known as digital inhalers or electronic monitoring devices, are inhalers with either integrated sensors or add-on sensors that can be attached to traditional inhalers or spacers. Over time, their functionality has evolved from relatively simple electronic dose counters with manual read-out to fully connected systems that support medication adherence, reduce short-acting beta-agonist (SABA) use, allow personalized inhaler technique training, predict exacerbations, and guide clinical decision-making in real time (8). Effectiveness of Smartinhalers can be assessed using different dimensions ranging from technical to therapeutic and socio-economic outcomes (Figure 3.1) (14). Generally, Smartinhalers have been shown to be effective in enhancing medication adherence (15), but their effects on clinical outcomes such as exacerbations and quality of life are less consistent. In the following sections, an overview of their different functionalities and evidence is provided, mostly focusing on their clinical benefit.

3.3.1 Support Medication Adherence

Around 60% of patients using ICS/LABA maintenance inhalers have poor adherence (16), making Charlotte's poor control not uncommon. The earliest clinical trials using Smartinhalers in adults and children with asthma demonstrated convincing effects on enhancing medication adherence (17–19). Notably, these trials used add-on devices to regular inhalers and provided audio-visual reminders to patients when a new dose was due. Inhaler usage was time-stamped and recorded. In a six-month paediatric trial (N = 220), median adherence was 84% in the intervention group and 30% in the control group, accompanied by some improvements in asthma control for the intervention group (19). In an Australian study performed in primary care (N = 146), similar results were observed regarding adherence in adults, with intervention patients having 73% adherence versus 46% in controls, and fewer severe exacerbations (18). In Charlotte's case, a Smartinhaler with reminders may thus be helpful, given she indicated that she "sometimes" forgets to take her inhaler.

3.3.2 Support Inhaler Technique

Over 70% of patients using inhalers have difficulties achieving correct inhaler technique (20). The latest and more advanced Smartinhalers are capable not only of recording adherence but also of measuring parameters related to inhaler technique such as handling and orientation of the device, time between actuation and start of inhalation, peak inspiratory flow, and inhaled volume. Sensors are used that can detect acoustics, air flow, or vibration (21–24). Using these data, patient inhaler education can be tailored to correct the inhalation errors made. Indeed, in an Irish study performed in community pharmacies using a Smartinhaler, the critical technique error rate was significantly lower in the intervention group versus usual care (17.5 vs. 36.1) at six months (25). Similar results were obtained with a personalized approach using data from a smart, digital spacer in the Netherlands, where inhaler technique errors dropped by around one-third (26).

3.3.3 Reduce SABA Use

Excessive use of SABA is associated with increased risk of exacerbations and mortality (27). Smartinhalers can reduce SABA use (19, 24, 28), probably due to optimization of inhaler technique, increased awareness of asthma

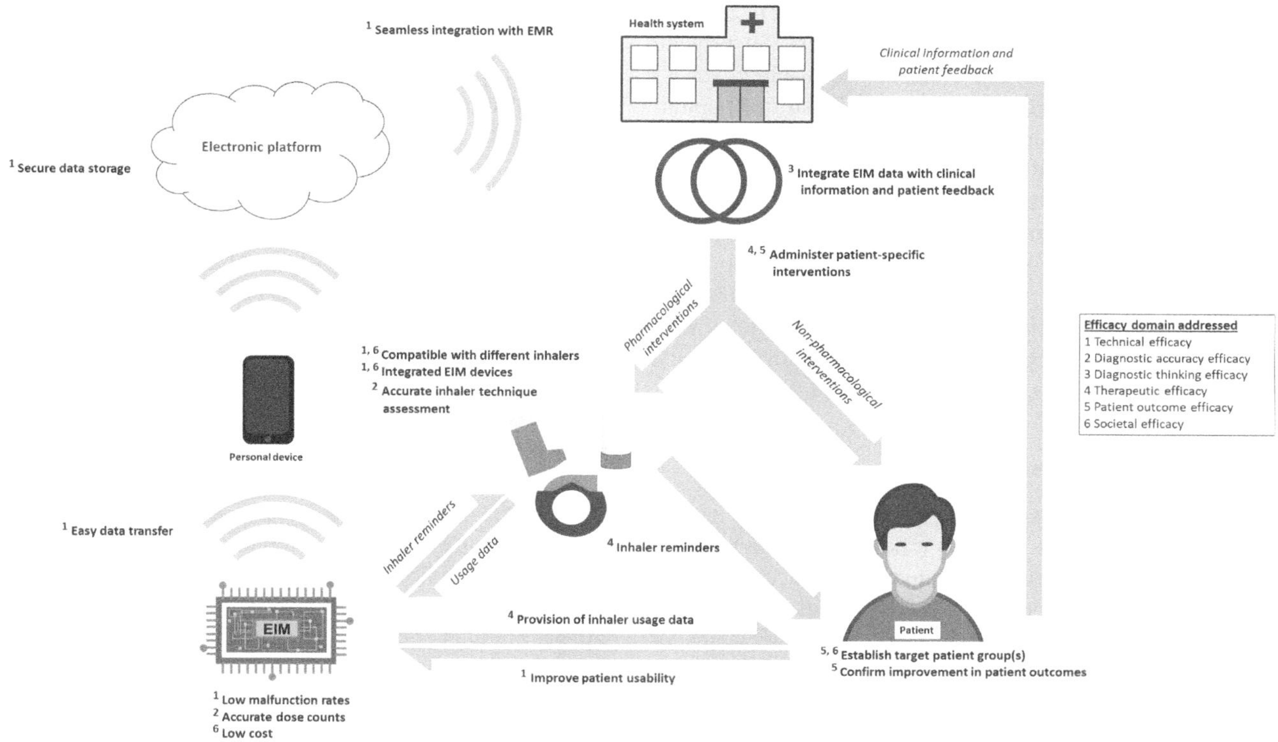

FIGURE 3.1 Effectiveness dimensions of Smartinhalers. EIM: Electronic inhaler monitoring. (Reused, with permission from [14].)

status, and improved adherence to maintenance inhaler regimens. For example, in a six-month paediatric trial in New Zealand, the median proportion of days with reliever usage was 9.5% in the Smartinhaler group versus 17.4% in the control group ($p = 0.002$) (19). Similarly, in a 12-week US study, the weekly number of SABA-free days increased from 3.4 to 4.6 after 12 weeks of Smartinhaler use (24).

3.3.4 Predict Exacerbations

One of the major treatment goals of asthma is to prevent exacerbations (6). Using data from a smart device that could measure SABA inhaler usage as well as technique, machine learning models have been developed that can predict an exacerbation up to five days in advance with an area under the receiver operating characteristic curve (AUROC) of 0.83 (29). The strongest predictive factors were the number of daily SABA inhalations in the four days prior to an exacerbation (47%), inhalation parameters (inhalation volume, peak inspiratory flow, inhalation duration) (11%), and comparison to baseline values of these parameters (14%). With such prediction models becoming more and more accurate and including more parameters (e.g. maintenance inhaler use, environmental triggers), asthma treatment could be shifting from reactive to proactive (self-)management.

3.3.5 Guide Clinical Decision-Making

Given the detailed and objective measurements collected by Smartinhalers, these data can be used to guide clinical decision-making. In particular, this is helpful to understand and manage difficult-to-treat asthma, which seems the case for Charlotte. Without objective data in this population, it is difficult to assess whether a patient with uncontrolled asthma on medium/high-dose ICS-LABA has severe (refractory) asthma or poor adherence and/or inhaler technique. Consequently, patients' treatment burden and costs may be unnecessarily increased, e.g. with step-up to higher-dose ICS, oral corticosteroids, and/or biologic therapy (21). In the INCA Sun trial, 213 patients with uncontrolled asthma were randomized to a Smartinhaler-based treatment strategy or usual care, with co-primary end-points being adherence and treatment burden. While adherence in the intervention group was higher over the 32-week trial period, only 11% were assessed as requiring biologic add-on treatment compared to 21% of control group patients. Additionally, patients in the intervention group were less likely to be advised to step up to high-dose ICS and more likely to step down to medium/low-dose ICS. Overall, the Smartinhaler-informed decision-making model resulted in cost savings of around €3,000 per patient (30).

3.3.6 Cost-Effectiveness

The additional functionality of Smartinhalers makes them more expensive than traditional inhalers. As such, proof of their added health economic value is essential to support the business case for wider implementation in daily clinical practice and healthcare systems (31). Indeed, several reviews have highlighted the need for robust cost-effectiveness analyses of digital inhalers (8, 32, 33). Charlotte and her doctor also wonder whether a Smartinhaler will provide them with value for money. Currently, cost-effectiveness evidence remains scarce for the overall asthma population; however, the economic value of digital inhalers in the subgroup of patients with difficult-to-treat asthma has been clearly demonstrated (34). In this population, economic gains due to Smartinhalers are mainly driven by a decreased proportion of patients requiring step-up treatment to biologic add-on therapies. In other populations, such as in patients initiating asthma therapy, patients with frequent exacerbations or those already on biologic therapy, more cost-effectiveness evidence is required (8).

3.4 TELEMEDICINE

The World Health Organization (WHO) defines telemedicine as "an interaction between a healthcare provider and a patient when the two are separated by distance"(35). This communication may be synchronous (as in telephone or video consultations) or asynchronous (as in exchange of monitoring data, questionnaire responses, and queries by e-mail or Short Message Service [SMS]) (36).

3.4.1 Potential of Telemedicine in Asthma

Asthma is a variable condition (6). Symptoms that vary in response to triggers are associated with changes in airflow obstruction causing attacks that are at best inconvenient but (as in Charlotte's case) can be severe enough to warrant hospital admission. It follows that all people with asthma should be aware of how to recognize deterioration and the prompt actions they should take. Traditionally delivered in a face-to-face review and summarized in a paper action plan (3), telemedicine can contribute to self-management support by providing access to online information (37), logging of clinical status (38, 39), and facilitating remote reviews (40).

3.4.2 Digital Monitoring

Charlotte is interested in a Smartinhaler that can not only support her adherence to regular preventive medication but offers the potential to monitor reliever inhaler use as an indicator of poor control. Patients allocated to using a digital SABA inhaler linked to a dashboard, checked weekly by their clinician, were more likely to achieve good control over the three-month study (24). Traditionally, self-monitoring is based on symptom questionnaires with peak flow monitoring, and this has been used in multiple apps that offer features for logging symptom scores and readings from smart peak flow meters (41).

Despite expressing interest in monitoring asthma status, patients rarely persist with logging symptoms or peak flows for more than a few weeks (Figure 3.2), even in the context of a research project (42).

With the broad range of sensors now available or under development, it may be possible to monitor stable asthma without any human input, alerting the patient if/when the monitoring suggests control may be slipping. For example:

- Smartinhalers can detect whether usage changes (especially nighttime use) or if inspiratory effort falls.
- Cough monitors could detect new symptoms.
- Voice assistants on mobile phones could detect a change in speech/breathing.

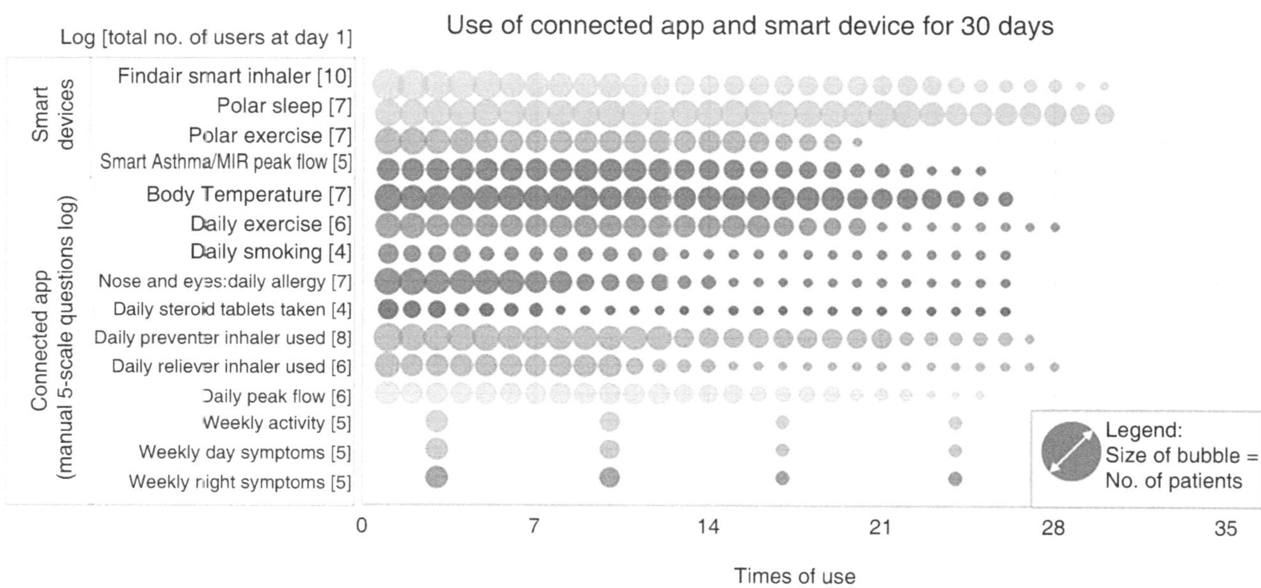

FIGURE 3.2 Use of connected apps and smart devices. (Reused with permission from [42].)

- Activity monitors could detect a change in gait or distances walked.
- Environmental sensors can detect poor air quality or pollen counts.

Combined with the potential of AI to interpret changes in parameters for individuals, such "passive" data may form the basis of future action plans.

3.4.3 Digital Action Plans

Supported self-management is a highly effective intervention (3, 43). Typically, however, apps are limited to monitoring and rarely include even basic algorithms for triggering advice as would be included in an action plan (41). This is currently a major limitation for digital asthma care, as monitoring without actions does not change outcomes: indeed multiple systematic reviews evaluating asthma telemonitoring have concluded that there is no consistent evidence of effectiveness (39, 40, 44). On the other hand, none of these reviews identified any harm, so Charlotte may be given the choice of whether she uses a monitoring app in conjunction with a Smartinhaler, though, in the absence of evidence of cost-effectiveness, it may not be reimbursed by the health service. Her doctor should check the features of the app and be prepared to provide her with a paper action plan (which she can photograph or scan and keep on her smartphone) if her monitoring logs suggest her asthma status is deteriorating. In contrast, a review of interventions that used combinations of tele-case management, telemonitoring, teleconsultations, reminders, and education concluded that such multifaceted interventions may be effective in improving quality of life (45).

3.4.4 Remote Consultations

Twenty years before the COVID-19 pandemic accelerated interest in remote consulting (46), telephone reviews for the routine review of people with asthma by asthma-trained primary care nurses were shown to cost-effectively improve access without compromising clinical outcomes (47, 48). On a practical level, opportunistic telephone reviews can establish contact with non-attenders (49) and enable assessment of control and risk of attacks so that the need for a face-to-face consultation can be assessed and discussed with the patient (50). A Cochrane review (n = 6 studies) confirmed that telephone reviews enabled more people to receive routine care, and, despite concerns about the limitations of telephone consultations, there was no evidence of deterioration in asthma control (51).

There is less evidence about the role of video-consulting to provide routine care for asthma, though the ability to observe a patient's clinical status, watch and correct inhaler technique, and screen-share to complete an action plan (52) suggests there may be practical advantages over telephone reviews. A video consultation may seem more "human" and improve rapport building (53), though the practicalities of inadequate infrastructure or unfamiliar technology proved challenging in the early days of the pandemic (54).

Even more "remote" than telephone or video consultations, asynchronous communication using validated control questionnaires are being promoted by primary care electronic systems and may prove to have utility as a means of triage, but there will be concerns about the quality of the asthma care that can be provided in this way.

3.5 ARTIFICIAL INTELLIGENCE

3.5.1 Definitions

Artificial intelligence (AI) is a set of machine algorithms that can learn from data and carry out the tasks that typically require human intelligence. It is generally categorized into three groups depending on how "intelligent" the algorithm is: (1) artificial narrow intelligence (ANI), (2) artificial general intelligence (AGI), and (3) artificial super-intelligence (ASI). ANI requires human intelligence to make the rules that the AI uses to make a decision. AGI and ASI have the intelligence to learn, think, and create the rules to make decisions on an action.

AI can also be categorized based on their learning abilities—for example: machine learning (ML) and deep learning. Machine learning is a subfield of AI where techniques are used to create an algorithm based on the observation of a pattern in a dataset to perform a "human" action. Humans are involved in supporting the machine to learn. Deep learning is a subset of ML, which uses advanced techniques, for example artificial neural networks, to reach an accurate conclusion without human support (55). The latest "real-life" AI application (generative AI) allows users to use natural language to produce a series of text instructions and to generate content like images, music, videos, document context, and program codes. The application is user friendly and easy to access online. It can enhance a dynamic interaction with patients and encourage the use of AGI and ASI to support personalized care but has also prompted concerns about its safety to patients. There are questions about who will ensure that the personalized advice is accurate and how to prevent bias and ensure unfair predictions from limited historical data generated in ethnic minorities and digitally disconnected groups of patients (56).

3.5.2 Overview of AI Applications in Asthma

Artificial intelligence can be applied across the spectrum of asthma care, ranging from prevention to diagnosis and treatment (12, 57). Most applications use asthma clinical guidelines to create rules that underpin diagnostic advice or self-management to patients, or use machine learning to categorize asthma control and predict the risk of exacerbations from electronic health records or patient-reported data. Machine learning techniques such as ANI and decision trees are commonly used in asthma research (57). Although studies are moving from ANI and AGI towards ASI, most are in the stage of testing the feasibility and technical accuracy of the AI decisions; few have been deployed in real time to evaluate the usability, clinical effectiveness, and safety for patients. Notably, a large amount of high-quality population-level asthma data (e.g. asthma control status, physiological parameters, treatments, and environmental exposure) is needed for a successful movement to ASI (57).

3.5.2.1 Diagnosis

Overdiagnosis and under-diagnosis is a well-known problem in asthma, where AI can potentially help (7). Indeed, rule-based algorithms in clinical decision support systems (CDSS) can identify patients who have a high probability of having asthma (58). Using retrospective EHR data, a CDSS can categorize confirmed and suspected asthma patients based on existing clinical guidelines. An increasing number of studies are using AI in a smartphone to support remote diagnosis. For example, a hidden Markov model and a wearable device to detect respiratory sounds and wheezing have been used to support a remote diagnosis of asthma with an accuracy of 95% (sensitivity 89%; specificity 96%) (59). These studies demonstrate the potential of AI to provide a diagnosis based on classifying auscultations without an in-person consultation. Indeed acoustic digital equipment detects wheezing earlier than a clinician with a stethoscope (60)—by the time wheeze is audible, lung function may have dropped by a third (61).

3.5.2.2 Classification of Asthma Severity, Asthma Phenotypes, and Treatment Stratification

Respiratory sounds, asthma control, and hospitalization data are commonly used in AI to help clinicians to classify asthma severity and control status (57). Notably, ML/deep learning techniques that link genomic data and patients' responses to medication have been used to identify phenotypes such as allergic or nonallergic asthma, or asthma endotypes in adult and paediatric asthma (62–64). Furthermore, using retrospective EHR/patient-reported datasets, rule-based algorithms could stratify patients based on their risk for safe discharge or to initiate readmission prevention (65, 66).

3.5.2.3 Self-Management and Exacerbation Prediction

In supporting patients' asthma self-management, AI has multiple applications. For example, AI can automatically detect adherence and inhalation technique using a wireless monitoring device mounted on the wall of the patient's home (67). Moreover, using connected data of multiple devices, such as personal wearable devices and Smartinhalers, AI can learn from individual patient data in order to provide timely advice to improve control or prevent exacerbations (29, 68, 69). For Charlotte, this may be an interesting feature, given she suffered from several exacerbations. ANI can be based on "rules'" derived from clinical guidelines, that identify high-risk patients and provide individualized evidence-based treatment advice (65, 66). AGI can learn from patients' past patterns of attacks and use these to predict the future likelihood of an asthma attack and provide personalized management advice based on an asthma action plan previously agreed with the clinician (57). ASI can use deep learning techniques to create rules based on its observations of patients' responses to their environmental triggers. Multiple, diverse, large population datasets/biobanks will be needed to increase accuracy ("intelligence") and enable tailor-made, dynamic treatment advice to be provided (70).

3.5.3 Performance of AI

AI can reduce the asthma under- or overdiagnosis rate and provide faster diagnosis decisions and treatment suggestions to patients than a traditional diagnostic process undertaken by clinicians (71–73). When AI is used to support patient self-management, the accuracy of its advice depends on the quality of the input data, e.g. by patient self-report or automatically detected by passive sensors. The former typically contain an inherent risk of bias because patients forget, feel too ill, or are not motivated to record their asthma measurements, and some may even manipulate their data. The latter can be used to collect patient data automatically and silently. Monitoring devices used to derive AI algorithms typically have a CE/UKCA marking certifying their technical accuracy under laboratory conditions where assessment of accuracy is based on the correct use of the device as instructed by the manufacturer. In reality, instructions for use may not be clear or understandable by patients, which may lead to misuse of the devices and inaccurate input data to the AI algorithm, causing incorrect advice to patients (74). Therefore, more evidence is needed in the implementation stage of AI to prove clinical effectiveness and safety and to understand a system's usability in the real-life setting (57).

3.6 IMPLEMENTATION BARRIERS AND FACILITATORS

The body of evidence for digital technologies in asthma is continuing to increase with compelling evidence of potential benefit. Yet successful implementation is complex, requiring understanding of the patient, professional, and organizational perspectives, as well as the political, regulatory, and socio-economic contexts (10).

3.6.1 Context

From a technology perspective, there are basic infrastructure prerequisites such as nationwide Wi-Fi coverage and a reliable electricity supply that need to be in place for digital technologies to work (75). The lack of a unified system to capture data and integrate with electronic medical records diminishes the benefits of digital monitoring. Successful multi-country implementation of innovative technology in daily practice is further hampered by diversity in healthcare systems, differential (or no) reimbursement pathways for eHealth, and inconsistent interpretation of digital policy regulations across countries. Given the potential for scale-up in the very near future, international harmonization of standards is urgently required, as are research evaluating cost-effectiveness and budget impact (76).

3.6.2 Organizational Challenges

Significant organizational changes are needed to establish and sustain digital healthcare (e.g. practical resources, skills training, proper reimbursement, integration with existing patient management systems, transferability of data across settings, privacy issues) (77, 78). Indeed, a practical challenge for people with asthma wanting to monitor their asthma, potential triggers, and environmental factors that influence their asthma is that this requires data from multiple sensors each with its own branded app so that patients and clinicians need to monitor multiple apps or dashboards. There are pilot projects seeking to launch device-agnostic connected platforms (79, 80), but current systems are not yet as simple as plug and play, which may be acceptable to technology-expert users but will discourage general adoption (42).

3.6.3 Leave No One Behind

Societal challenges to be considered are the potential of digital technology to increase inequities in access to healthcare due to age or gender, rurality, deprivation, limited (or no) access to technology, or poor eHealth literacy (81). The principles of fairness in digital healthcare provision mean engaging with potentially marginalized groups (socio-economically deprived communities, ethnic minority groups, elderly, and those with poor access to technology or limited eHealth literacy) throughout the development process to ensure user interfaces are designed to be inclusive (79) and able to be used on basic, affordable technology (82). These considerations are particularly pertinent in low- and middle-income countries where over 90% of asthma deaths occur (83).

3.6.4 Ethical Challenges of AI

AI has its potential for clinical asthma care, education, and research, yet its wider application needs to consider several ethical implications. Amongst others, these considerations include (1) informed consent to use data to inform AI; (2) safety, transparency, and fairness of algorithms used to avoid bias; (3) trustworthiness including accuracy in input data and reliability of outcomes; (4) data privacy, especially regarding sensitive health data; and (5) agreement on the data owner and responsible party (84).

3.6.5 Patient Engagement

When considering the implementation of digital asthma care, involving all stakeholders' views is of paramount importance. Among these stakeholders, patients (and/or their caretakers) and clinicians are particularly important given their roles as end users. More widely, stakeholders include healthcare policymakers, insurers, and industry (85). Patients attending European Lung Foundation digital health workshops were keen to use apps to monitor and learn about their condition, access timely advice, and reduce travel time for consultations (58). In two qualitative studies on the use of digital inhalers, similar findings were observed, with patients highlighting that additional functionalities, good usability, clarity on data accessibility, and support of the digital tools by their clinicians would be facilitators for their use. In contrast, lack of compatibility, lack of reimbursement, and lack of insight into data privacy and security were some of the barriers (85, 86).

Regarding AI, in a qualitative study performed among 12 patients (≥16 years) and 12 clinicians, both groups expressed concerns about trusting AI. Patients saw potential in digital monitoring to support their self-management but were not ready to accept that AI could provide novel advice without the interpretation of their clinicians (76). Similar views were expressed by 295 parents of children with asthma being treated in one of four paediatric hospitals asking their opinion regarding the use of AI in clinical decision support for the care of their children (87). Two-thirds agreed that AI could be useful in asthma diagnosis and monitoring, but only 15% thought that it could replace physicians in this task, and none supported the idea that AI could make decisions on its own. Of note, this study also revealed large differences in parents' opinions on AI, with appreciation of the physician–patient relationship, the number of digital devices owned, as well as socio-economic status being some of the drivers of differences.

Children's views on adoption of AI-based asthma care have been investigated using semi-structured interviews in 104 children aged 8–17 (88). Children generally valued the possibility of support, especially at home and in real time, but mentioned technical issues and loss of "humanness" as major drawbacks. Just over half would like to use AI-based support if it were as effective as traditional care, while 93% would use it if it were more effective. Those with more computer skills tended to be more positive in their opinion of AI; prior experience of a good clinician–patient relation was a negative factor.

3.6.6 Healthcare Professional Engagement

Healthcare professionals embraced remote consulting for reasons of infection control in the pandemic, and many have been convinced of the utility (though not necessarily the time/cost efficiency) of telephone/video consultations (89). Both patients and professionals raised concerns that remote consultations were less "human" and lacked the

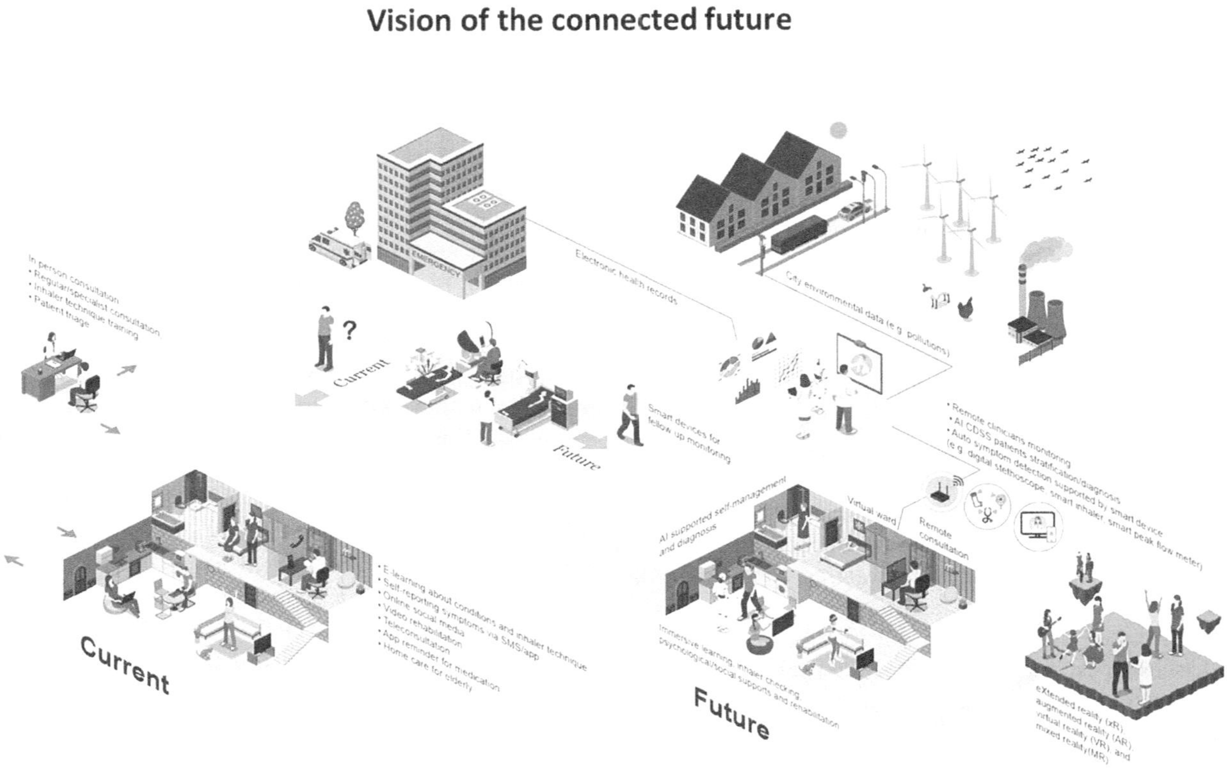

FIGURE 3.3 Envisioned future of asthma care. (Reused, with permission from [10].)

empathy that could be built in a face-to-face meeting (90), though this could be mitigated if the remote consultation was built on existing relationships (91). Video-consulting was seen as having a potential advantage in enabling rapport (92). Clinicians wanted "solid evidence" of the effectiveness and safety of AI before they were prepared to trust decisions (76).

3.7 VISION OF THE FUTURE OF ASTHMA CARE

It seems highly likely that digital technologies are here to stay, and their further uptake will transform the way we deliver asthma care (Figure 3.3), though the speed at which this digital transformation will take place and demonstration of its effectiveness are uncertain. The bottleneck is not the pace at which technology is being developed; rather it is dependent on system barriers within the healthcare community, verifiable accuracy of data, lack of policy-driven infrastructure, as well as acceptance by and suitability for patients (10). In a vision of the future, asthma diagnoses could be supported by AI, reducing under-, over-, and misdiagnoses. Physical consultations could be replaced by patient feedback and decision support that is personalized using AI. This feedback will be informed by the patient's own data, collected using remote telemonitoring of clinical parameters (e.g. peak expiratory flow), environmental data (e.g. air quality, pollen), and behavioural data (e.g. medication adherence), supplemented by periodic patient-reported outcomes.

This new way of delivering asthma management will not replace healthcare professionals but will require healthcare professionals to adapt to these new models of decentralized digital asthma care delivery. In doing so, more patients could be served with a smaller healthcare workforce, thereby easing the growth in healthcare demands in an increasingly ageing population. Importantly, user-friendly design should enable most people to benefit from this digital transformation, but care will be needed to ensure that no one is left behind. Initially there will need to be a slow progression to hybrid models, with some patients being digitally supported and others still using some traditional care. Over time, the latter share will reduce, while the former will become the new standard of care. The speed at which this occurs may differ across the globe, yet that this digital transformation eventually becomes the "new norm" seems inevitable (46).

3.8 CONCLUSION

Digital technologies such as Smartinhalers, telemedicine, and AI are increasingly being developed and validated yet slowly implemented in asthma care. While evidence is accumulating and several system challenges are yet to be overcome, these technologies hold great promise in shaping the future of asthma care. However, implementation needs to take into account that nobody is left behind, ensuring optimal asthma care for all across the globe. Digital asthma care is envisioned to advance and complement, not replace, traditional asthma care, and healthcare professionals are encouraged to embrace these developments.

REFERENCES

(1) Adams NP, et al. Inhaled beclomethasone versus placebo for chronic asthma. *Cochrane Database Syst Rev* 2005;(1):CD002738.

(2) Lavorini F, et al. New inhaler devices—the good, the bad and the ugly. *Respiration* 2014;88(1):3–15.

(3) Pinnock H, et al. Systematic meta-review of supported self-management for asthma: a healthcare perspective. *BMC Med* 2017;15(1):64–67.

(4) Pavord ID, et al. After asthma: redefining airways diseases. *Lancet* 2018;391(10118):350–400.

(5) Normansell R, et al. Omalizumab for asthma in adults and children. *Cochrane Database Syst Rev* 2014;(1):CD003559.

(6) Yorgancioglu A, et al. Global initiative for asthma: 30 years of promoting evidence-based asthma care. *Allergy* 2023;78(7):1737–1739.

(7) Aaron SD, et al. Underdiagnosis and overdiagnosis of asthma. *Am J Respir Crit Care Med* 2018;198(8):1012–1020.

(8) Jansen EM, et al. Global burden of medication non-adherence in chronic obstructive pulmonary disease (COPD) and asthma: a narrative review of the clinical and economic case for smart inhalers. *J Thorac Dis* 2021;13(6):3846–3864.

(9) Price D, et al. Asthma control and management in 8,000 European patients: the Recognise Asthma and Link to Symptoms and Experience (REALISE) survey. *NPJ Prim Care Respir Med* 2014;24:14009.

(10) Pinnock H, et al. Implementation of digital home monitoring and management of respiratory disease. *Curr Opin Pulm Med* 2023;29(4):302–312.

(11) Khoury P, et al. A framework for augmented intelligence in allergy and immunology practice and research-a work group report of the AAAAI health informatics, technology, and education committee. *J Allergy Clin Immunol Pract* 2022;10(5):1178–1188.

(12) Khanam UA, et al. A scoping review of asthma and machine learning. *J Asthma* 2023;60(2):213–226.

(13) Kraman SS, et al. Smart devices are poised to revolutionize the usefulness of respiratory sounds. *Chest* 2023;163(6):1519–1528.

(14) Tay TR, et al. Electronic inhaler monitoring for chronic airway disease: development and application of a multidimensional efficacy framework. *J Allergy Clin Immunol Pract* 2022;10(5):1189–1201.

(15) Chan A, et al. Digital interventions to improve adherence to maintenance medication in asthma. *Cochrane Database Syst Rev* 2022;6(6):CD013030.

(16) van Boven JFM, et al. Trajectory analyses of adherence patterns in a real-life moderate to severe asthma population. *J Allergy Clin Immunol Pract* 2020;8(6):1961–1969.

(17) Vasbinder EC, et al. e-Monitoring of asthma therapy to improve compliance in children (e-MATIC): a randomised controlled trial. *Eur Respir J* 2016;48(3):758–767.

(18) Foster JM, et al. Inhaler reminders improve adherence with controller treatment in primary care patients with asthma. *J Allergy Clin Immunol* 2014;134(6):1260–1268.

(19) Chan AHY, et al. The effect of an electronic monitoring device with audiovisual reminder function on adherence to inhaled corticosteroids and school attendance in children with asthma: a randomised controlled trial. *Lancet Respir Med* 2015;3(3):210–219.

(20) Price DB, et al. Inhaler errors in the CRITIKAL study: type, frequency, and association with asthma outcomes. *J Allergy Clin Immunol Pract* 2017;5(4):1071–1081.

(21) Sulaiman I, et al. A randomised clinical trial of feedback on inhaler adherence and technique in patients with severe uncontrolled asthma. *Eur Respir J* 2018;51(1):1701126.

(22) Sportel ET, et al. Does immediate smart feedback on therapy adherence and inhalation technique improve asthma control in children with uncontrolled asthma? A study protocol of the IMAGINE I study. *Trials* 2020;21(1):801–804.

(23) Dierick BHJ, et al. Can electronic monitoring with a digital smart spacer support personalised medication adherence and inhaler technique education in patients with asthma?: Protocol of the randomised controlled OUTERSPACE trial. *BMJ Open* 2022;12(6):e059929.

(24) Hoyte FCL, et al. Effectiveness of a digital inhaler system for patients with asthma: a 12-week, open-label, randomized study (CONNECT1). *J Allergy Clin Immunol Pract* 2022;10(10):2579–2587.

(25) O'Dwyer S, et al. Personalized biofeedback on inhaler adherence and technique by community pharmacists: a cluster randomized clinical trial. *J Allergy Clin Immunol Pract* 2020;8(2):635–644.

(26) Dierick BJH, et al. Electronic monitoring with a digital smart spacer to support personalized inhaler use education in patients with asthma: The randomized controlled OUTERSPACE trial. *Respir Med* 2023;218:107376.

(27) Nwaru BI, et al. Overuse of short-acting beta (2)-agonists in asthma is associated with increased risk of exacerbation and mortality: a nationwide cohort study of the global SABINA programme. *Eur Respir J* 2020;55(4):1901872.

(28) Mosnaim GS, et al. The impact of patient self-monitoring via electronic medication monitor and mobile app plus remote clinician feedback on adherence to inhaled corticosteroids: a randomized controlled trial. *J Allergy Clin Immunol Pract* 2021;9(4):1586–1594.

(29) Lugogo NL, et al. A predictive machine learning tool for asthma exacerbations: results from a 12-week, open-label study using an electronic multi-dose dry powder inhaler with integrated sensors. *J Asthma Allergy* 2022;15:1623–1637.

(30) Hale EM, et al. Use of digital measurement of medication adherence and lung function to guide the management of uncontrolled asthma (INCA Sun): a multicentre, single-blinded, randomised clinical trial. *Lancet Respir Med* 2023;11(7):591–601.

(31) van Boven JFM, et al. Making sense of cost-effectiveness analyses in respiratory medicine: a practical guide for non-health economists. *Eur Respir J* 2019;53(3):1801816.

(32) Chrystyn H, et al. Real-life inhaler adherence and technique: time to get smarter! *Respir Med* 2019;158:24–32.

(33) Mosnaim GS, et al. Digital inhalers and remote patient monitoring for asthma. *J Allergy Clin Immunol Pract* 2022;10(10):2525–2533.

(34) van de Hei SJ, et al. Long-term cost-effectiveness of digital inhaler adherence technologies in difficult-to-treat asthma. *J Allergy Clin Immunol Pract* 2023. https://doi.org/10.1016/j.jaip.2023.06.051

(35) World Health Organization. *Global diffusion of eHealth: making universal health coverage achievable. Report of the third global survey on eHealth.* World Health Organization, 2016.

(36) World Health Organization. *Telemedicine: opportunities and developments in Member States: Report on the second global survey on eHealth*. World Health Organization, 2009.
(37) Rikkers-Mutsaerts ERVM, et al. Internet-based self-management compared with usual care in adolescents with asthma: a randomized controlled trial. *Pediatr Pulmonol* 2012;47(12):1170–1179.
(38) Marcano Belisario JS, et al. Smartphone and tablet self management apps for asthma. *Cochrane Database Syst Rev* 2013;(11):CD010013.
(39) Hui CY, et al. The use of mobile applications to support self-management for people with asthma: a systematic review of controlled studies to identify features associated with clinical effectiveness and adherence. *J Am Med Inform Assoc* 2017;24(3):619–632.
(40) Kew KM, Cates CJ. Home telemonitoring and remote feedback between clinic visits for asthma. *Cochrane Database Syst Rev* 2016;(8):CD011714.
(41) Huckvale K, et al. The evolution of mobile apps for asthma: an updated systematic assessment of content and tools. *BMC Med* 2015;13:58-x.
(42) Hui CY, et al. Assessing the technical feasibility of a flexible, integrated Internet-of-things connected for asthma (C4A) system to support self-management: a mixed method study exploring patients and healthcare professionals perspectives. *JAMIA Open* 2022;5(4):ooac110.
(43) Hodkinson A, et al. Self-management interventions to reduce healthcare use and improve quality of life among patients with asthma: systematic review and network meta-analysis. *BMJ* 2020;370:m2521.
(44) Snoswell CL, et al. A systematic review and meta-analysis of change in health-related quality of life for interactive telehealth interventions for patients with asthma. *Value Health* 2021;24(2):291–302.
(45) Chongmelaxme B, et al. The effects of telemedicine on asthma control and patients' quality of life in adults: a systematic review and meta-analysis. *J Allergy Clin Immunol Pract* 2019;7(1):199–216.
(46) Pinnock H, et al. Telemedicine and virtual respiratory care in the era of COVID-19. *ERJ Open Res* 2022;8(3):00111-2022.
(47) Pinnock H, et al. Cost-effectiveness of telephone or surgery asthma reviews: economic analysis of a randomised controlled trial. *Br J Gen Pract* 2005;55(511):119–124.
(48) Pinnock H, et al. Accessibility, acceptability, and effectiveness in primary care of routine telephone review of asthma: pragmatic, randomised controlled trial. *BMJ* 2003;326(7387):477–479.
(49) Pinnock H, et al. Accessibility, clinical effectiveness, and practice costs of providing a telephone option for routine asthma reviews: phase IV controlled implementation study. *Br J Gen Pract* 2007;57(542):714–722.
(50) Gruffydd-Jones K, et al. Targeted routine asthma care in general practice using telephone triage. *Br J Gen Pract* 2005;55(521):918–923.
(51) Kew KM, Cates CJ. Remote versus face-to-face check-ups for asthma. *Cochrane Database Syst Rev* 2016;4(4):CD011715.
(52) Hamour O, et al. Completing asthma action plans by screen-sharing in video-consultations: practical insights from a feasibility assessment. *NPJ Prim Care Respir Med* 2020;30(1):48–88.
(53) Donaghy E, et al. Acceptability, benefits, and challenges of video consulting: a qualitative study in primary care. *Br J Gen Pract* 2019;69(686):e586–e594.
(54) Car J, et al. Video consultations in primary and specialist care during the covid-19 pandemic and beyond. *BMJ* 2020;371:m3945.
(55) Singapore Computer Society. Overview of artificial intelligence, machine and deep learning. Available at: https://www.scs.org.sg/articles/machine-learning-vs-deep-learning.
(56) Johnson KB, et al. Precision medicine, AI, and the future of personalized health care. *Clin Transl Sci* 2021;14(1):86–93.
(57) Exarchos KP, et al. Artificial intelligence techniques in asthma: a systematic review and critical appraisal of the existing literature. *Eur Respir J* 2020;56(3):2000521.
(58) Canny A, et al. Patient views on asthma diagnosis and how a clinical decision support system could help: a qualitative study. *Health Expect* 2023;26(1):307–317.
(59) Oletic D, Bilas V. Asthmatic wheeze detection from compressively sensed respiratory sound spectra. *IEEE J Biomed Health Inform* 2018;22(5):1406–1414.
(60) Levy ML, et al. Wheeze detection: recordings vs. assessment of physician and parent. *J Asthma* 2004;41(8):845–853.
(61) McFadden ERJ, et al. Acute bronchial asthma. Relations between clinical and physiologic manifestations. *N Engl J Med* 1973;288(5):221–225.
(62) Krautenbacher N, et al. A strategy for high-dimensional multivariable analysis classifies childhood asthma phenotypes from genetic, immunological, and environmental factors. *Allergy* 2019;74(7):1364–1373.
(63) Wu W, et al. Multiview cluster analysis identifies variable corticosteroid response phenotypes in severe asthma. *Am J Respir Crit Care Med* 2019;199(11):1358–1367.
(64) Ross MK, et al. Discovering pediatric asthma phenotypes on the basis of response to controller medication using machine learning. *Ann Am Thorac Soc* 2018;15(1):49–58.
(65) Tsai C, et al. Risk stratification for hospitalization in acute asthma: the CHOP classification tree. *Am J Emerg Med* 2010;28(7):803–808.
(66) Noble M, et al. Predicting asthma-related crisis events using routine electronic healthcare data: a quantitative database analysis study. *Br J Gen Pract* 2021;71(713):e948–e957.
(67) Zhao M, et al. Assessment of medication self-administration using artificial intelligence. *Nat Med* 2021;27(4):727–735.
(68) Finkelstein J, Jeong IC. Machine learning approaches to personalize early prediction of asthma exacerbations. *Ann N Y Acad Sci* 2017;1387(1):153–165.
(69) Zein JG, et al. Novel machine learning can predict acute asthma exacerbation. *Chest* 2021;159(5):1747–1757.
(70) Subramanian M, et al. Precision medicine in the era of artificial intelligence: implications in chronic disease management. *J Transl Med* 2020;18(1):472–475.
(71) Moslemi A, et al. Differentiating COPD and asthma using quantitative CT imaging and machine learning. *Eur Respir J* 2022;60(3):2103078.
(72) Kaplan A, et al. Artificial intelligence/machine learning in respiratory medicine and potential role in asthma and COPD diagnosis. *J Allergy Clin Immunol Pract* 2021;9(6):2255–2261.
(73) Topalovic M, et al. Artificial intelligence outperforms pulmonologists in the interpretation of pulmonary function tests. *Eur Respir J* 2019;53(4):1801660.
(74) Fraser AG, et al. The need for transparency of clinical evidence for medical devices in Europe. *Lancet* 2018;392(10146):521–530.
(75) Hui CY, et al. Mapping national information and communication technology (ICT) infrastructure to the requirements of potential digital health interventions in low- and middle-income countries. *J Glob Health* 2022;12:04094.

(76) Hui CY, et al. Patients' and clinicians' perceived trust in internet-of-things systems to support asthma self-management: qualitative interview study. *JMIR Mhealth Uhealth* 2021;9(7):e24127.
(77) Shaw SE, et al. Achieving spread, scale up and sustainability of video consulting services during the COVID-19 pandemic? Findings from a comparative case study of policy implementation in England, Wales, Scotland and Northern Ireland. *Front Digit Health* 2021;3:754319.
(78) James HM, et al. Spread, scale-up, and sustainability of video consulting in health care: systematic review and synthesis guided by the NASSS framework. *J Med Internet Res* 2021;23(1):e23775.
(79) Bui AAT, et al. Biomedical REAl-Time Health Evaluation (BREATHE): toward an mHealth informatics platform. *JAMIA Open* 2020;3(2):190–200.
(80) Venkataramanan R, et al. Determination of personalized asthma triggers from multimodal sensing and a mobile app: observational study. *JMIR Pediatr Parent* 2019;2(1):e14300.
(81) Latulippe K, et al. Social health inequalities and eHealth: a literature review with qualitative synthesis of theoretical and empirical studies. *J Med Internet Res* 2017;19(4):e136.
(82) Hernandez K, et al. *Leaving no one behind in a digital world. K4D emerging issues report.* Institute of Development Studies, 2018.
(83) GBD Chronic Respiratory Disease Collaborators. Prevalence and attributable health burden of chronic respiratory diseases, 1990–2017: a systematic analysis for the global burden of disease study 2017. *Lancet Respir Med* 2020;8(6):585–596.
(84) Satapathy P, et al. Artificial intelligence in respiratory therapy: opportunities and ethical challenges. *Respir Med* 2023;217:107342.
(85) van de Hei SJ, et al. Anticipated barriers and facilitators for implementing smart inhalers in asthma medication adherence management. *NPJ Prim Care Respir Med* 2023;33(1):22.
(86) Adejumo I, et al. Qualitative study of user perspectives and experiences of digital inhaler technology. *NPJ Prim Care Respir Med* 2022;32(1):57–59.
(87) Abdoul C, et al. Parents' views on artificial intelligence for the daily management of childhood asthma: a survey. *J Allergy Clin Immunol Pract* 2021;9(4):1728–1730.e3.
(88) Gonsard A, et al. Children's views on artificial intelligence and digital twins for the daily management of their asthma: a mixed-method study. *Eur J Pediatr* 2023;182(2):877–888.
(89) Campbell JL, et al. Telephone triage for management of same-day consultation requests in general practice (the ESTEEM trial): a cluster-randomised controlled trial and cost-consequence analysis. *Lancet* 2014;384(9957):1859–1868.
(90) Boers SN, et al. SERIES: eHealth in primary care. Part 2: Exploring the ethical implications of its application in primary care practice. *Eur J Gen Pract* 2020;26(1):26–32.
(91) Orlando JF, et al. Systematic review of patient and caregivers' satisfaction with telehealth videoconferencing as a mode of service delivery in managing patients' health. *PLOS ONE* 2019;14(8):e0221848.
(92) Funderskov KF, et al. Telemedicine in specialised palliative care: Healthcare professionals' and their perspectives on video consultations-A qualitative study. *J Clin Nurs* 2019;28(21–22):3966–3976.

4 Endotypes and Asthma

Sarah Diver, Richard Russell, and Pranabashis Haldar

CASE STUDY

A 44-year-old Caucasian woman was referred to the asthma clinic with daily episodes of exertional breathlessness associated with wheeze, chest tightness, and a non-productive cough. Two years previously, her primary care physician had diagnosed her with asthma, but her symptoms failed to respond satisfactorily to an escalating regime of asthma medication. At the time of referral, she was prescribed regular inhaled corticosteroids (1600 mcg/day beclomethasone equivalent), a long-acting beta-2 adrenergic agonist, theophylline, maintenance oral prednisolone (10 mg daily), and an as-needed short-acting beta-2 adrenergic agonist. She reported no childhood or family history of asthma but suffered with seasonal allergic rhinitis. She previously worked as a librarian and was a lifelong non-smoker. She lived alone and kept no domestic pets.

A detailed assessment in the asthma clinic identified that she was clinically obese with a body mass index (BMI) of 36 kg/m^2. She had a respiratory rate of 24 breaths per minute at rest and breathed predominantly through her mouth. Respiratory examination identified mild expiratory wheeze with symmetrically reduced breath sounds. Spirometry demonstrated airways obstruction (forced expiratory volume in 1 second [FEV_1] 66% predicted, FEV_1/forced vital capacity [FVC] ratio 0.6), with an 8% improvement in FEV_1 after 400 mcg of inhaled albuterol. Bronchial provocation testing with methacholine (PC20) was positive at 6.4 mg/mL. Laboratory investigations, including total immunoglobulin E (IgE) and specific IgE for common allergens and moulds, were unremarkable. Chest radiograph was normal. Fractional nitric oxide concentration in exhaled breath (FeNO) was normal at 8 parts per billion, and induced sputum quantitative cell count comprised 74% neutrophils, 24% macrophages, 2% lymphocytes, and 0% eosinophils. She reported a high score of 28 on the Nijmegen Questionnaire, suggesting hyperventilation.

Based on this assessment, she was deemed to have non-eosinophilic (T2-low) asthma, with a breathing pattern disorder and obesity contributing significantly to her symptom burden. Her oral prednisolone dose was weaned down and eventually stopped. She was referred to a dietician for weight reduction advice and was seen by a physiotherapist for breathing retraining. Serial-induced sputum for quantitative cell counts remained non-eosinophilic after withdrawal of oral glucocorticoid therapy. With time, she was able to lose weight, and her symptoms improved significantly.

4.1 INTRODUCTION

> Surely it is hard to believe that the wheeze which comes to the young school girl for a day or two in the middle of the ragweed season is the same disease as that which develops suddenly in the tired businessman or in the harassed housewife and pushes them down to the depths of depletion and despair. The problem is still wide open: the approach to it is not at all clear.
>
> **Rackemann 1948 [1]**

Asthma is a highly heterogeneous condition characterised by considerable variability in patterns of airway pathology, physiological disturbance, clinical symptoms, and response to therapy. Some asthma guidelines have typically recommended a one-size-fits-all approach to management that is frequently ineffective and, as the case study illustrates, may contribute to iatrogenic harm. This chapter will discuss asthma heterogeneity and the rationale for characterising distinct asthma phenotypes and endotypes to inform and support patient-oriented clinical care.

4.2 HETEROGENEITY IN ASTHMA

The absence of a disease-specific marker for asthma compromises diagnostic rigor, and there are several accepted approaches to securing an asthma diagnosis [2]. As such, heterogeneity in asthma is multifactorial and reflects both complex multi-scale pathophysiology and the likely inclusion of different diseases under a common umbrella (summarised in Figure 4.1).

Clinical heterogeneity is further compounded by a number of associated comorbidities. These represent both overlapping and unrelated pathologies that coexist to either mimic or exacerbate asthma symptoms. In common with other chronic diseases, the clinical expression of asthma is also often associated with a variable psychosocial component, which is frequently overlooked and may be difficult to quantify [4]. Finally, heterogeneity in the response to asthma pharmacotherapy is complex, multifactorial, and a critical determinant of individualising management in patients with refractory asthma.

DOI: 10.1201/9781003287209-5

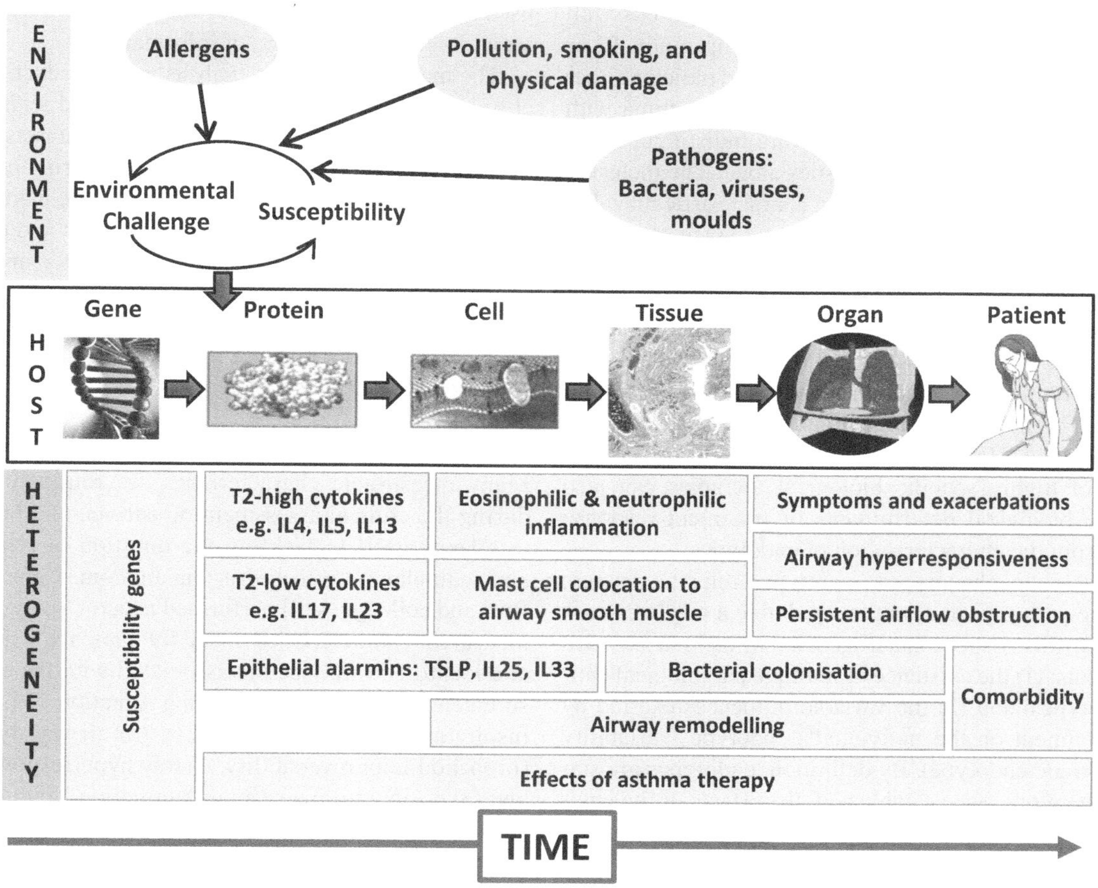

FIGURE 4.1 Examples of asthma heterogeneity across scales of disease from gene to patient. Comorbidity includes many features including obesity, inducible laryngeal obstruction, breathing pattern disorder, smoking, and psychosocial factors. (Adapted from [3].)

4.2.1 Importance of Characterising Asthma Heterogeneity

Heterogeneity impacts both the clinical care and scientific understanding of asthma. From a clinical standpoint, awareness and understanding of heterogeneity have focussed primarily on patients with difficult or refractory asthma, in whom conventional management, including glucocorticoids, is suboptimal or ineffective. In these patients, heterogeneity reflects the different aetiologies contributing to poor clinical control. Management requires systematic evaluation to characterise this heterogeneity and guide a multidisciplinary patient-oriented approach to address the factors identified.

From a scientific perspective, heterogeneity increases the likelihood of type II errors in genetic and molecular association studies. This is especially pertinent for gene-association studies where functional single nucleotide polymorphisms have a very low, independent attributable risk (less than 5%) [5]. Biologic therapies targeting specific immune pathways have been developed in recent years and have revolutionised the treatment of severe uncontrolled asthma [6]. Successful development of these drugs has been underpinned by clinical trials that have targeted subgroups of patients in whom these immune pathways are implicated in their disease [7]. These therapies are also providing invaluable *in vivo* data characterising the heterogeneity in human asthma immunobiology.

4.3 DEFINING PHENOTYPES AND ENDOTYPES

The purpose of characterising heterogeneity is to identify clinically and biologically meaningful subpopulations defined by shared aetiology, immunopathology, clinical expression, and treatment response. These subpopulations are often referred to as distinct phenotypes. In biology, a phenotype is defined as "the observable properties of an organism arising as a product of the interaction of their genotype with the environment." As this utilises *observable* characteristics, it is inherently a convenient way to describe clinical phenotypes based on routinely collected clinical variables. When the observations are extended to represent multiple aspects of the disease, there is a greater likelihood of identifying stable and meaningful phenotypes that share a mechanistic relationship. This is important, as a limitation of phenotypes based on clinical observations alone is the risk of grouping together biologically distinct groups with similar clinical disease expression. For example, non-T2 or T2-low asthma (discussed further later) could indicate either a distinct phenotype or T2-high eosinophilic asthma with good inflammatory control. The two are indistinguishable based on inflammatory characteristics alone. The inclusion of clinical symptom expression as a characteristic may distinguish these groups by revealing concordance of expression (few symptoms) with well-controlled T2-high asthma and discordance (high symptoms) in the T2-low phenotype driven by other disease mechanisms. Furthermore, such a system would correctly classify poorly and well-controlled T2-high asthma as the same phenotype across a spectrum of severity (high markers of T2 inflammation + high symptoms versus low T2 markers + few symptoms, respectively). The use of highly specific biological therapies can also reveal the biological determinants of treatment response that underpin the characterisation of endotypes.

In contrast to phenotypes, endotypes refer to discrete pathogenic pathways that, in theory, define a single disease process. In this respect, heterogeneity in asthma has two key elements: (1) the existence of multiple pathological entities (endotypes) and (2) the variable influences exerted by the environment on the individual's endotype (variability within a single endotype). By definition, endotypes are stable, and therefore, once established, the effects of the environment may be better understood.

4.4 CAPTURING HETEROGENEITY IN ASTHMA: MULTIVARIATE STATISTICAL TECHNIQUES

Several mathematical techniques have been widely applied across medicine to capture heterogeneity within groups of patients with overarching diagnoses, based on relevant variables. Factor analysis and cluster analysis are multivariate techniques that have been increasingly used to characterise heterogeneity. Although conceptually similar, the two techniques differ in the algorithms that they employ, with implications for their respective suitability to different classification tasks. Both techniques identify patterns within data that provide information on the likely underlying structure of the dataset. A consideration of these methods, and their underpinning principles, remains relevant, as they are empirical to the rapidly evolving application of machine learning methods in asthma.

4.4.1 Factor Analysis

Factor analysis includes a group of algorithms primarily used to identify patterns of variability and the correlation between variables within a dataset. In brief, variables that are grouped together are represented by a factor, calculated as the vectorial sum of the contributions from each component variable. The factor, therefore, represents a weighted sum of data from all the grouping variables and may be used in place of the individual variables in a further analysis without significant loss of information.

The main use of factor analysis is data reduction, which eliminates some of the problems associated with applying classical statistical techniques to complex datasets. Through the identification of groups of variables sharing related patterns of expression, statistical inferences are made that can provide insight into underlying mechanisms and processes. However, the relationships defined by factor analysis are mathematical and not biological; therefore the identified patterns should be considered hypothesis generating. Factor analysis should not be used in isolation to draw biological conclusions.

4.4.1.1 Factor Analysis in Asthma

Many measurable characteristics are routinely recorded during the clinical assessment of asthma, and factor analysis lends itself to tackling the question of relationships and redundancy of these various outcomes. For example, Rosi and colleagues [8] performed a factor analysis of eight measured characteristics from 99 patients with asthma and identified three factors associated with the eight measurements, representing (1) lung function (FEV_1, FVC, inspiratory vital capacity [IVC]); (2) airway dysfunction (bronchodilator reversibility, airway hyperresponsiveness); and (3) eosinophilic airway inflammation (sputum eosinophils, eosinophil cationic protein [ECP]), respectively. The factor model presents a view of the independent components or domains that contribute to clinical phenotypes. These domains may also have clinical utility as "treatable traits," where treatments that improve specific outcomes are available.

4.4.2 Cluster Analysis

Cluster analysis is a generic term for a group of statistical methods designed primarily to identify groups or clusters of homogeneous observations within heterogeneous multivariate datasets [9]. In mathematical terms, a cluster refers to a collection of items that exhibits "internal cohesion" (within-group homogeneity) and "external isolation" (between-group separation). Whereas factor analysis classifies the patterns of expression of variables, cluster analysis is more appropriately utilised to perform the classification of the population based on patterns of expression for specified variables. Conceptually, the identification of risk groups rather than risk factors in this way may be a better approach for studying complex, multifactorial outcomes.

4.4.2.1 Cluster Analysis in Asthma

Cluster analysis techniques have been widely applied in asthma, with notable studies outlined in Table 4.1. In addition to the cluster analysis performed by Haldar et al. [10], unsupervised clustering based on clinical variables has also been performed on large cohorts including SARP [11] and U-BIOPRED [12], with results supportive of the clinical phenotypes described in this chapter. Although there are

TABLE 4.1
Key Studies Utilising Unsupervised Clustering to Identify Clinical Phenotypes in Asthma

Study or Cohort	Clustering Methodology	Sample Size	Description of Clusters
Leicester, UK [10]	Unsupervised K-means clustering based on atopic status, PEF variability, induced sputum eosinophil count, ACQ-5	Primary care = 184 Secondary care = 187 Longitudinal cohort = 68	**Early-onset allergic:** airway dysfunction, high symptom scores, eosinophilic inflammation, exacerbations **Late-onset non-eosinophilic:** obese, female preponderance, high symptom scores **Late-onset eosinophilic:** male preponderance, eosinophilic inflammation, lower symptom scores **Early-onset symptom predominant:** high symptom scores, minimal eosinophilic inflammation
U-BIOPRED [12]	Unsupervised partition-around-medoids clustering of clinical features based on: age of onset, pack years smoking history, BMI, FEV_1, FEV_1/FVC, ACQ-5, self-reported exacerbations in the previous year, daily dose of prednisolone or equivalent	Training = 266 Validation = 152	**Moderate to severe allergic:** normal lung function, low eosinophils, low OCS use **Severe late-onset non-allergic eosinophilic:** obese, smokers, poor control, severe airflow obstruction **Severe late-onset allergic eosinophilic:** non-smokers, lower BMI, severe airflow obstruction **Severe symptom-high:** obese, female preponderance, frequent exacerbations, poor quality of life, normal or mildly reduced lung function
SARP [11]	Ward minimum-variance unsupervised hierarchical clustering based on 34 variables relating to demographics, lung function, atopic status, medication use, symptoms, comorbidities, healthcare utilisation, lifestyle factors, and family history	Total = 726 (mild = 260, moderate = 157, severe = 304)	**Mild early-onset allergic:** normal lung function, minimal medication use, minimal healthcare utilisation **Moderate early-onset allergic:** similar to preceding but with more medication use, worse symptoms, worse (although reversible) lung function **Late-onset non-allergic obese:** reduced lung function, high symptom scores, high burden of treatment **Severe early-onset allergic:** reversible airflow obstruction, high burden of treatment, high symptom scores, reduced quality of life **Severe late-onset non-allergic:** female preponderance, limited bronchodilator reversibility
Amelink et al. [13]	K-means non-hierarchical clustering based on 11 factors: gender, occupational asthma, home environmental influences, family atopy, smoking pack years, NSAID intolerance, prednisolone dependency, FEV_1, total IgE, sputum eosinophils, AQLQ	200 (adult-onset asthma)	**Severe eosinophilic inflammation-predominant:** female preponderance, persistent airflow obstruction, increased FeNO, increased sputum eosinophils **Symptom-high, frequent healthcare utilisation non-eosinophilic:** obese female preponderance, highest symptom scores, GORD, no airflow obstruction or eosinophilic inflammation but disproportionate healthcare utilisation **Mild to moderate well-controlled asthma:** male preponderance, aspirin sensitivity, low healthcare utilisation
COREA and SCH cohorts [14]	Wards hierarchical clustering then K-means clustering based on: FEV_1, BMI, age at onset, atopic status, smoking history, exacerbations requiring hospital visit	COREA = 724 SCH = 1843	**Smoking asthma:** 97% male, well-preserved lung function **Severe obstructive asthma:** lowest lung function with greatest bronchodilator reversibility, high proportion with severe exacerbations **Early-onset atopic asthma:** minimal smoking history, youngest age of onset **Late-onset mild asthma:** preserved lung function
UK Severe Asthma Registry [15]	Two-way cluster/mixture analysis model based on 23 variables relating to demographics, smoking status, atopic status, healthcare utilisation, comorbidities, lung function, blood eosinophils, medication use, and recruiting centre	349	**Early-onset allergic asthma:** frequent and severe exacerbations, poor lung function (but high bronchodilator reversibility), high OCS use **Late-onset obese asthma:** frequent exacerbations, high burden of treatment, normal lung function, high rates of depression **Normal lung function, least severe:** non-atopic, normal lung function, few exacerbations, low burden of treatment **Late-onset eosinophilic:** frequent exacerbations **Airflow obstruction:** worst lung function, highest OCS use, low frequency of exacerbations

some differences in the way these analyses are performed, broad similarities in the phenotypes reported and wide recognition of a number of subgroups are reported: (1) early onset, mild, allergic asthma; (2) early onset, moderate to severe asthma with remodelling; (3) late onset, non-allergic, eosinophilic asthma (high levels of airway inflammation and few symptoms); and (4) late onset, non-allergic non-eosinophilic asthma (female patients with obesity and a high symptom burden, despite low or absent markers of T2 inflammation). As research methodologies have progressed, cluster analysis has been performed in asthma using increasingly complex 'omics datasets to provide insight into pathophysiology.

4.4.3 Limitations of Multivariate Methods

The multivariate techniques described, along with other exploratory statistical methods that examine the structure and shape of data such as topological data analysis (TDA) [16, 17], have a growing application in the applied sciences. However, the idea that these numerical approaches yield results that are objective and free of *a priori* bias should not be considered dogma. Applying multivariate techniques to biological disciplines relies appropriately on subject-specific expertise, for example, in deciding the factors for inclusion in an analysis, selecting the optimal number of clusters, and interpreting the results. All of these aspects have a significant subjective weighting. In an exploratory context, multivariate techniques are, perhaps, better considered as offering a quantitative solution to a qualitative problem. From a methodological perspective, there is no accepted standardised approach, and far from being "black-box" techniques, analyses can be customised in accordance with the study and the subject-specific aims. Variability is also compounded by differences in the composition of the populations sampled, and the outcome of an analysis at a single centre would require replication at others for validation. Additionally, these techniques do not include the dimension of time, and reassessment of the same subjects over time may yield different results. Until a validated and standardised methodology is available, conclusions derived from the outcomes of such studies require cautious interpretation and extrapolation.

With the growing appreciation of the heterogeneity and complexity of conditions such as asthma, there is acknowledgement of the imprecision of the phenotyping approaches described [18, 19]. This has precipitated a drive to identify more robust methods that fulfil the goal of "precision medicine" and the "right treatment (s) for the right patient at the right time" [20]. Capturing dynamic changes in the lungs, in parallel with interactions between the host and their external and internal environments, is more likely to provide mechanistic insights that yield therapeutic targets and biomarkers but that require multiscale 'omic datasets across spatial scales with many complex interacting components. Therefore, the future may hold a shift towards integrative systems bioinformatics rather than the traditional reductionist approaches [21, 22].

4.4.4 Conclusions

Despite their limitations, multivariate statistical approaches are widely applied to characterise heterogeneity in asthma, with phenotypes that are reproduced or overlap across multiple large cohorts and studies. These methods provide complementary information and have frequently been used in tandem: factor analysis to define distinct domains or dimensions of the asthma phenotype and cluster analysis to study distinct patterns of domain co-expression within the asthma population. As computing capabilities continue to expand, integrative bioinformatics approaches to analyse multiscale 'omics data are now being explored. However, the practical implementation of artificial intelligence and machine learning techniques to support these will bring new challenges.

4.5 ENDOTYPES OF ASTHMA

Although more readily tractable, the importance of characterising clinical phenotypes to inform clinical care is being superseded by the relevance of identifying the T2 endotype, which better associates with response to corticosteroids and the newer monoclonal antibody therapies. Nonetheless, the presence or absence of allergy remains a useful phenotypic marker to identify patients in whom anti-IgE therapy could improve disease control, a therapy now associated with a wealth of safety data [23].

The concept of endotypes has grown alongside the development of monoclonal antibodies targeting T2-specific cytokines, which clearly and consistently improve asthma exacerbation rates and corticosteroid dependence. However, even in carefully selected trial populations with elevated T2 biomarkers, responses are variable and incomplete. This suggests that other factors may influence treatment efficacy or that multiple mechanisms responsible for disease expression may coexist within an individual. Integrating clinical, biological, and metabolic data to identify more specific biomarkers will be helpful in future, as will performing unbiased analyses at exacerbation [24] and during periods of clinical instability. Ideally, well-conducted longitudinal analyses will inform endotype stability in due course.

4.5.1 T2-High Endotype

4.5.1.1 Pathophysiology

T2-mediated eosinophilic inflammation is the most common inflammatory endotype, demonstrated in 80% of corticosteroid-naïve [25] and 50% of corticosteroid-treated patients [26], potentially an underestimate due to the T2-suppressive effects of treatment. With childhood-onset disease in particular, it is often associated with allergy.

In allergic asthma, dendritic cells stimulate T-helper 2 (Th2) cells in the presence of coactivators such as epithelial-derived thymic stromal lymphopoietin (TSLP), with subsequent production of the characteristic T2 cytokines interleukin (IL)4, IL5, and IL13. TSLP, along with the other epithelial "alarmins" IL25 and IL33, activates type 2

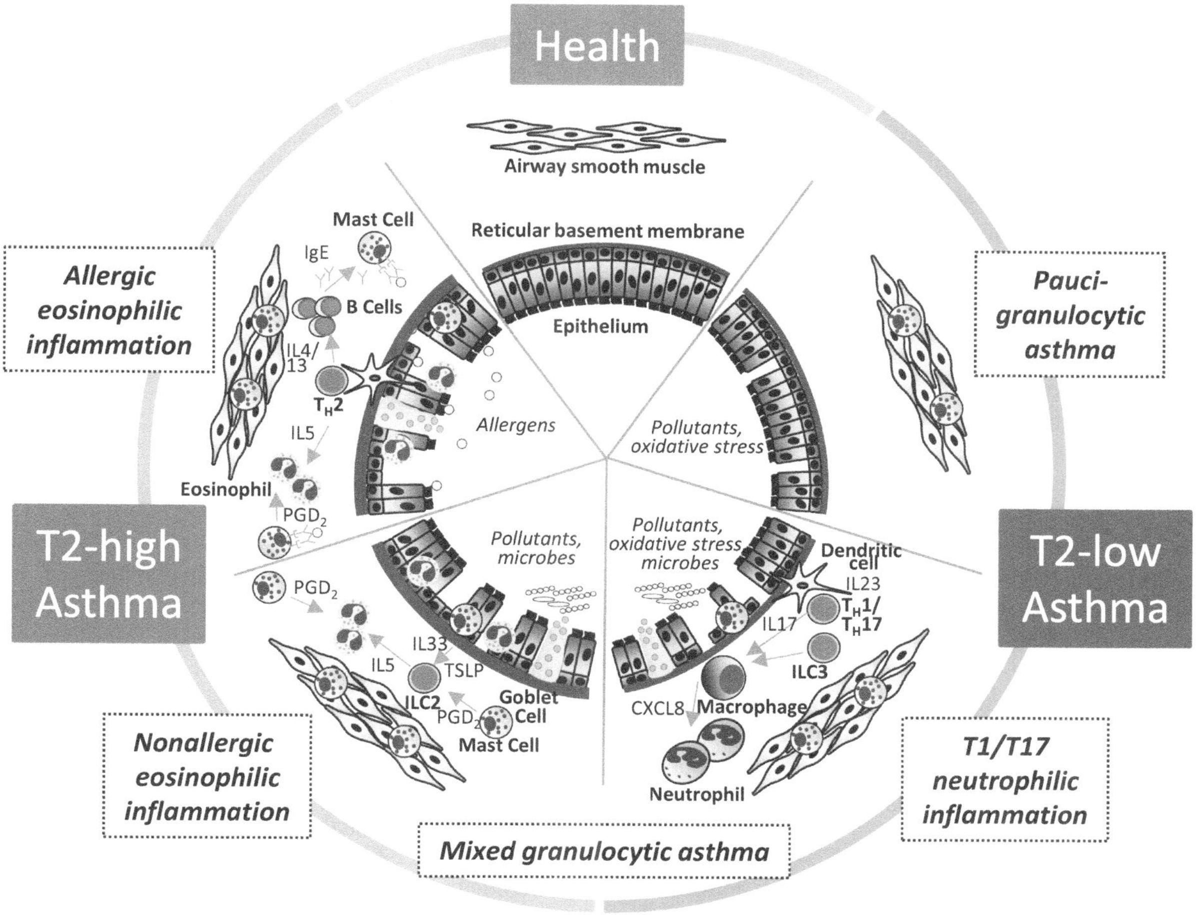

FIGURE 4.2 Heterogeneity of asthma immunopathology segmented into example endotypes based on inflammatory mechanisms: T2-high encompasses both allergic and nonallergic eosinophilic inflammation, and T2-low encompasses neutrophilic and pauci-granulocytic asthma, with a mixed endotype demonstrating features of both. (Adapted from [3].)

innate lymphoid cells (ILC2) promoting T2 inflammation and upregulating IL5 and IL13 (but not IL4) in response to epithelial insult in non-allergic disease. IL5 is an integral cytokine involved in recruitment, maturation, and survival of eosinophils. IL4 and IL13 facilitate eosinophil trafficking into tissues via upregulation of adhesion receptors on the vascular endothelium. Eosinophils are recruited to the lung mucosa under the influence of chemokines acting via the CC-chemokine type 3 receptor and by activation of prostaglandin D2 type 2 receptor (DP2), also termed "chemoattractant receptor-homologous molecule" expressed on Th2 cells (CRTH2). DP2 is also expressed by T2-lymphocytes, ILC2, and mast cells. Release of eosinophil products causes damage directly to the bronchial epithelium and may also cause bronchoconstriction through the release of cysteinyl leukotrienes. IL4 promotes B cell production of immunoglobulin E (IgE) following B cell class switching. IgE then binds with high affinity to mast cells, which, following allergen cross-linking, results in degranulation with release of granule products, eicosanoids, and cytokines. These contribute to the overall inflammatory milieu and activation of bronchial epithelium cells, mucous glands, goblet cells, and airway smooth muscle. IL13 also increases the airway smooth muscle response and is involved in mucus hypersecretion [3, 6]. The expression of three genes inducible with IL13 (*POSTN*, *CLCA1*, and *SERPINB2*) has been utilised to provide molecular validation of the T2 endotype [27] (Figure 4.2).

4.5.1.2 Biomarkers

Evaluation of three biomarkers is now recommended in international asthma guidance [28] to indicate the possibility of refractory T2 airway inflammation: (1) peripheral blood eosinophil count ≥150/μl, (2) FeNO ≥20ppb, and/or (3) sputum eosinophils ≥2%. Sputum eosinophils have historically been considered the gold standard. However, there is growing evidence supporting the use of FeNO and blood eosinophils as robust biomarkers of exacerbation risk that are cheaper and more widely accessible [29–31]. Biomarker levels can be indicative of response to T2 biologics and corticosteroids, with FeNO demonstrating a specific clinical utility for evaluating nonadherence to inhaled corticosteroids in severe asthma [32].

Analysis of 'omics datasets provide the opportunity to identify more specific biomarkers associated with T2-driven disease. Transcriptomic [33] and proteomic [34] approaches have suggested biomarkers associated with eosinophilic or allergic disease; however, until more is known about the outcomes associated with these highly specific biomarkers, it is unclear whether these could support patient management in a real-world setting.

4.5.1.3 Important Clinical Characteristics

Response to Biologics: Multiple biologic agents are now licensed in severe asthma for those with evidence of allergic or T2-driven disease. The biomarker level considered diagnostic of the T2 endotype is subject to discussion, and therefore inclusion criteria for pivotal RCTs of T2-targeted agents have varied. While there is little dispute about prescribing these agents for those with the highest biomarker levels, the lowest biomarker level associated with a response adequate to justify treatment is less clear and may vary at an individual level.

Glucocorticoid Response: Presence of T2 eosinophilic airway inflammation is accepted to be a determinant of the clinical response to glucocorticoid therapy, as evidenced by various studies [35, 36]. Similar differential responses in those with and without evidence of eosinophilia has been reported in chronic obstructive pulmonary disease (COPD) [37] and in subjects without a specific respiratory diagnosis presenting with new symptoms of airways disease [38]. In this context, T2-driven eosinophilic inflammation may be viewed more generally as a phenotypic determinant of airways disease.

Severe Exacerbations: RCTs of T2-targeted biologics have consistently demonstrated a significant reduction in asthma exacerbations, whilst the impact on other clinical outcomes has been more modest [6], providing evidence of the link between this clinical outcome and T2 airway inflammation.

4.5.2 T2-Low Endotype

In contrast with T2-high asthma, T2-low asthma is poorly specific, encompassing all subgroups of disease without evidence of active T2 inflammation at the time of assessment. In this respect, the T2-low endotype is perhaps an oxymoron, with clinical utility predominantly related to the implication of a lack of response to corticosteroids or T2-targeted biologics. Both neutrophilic and paucigranulocytic patterns of sputum inflammation are recognised, supporting the existence of significant heterogeneity within this group.

T2-low, non-eosinophilic asthma has previously been reported in up to 50% of asthma patients [36], although glucocorticoid optimisation studies in severe disease suggest that a significant proportion of this group have underlying T2 inflammation when this is not iatrogenically suppressed [39]. The mechanisms driving persisting asthma symptoms and physiological changes in those with controlled T2 inflammation are not well understood, and reduced responsiveness of these clinical end-points to T2-targeted biologic therapies, compared with asthma exacerbations, suggests these outcomes are dissociated. The landscape is further complicated by the observation that 50% of exacerbations in a cohort of severe eosinophilic asthmatics on mepolizumab were not associated with sputum eosinophilia [40]. This is consistent with the observation that anti-eosinophil therapies achieve an overall 50% reduction in exacerbation frequency. Therefore, non-T2 events and mechanisms are also clinically relevant in those with documented T2-high disease. At an individual level, evaluation to understand the contribution of processes beyond T2 inflammation can support personalised treatment and clinical management decisions. Recognition of this has led to the development of the so-called treatable traits approach, discussed later in this chapter [41].

4.5.2.1 Pathophysiology

T2-Low Inflammation: Compared to T2-high eosinophilic inflammation, T2-low inflammation is less well-characterised (Figure 4.2). Inflammation can be neutrophilic in response to increased CXC chemokine receptor 1/2 (CXCR1/2) chemokines such as CXC Motif Chemokine Ligand 8 (CXCL-8) [3]. T1/T17 pathways have been implicated in T2-low disease, but these are not fully defined, although a previous study of T17 and T2 epithelial gene expression signatures suggests upregulation of these pathways is mutually exclusive in individual samples [42]. Pathways may be shared upstream of differentiation to T2-high and T2-low mediated inflammation; therefore, the epithelial "alarmins"; TSLP, IL33, and IL25 may drive airway inflammation independent of T2 status [43]. Despite evidence implicating certain mediators in T2-low inflammation, targeted therapies, including anti-TNFα, anti-CXCR2, and anti-IL17 have demonstrated very limited effect [44–46]. Targeting IL23 even hastened time to asthma worsening, possibly caused by T17 pathway suppression leading to reciprocal T2 upregulation [47]. The anti-TSLP agent tezepelumab reduces exacerbations in T2-low asthma; however, efficacy increases with higher blood eosinophil counts, and the mechanism of action in T2-low disease is not clearly defined [48, 49].

Pathogens: It is well recognised that bacteria, viruses, and fungi may impact on disease course in severe asthma. Subgroups with bacterial disease drivers during clinical stability and at exacerbation [24, 50] may be distinct from subgroups with other biological drivers, which may be related to predominance of key pathogens such as Proteobacteria and, more specifically, *Haemophilus influenzae* [51], within the airway microbiome. Viral infection, particularly rhinovirus, is a well-recognised aetiological factor in asthma exacerbations and is associated with suboptimal interferon responses [52], whilst fungal sensitisation is reported in up to 50% with severe asthma [53].

Airway Remodelling: Airway remodelling describes changes in airway structure, including epithelial thickening or loss of integrity, airway smooth muscle (ASM) hyperplasia and hypertrophy, subepithelial fibrosis, mucus gland and goblet cell hyperplasia, and neoangiogenesis [54]. Remodelling can occur in both child and adult asthma, indicating an independent disease mechanism rather than simply the cumulative temporal consequence of chronic inflammation [55]. Increased ASM predicts airflow obstruction and, with epithelial thickness, is associated with reduced luminal area on quantitative computed tomography, whilst airway vascularity predicts air trapping [56].

Airway Hyperresponsiveness: Airway hyperresponsiveness (AHR) reflects airway narrowing in response to direct or indirect stimuli and is a consequence of augmented ASM contractility, occurring independently of inflammatory profile. Mast cells are co-located to the ASM bundle, and, through production of cytokines, they promote ASM survival, activation, and contractility, and their number is associated with the degree of AHR [57]. High-mobility group box 1 (HMGB1) has been shown to be upregulated in severe asthma and potentiates ASM contraction via toll-like receptor 4, which may lead to ASM dysfunction and AHR through a reduced capacity to generate reactive oxygen species (ROS) [58]. Animal studies have demonstrated that metallothionein-2 (MT-2) can relax ASM and reduce pulmonary resistance via transgelin-2 (TG2) [59].

Oxidative Stress: Oxidative stress reflects biological damage and interruption of cell signalling that occurs due to the presence of excessive reactive oxygen and nitrogen species (ROS and RNS) relative to protective antioxidants (a redox imbalance). In asthma, there is evidence of both airway and systemic oxidative stress, which increases with disease severity. Quantification of oxidative stress directly is difficult; however, extensive work has characterised indirect biomarkers of oxidative stress including those representing the effects of ROS on proteins, lipids, and DNA [60].

4.5.2.2 Important Clinical Characteristics

Glucocorticoid Resistance: In contrast to those with T2-high, eosinophilic disease, glucocorticoid therapy has failed to demonstrate objective improvements in subgroups with T2-low, non-eosinophilic disease, despite similar bronchodilator response to short-acting beta-agonists [61, 62]. The mechanism driving this characteristic is not fully elucidated but may result from bacterial and viral respiratory infections, obesity, and increased dietary fat intake [63].

Obesity: Whilst obesity has been associated with both eosinophilic and non-eosinophilic asthma, the obese, highly symptomatic, non-eosinophilic phenotype with poor response to glucocorticoids is widely recognised by clinicians. Polymorphisms in genes involved in IL6 signalling are associated with asthma. The IL6 pathway is associated with metabolic dysfunction and low-grade systemic inflammation in a subgroup of obese patients who demonstrate an increased frequency of exacerbations and lower lung function, along with elevated blood neutrophils and CRP. Obese patients may also demonstrate changes in L-arginine and nitric oxide metabolism, mitochondrial dysfunction, insulin resistance, and immune dysregulation, which are associated with diet and lipid metabolism and have the potential to affect airway function through mechanisms including impaired bronchodilation, increased oxidative stress, and T1 polarisation [64].

Airway Pathogens: The airway microbiome differs between inflammatory phenotypes with reduced alpha-diversity and more *Haemophilus* and *Moraxella* in T2-low, neutrophilic disease [50, 65], with the presence of anti-bacterial signatures in the transcriptome suggesting these organisms are phenotypic drivers [66]. Whilst maintenance macrolide use has been shown to reduce exacerbations across both eosinophilic and non-eosinophilic asthma [67], the response was most marked in those with positive bacterial culture, and *post hoc* analyses have suggested the airway load of *H. influenzae* to be predictive of treatment response [51]. Identification of specific bacterial pathogens affecting clinical outcomes will allow the development of strategies that reduce the burden of antimicrobial use in T2-low disease. One example of this has been the use of phage therapy to reduce bacterial load and associated inflammatory responses in an acute mouse infection model with *P. aeruginosa* [68]. Alternatively, reflecting our understanding of the gut microbiome, future interventions could focus on maintenance or promotion of a healthy airway microbial community.

4.5.3 Use of 'Omics Data to Identify Asthma Endotypes

There is increasing interest in the use of 'omics data to provide highly granular molecular data for characterising highly specific asthma endotypes [69]. The most notable contribution thus far has been with transcriptomics, characterising gene signatures that differentiate between T2-high and T2-low endotypes [27]. Subsequent cluster analysis of data from the U-BIOPRED cohort has suggested three transcriptome clusters in severe asthma, and the lack of clean separation between these and commonly recognised inflammatory phenotypes based on sputum cell counts has provided important pathophysiological insights [70].

More recently, microbiome data has also been used to identify subgroups of disease [16, 71], although less is understood about the interaction between host and airway microbial community and how this leads to clinical expression of disease. Study of volatile organic compounds (VOCs) in exhaled breath to characterise the metabolome is an innovative approach, with some highly attractive features including ease of patient sampling [17]. Small studies suggest the ability to differentiate disease features including inflammatory phenotype and glucocorticoid responsiveness in asthma [72, 73]. Evaluation of the proteome in patients with severe asthma indicated 10 proteotypes, and subsequent integration with clinical data have suggested multiple distinct mechanisms contributing to the T2 endotype [74].

In conclusion, the understanding of asthma pathophysiology is likely to be strengthened by combined analysis of multiple 'omics datasets collected across patient cohorts. New insights could be invaluable for the development of novel biomarkers and therapeutic agents that contribute to advancing the longer-term goals of asthma remission and cure.

4.6 THE TREATABLE TRAITS APPROACH

In contrast to the use of disease labels such as asthma or COPD that fail to capture complex heterogeneity at the patient level, the treatable traits approach aims to identify specific observable features of disease (Figure 4.4) that relate to meaningful clinical outcomes, with associated treatments. These may be present alone or in combination in the individual patient [75]. These traits should be associated with validated biomarkers, which may include not only specific molecules and cells but lung function abnormalities, imaging, or patient-reported measures. For example, T2 inflammation is a trait related to exacerbation risk, identifiable by biomarkers such as FeNO and blood eosinophil counts, and treatable with steroids or biologics. Another example is gastro-oesophageal reflux, related to exacerbations and quality of life, identifiable from evaluation of symptoms or oesophageal manometry, and treatable either medically, with medications including proton-pump inhibitors, or surgically, with fundoplication [76]. Traits have been categorised into pulmonary, extra-pulmonary, or lifestyle and behavioural domains, as shown in Figure 4.3.

Whilst this provides clinicians with a framework to deliver personalised clinical management, there are a number of limitations [75]. This approach assumes a broad stability in specific traits, which evidence suggests may not be the case. For example, the occurrence of T2-low exacerbations in those with T2-high disease, means that using biologics alone as a solution for exacerbations is likely to lead to incomplete disease control [40]. Similarly, problems are associated with traits such as airway infection. Sputum culture is certainly an imperfect biomarker, and evidence for molecular biomarkers of infection is currently lacking. Additionally, there is a paucity of longitudinal microbiome data in asthma to characterise the behaviour of this trait over time, which might provide valuable information directing the use of targeted interventions. For example, the optimal length of time that macrolide therapy should be administered for is not known. Other therapies, such as anti-TSLP or as required ICS/LABA, have demonstrated efficacy "across traits" or inflammatory endotypes. Development of future therapies that are efficacious regardless of trait may negate the treatable traits approach.

There are also practical issues with the treatable traits approach. With a median of almost seven traits identified in an individual with severe asthma, it is not at all clear which traits should be prioritised or how effective proposed treatments are likely to be. For example, treatment of comorbidities such as obesity or depression can be complex and prolonged with variable efficacy.

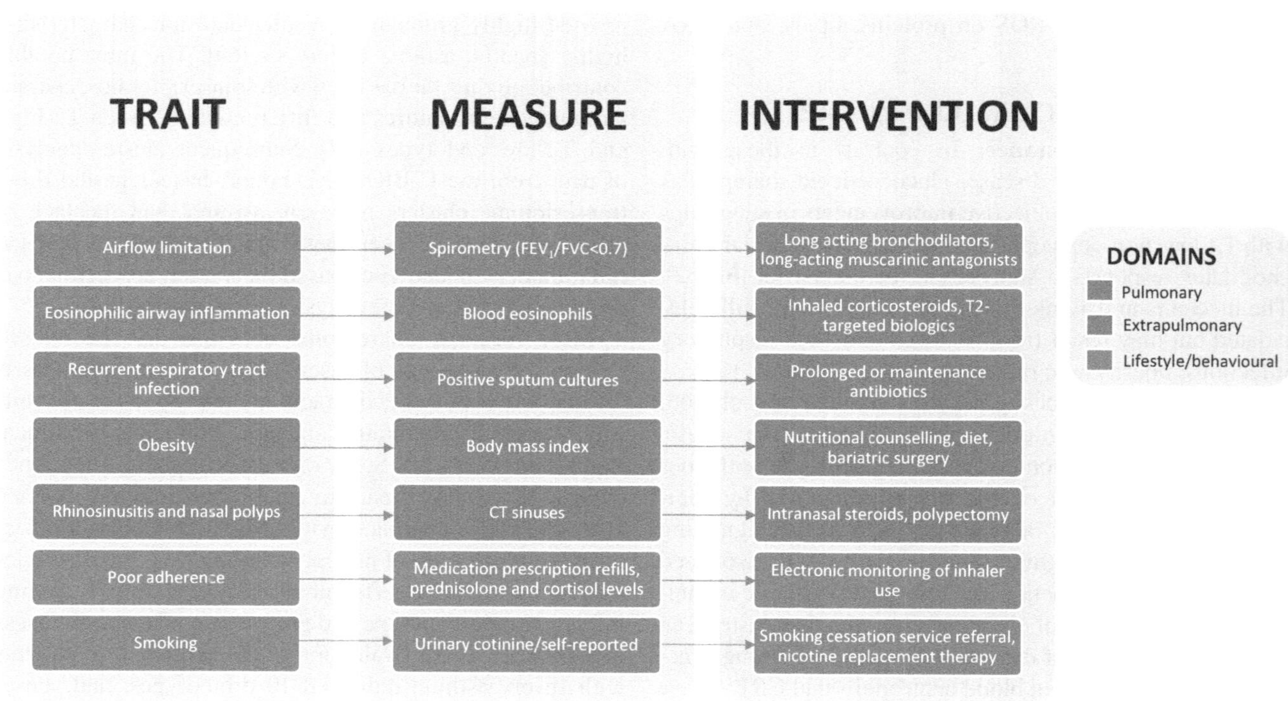

FIGURE 4.3 Examples of treatable traits within pulmonary, extra-pulmonary, and behavioural/lifestyle domains, with corresponding methods of identification and treatment.

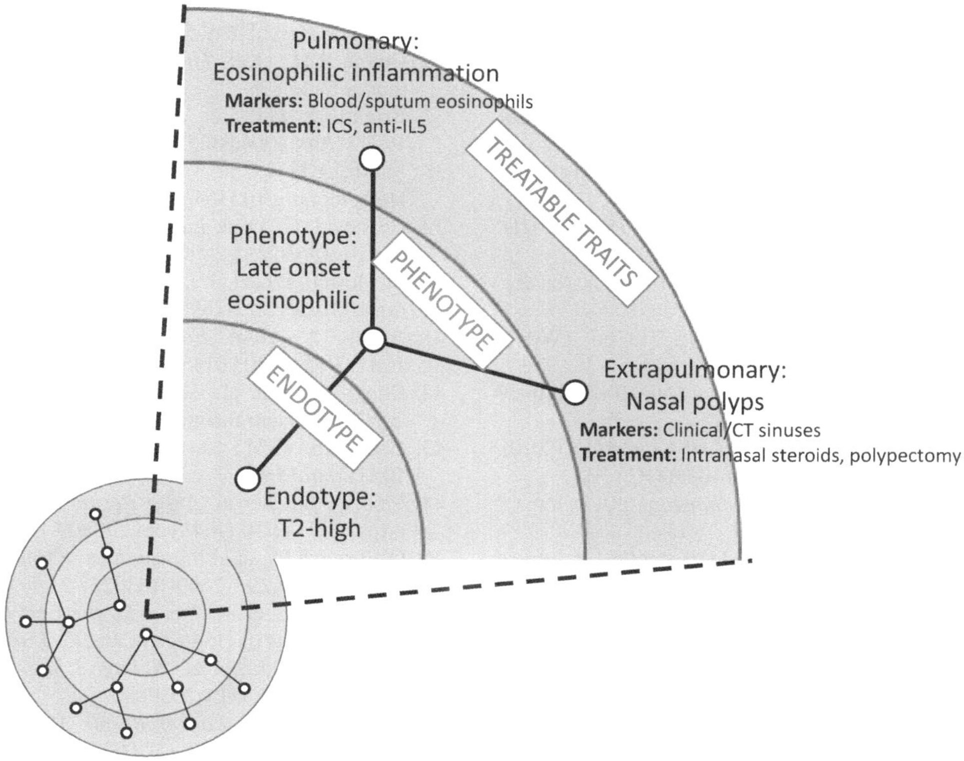

FIGURE 4.4 Schematic representation of the relationship between endotypes, phenotypes, and treatable traits.

4.7 CONCLUSIONS

Heterogeneity in asthma is multifactorial and highly relevant to clinical practice, as it is a major determinant of effective approaches to treatment. An individual patient may get no benefit from a treatment that is transformative in the asthma control of another patient. As such, personalised treatment informed by the factors driving poor asthma control is a necessity rather than an ideal for the provision of effective clinical care.

Multiple approaches have been taken to categorising asthma heterogeneity, with variable clinical utility. Observable disease and patient characteristics have been used to construct phenotypes, but this approach does not necessarily inform the underlying pathobiology that is a key determinant of effective and rational therapeutic strategies.

Categorisation based on underlying pathophysiological mechanisms defines endotypes, which more precisely characterise disease on the basis of whether there is measurable T2 inflammation using well-validated clinical biomarkers. While this has revolutionised clinical asthma management, enabling targeted provision of novel biological therapies, inter-patient variations in response highlight limitations of this approach and our broader understanding of the drivers of clinical disease expression. This is most notable for the T2-low endotype for which multiple pathobiological mechanisms are responsible for similar patterns of clinical expression.

The treatable traits model provides an attractive framework for clinicians to address the complex contribution of comorbidities and disease mechanisms beyond T2 inflammation in the individual patient. Yet traits are not always stable, and their contribution to disease expression may vary longitudinally, making regular re-evaluation of the patient key.

The evolution in characterising asthma heterogeneity through phenotypes to endotypes, and subsequently treatable traits, reflects adaptation both to growing insight of underlying pathophysiology and the need to apply this knowledge in a clinically meaningful framework. To date, multivariate statistical techniques have been integral to the progress made so far. With ever-increasing computer processing power, new opportunities to analyse and integrate multiscale 'omics approaches will likely yield more granular and robust categorisation of the asthma spectrum to support novel mechanistic insights and approaches to targeted intervention that will lead us further towards the goal of personalised and optimal care for all.

REFERENCES

1. Rackemann, F.M. *Am J Med* (1947). https://doi.org/10.1016/0002-934347)90204-0(
2. British Thoracic Society/Scottish Intercollegiate Guidelines Network. (2019). https://www.brit-thoracic.org.uk

3. Russell, R.J., et al. *Clin Sci (Lond)* (2017). https://doi.org/10.1042/cs20160253
4. Harrison, B.D. *Thorax* (1998). https://doi.org/10.1136/thx.53.6.519
5. Anderson, G.P. *Lancet* (2008). https://doi.org/10.1016/s0140-6736(08)61452-x
6. Diver, S., et al. *Clin Exp Allergy* (2018). https://doi.org/10.1111/cea.13086
7. Pavord, I.D., et al. *J Allergy Clin Immunol Pract* (2021). https://doi.org/10.1016/j.jaip.2020.08.039
8. Rosi, E., et al. *J Allergy Clin Immunol* (1999). https://doi.org/10.1016/s0091-6749(99)70496–3
9. Everitt, B.S., et al. *Cluster Analysis*. 5th ed. (Wiley, 2011).
10. Haldar, P., et al. *Am J Respir Crit Care Med* (2008). https://doi.org/10.1164/rccm.200711-1754OC
11. Moore, W.C., et al. *Am J Respir Crit Care Med* (2010). https://doi.org/10.1164/rccm.200906-0896OC
12. Lefaudeux, D., et al. *J Allergy Clin Immunol* (2017). https://doi.org/10.1016/j.jaci.2016.08.048
13. Amelink, M., et al. *J Allergy Clin Immunol* (2013). https://doi.org/10.1016/j.jaci.2013.04.052
14. Kim, T.B., et al. *Eur Respir J* (2013). https://doi.org/10.1183/09031936.00100811
15. Newby, C., et al. *PLOS ONE* (2014). https://doi.org/10.1371/journal.pone.0102987
16. Diver, S., et al. *Allergy* (2020). https://doi.org/10.1111/all.14058
17. Ibrahim, W., et al. *Sci Transl Med* (2022). https://doi.org/10.1126/scitranslmed.abl5849
18. Fleming, L., et al *Thorax* (2012). https://doi.org/10.1136/thoraxjnl-2011-201064
19. Kermani, N.Z., et al. *Eur Respir J* (2021). https://doi.org/10.1183/13993003.01836-2020
20. Chung, K.F., et al. *Allergy* (2019). https://doi.org/10.1111/all.13771
21. Thamrin, C., et al. *Am J Respir Crit Care Med* (2016). https://doi.org/10.1164/rccm.201511–2288PP
22. Li, C.X., et al. *Eur Respir J* (2018). https://doi.org/10.1183/13993003.01930-2017
23. Normansell, R., et al. *Cochrane Database Syst Rev* (2014). https://doi.org/10.1002/14651858.CD003559.pub4
24. Ghebre, M.A., et al. *J Allergy Clin Immunol* (2018). https://doi.org/10.1016/j.jaci.2018.04.013
25. Eltboli, O., et al. *Expert Rev Respir Med* (2013). https://doi.org/10.1586/ers.12.81
26. Douwes, J., et al. *Thorax* (2002). https://doi.org/10.1136/thorax.57.7.643
27. Woodruff, P.G., et al. *Am J Respir Crit Care Med* (2009). https://doi.org/10.1164/rccm.200903-0392OC
28. Global Initiative for Asthma (GINA). (2024). http://www.ginasthma.org
29. Pavord, I.D., et al. *Lancet Respir Med* (2020). https://doi.org/10.1016/s2213-2600(20)30053–9
30. Shrimanker, R., et al. *Am J Respir Crit Care Med* (2019). https://doi.org/10.1164/rccm.201903-0599LE
31. Kraft, M., et al. *Eur Respir J* (2021). https://doi.org/10.1183/13993003.00413-2021
32. Heaney, L.G., et al. *Am J Respir Crit Care Med* (2019). https://doi.org/10.1164/rccm.201806-1182OC
33. Kuo, C.S., et al. *Am J Respir Crit Care Med* (2017). https://doi.org/10.1164/rccm.201512-2452OC
34. Nieto-Fontarigo, J.J., et al. *Allergy* (2020). https://doi.org/10.1111/all.14406
35. Green, R.H., et al. *Lancet* (2002). https://doi.org/10.1016/s0140-6736(02)11679-5
36. Green, R.H., et al. *Thorax* (2002). https://doi.org/10.1136/thorax.57.10.875
37. Brightling, C.E., et al. *Thorax* (2005). https://doi.org/10.1136/thx.2004.032516
38. Smith, A.D., et al. *Am J Respir Crit Care Med* (2005). https://doi.org/10.1164/rccm.200411-1498OC
39. Heaney, L.G., et al. *Lancet Respir Med* (2021). https://doi.org/10.1016/s2213-2600(20)30397-0
40. McDowell, P.J., et al. *Lancet Respir Med* (2021). https://doi.org/10.1016/s2213-2600(21)00004-7
41. Agusti, A., et al. *Eur Respir J* (2016). https://doi.org/10.1183/13993003.01359-2015
42. Choy, D.F., et al. *Sci Transl Med* (2015). https://doi.org/10.1126/scitranslmed.aab3142
43. Gauvreau, G.M., et al. *Allergy* (2023). https://doi.org/10.1111/all.15609
44. Wenzel, S.E., et al. *Am J Respir Crit Care Med* (2009). https://doi.org/10.1164/rccm.200809-1512OC
45. O'Byrne, P.M., et al. *Lancet Respir Med* (2016). https://doi.org/10.1016/s2213-2600(16)30227-2
46. Busse, W.W., et al. *Am J Respir Crit Care Med* (2013). https://doi.org/10.1164/rccm.201212-2318OC
47. Brightling, C.E., et al. *N Engl J Med* (2021). https://doi.org/10.1056/NEJMoa2030880
48. Diver, S., et al. *Lancet Respir Med* (2021). https://doi.org/10.1016/s2213-2600(21)00226-5
49. Menzies-Gow, A., et al. *N Engl J Med* (2021). https://doi.org/10.1056/NEJMoa2034975
50. Green, B.J., et al. *PLOS ONE* (2014). https://doi.org/10.1371/journal.pone.0100645
51. Taylor, S.L., et al. *Eur Respir J* (2020). https://doi.org/10.1183/13993003.00194-2020
52. Wark, P.A., et al. *J Exp Med* (2005). https://doi.org/10.1084/jem.20041901
53. O'Driscoll, B.R., et al. *BMC Pulm Med* (2005). https://doi.org/10.1186/1471-2466-5-4
54. Berair, R., et al. *Drugs* (2014). https://doi.org/10.1007/s40265-014-0250-4
55. O'Reilly, R., et al. *J Allergy Clin Immunol* (2013). https://doi.org/10.1016/j.jaci.2012.08.044
56. Berair, R., et al. *Eur Respir J* (2017). https://doi.org/10.1183/13993003.01507-2016
57. Brightling, C.E., et al. *N Engl J Med* (2002). https://doi.org/10.1056/NEJMoa012705
58. Di Candia, L., et al. *J Allergy Clin Immunol* (2017). https://doi.org/10.1016/j.jaci.2016.11.049
59. Yin, L.M., et al. *Sci Transl Med* (2018). https://doi.org/10.1126/scitranslmed.aam8604
60. Michaeloudes, C., et al. *Mol Aspects Med* (2022). https://doi.org/10.1016/j.mam.2021.101026
61. McGrath, K.W., et al. *Am J Respir Crit Care Med* (2012). https://doi.org/10.1164/rccm.201109-1640OC
62. Berry, M., et al. *Thorax* (2007). https://doi.org/10.1136/thx.2006.073429
63. Wadhwa, R., et al. *Eur Respir Rev* (2019). https://doi.org/10.1183/16000617.0096-2019
64. Fitzpatrick, A.M., et al. *J Allergy Clin Immunol Pract* (2020). https://doi.org/10.1016/j.jaip.2019.11.006
65. Taylor, S.L., et al. *J Allergy Clin Immunol* (2018). https://doi.org/10.1016/j.jaci.2017.03.044
66. Singhania, A., et al. *Am J Respir Cell Mol Biol* (2018). https://doi.org/10.1165/rcmb.2017-0162OC

67. Gibson, P.G., et al. *Lancet* (2017). https://doi.org/10.1016/s0140-6736(17)31281-3
68. Waters, E.M., et al. *Thorax* (2017). https://doi.org/10.1136/thoraxjnl-2016-209265
69. Tyler, S.R., et al. *J Allergy Clin Immunol* (2019). https://doi.org/10.1016/j.jaci.2019.05.015
70. Kuo, C.S., et al. *Eur Respir J* (2017). https://doi.org/10.1183/13993003.02135-2016
71. Abdel-Aziz, M.I., et al. *J Allergy Clin Immunol* (2021). https://doi.org/10.1016/j.jaci.2020.04.018
72. Ibrahim, B., et al. *Thorax* (2011). https://doi.org/10.1136/thx.2010.156695
73. van der Schee, M.P., et al. *Eur Respir J* (2015). https://doi.org/10.1183/09031936.00044414
74. Schofield, J.P.R., et al. *J Allergy Clin Immunol* (2019). https://doi.org/10.1016/j.jaci.2019.03.013
75. Melhorn, J., et al. *Ann Allergy Asthma Immunol* (2022). https://doi.org/10.1016/j.anai.2022.02.005
76. Cheung, T.K., et al. *Chest* (2009). https://doi.org/10.1378/chest.08-1702

Section II

Diagnosis of Asthma

5 Guidelines in Asthma

Krystelle Godbout and Louis-Philippe Boulet

GUIDELINES INTEGRATION INTO CARE: CASE STUDY

A 28-year-old man consults for persistent respiratory symptoms suggestive of asthma. He is currently on no regular treatment and has never exacerbated. Remembering a recent conference about the new asthma guidelines, the clinician decides to prove the diagnosis of asthma before initiating long-term treatment. Spirometry is ordered that comes back showing a fully reversible airway obstruction (forced expiratory volume in one second (FEV_1), reversibility of 15%, and 560 ml up to 90% predicted) supporting the suspected diagnosis. The physician then evaluates asthma control and confounding factors using its PRESTINE integrated tool synced with the latest guidelines in his electronic medical record system. He concludes that the patient is uncontrolled without therapy and has an allergic rhinitis that contributes to the symptoms.

Wanting to start asthma treatment for his uncontrolled asthma, the physician wonders whether this young man could benefit from the new budesonide/formoterol as-needed strategy (anti-inflammatory reliever [AIR] strategy) he has heard about. To guide him, he consults the local asthma guidelines pocket guide. He notes that his local guidelines do not recommend this strategy if the patient can adhere to regular inhaled corticosteroids (ICS) as it provides better symptomatic control. Therefore, he makes a prescription for a regular ICS and sends him for asthma education to help him adhere to regular therapy. The asthma educator contacts him upon evaluating the patient as no written action plan (WAP) was given to the patient. The physician realizes his oversight and prescribes a four-fold increase in ICS in the event of a loss of asthma control. The educator provides these written instructions to the patient.

Upon follow-up three months later, the patient fails to adhere to regular ICS therapy despite the education provided. He, however, takes his short-acting beta-agonist (SABA) reliever two to three times a week. The physician confirms with his asthma guidelines pocket guide that he is now a good candidate for the AIR strategy and modifies his treatment to budesonide/formoterol as needed.

5.1 INTRODUCTION

Asthma is a common disease, which, despite our progress in its understanding and treatment, still causes significant morbidity, quality of life impairment, and, even nowadays, mortality, particularly in low- to middle-income countries.[1,2] About four decades ago, in response to the increasing asthma-related deaths, experts reunited to create guidelines and provide clinicians with recommendations on the best practices in asthma care.[3] Since then, numerous clinical practice guidelines (CPGs) have been issued at the national and international levels, offering scientifically developed recommendations to guide decision-making and inform healthcare providers and administrators about what should be considered optimal care.[4–6] Most guidelines are sponsored by national or regional medical organizations while the Global Initiative for Asthma (GINA), which is not a "traditional" guideline but is often considered as such, has been developed by independent experts with an international scope.[7]

Clinical practice guidelines production methodology varies but usually involves a synthesis of the current knowledge on asthma and its management, following the review of the most recent pertinent studies. Efforts are made for the ensuing recommendations to be evidence-based, but experts' consensus opinions are inevitable due to the lack of sufficient data on certain aspects of asthma care (e.g. optimal oral corticosteroid regimen during severe flare-ups, comparative efficacy of biologics etc.[8] As a result, despite improvement and standardization in CPGs development methodologies, differences in recommendations are found between guidelines, reflecting different interpretation of evidence, or consideration of different outcomes' determinants.[9, 10] However, the basic key concepts and treatment strategies are usually not too different.

To avoid biases in guidelines recommendations, important steps have been taken in the early 2000s with the development of new standardized methodologies such as GRADE (Grading of Recommendations, Assessment, Development, and Evaluations), PICO questions (Population, Intervention, Comparison, and Outcome), and AGREE (Appraisal of Guidelines for Research & Evaluation).[11–13] Prior guidelines used unvalidated methods for grading the quality of evidence and the strength of recommendations. The GRADE Working Group was the first to develop a robust approach to grading evidence and recommendations, which is still much in use today. Furthermore, for assessing methodological

DOI: 10.1201/9781003287209-7

quality of clinical practice guidelines, AGREE is a preferred tool.[14]

However, these recent tools require much time, resources, and energy to update current evidence and formulate recommendations, limiting the frequency of guidelines updates. The very specific recommendations may also be difficult to integrate in a general framework of asthma management. As a result, alternative evidence-based methodologies have been used to make clinical guidance, as used in the annually updated GINA reports.[7]

Despite all the efforts deployed in asthma guidelines, major care gaps remain, due in part to insufficient implementation of recommendations.[15] Barriers and facilitators to their application in current care, particularly at the primary care level, have been identified and will be further reviewed in this chapter. Among other things, intrinsic implementability of the guidelines should be improved, and implementation tools and strategies should be offered to clinicians.[16, 17]

This chapter provides an overview of the production of asthma guidelines and their main recent recommendations and offers potential solutions on how to facilitate their implementation.

5.2 GUIDELINES DEVELOPMENT

5.2.1 Establishing the Scope of the Guidelines

The development of a CPG starts with the identification of a significant problem or condition for which management guidance is required. A guideline working group, ideally multidisciplinary, is then formed and settles on an operative scheme. This plan includes the scope of the project, the population targeted, the methodology selected, how the systematic literature review will be conducted, and how a consensus will be achieved in order to ensure quality recommendations while mitigating biases. Once completed, the document should be revised by relevant experts and stakeholders, for potential clarifications or improvements. Closely associated with the process of CPG making, dissemination activities and promotion of implementation into current care, considering local factors, are planned for in the initial developmental steps.

5.2.2 Evaluating the Evidence and Strength of Recommendations

5.2.2.1 PICO Questions

Generating specific questions that will be addressed with a systematic literature review is one of the first steps in CPG production.[18, 19] A commonly used method is the making of PICO questions that systematically consider the Population(s) at risk, Intervention(s), Comparator(s), and Outcome(s). A pilot study suggested that using PICO questions increased the precision and relevancy of literature search results.[20] There is, however, no established approach for the development of these key clinical questions, although some attempts have been made. Chakraborty et al. created a protocol by integrating best-practice approaches and clinically relevant qualitative research studies. This best-practice protocol was then successfully used to develop the key clinical questions of a new guideline on mental health.[21] Therefore, although more work is needed on the optimal way to achieve relevant questions for CPGs, the current PICO method offers a standardized way to construct them.

Indeed, by focusing on well-defined aspects of care, PICO questions lead to a better assessment of the evidence. It, however, limits the scope of the review, and it may become difficult to integrate new evidence in the overall scheme of treatment. For example, an extensive report such as the one produced by GINA would require more than 200 PICO questions to cover the whole set of recommendations and probably quite a few years of work. Its different methodology, addressed later in the chapter, allows for an evidence-based annually updated clinical strategy.

5.2.2.2 GRADE Methodology

A variety of quality assessment tools for CPGs exists, but GRADE is probably the most used (Figure 5.1).[22] It is not limited to guidelines and also uses systematic reviews and health technology assessments. Originating from a desire for an unbiased literature search and grading system, the GRADE Working Group first started as an informal collaboration.[11, 12, 23, 24] The subsequently developed GRADE approach provides guidance on how to grade the quality of evidence and strength of recommendations. It includes a comprehensive set of criteria to grade evidence as high, moderate, low, or very low according to factors such as the study methodology, consistency, and precision of the results, and directness of the evidence with an acknowledgement of values and preferences. A pragmatic interpretation of strong versus weak recommendations for clinicians, patients, and policymakers can also be found. This unbiased process mitigates potential biases and makes the remaining ones more transparent.[25] Although excellent for grading the quality of evidence, GRADE follows a stringent process using specific terminology that requires a significant amount of work. Furthermore, it faces significant difficulties in the evaluation of complex interventions, choice of outcomes, and outcome measures and discrimination of different observational studies.[26]

5.2.2.3 AGREE

The AGREE (Appraisal of Guidelines for Research & Evaluation) instrument was originally developed in 2001 and subsequently refined to assess the methodological rigour and transparency in which a guideline is developed.[13, 16, 27] The most recent tools, AGREE II and AGREE REX, respectively address CPG development process and recommendations.[28–29] AGREE II is widely used and focused on guidelines development, involving 23 items grouped in six domains: scope and purpose, stakeholder involvement, rigour of development, clarity of presentation, applicability, and editorial independence.[28] The AGREE REX contains

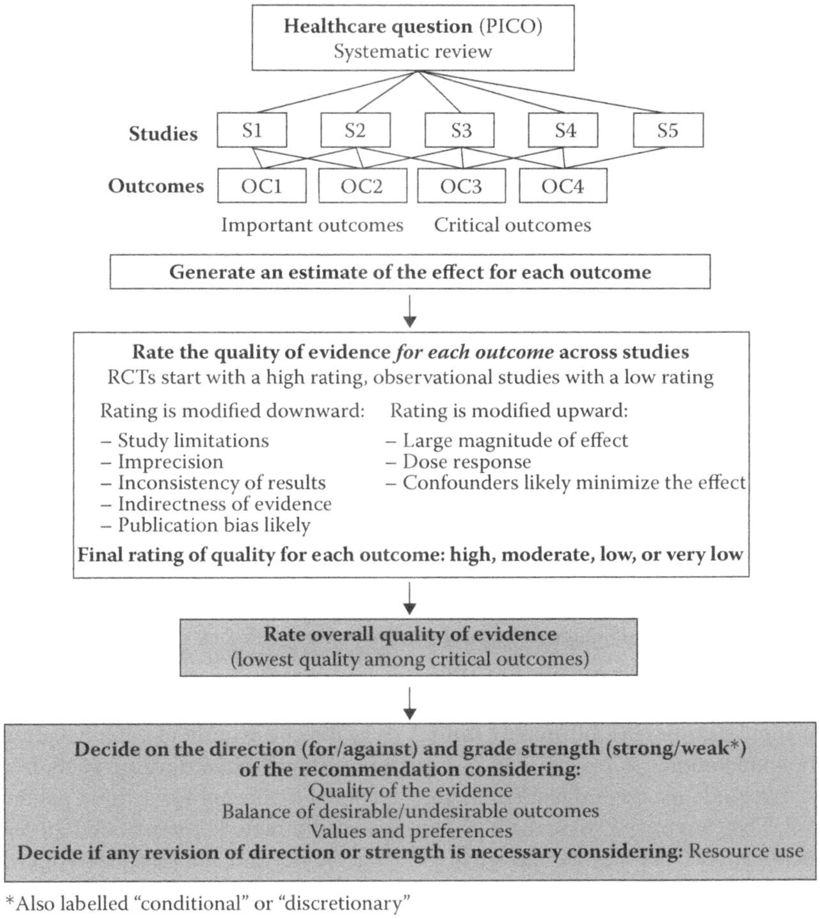

FIGURE 5.1 Schematic view of the GRADE process for developing recommendations. Abbreviation: RCT, randomized controlled trials. (From Guyatt G.H. et al. *J Clin Epidemiol* (2011), PMID: 21195583/https://doi.org/10.1016/j.jclinepi.2010.04.026. With permission.)

nine items within three guideline recommendation quality domains: clinical applicability, values and preferences, and implementability.[29] Both tools are available on the AGREE Enterprise website (www.agreetrust.org) as an open access resource to support practice guidelines.

AGREE was developed to address the issue of variability in guideline quality using a checklist for their assessment. The relative importance and subjectivity of some proposed criteria may, however, influence the results. Missing information in the assessed guidelines may also impair proper assessment. Nevertheless, it offers a structured method for the evaluation of these documents, reducing the variability in appraisal.

5.2.3 Updating Guidelines

Most national and international guidelines are regularly updated, although the process usually takes months to years, and only some specific questions are usually addressed. The whole document may be revised only after five years or more, questioning the value of some recommendations in front of more recent developments. Although it is difficult to speed up the production of guidelines, some groups such as the GINA choose different methods to allow for a yearly update. More effective timely methods for revising current guidelines should be developed to make them more up-to-date, living documents.

5.3 USEFULNESS AND LIMITATIONS OF GUIDELINES

5.3.1 Usefulness

Clinical practice guidelines have become essential tools for clinicians. They standardize and organize current knowledge and provide evidence-based recommendations for healthcare professionals. Although this should translate into an improvement in patient care, such evidence is limited.

The best testimony to guidelines impact in asthma is perhaps the major decrease in hospital admission and asthma-related deaths since their first publications in the late 1980s. However, when looking more precisely at studies of guidelines implementation, mixed results are found.[30] Uptake of the interventions is often poor, which mitigates potential results. Still, improvement in asthma outcome and medical management has been seen in a few studies, suggesting potential benefits when implementation is successful. Such is the case of Europe in which numerous successful local implementations programmes of key recommendations from guidelines have been reported improving patients' clinical condition while reducing direct and indirect costs.[31] Similarly, using more expensive medications to achieve better asthma control paradoxically leads to a reduction in direct asthma costs by reducing work absenteeism and acute care or hospital admissions.[32] Better documentation of asthma guidelines impacts and addressing gaps in their implementation is required to better improve asthma care in routine practice.

5.3.2 Challenges and Limitations

Although important for clinical practice, guidelines may also be a source of frustration and confusion for clinicians. Current asthma CPGs are all based on evidence after a rigorous examination process, but the recommendations are limited to the available evidence, leaving many questions unanswered. Moreover, the methodologies used to produce recommendations and knowledge gaps lead to inconsistencies between guidelines. These discrepancies highlight the regional specificities and the preference given to the different treatment considerations by the working group. They may, however, be confusing for clinicians, ultimately limiting proper guideline implementation.

It is important to note that guideline recommendations are made at a population level. They are issued when the benefits outweigh the risks for most patients, but they cannot apply to every situation encountered in clinical practice. Some recommendations may not have the adaptability and individualization that is frequently needed by clinicians. Treatment cost, access, patient's preference and comorbidities, and disease phenotype may make a less recommended treatment preferable in an individual patient, such as using montelukast over ICS or increasing the dose of ICS over adding a long-acting beta-2 agonist (LABA), although asthma control should be checked to determine if these are sufficient.

The development of guidelines is a lengthy process that takes years to come to fruition. This delays the inclusion of new evidence into the recommendations, leaving clinicians with an uncertainty in "if or how" to integrate novelties into their practice for years. That may explain, in addition to their succinct and clinically targeted content in all domains of medicine, the popularity of *online* and regularly revised evidence-based clinical resources such as UpToDate or DynaMed.[33, 34]

5.4 GUIDELINES IN ASTHMA

5.4.1 General Asthma

With asthma being the most common inflammatory airway disease worldwide, many national respiratory societies or institutes have developed their own guidelines to help professionals care for asthma patients (Table 5.1).[35–41] They generally include recommendations on diagnosis and pharmacologic and nonpharmacologic management, although

TABLE 5.1
Guidelines in Asthma

	GINA	BTS/SIGN	NICE	NAEPP	CTS	ERS	ATS/ERS
Current guidelines	2022 Updated annually	2019	2017 Minor pediatric update in 2021	2007 Update on 6 topics in 2020	2021 2017 for severe asthma	2022	2014 2019 update on management
Target population	Paediatrics Adolescents Adults	Paediatrics Adolescents Adults	Paediatrics Adolescents Adults	Paediatrics Adolescents Adults	Paediatrics Adolescents Adults	Adults	Adolescents Adults
Target region	International	United Kingdom	United Kingdom	United States	Canada	Europe	United States Europe
Recommendations strength	No	GRADE methodology	No	GRADE methodology	GRADE methodology	GRADE methodology	GRADE methodology
Level of evidence	A to D where applicable		GRADE				
Asthma diagnosis	X	X	X	2007 FeNO 2020	X	X	–
Asthma management	X	X	X	2020	X	–	–
Acute asthma	X	X		2007	–	–	–
Severe asthma	Specific section	No specific section but included throughout	–	–	2017 specific guidelines	–	Severe asthma-specific guidelines

Abbreviations: ATS: American Thoracic Society, BTS: British Thoracic Society, CTS: Canadian Thoracic Society, ERS: European Respiratory Society, GINA: Global Initiative for Asthma, GRADE: Grading of Recommendations, Assessment, Development and Evaluation, NAEPP: National Asthma Education and Prevention Program, NICE: National Institute for Care and Health Excellence, SIGN: Scottish Intercollegiate Guidelines Network they may look at specific aspects of asthma management such as the recent European Respiratory Society (ERS) task force report focusing solely on diagnosis.[41] Although most guidelines are intended for professionals of their own country, one noteworthy exception is the GINA report.[35] First established in 1993, the GINA scientific committee includes physicians from diverse geographic regions and is independent of respiratory societies, making it the only true asthma international strategy. CPGs are periodically updated, usually through new PICO questions focused on evolving topics. This lengthy process may, however, take years to come to fruition, limiting the responsiveness of guidelines to new evidence. By choosing not to use the PICO questioning or GRADE methodology to produce recommendations, GINA has allowed a prompt integration of emerging evidence into its annual report. Its methodology, detailed on the GINA website (www.ginaasthma.org), involves a twice yearly update of evidence with new publications exempt of quality issues being individually reviewed and then discussed in a Science Committee meeting. Upon this discussion, a decision is made on inclusion of the publication in the main report and possible related recommendations adjustments.[35] This always up-to-date material makes the GINA guideline a worldwide favourite among asthma caregivers.

5.4.2 Severe Asthma

The field of severe asthma has dramatically evolved in the past 10 years. The new targeted therapies available have made the use of precision medicine essential in the clinical management of severe asthmatics. As this treatment approach differs from the care of non-severe asthma in which incremental treatment steps are used in a one-size-fits-all manner, specific guidance in severe asthma was needed. Of note, however, in non-severe asthma, these steps can be modulated according to patients' characteristics and preferences, offering some form of treatment individualization. Nevertheless, CPGs focused on the diagnosis and management of severe asthma were then created. For example, GINA, ATS/ERS, and the Canadian Thoracic Society (CTS) produced such specific guidance, although only GINA updates it annually (Table 5.1).[35, 42–44]

5.5 CURRENT ASTHMA RECOMMENDATIONS

It is beyond the scope of this chapter to review in detail the different guidelines-based recommendations in the diagnosis and management of asthma, which will be addressed by the other chapters in this book. The general principles and differences that can be found in the aforementioned guidelines will, however, be highlighted in the following sections.

5.5.1 General Asthma

5.5.1.1 Definition and Diagnosis

The definition of asthma has not significantly changed in the last two decades and highlights the inflammatory nature of the disorder together with the physiological hallmarks of asthma: variable airway obstruction and airway hyperresponsiveness. There have, however, been some developments in asthma diagnosis. As incorrect clinical diagnosis is common, all consensuses stress the importance of an objective diagnosis,[45] with reversible airway obstruction on spirometry as the preferred method. It is however, acknowledged that spirometry is frequently normal in asthma and that alternative methods are needed.[46] These include bronchoprovocation challenges with methacholine, exercise challenge, mannitol, or other agents, or peak expiratory flow measurements. Fractional exhaled nitric oxide (FeNO) was recently included as an adjunct diagnostic tool by some CPGs (BTS/SIGN, NICE, NAEPP, and ERS).[36, 37, 39, 41] A measure >40–50 ppb has indeed shown a high specificity (75–95%) to rule in the diagnosis of asthma.[41, 47, 48] Its sensitivity is, however, much lower (19–56%), and a normal value does not exclude asthma.

It is important to note that no diagnostic test is specific for asthma and that many diseases such as COPD, allergic rhinitis, and bronchiectasis can lead to falsely positive "asthma tests." This is reflected in some CPGs criteria for diagnosis. For example, the NICE guideline advises a combination of two positive tests and the BTS/SIGN a response to treatment to establish a diagnosis of asthma with confidence.[36, 37]

Diagnosis of asthma in children under six years old is often challenging, as pulmonary function tests are unreliable at that age. Most CPGs recommend a compatible clinical evaluation together with a trial of treatment to establish diagnosis at that age.[35, 40]

5.5.1.2 Goal of Therapy

Asthma is a chronic disease that can only be controlled, not cured. Guidelines align in their goals for treatment that are to mitigate current impairments and prevent future risks caused by the disease or its treatment. There is, however, much variation in the definitions of asthma control between guidelines, which involve a set of clinical and physiological criteria (Table 5.2). Biomarkers have shown promise to assess asthma control, but, except for the CTS guideline, they have yet to make their way into guidelines.[40] Because of its value as a marker and target to prevent exacerbations, sputum eosinophils count has been included by the CTS as a criterion for control. Its limited availability, however, restricts its use in clinical practice.

With many asthmatic patients being low perceivers, most CPG use FEV_1 as a criterion to assess asthma control. Not considering lung function has indeed been linked to an overestimation of control.[49] The variable nature of asthma, however, does not rule out uncontrolled asthma in the face of a normal FEV_1. GINA no longer uses a specific lung function criterion and instead highlights low FEV_1 as a risk factor for future exacerbations.[35] By doing so, it dilutes the importance of measuring FEV_1 in many (more than 20) other factors of future risk, making physicians more likely to overlook it.

Prevention of future risks include minimization of exacerbations, hospital admissions and deaths, permanent

TABLE 5.2
Criteria for Control

		GINA	BTS/SIGN	NICE	NAEPP	CTS
Current impairment	**Daytime symptoms**	≤ 2 days/week	No	< 3 days/week	≤ 2 days/week	≤ 2 days/week
	Nighttime awakening	No	No	< 1 night/week	≤ 2 nights/month	< 1 night/week and mild
	Reliever use	SABA ≤ 2 dose/week	No need	SABA < 2 days/week	SABA ≤ 2 days/week	SABA or bud/form ≤ 2 doses/week
	Activity	No limitation	No limitation	–	No interference with normal activity	Normal
	Lung function	–	FEV_1 or PEF >80%	–	FEV_1 or PEF >80%	FEV_1 or PEF >90%
Future risks	**Exacerbation**	Assess risk factors	No	–	0–1/year	Mild (no OCS) and infrequent
	Loss of lung function	Assess risk factors		–	Longitudinal assessment	–
	Side effect of medication	Assess risk factors	Minimal	–	To be considered	–
	Other	–	–	–	ATAQ 0 ACQ ≤0.75 ACT ≥20	No absence from work or school due to asthma PEF diurnal variation <10–15% Sputum eosinophils <2–3%

Abbreviations: ACQ: Asthma Control Questionnaire, ACT: Asthma Control Test, ATAQ: Asthma Therapy Assessment Questionnaire, BTS: British Thoracic Society, bud-form: budesonide-formoterol, CTS: Canadian Thoracic Society, FEV_1: forced expiratory volume in the first second, GINA: Global Initiative for Asthma, NAEPP: National Asthma Education and Prevention Program, NICE: National Institute for Care and Health Excellence, OCS: oral corticosteroid, PEF: peak expiratory flow, SABA: short-acting beta-agonist, SIGN: Scottish Intercollegiate Guidelines Network

loss of lung function, and treatment-related adverse effect. Prevention of exacerbations is especially important in asthma, as they lead to accelerated lung function decline, and the often-needed oral corticosteroids (OCS) are responsible for significant side effects.[50–52] Almost all guidelines agree that even one OCS-treated exacerbation should trigger a revaluation of therapy.

5.5.1.3 Patient Education

All CPGs stress education as an essential element of asthma management. It should be performed as soon as the diagnosis is made and integrated afterward into all aspects of care. Some consensuses go further into details of the components of an asthma education programme, whose goal is to provide the patient and the family with self-management skills.[35, 38, 40] Notions about asthma pathophysiology and triggers, self-management skills with a written action plan (WAP) and inhaler technique education and training are all essential elements of such a programme but should be agreed and adapted to the patient's needs and situation.

5.5.1.4 Asthma Management Principles

Pharmacological treatment is one of the multiple components involved in the management of asthma. Many factors impact control and should therefore be addressed as part of asthma care, frequently prior to escalation of therapy. All CPGs agree on this.

The nonpharmacological management steps first include ensuring that symptoms are of asthmatic origin, as overdiagnoses are common.[45] Identifying and addressing contributory factors such as nonadherence, poor inhaler technique, triggers, and comorbidities then follow. Triggers include domestic and occupational environmental exposures, smoking, and, in some patients, medications. Allergen mitigation strategies are, however, mostly unsupported by evidence and expensive and should therefore be tailored to the patient's symptoms, sensitization, and exposure. GINA and NAEPP agree that allergen avoidance should not necessarily be used as a routine strategy in asthma but that reduction of mould, house-dust mites, and pests (cockroaches and rodents) strategies have proven the most beneficial, especially for children.[35, 39] Comorbidities to be addressed in asthma vary across guidelines but most frequently involve rhinosinusitis, gastro-oesophageal reflux, obesity, obstructive sleep apnoea, and psychological conditions.

5.5.1.5 Pharmacological Treatment

Medications given in asthma are divided in two categories: controllers and relievers. Controllers serve to prevent symptoms and exacerbations and are either anti-inflammatory medications or long-acting bronchodilators. Relievers are used as needed to swiftly alleviate intermittent symptoms. They include fast-acting bronchodilators like short-acting beta-2 agonists (SABA) or formoterol and long-acting beta-2 agonists (LABA) with a rapid onset of action.

Most guidelines present asthma treatment as incremental steps, in which the controller is progressively increased until control is achieved. ICS are the mainstay of treatment to which long-acting beta-2 agonists (LABA) are then added before the ICS dose is increased. Long-acting beta-2 agonists should not be used as monotherapy in asthma, as they do not improve airway inflammation and have been linked to an excess in mortality.[53] Leukotriene-receptors antagonist (LTRA) can be used as a second-choice add-on therapy to any treatment steps in most guidelines. The NICE, however, positions it before LABAs, as the first add-on option to ICS, contrary to other CPGs.[37] Caution should be taken with LTRA as they have been related to behaviour and mood-related changes, leading to a Food and Drug Administration (FDA) black box warning. More recent guidelines (GINA and NAEPP) also added long-acting antimuscarinic antagonists (LAMA) as an add-on option to medium- or high-dose regular ICS/LABA to reduce exacerbation and increase lung function.[35, 39]

ICSs are introduced early in the course of the disease as they target the inflammation causing the disease and have been shown to improve lung function and airway hyperresponsiveness, reduce asthma symptoms, and prevent exacerbations.[53] They have been used as regular medication for decades, but recent studies led to a re-evaluation of this paradigm. Four clinical trials studying budesonide/formoterol as-needed in mild asthmatics showed that this approach decreased exacerbations and hospital admissions when compared to as-needed SABA and was comparable to ICS taken regularly.[54–57] It was GINA to first introduce the *as-needed* ICS/formoterol controller option in their 2019 report and decided to position it as the preferred treatment option, over regular ICS, not only in mild but also in very mild asthmatic patients, a population in which data is still lacking. By doing so, the use of as-needed SABA alone in asthma was no longer an option. This decision was supported by the poor adherence to ICS and overuse of SABA in asthma, two risk factors of severe exacerbations and asthma-related deaths. The other guidelines were more conservative in their recommendations of as-needed ICS/formoterol. Only the CTS recommended its use in their 2021 algorithm for a very selected population: mild asthmatics unable to adhere to regular ICS therapy despite substantial education and support or as an alternative to ICS in very mild asthmatics well-controlled on as-needed SABA alone but at high risk of exacerbations.[40] The NAEPP evaluated the approach but decided there was still no place for ICS/formoterol in their algorithm, as it is no better than ICS taken regularly and is more costly than as-needed ICS and SABA taken concomitantly.[39] They, however, recommended this last option as an alternative to regular ICS in their 2020 guidelines (conditional recommendation). Consequently, except for GINA, all guidelines still recommend as-needed SABA alone in a selected population of asthmatic patients, well-controlled without regular treatment. GINA places PRN SABA only in conjunction with ICS as a "less-preferred option." It should, however, be pointed out that even well-controlled asthma can experience a severe exacerbation and that a rapid introduction of ICS may be needed.

Budesonide-formoterol can also be used as a reliever, in lieu of SABA, in patients already on the medication as a regular controller (called maintenance and reliever therapy [MART]), a strategy that has been shown to decrease severe exacerbations[58] This option is recommended by all guidelines, but the GINA, NICE, and NAEPP position it as the preferred approach in moderate asthma.[35, 37, 39]

Treatment options are more limited in paediatric asthma. Although the treatment steps usually resemble that of adults in children 6–11 years old, in younger children an increase in ICS is preferred over adding a LABA. It is also recommended to consider a LTRA, which is more effective in children and may be used as an alternative, rather than an add-on, to regular ICS. One should, however, balance the neuropsychiatric risks associated with LTRAs when choosing this therapy as a first-line option in children.

5.5.1.6 Monitoring

Asthma follow-up is centred around the clinical evaluation and measurement of airway obstruction. Criteria for the control and probability of future risks should be assessed at each visit, and spirometry performed regularly. Validated questionnaires such as the Asthma Control Questionnaire (ACQ) and Asthma Control Test (ACT) may also be used. Inflammation-guided treatment (sputum eosinophils or FeNO) has been shown to reduce exacerbations in moderate to severe asthma, but the limited access to these measures prevents the approach to be widely adopted and recommended. Currently, only the GINA and NAEPP recommend the strategy as an option, when available.[35, 39] All guidelines align on the fact that a treatment step down should be attempted when the disease is perfectly controlled, although such degree of control is not defined in many.

5.5.1.7 Management of Exacerbations

A few guidelines include a section on the specific management of acute asthma (Table 5.1), but all position the use of a written action plan (WAP) as a self-management strategy for home treatment of non-severe exacerbations. Except for the NAEPP, all CPGs recommend a four- or five-fold increase in ICS in the face of acute symptoms or PEF worsening, indicating an exacerbation onset. The NAEPP support their decision against the increase in ICS on their negative systematic review report and poor adherence to ICS in the positive pivotal 2018 study.[59] They, however, consider the strategy reasonable if adherence to ICS is uncertain or known to be poor.[39]

In the acute care setting, the treatment intensity and decision to admit should be based on clinical signs and lung function assessment (spirometry of PEF) at presentation and after initial management. Short-acting bronchodilators are the basis of initial management and systemic corticosteroids added in the face of a FEV_1 or PEF below 40–50% or not improving after initial bronchodilator administration.[35, 36, 38]

There is currently a lack of proper guideline for acute asthma management in the intensive care unit (ICU), although some relevant information can be found in the NAEPP and BTS/SIGN guidelines.[33, 35] While both address advanced treatments such as heliox or intravenous magnesium sulfate, only NAEPP discusses some ventilator strategies, but in a very limited fashion.

5.5.2 Severe Asthma

5.5.2.1 Definition and Diagnosis

It is important to highlight that the severity of symptoms does not define the severity of asthma, which is rather based on the amount of treatment needed to control the disease, reflecting the severity of the intrinsic mechanisms leading to the clinical phenotype.[42] Severe asthma benefits from its own definition, which is agreed upon by all guidelines. It is defined as the need for high-dose ICS and a second controller (usually LABA) or systemic glucocorticoids for 50% of the previous year to prevent asthma from becoming uncontrolled or remaining uncontrolled despite this therapy.[43] All guidelines also stress the crucial step of differentiating severe asthma from difficult-to-treat asthma, which is asthma that improves with optimal adherence to asthma treatment or after diagnosis and management of potential comorbidities or confounders.

5.5.2.2 Phenotyping

Asthma is a heterogeneous disease, and severe asthma is not different. However, many severe asthma treatments target specific pathways and are therefore effective in only a subset of patients. To select the most appropriate treatment, all guidelines recommend phenotyping as an initial management step in severe asthma. At present, the most useful phenotypes are those involving type 2 (T2) inflammation, allergic, and/or eosinophilic. Biomarkers are important tools to uncover T2 inflammation, but clinical markers such as age of onset, comorbidities, allergen-driven symptoms, or OCS dependency are also important indicators. Currently available T2 biomarkers include blood eosinophils, IgE, sputum eosinophils, and FeNO. And because T2 inflammation may be dynamic or influenced by OCS treatment, GINA recommend considering the measurement of FeNO and blood eosinophils up to three times, on the lowest OCS dose possible, before concluding a non-T2 asthma phenotype.[35]

5.5.2.3 Pharmacological Treatment

Treatment options in severe asthma include biologic therapy (anti-IgE, anti-IL5/IL5R, anti-IL4R, and anti-TSLP), low-dose azithromycin, LAMAs, LTRAs, OCS, and bronchial thermoplasty. Long considered the only effective treatment in severe asthma, OCSs are now recommended as a last option. They have been mostly replaced by monoclonal antibodies targeting various cytokines of the inflammatory cascade, which have been shown very effective with a better safety profile. GINA recommend their use above any other add-on treatment, if available, when there is evidence of uncontrolled T2 inflammation.[35] Guidance on biologic selection may, however, be confusing for clinicians. The ERS/ATS, GINA, and CTS identify predictors of response for every biologic class available (Table 5.3), but many predictors overlap, and the evidence to support more precise selection is lacking.[35, 42, 44] For example, blood eosinophil count is a predictor of response to every biologic in severe asthma and is therefore of little value to select between therapies.

Non-T2 asthma is a more challenging phenotype to treat. LAMA and low-dose azithromycin are recommended by the ATS/ERS, GINA, and CTS as potential add-on treatment to high-dose ICS/LABA to decrease exacerbations and symptoms and are therefore frequently used.[35, 42, 44] Two monoclonal antibodies have also shown some effect in non-T2 asthma, although the benefits are less impressive than in patients displaying eosinophilic inflammation. Dupilumab, an anti-ILR antibody, is recommended in non-eosinophilic patients on maintenance OCS.[35, 44] Because the anti-TSLP tezepelumab has only been recently developed, only GINA addresses its use. It is positioned, as every other biologic, mainly in T2 asthma, although consideration may be given in low or non-T2 asthma.[35] Bronchial thermoplasty is discussed in every severe asthma guideline, but because of the low quality of evidence currently available, the limited facilities providing the treatment, and its relative invasiveness, its use is only recommended in the context of a clinical trial or registry or in highly specialized centres.[35, 43] It should be remembered that these therapies are all initially prescribed as "therapeutic trials" and should be stopped if asthma control and risk factor parameters fail to show significant improvement at follow-up.

5.6 ADHERENCE TO ASTHMA GUIDELINES

5.6.1 Adherence

Knowledge of current asthma guidelines is often poor among clinicians, particularly in primary care.[56] Specialists (respirologists, allergists, paediatricians, and internists) are indeed more knowledgeable about asthma, more likely to confirm a diagnosis of asthma by objective measures, and follow national asthma guidelines in addition to being more likely to provide patients with written asthma action plans.[15, 60–64] Looking at implementation of the NAEPP guideline using the National Asthma Survey of Physicians: National Ambulatory Medical Care Survey, Akinbami et al. also found that US paediatricians were more likely to provide asthma action/treatment plans than primary care physicians and internists.[65] Self-efficacy and frequent referral were associated with adherence, which was higher for

TABLE 5.3
Recommendation for Therapies in Severe Asthma

		GINA 2022	ATS/ERS 2014 and 2019	CTS 2017
	LAMA	Medium- or high-dose ICS/LABA and exacerbation	Medium- or high-dose ICS/LABA and exacerbation	Uncontrolled severe asthma
	Macrolides	Persistent symptoms despite high-dose ICS/LABA	Persistent symptoms or uncontrolled despite high-dose ICS/LABA	Severe asthma and exacerbation
	Bronchial thermoplasty	In severe asthma in the context of a clinical trial or registry	In severe asthma in the context of a clinical trial or registry	Limited role in highly specialized centre
Guidance for selection	**Anti-IgE**	SEVERE ALLERGIC ASTHMA Blood eosinophils ≥260/μL FeNO ≥20 ppb Allergen-driven symptoms Childhood-onset asthma	Blood eosinophils ≥260/μL FeNO ≥19.5 ppb	Blood eosinophils ≥260–300/μL
	Anti-IL5/5R	SEVERE EOSINOPHILIC ASTHMA Higher blood eosinophils More exacerbation Adult-onset asthma Nasal polyposis	Blood eosinophils ≥150/μL and exacerbation	Blood eosinophils Mepolizumab: ≥150/μL at initiation or 300/μL in the last year Benralizumab: ≥300/μL Reslizumab: ≥400/μL
	Anti-IL4R	SEVERE EOSINOPHILIC/TYPE 2 ASTHMA Higher blood eosinophils Higher FeNO MAINTENANCE OCS REGARDLESS OF BLOOD EOSINOPHILS	–	–
	Anti-TSLP	SEVERE ASTHMA Higher blood eosinophils Higher FeNO Consider in non-type 2 asthma	–	–

Abbreviations: ATS: American Thoracic Society, CTS: Canadian Thoracic Society, ERS: European Respiratory Society, FeNO: forced exhaled nitric oxide, GINA: Global Initiative for Asthma, ICS: Inhaled corticosteroid, IL: interleukin, LABA: long-acting $beta_2$-agonists, LAMA: long-acting antimuscarinic antagonists, TSLP: thymic stromal lymphopoietin

history-taking recommendations and lower for recommendations involving patient education, equipment, and expertise.

Large variations have been observed in the effective translation of current asthma guidelines recommendations into care.[66, 67] A success story often cited is from Finland, where the national program launched in the 1990s resulted in the widespread adoption of national guidelines.[68] Local asthma coordinators that ensured high quality of asthma management in primary care were considered a key factor of this success.[69] Many aspects of the CPGs are still insufficiently implemented into clinical practice, particularly regarding the use of SABAs, the provision of a WAP, and the referral for asthma education.[70] Discrepancies were also found in children between the pharmacological prescriptions and current asthma guidelines, especially on use of bronchial anti-inflammatory therapy. Likewise, low adherence to guidelines was shown with the Physician Practice Assessment Questionnaire (PPAQ), a standardized questionnaire to assess Canadian asthma and chronic obstructive pulmonary disease (COPD) guidelines implementation by primary care physicians.[71] In asthma, a low score (application of recommendations in less than 50% of patients) was seen in referral for patient education, provision of a written action plan, regular assessment of inhaler technique, and referral to a specialist for difficult to control asthma or uncertain diagnosis.[72] Although this showed suboptimal implementation of many CPG recommendations, more studies are needed to assess the true current uptake of guidelines and the influence of initiatives to promote their use.

Despite poor uptake of recommendations, clinicians usually recognize that guidelines help to standardize medical practice and benefit the patient. They, however, need guidance on how to implement them in addition to better access to asthma educators and other asthma resources (e.g. medication, spirometry).

5.6.2 Factors Limiting Implementation

There are many barriers to effective asthma guidelines implementation.[73] Some are at the level of clinicians, but others are related to the patient's behaviour and agreement with recommendations.

5.6.2.1 Healthcare Professional Level

Guidelines are usually helpful to improve practice. Physicians are, however, faced with many different guidelines on various diseases, making it difficult to read and assimilate them all. Implementation into routine care is even more problematic and requires strategies adapted to the clinician's context and resources, including socio-economic and organizational factors. Adaptation of guidelines to cultural and socio-economic settings may improve uptake.[74]

Guidelines are often lengthy and considered complex by general practitioners.[75, 76] The translation of their recommendations into care is influenced by their level of knowledge, attitudes, skills, beliefs, and values.[75–77] The lack of time or resources and uncertainties regarding applications for a given patient may also impair implementation and need to be addressed.[78, 79]

A few studies looked at the barriers to implementation of guidelines recommendation. Wiener-Ogilvie et al. audited compliance with three key recommendations of British guidelines and found that about two-thirds of patients were treated appropriately with add-on therapy, while only 23% had been given an asthma action plan.[80] Barriers identified by clinicians were doubtful about the care being evidenced-based and relevance to primary care, lack of knowledge and skills, and lack of time and resources. Although most physicians were aware of the key recommendations, less were persuaded that they were helpful, and many considered that a reorganization of local care would be needed to adequately implement those. Another study surveyed New York providers about self-reported adherence to five NAEPP asthma guideline components.[81] Although not optimal, adherence to ICS use (62%) and influenza vaccinations (73%) was better than for peak flow monitoring (34%), asthma action plan use (9%), and allergy testing (10%). Potential barriers included lack of agreement with guidelines, lack of self-efficacy, lack of outcome expectancy, and external barriers.

Pharmacists have an important role in guidelines implementation as their direct and frequent contacts with patients offer an opportunity to reinforce key messages. Specific pharmaceutical care guidelines have been produced and studied. Kuipers et al. evaluated community pharmacists' adherence to such recommendations in the Netherlands.[82] They found that questions regarding the type of lung disease and patients' expectations, wishes, and concerns were often not collected and that inhalation instructions were less provided at refill dispensing. More studies are needed to evaluate the role and guideline recommendations implementation in pharmacies.

5.6.2.2 Patient Level

Patients' acceptance of healthcare providers' suggestions depends on various personal characteristics and motivation for behaviour change. Questionnaires such as the SABA Reliance Questionnaire (SRB) may elicit beliefs preventing patient's uptake of recommentations.[83] Good communication between the patient and caregivers is of importance as poor professional–patient communication often explains the poor uptake of guideline recommendations in primary care.[84] Key communication skills, required for an effective professional–patient partnership, should be developed and applied. Methods such as the "shared decision-making" and "motivational interviews" may help improve patient adherence to recommendations.[85, 86]

5.7 INTEGRATING ASTHMA GUIDELINES INTO CARE

Guidelines implementation starts with the built-in features of the reports. A specific framework developed by Gagliardi et al. proposed ways to improve guidelines organized in the domains of adaptability, usability, validity, applicability, communicability, accommodation, implementation, and evaluation.[87] Providing necessary resources and provider-focused education may also improve best practice and facilitate healthcare workers' adherence.[88] Decision support tools, feedback and audit, and clinical pharmacy support are likely to improve adherence to asthma guidelines. There is, however, a need to evaluate healthcare provider-targeted interventions with standardized outcomes.[89]

The dissemination of guidelines through medical/scientific publications, mailings, continuing professional development (CPD), workshops, and symposia may not be sufficient to change medical practice.[83] A multidisciplinary approach should be promoted, and the implementation of guidelines should be tailored to the environment and resources available.[74, 90]

5.7.1 Knowledge-to-Action Plan

Knowledge translation strategies have been refined in the last decades, and models such as the Knowledge-to-Action framework have been developed to structure the interventions (Figure 5.2).[91] This model first starts with knowledge synthesis and creation of tools to effectively communicate the information. To achieve appropriate use of the created knowledge, a continuous action cycle is then entered. Knowledge is chosen and adapted to the identified context, and barriers to its use are assessed to select and implement tailored interventions. Next, the quality of the intervention is assessed through its impact on patient's outcomes, and the overall process is then reviewed and updated. An effective knowledge translation process will generate implementation tools adapted to the user's needs and preferences and facilitate the application of recommendations into current care, while ensuring a personalized management of the condition.

5.7.2 How to Improve Implementation: The Role of Implementation Tools

Many publications have discussed how to improve the implementation of CPGs. Interactive strategies, practice

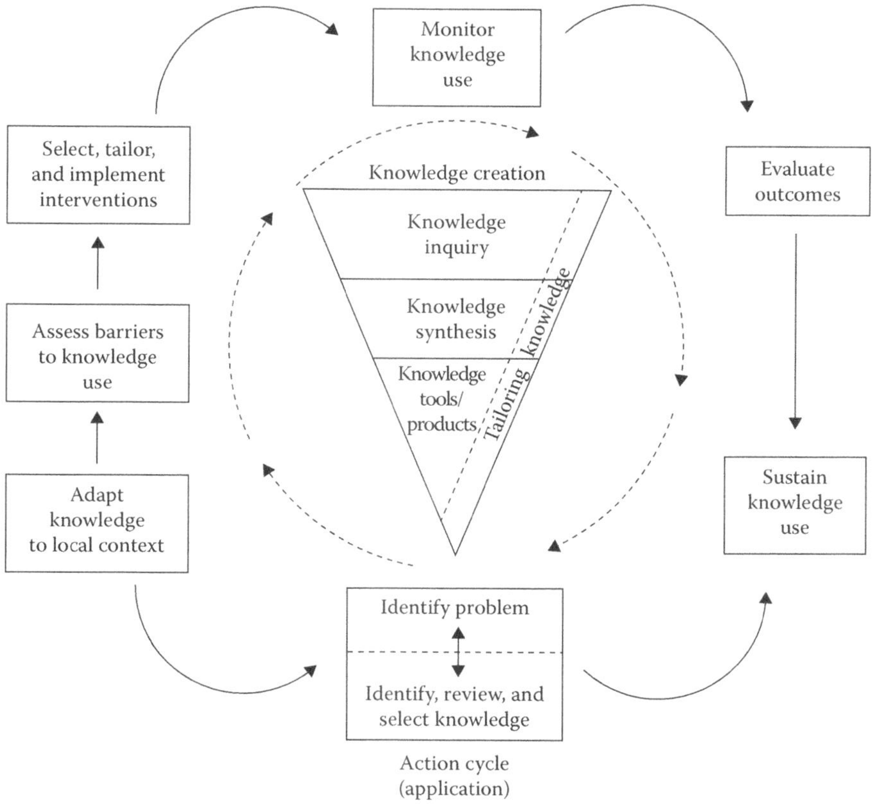

FIGURE 5.2 Knowledge-to-Action framework. (Knowledge-to-Action Model from Graham ID et al., *J Contin Educ Health Prof* (2006) PMID: 16557505/https://doi.org/10.1002/chp.47. With permission.)

aids, reminders, algorithms, and summaries, particularly using new electronic tools, have been considered useful to facilitate the translation of guideline recommendations into clinical practice.[74, 92] Applying the principles of intrinsic implementability of guidelines/reports with tables, figures, and algorithms may also help the uptake of recommendations.[93]

Guideline developers have now produced summaries of their key recommendations, for example Slim Jims of the CTS or GINA's *Pocket Guide for Asthma Management and Prevention*.[94] These documents help to quickly review the main features of a guideline while referencing the core document if needed. Patients' guideline summaries are also becoming increasingly available.[95] Toolboxes for guideline development, implementation, revision, and evaluation have been published, but many have not been fully integrated into guideline reports yet.

Assessment tools such as the Guideline Implementability Appraisal (GLIA) help assess the implementability of guidelines.[93] GLIA includes 31 items, categorized into 10 dimensions, nine being applied individually to each recommendation of the guideline. Decidability and executability are key dimensions, while the others are global: presentation and formatting, measurable outcomes, apparent validity, flexibility, effect on process of care, novelty/innovation, and computability. Forums such as the Guidelines International Network (G-I-N) can also help exchange ideas on the best methods to effectively translate guidelines.[96]

Guidelines integration to electronic medical records (EMR) is increasingly available and can help improve access to recommendations at the point of care. Initiatives such as the Canadian PRESTINE project have been developed to help standardize EMR content and should help implement current guidelines.[97]

5.7.3 From the Perspective of Healthcare Systems

Various programmes exist at local or regional levels to help improve guideline implementation. Many of those have been proposed and some evaluated. Here are a few examples of such large-scale programmes:

1. An emergency department (ED) and standardized ED asthma care pathway (ACP) programme have been developed to improve asthma management guidelines and patient outcomes in Canada.[98] It resulted in an improved use of metered-dose inhalers (MDIs), ICS, referrals, oxygen, and documentation of teaching and increased patient recollection of teaching compared to the control sites.
2. Some benefits were also seen from an ED programme aimed at improving referral to asthma educators.[99]
3. A similar initiative was aimed at introducing the Paediatric Acute Asthma Management Guideline (PAMG) to the ED of a paediatric tertiary care hospital.[100] During the implementation of the

PAMG, patients who visited the ED were more likely to receive OCS and oxygen saturation reassessment before ED discharge. Improvements in asthma education and discharge planning were noted, although the changes were not statistically significant.

These observations suggest, among many others, that systematically induced changes can result in a significant improvement in care delivery. It also illustrates the difficulties in changing practice behaviours and integrating tools to help implement guidelines and standardize care. Furthermore, the sustainability of the changes when the resources allocated to the programme are reduced or stopped are unknown. Studying barriers to guidelines recommendations should help offer better support.

5.7.4 Guidelines Implementation in Low- to Middle-Income Countries

Guidelines implementation in low- to middle-income countries (LMIC) is a significant challenge. Many care gaps, detailed in the publication by Meghji et al., persist in these countries.[2] This situation is exacerbated by the difficult access to care and essential resources, including the basic medications required to control the disease.[101] In this regard, the GINA annual report attempted to provide alternatives for LMIC in case of challenging access to care or unavailable preferred strategies, and the World Health Organization affiliated group GARD (Global Alliance against Chronic Respiratory Diseases) are involved in initiatives to help address this urgent problem.[102]

5.8 FUTURE OF ASTHMA GUIDELINES

Although current asthma guidelines have been improved in the last decades with the help of standardized methodologies and evidenced-based applications, research is still needed to further refine their content and implementation into clinical care. More resources should be made available to accomplish these goals. New communication tools such as smartphones, tablet computers, and user-friendly websites offer innovative ways to help not only clinicians integrate guideline recommendations into their practice but also patients to advocate for better care.

It was recently stressed that asthma key management decisions are mostly made at the non-specialist level, where management is mainly symptom-guided, with insufficient use of spirometry and little attempt made to personalize management.[103] However, making a diagnosis of asthma in primary care can be challenging due to the poor specificity of symptoms and low sensitivity of lung function tests, while important features such as airway inflammation are usually not considered in therapeutic choices. A different management approach has been proposed in which treatment decisions are driven by the identification of key treatable mechanistic traits, called treatable traits.[104] This approach, particularly adapted for severe asthma, may help tailor asthma care in less severe patients.[105] This concept has already made its way in some guidelines and is likely to be of increased use. For example, assessment of airway eosinophilia as a control criterion has been included in CTS guidelines for more than a decade, and T2 and non-T2 asthma are commonly used terms in severe asthma guidelines.

Guidelines still have an important role to play in helping clinicians optimally manage asthma in populations and individuals. They improve knowledge, define optimal management, and position new therapies. They also address the many care gaps remaining in asthma. CPGs should, however, have clear and implementable recommendations and tools to facilitate application in clinical care. The work translating recommendations into practice should begin as soon as the guidelines are produced. Patient engagement should also be promoted through guideline patient tools.

5.9 CONCLUSION

Evidence-based guidelines help optimize medical practice, but efforts should be made to better implement them. Standardized methods to produce, assess, and translate guidelines more effectively have been developed. Patients are now increasingly involved at all steps of guidelines production and implementation. Among the first practice guidelines to be produced, asthma CGPs have been constantly updated since. Although some contradictions still exist between guidelines, recommendations are now more consistent. The main principles reside on confirming the diagnosis objectively, achieving and maintaining control defined by a set of criteria, and using nonpharmacological and pharmacological interventions to achieve this goal. Attention should be given to persistent care gaps and improving the tools as well as the initiatives developed and promoted to address them. New electronic tools should help disseminate and integrate guideline evidence-based recommendations into care while personalizing asthma assessment and therapy.

REFERENCES

1. Rabe KF et al., *J Allergy Clin Immunol* (2004) PMID: 15241342/https://doi.org/10.1016/j.jaci.2004.04.042
2. Meghji J et al., *Lancet* (2021) PMID: 33631128/https://doi.org/10.1016/S0140-6736(21)00458-X
3. Sears MR., *Eur J Respir Dis Suppl* (1986) PMID: 2876911
4. Boulet LP in Middleton's Allergy: Principles and Practice, Chapter 70 (2003)
5. Hargreave FE et al., *J Allergy Clin Immunol* (1990) PMID: 2355155/https://doi.org/10.1016/0091-6749(90)90056-a
6. British Thoracic Society, Research Unit of the Royal College of Physicians of London, King's Fund Centre, National Asthma Campain. *BMJ* (1990) PMID: 1977482/https://doi.org/10.1136/bmj.301.6753.651
7. Boulet LP et al., *Eur Respir J* (2019) PMID: 31273040/https://doi.org/10.1183/13993003.00598-2019
8. Kroegel C et al., *Drugs* (2009) PMID: 19537836/https://doi.org/10.2165/00003495-200969090-00004.

9. Gupta S et al., *Can Respir J.* (2016) PMID: 27445525/https://doi.org/10.1155/2016/3085065
10. Tan LD et al., *Curr Opin Pulm* Med (2022) PMID: 35190509/https://doi.org/10.1097/MCP.0000000000000867
11. Guyatt GH et al., *BMJ* (2008) PMID: 18436948/https://doi.org/10.1136/bmj.39489.470347.AD
12. Guyatt GH et al., *BMJ* (2008) PMID: 18467413/https://doi.org/10.1136/bmj.39493.646875.AE
13. Brouwers MC et al., *BMJ* (2016) PMID: 26957104/https://doi.org/10.1136/bmj.i1152
14. AGREE (2022) <https://www.agreetrust.org/agree-ii/>
15. Boulet LP et al., *Can Respir J* (2006) PMID: 16552449/https://doi.org/10.1155/2006/810978
16. Gagliardi AR et al., *Implement Sci* (2009) PMID: 19573246/https://doi.org/10.1186/1748-5908-4-36
17. Kastner M et al., *BMC Fam Pract* (2014) PMID: 24476491/https://doi.org/10.1186/1471-2296-15-19
18. Straus SE et al., *Evidence-based medicine: how to practice and teach EBM*. 3rd ed. (Elsevier, 2005)
19. Huang X et al., *AMIA Annu Symp Proc* (2006) PMID: 17238363
20. Schardt C et al., *BMC Med Inform Decis Mak* (2007) PMID: 17573961/https://doi.org/10.1186/1472-6947-7-16
21. Chakraborty S et al., *Health Res Policy Syst* (2020) PMID: 32993665/https://doi.org/10.1186/s12961-020-00628-3
22. Zeng X et al., *J Evid Based Med* (2015) PMID: 25594108/https://doi.org/10.1111/jebm.12141
23. Guyatt G et al., *J Clin Epidemiol* (2011) PMID: 21195583/https://doi.org/10.1016/j.jclinepi.2010.04.026
24. Guyatt GH et al., *J Clin Epidemiol* (2011) PMID: 21185693/https://doi.org/10.1016/j.jclinepi.2010.09.011
25. Brozek JL et al., *Allergy* (2009) PMID: 19210357/https://doi.org/10.1111/j.1398-9995.2009.01973.x
26. Hilton Boon M et al., *J Clin Epidemiol* (2021) PMID: 33476768/https://doi.org/10.1016/j.jclinepi.2021.01.001
27. Brouwers MC et al., *CMAJ* (2010) PMID: 20513780/https://doi.org/10.1503/cmaj.091714
28. Brouwers MC et al., *Semin Nucl Med* (2019) PMID: 30819394/https://doi.org/10.1053/j.semnuclmed.2018.11.001
29. Brouwers MC et al., *J Clin Epidemiol* (2020) PMID: 32473992/https://doi.org/10.1016/j.jclinepi.2020.05.025
30. Podjasek JC et al., *Curr Opin Allergy Clin Immunol* (2013) PMID: 23571409/https://doi.org/10.1097/ACI.0b013e32836093c3
31. Selroos O et al., *Eur Respir Rev* (2015) PMID: 26324809/https://doi.org/10.1183/16000617.00008114
32. Sadatsafavi M et al., *Allergy* (2016) PMID: 26529357/https://doi.org/10.1111/all.12803
33. Uptodate (2022). <https://www.uptodate.com/>
34. Bradley-Ridout G et al., *J Med Libr Assoc* (2021) PMID: 34629966/https://doi.org/10.5195/jmla.2021.1176
35. Global Initiative for Asthma. (2022).<https://ginasthma.org>
36. British Thoracic Society & Scottish Intercollegiate Guidelines Network (2019) <https://www.sign.ac.uk/our-guidelines/british-guideline-on-the-management-of-asthma/>
37. National Institute for Health and Care Excellence (NICE) (2021) <https://www.nice.org.uk/guidance/ng80>
38. National Asthma Education and Prevention Program. *J Allergy Clin Immunol* (2007) PMID: 17983880/https://doi.org/10.1016/j.jaci.2007.09.043
39. National Asthma Education and Prevention Program Coordinating Committee Expert Panel Working Group. *J Allergy Clin Immunol* (2020) PMID: 33280709/https://doi.org/10.1016/j.jaci.2020.10.003
40. Yang CL et al., *Can J Respir Crit Care Sleep Med* (2021) doi: 10.1080/24745332.2021.1945887
41. Satia LR et al., *Eur Respir J* (2022) PMID: 35169025/https://doi.org/10.1183/13993003.01585–2021
42. FitzGerald JM et al., *Can J Respir Crit Care Sleep Med* (2017) https://doi.org/10.1080/24745332.2017.1395250
43. Chung KF et al., *Eur Respir J* (2014) PMID: 24337046/https://doi.org/10.1183/09031936.00202013
44. Holguin F et al., *Eur Respir J* (2020) PMID: 31558662/https://doi.org/10.1183/13993003.00588–2019
45. Aaron SD et al., *JAMA*. (2017) PMID: 28114551/https://doi.org/10.1001/jama.2016.19627.
46. National Institute for Health and Care Excellence (NICE); 2021 Mar 22. (NICE Guideline, No. 80.) Available from: https://www.ncbi.nlm.nih.gov/books/NBK560178/
47. Karrasch S et al., *Thorax* (2017) PMID: 27388487/https://doi.org/10.1136/thoraxjnl-2016–208704
48. Nekoee H et al., *ERJ Open Res* (2020 PMID: 32714964/https://doi.org/10.1183/23120541.00169-2020.
49. Dostaler SM et al., *J Asthma* (2011) PMID: 22091743/https://doi.org/10.3109/02770903.2011.631243
50. Bai TR et al., *Eur Respir J* (2007) PMID: 17537763/https://doi.org/10.1183/09031936.00165106
51. Price DB et al., *J Asthma Allergy* (2018) PMID: 30214247/https://doi.org/10.2147/JAA.S176026.
52. Nelson HS et al., *Chest* (2006) PMID: 16424409/https://doi.org/10.1378/chest.129.1.15
53. Barnes PJ et al., *J Allergy Clin Immunol* (1998) PMID: 9802359/https://doi.org/10.1016/s0091-6749(98)70268-4
54. O'Byrne PM et al., *N Engl J Med* (2018) PMID: 29768149/https://doi.org/10.1056/NEJMoa1715274
55. Bateman ED et al., *N Engl J Med* (2018) PMID: 29768147/https://doi.org/10.1056/NEJMoa1715275
56. Beasley R et al., *N Engl J Med* (2019) PMID: 31112386/https://doi.org/10.1056/NEJMoa1901963
57. Hardy J et al., *Lancet* (2019) PMID: 31451207/https://doi.org/10.1016/S0140-6736(19)31948-8
58. O'Byrne PM et al., *Am J Respir Crit Care Med* (2005) PMID: 15502112/https://doi.org/10.1164/rccm.200407-884OC
59. McKeever T et al., *N Engl J Med* (2018) PMID: 29504499/https://doi.org/10.1056/NEJMoa1714257
60. Janson S et al., *J Asthma* (2004) PMID: 15260468/https://doi.org/10.1081/jas-120026093
61. Partridge MR et al., *Eur Respir J Suppl* (2003) PMID: 12572698/https://doi.org/10.1183/09031936.0.00054503
62. Rabe KF et al., *Eur Respir J* (2000) PMID: 11153575/https://doi.org/10.1183/09031936.00.16580200
63. Lai CK et al., *J Allergy Clin Immunol* (2003) PMID: 12589343/https://doi.org/10.1067/mai.2003.30
64. Fuhlbrigge AL et al., *Am J Respir Crit Care Med* (2002) PMID: 12379546/https://doi.org/10.1164/rccm.2107057
65. Akinbami LJ et al., *J Asthma* (2020) PMID: 30821526/https://doi.org/10.1080/02770903.2019.1579831
66. Price C et al., *BMJ Open* (2019) PMID: 30696669/https://doi.org/10.1136/bmjopen-2018-022506
67. Boulet LP et al., *Can Respir J* (2013) PMID: 23936884/https://doi.org/10.1155/2013/496923
68. Pakkasela J et al., *Eur Clin Respir J* (2022) PMID: 36457457/https://doi.org/10.1080/20018525.2022.2149918
69. Haahtela T et al., *Thorax* (2006) PMID: 16877690/https://doi.org/10.1136/thx.2005.055699
70. Jin R et al., *Can Respir J* (2000) PMID: 11121090/https://doi.org/10.1155/2000/587151.
71. Boulet LP et al., *Respir Med* (2011) PMID: 20797841/https://doi.org/10.1016/j.rmed.2010.07.022.
72. Yawn BP et al., *Mayo Clin Proc* (2016) PMID: 26944837/https://doi.org/10.1016/j.mayocp.2016.01.010

73. Tan WC et al., *Int J Tuberc Lung Dis* (2006) PMID: 16848330
74. Harrison MB et al., *CMAJ* (2010) PMID: 19969563/https://doi.org/10.1503/cmaj.081232
75. Baiardini I et al., *Curr Opin Allergy Clin Immunol* (2009) PMID: 19390434/https://doi.org/10.1097/ACI.0b013e32832b4651
76. Kitson AL, Strauss S., *Knowledge Translation in Health Care: Moving from Evidence to Practice.* Section 3 (BMJ Books) (2009)
77. Grol R et al., *Lancet* (2003) PMID: 14568747/https://doi.org/10.1016/S0140-6736(03)14546–1
78. Partridge MR et al., *Eur Respir J* (2000) PMID: 10706483/https://doi.org/10.1034/j.1399-3003.2000.15b01.x
79. Grimshaw JM et al., *Qual Health Care* (1994) PMID: 10136260/https://doi.org/10.1136/qshc.3.1.45
80. Wiener-Ogilvie S et al., *Prim Care Respir J* (2007) PMID: 18026674/https://doi.org/10.3132/pcrj.2007.00074
81. Wisnivesky JP et al., *Ann Allergy Asthma Immunol* (2008) PMID: 18814449/https://doi.org/10.1016/S1081-1206(10)60491-7
82. Kuipers E et al., *NPJ Prim Care Respir Med* (2019) PMID: 31296863/https://doi.org/10.1038/s41533-019-0139-5
83. Chan AHY et al., *J Allergy Clin Immunol Pract* (2020) PMID: 32702517/https://doi.org/10.1016/j.jaip.2020.07.014
84. Moffat M et al., *Fam Pract* (2007) PMID: 17158184/https://doi.org/10.1093/fampra/cml062
85. Légaré F et al., *Cochrane Database Syst Rev* (2010) PMID: 20464744/https://doi.org/10.1002/14651858.CD006732.pub2
86. Lavoie KL et al.. *Patient Prefer Adherence* (2014) PMID: 25422587/https://doi.org/10.2147/PPA.S66966
87. Gagliardi AR et al., *Implement Sci* (2011) PMID: 21426574/https://doi.org/10.1186/1748-5908-6-26
88. Pudasainee-Kapri S., *J Pediatr Nurs* (2021) PMID: 33212342/https://doi.org/10.1016/j.pedn.2020.09.020
89. Okelo SO et al., *Pediatrics* (2013) PMID: 23979092/https://doi.org/10.1542/peds.2013-0779
90. Burgers J et al., *Improving Patient Care. The Implementation of Change in Clinical Practice, Ch. 6* (2005)
91. Graham ID et al., *J Contin Educ Health Prof* (2006) PMID: 16557505/https://doi.org/10.1002/chp.47
92. Tomaszewski W., *Acta Bioeng Biomech* (2012) PMID: 22741924
93. Shiffman RN et al., *BMC Med Inform Decis Mak* (2005) PMID: 16048653/https://doi.org/10.1186/1472-6947-5-23.
94. Flodgren G et al., *Cochrane Database Syst Rev* (2016) PMID: 27546228/https://doi.org/10.1002/14651858.CD010669.pub2
95. Global Initiative for Asthma. (2022). <https://ginasthma.org/gina-patient-guide-you-can-control-your-asthma/>
96. Qaseem A et al., *Ann Intern Med* (2012) PMID: 22473437/https://doi.org/10.7326/0003-4819-156-7-201204030-00009
97. Lougheed MD et al., *Can Respir J* (2012) PMID: 22536581/https://doi.org/10.1155/2012/870357
98. Lougheed MD et al., *CJEM* (2009) PMID: 19523270/https://doi.org/10.1017/s1481803500011234
99. Robichaud P et al., *Chest* (2004) PMID: 15539718/https://doi.org/10.1378/chest.126.5.1495
100. To T et al., *Respir Med* (2010) PMID: 20434896/https://doi.org/10.1016/j.rmed.2010.03.028
101. Dubaybo BA., *Res Rep Trop Med* (2021) PMID: 33727880/https://doi.org/10.2147/RRTM.S247716
102. Khaltaev N., *J Thorac Dis* (2017) PMID: 29268538/https://doi.org/10.21037/jtd.2017.11.91
103. Shaw DE et al., *Lancet Respir Med* (2021) PMID: 33639099/https://doi.org/10.1016/S2213-2600(21)00021-7
104. Agusti A et al., *Respir Med* (2021) PMID: 34478992/https://doi.org/10.1016/j.rmed.2021.106572
105. McDonald VM et al., *Respirology* (2019) PMID: 30230137/https://doi.org/10.1111/resp.13389

6 Diagnosis of Asthma in Preschool Children

Liesbeth Duijts and Tarik Karramass

CASE PRESENTATION

Noa is a two-year-old boy who, accompanied by his parents, visits your paediatric outpatient clinic due to recurrent wheezing symptoms. Two days ago, he presented at the emergency department because of gradual worsening of symptoms of wheeze and shortness of breath without a fever or cold for a few days, which has kept him awake during the night. He was successfully treated with nebulized albuterol and sent home. The parents also mention that Noa had experienced three episodes of wheezing since the age of one year while having a cold or when walking in the countryside in the spring. Between episodes, he has a dry cough at night once a week and often sneezes. He has never received a course of oral steroids and has not been hospitalized for wheezing symptoms. Noa was born after an uncomplicated pregnancy but at 33 weeks of gestational age due to sudden maternal premature rupture of membranes. He had a good start and a normal birth weight. He was fully breastfed until the age of four months and has tolerated his diet of solid food well with no apparent signs of food allergies. He is exposed to parental environmental tobacco smoke, and two cats take part in their household. Noa's father has a history of childhood asthma and eczema. You performed percutaneous skin testing for a limited panel of aeroallergens and find that Noa is sensitized to cat dander and pollens. The parents have the following questions about the respiratory symptoms of Noa:

1. *"Does Noa have asthma?"*
2. *"If so, will he 'grow out of it,' or could we cure it?"*
3. *"Is it necessary to start daily treatment?"*

6.1 INTRODUCTION

Asthma symptoms often begin in early life.[1] Asthma symptoms may present heterogeneously, but wheezing is mostly considered the hallmark symptom. The prevalence of wheezing at preschool age (<5 years) has increased immensely in the past 30 years, and up to a half of all preschool children have experienced wheezing before the age of six years. Preschool children with recurrent wheezing experience twice the rate of outpatient physician visits and emergency department visits and five times the rate of hospitalization as compared to preschool children without wheezing, with all the associated economic consequences.[2] However, only a third of the children with asthma symptoms at preschool age will eventually develop asthma at school age. A large proportion of preschool children have asthma symptoms that are transient over time, and they might therefore have unnecessary drug treatment with potential side effects. Concurrently, 20% of the children with asthma at school age are asymptomatic in early life.[3, 4] This emphasizes the importance of properly diagnosing asthma in preschool children. Despite the large burden and extensive presence of children with wheezing, the diagnosis of asthma in preschool children is a challenging endeavour and differs from the diagnosis in school-age children, adolescents, and adults for numerous reasons. Firstly, episodic respiratory symptoms such as wheezing and cough are commonly present in children without asthma, particularly in those who are 1–2 years old.[5, 6] In addition, the difficulties inherent in diagnosing asthma in older children and adults are magnified in preschool children. Diagnostic studies such as spirometry, bronchial challenge testing, and exhaled nitric oxide (FeNO) that are used to support the diagnosis of asthma are often not feasible in preschool children. Thus, when considering an asthma diagnosis in younger children, one must rely on many aspects of their present and past medical history, their demographic, behavioural and environmental history, and family history.[7, 8] Finally, the diagnosis of asthma in preschool children is difficult to make because there is no clear definition. Numerous classifications have been used for the manifestation of wheezing in preschool children, and this is frequently the source of confusion for clinicians, scientists, and the families of the patients we treat. We also lack clarity in a definition for asthma in preschool children because we understand very little about the underlying inflammatory and pathological processes in this age group, which is likely to be complex and multifactorial, and because no single test establishes the diagnosis. This chapter will accordingly use the term "asthma in preschool children" and describes the current understanding of the

DOI: 10.1201/9781003287209-8

diagnosis of asthma in preschool children, which is divided into main sections on the patient's history, physical examination, and testing options.

6.2 MEDICAL HISTORY

When considering an asthma diagnosis in preschool children, one must rely on many aspects of their presenting respiratory symptoms, demographic, behavioural and environmental history for risk factors, past medical history including signs of previous or concurrent allergy and eczema, and family history. Findings of physical examination and additional testing may additionally support a diagnosis, but differential diagnoses should be considered. In the following paragraphs, each topic is described in more detail.

6.2.1 Important Aspects of the History of Present Illness

A diagnosis of asthma in preschool children should be promptly considered if recurrent or persistent respiratory symptoms such as wheeze, cough, difficulty breathing, or shortness of breath occur.

Recurrent wheeze (more than one episode) is the most frequent presenting symptom that is associated with asthma in preschool children. Wheeze is a high-pitched noise coming from the chest and not the throat. Wheeze is also often present during viral respiratory tract infections and occur around six to eight times per year in preschool children, most frequently in children below the age of three years.[5, 9, 10] Additionally, respiratory tract infections are strongly associated with asthma, and particularly respiratory syncytial virus and rhinovirus are suggested to have a role in asthma development.[11, 12] Use of recurrent wheeze symptoms alone for diagnosing asthma in preschool children remains therefore difficult. However, a wheeze or other respiratory symptoms such as cough and shortness of breath that occur recurrently, during sleep, or with triggers such as activity, laughing, crying, or exposure to tobacco smoke or furred or feathered animals is suggestive for asthma. Since parents may confuse wheeze with upper airway congestion or noise, previous physician-documented wheeze is helpful in confirming the presence of true wheeze.[13, 14]

Several classification systems of preschool wheeze have been proposed, such as atopic versus non-atopic wheeze, episodic viral wheeze versus multiple-trigger wheeze, or mild and infrequent wheeze versus severe or frequent wheeze. None of these classification systems is universally accepted, given the limited evidence on which they are based, and therefore no consensus on the preferred terminology of wheeze exists.

Cough at preschool age is extremely common, particularly during viral respiratory tract infections, which resolves in 10 days for 50% and up to 25 days for 90% of children. More characteristic for an asthma symptom, the cough is recurrently and persistently present, apart from a viral respiratory tract illness, generally dry and non-productive and often will respond to bronchodilator therapy. A frequent nocturnal cough may be associated with a more severe disease. Triggering factors for cough in the context of asthma could be the same as for wheeze.[6, 15–17]

Difficulty of breathing or shortness of breath that occurs during exercise or activity increases the likelihood of the diagnosis of asthma in preschool children. Activity in infants and toddlers also include crying and laughing, which are equivalent to exercise in older children. To avoid these symptoms, children often abstain from playing or exercise, which may not be easily noticeable by parents or caregivers.[18]

The number of unscheduled visits to the primary physician, emergency or urgent care centre visits, and hospitalizations secondary to wheezing episodes can help determine the severity of the symptoms. Finally, a good response to a trial period of therapies, including inhaled bronchodilators and corticosteroids, is helpful in assessing the aetiology of respiratory symptoms because simple upper respiratory tract infections without associated bronchospasm will not improve with the use of inhaled therapy.[19]

6.2.2 Important Aspects of Demographic, Behavioural, and Environmental History

A history on risk factors for the development of asthma in preschool children focused on demographic, behavioural, and environmental factors should be obtained.

The most prominent **sociodemographic factors** are the child's sex and ethnicity and parental socio-economic factors. Boys tend to have an up to 3.2-fold higher risk of recurrent wheeze in the first years of life.[20–22] This seems to change around pubertal age where girls, and in later life adult women, have a higher risk of asthma.[23, 24] Children of Black descent or Hispanic and African American ethnicities, and of a household with a low socio-economic status, have higher risks of recurrent wheezing in the first three years of life.[7] The underlying biological pathways need to be elucidated.

Of all **behavioural factors**, exposure to tobacco smoke exposure remains the most important and consistent factor associated with an increased risk of wheezing in preschool children. Meta-analyses of birth cohort data from the 1990s onwards have shown that both maternal smoking during pregnancy and smoke exposure after birth are associated with a 24% increased risk of wheeze and in a dose-dependent way.[25, 26] Maternal psychological stress may also contribute to the development and severity of wheezing in children irrespective of other risk factors or those with a family history of asthma.[27] A large body of research has been performed on maternal dietary patterns and supplement use during pregnancy and the risk of recurrent wheezing in the first year of life. Potential beneficial effects of, for example, a Mediterranean or anti-inflammatory diet, intake of potentially allergenic food such as milk, peanuts, tree nuts, and/or fish, supplement the use of fish oil; vitamin D and vitamin E are not yet conclusive.

Exposure to **environmental factors** that may affect the risk of asthma in preschool children are respiratory infections, air pollution, season, and living conditions. Multiple studies have demonstrated that lower respiratory tract infections in the first years of life are associated with an increased risk of wheezing and asthma. Specifically, human rhino virus (HRV), respiratory syncytial virus (RSV), or bronchiolitis in the first years of life are associated with an up to 3.5-fold increased risk of recurrent wheezing in preschool children. Recent developments enable examination of the microbiome, that is, the full community of microorganisms in the human body, and propose that colonization of some airway or gut microbiota are associated with increased risk of wheezing in preschool children. Future studies are needed to better understand the microbial mechanisms involved, the possibility of bidirectional associations, and are thus not yet of clinical use. Multiple indoor and outdoor air pollutants and their relationship with later development of asthma in preschool children have been examined. A meta-analysis showed that exposure to gas cooking and indoor NO_2 are associated with a 1.15-fold increased risk of current wheeze in children.[28] Meta-analyses of birth cohorts observed no cross-sectional associations of $PM_{2.5}$ and NO_2 with asthma at the age of four years,[29] while others reported an association of NO_2, SO_2, and PM10 exposure during pregnancy with childhood wheeze.[30] Climate and living conditions show that severe wheezing is more prominent in winter periods and less prevalent if there is a residential proximity to green spaces.[31] Housing conditions may contain the presence of potential allergens such as dust mites and pets.[32] Early sensitization and exposure to an indoor aeroallergen such as dog or cat dander, dust mites, mould, or cockroach allergens are strong predictors of subsequent persistent asthma in preschool children with recurrent wheeze. Thus, information such as the types of family pets, both furred and feathered, whether the pets are indoor or outdoor, and whether they sleep in the child's bedroom should be ascertained. Additional questions should address dampness and presence of mould in the home. Sensitization to mould species such as *Aspergillus* and *Penicillium* has been shown to be associated with an asthma diagnosis.[33] A recent meta-analysis assessing the health effects of indoor dampness or mould exposure in 31,742 children from eight ongoing European birth cohorts revealed that a home environment with mould in early life is associated with an increased risk of asthma in young children and allergic rhinitis symptoms in school-age children.[34] Previous studies have also shown that children who are sensitized to house-dust mite allergens and to mould are more likely to have asthma as documented by bronchial hyperresponsiveness.[34]

6.2.3 Important Aspects of Medical History

The general medical history should include details about the mode of delivery, gestational age at birth, birth weight, weight status at preschool age, and history of past or current medical conditions that are relevant to asthma development.

Elective caesarean delivery has been associated with altered gut microbiome development in infants, which may impact immune system regulation and may contribute to the development of asthma.[35] The relative risk of asthma at preschool age and school age for term-born children born via elective caesarean delivery, compared to those born through vaginal delivery, was 1.17 and 1.49, respectively.[35, 36]

Earlier gestational age at birth has been associated with higher risks of preschool wheezing according to a meta-analysis of almost 147,252 children of 31 birth cohorts.[37] Almost all children born before a gestational age of 40.0 weeks had an increased risk of preschool wheezing, but those born before 28 weeks of gestation had the highest risk of preschool wheezing as compared to term-born children (odds ratio [OR] [95% CI]: 3.87 [2.70, 5.53]). Around 30% of children born preterm also develop prematurity-related lung disease/bronchopulmonary dysplasia, of whom some also have airway hyperresponsiveness, a characteristic feature of asthma.[38] Low birth weight is often related to increased risk of asthma in preschool children (OR,1.10) (1.00, 1.21), but inverse associations of birth weight with childhood asthma are often explained by gestational age at birth. Furthermore, most infants with a low birth weight show catch-up growth in infancy. Catch-up growth and increased infant weight gain, independent of birth weight, are associated with an increased risk of wheezing at preschool age and asthma at school age.[39–41] Weight status including overweight and obesity in preschool children are also linked to asthma. While a clear mechanism has not yet been established, studies suggest that this link is due to intrathoracic and abdominal visceral fat, which reduces pulmonary vital capacity, increased obstruction-related respiratory resistance, and immune modulation due to production of pro-inflammatory adipokines produced by adipose tissue or airway dysanapsis.[42–44]

Children in the general population with early transient and persistent eczema have increased risks for developing asthma,[45] and this condition is considered a major risk factor in predicting the likelihood of asthma.[46] Eczema, often also called atopic eczema or atopic dermatitis, usually presents under the age of two years and with a chronic itchy rash, which in preschool children is often located on the cheeks, forehead, and/or extensor side of limbs. A history of food allergy or early allergic sensitization to aeroallergens such as dust mites, cats, and dogs have been associated with an increased risk of recurrent wheezing in preschool children and increase the likelihood that a wheezing child will develop persistent asthma.[32, 47, 48] Symptoms of allergic rhinitis could be similar to those of an upper respiratory infection. Allergic rhinitis is usually defined as nasal symptoms that last longer than 14 days and that also occur when the child does not have a cold. Other classic symptoms of allergic rhinitis or hay fever are nasal congestion, nasal itch, rhinorrhoea, and sneezing.

The history of other medical conditions that might present with asthma symptoms but require different diagnostics and treatment should also be addressed (Table 6.1).

TABLE 6.1
Differential Diagnosis of Recurrent Wheezing

Upper Airway Conditions
Allergic rhinitis
Sinusitis
Adenoidal hypertrophy
Large Airway Conditions
Laryngotracheomalacia
Foreign body aspiration
Vascular rings, laryngeal webs
Tracheoesophageal fistula
Vocal cord paresis/paralysis
External mass compressing airway (e.g. tumour, enlarged lymph nodes, or congenital heart disease)
Vocal cord dysfunction (rare in young children)
Small Airway Conditions
Viral bronchiolitis (e.g. RSV and RV)
Bronchopulmonary dysplasia
Bronchiolitis obliterans
Diseases associated with bronchiectasis
Cystic fibrosis
Immune deficiency disorders
Child interstitial lung disease (cILD)
Alpha-1-antitrypsin deficiency
Primary ciliary dyskinesia
Congenital lung malformations
Other
Gastro-oesophageal reflux disease

6.2.4 Important Aspects of Family History

Family studies have shown that lung function is a heritable trait in 30–50% of individuals, and for asthma this rises to 75%.[49] Genetic origins of asthma on a population-based level are less clear. Genome-wide association studies (GWAS) have enabled examination of disease associations with millions of common genetic variants, known as single nucleotide polymorphisms (SNPs). Recent GWAS have identified many common genetic variants associated with asthma-related outcomes, including childhood onset asthma, adult asthma, impaired lung function, and atopy. Overall, current studies have identified >400 different genetic variants associated with asthma.[50] Functional interpretation of these polymorphisms has enabled the proposal of at least 160 possible drug targets for asthma. Several of these are already targeted by existing asthma drugs. However, these identified genetic variants explain only up to 10% of the variance of disease and are not used in clinical practice.

Epigenetic mechanisms, mitotically heritable changes to the DNA that do not affect the DNA sequence but may influence its function, could link the role of environmental exposures with the genetically unexplained heritability for asthma.[51] Indeed, some studies have shown that adverse exposures in foetal life, for example maternal smoking during pregnancy, may impact DNA methylation, gene expression, and subsequent respiratory development, predisposing individuals to obstructive airway diseases throughout the life course.[52–54]

6.3 PHYSICAL EXAMINATION

Several portions of the physical examination may support asthma in preschool children. Starting from head to toe, or in another order depending on the cooperation of the child, creases under the lower eyelids (Denny Morgan folds) and dark circles under the eyes ("allergic shiners") indicate an atopic constitution and are mostly related to atopic dermatitis. Typical findings consistent with allergic rhinitis are the allergic salute shown as wiping and/or rubbing the nose in an upwards or transverse manner with the fingers, palm, or back of the hand. Examination of the nose will often reveal oedema and rhinorrhoea and of the throat a postnasal drip, but these signs are difficult to differentiate allergic rhinitis from viral upper respiratory illnesses. When performing a lung examination on a child who appears well, the oxygen saturation, respiratory rate, inspiratory-to-expiratory phase ratio, and auscultation will likely be normal. As such, a normal lung examination during a time when a child is well does not rule in or rule out the diagnosis of asthma. During an acute episode, a lung examination will be most helpful. The documentation of retractions, hypoxia, tachypnoea, and/or predominantly expiratory wheezing is important in characterizing the symptoms and the severity of an episode. A skin examination is important in determining whether the child has any concomitant eczema, which could present with erythema, excoriations, thickening, or lichenification. In the preschool-age group, the distribution of eczema may include the face and the extensor regions as seen in infancy, or it may be transitioning to the flexor regions as seen in the older age groups.

6.4 TESTING OPTIONS

6.4.1 Laboratory and Imaging Tests in Preschool Children

For allergic sensitization testing in preschool children with wheeze, the most useful additional test is either a skin prick test or blood sampling to measure specific IgE to a panel of (aero)allergens to identify allergic sensitization. Although allergic sensitization is a strong predictor for asthma, absence of sensitization to common aeroallergens does not rule out a diagnosis of asthma in preschool children. For example, more than 50% of children with onset of wheezing and atopy in infancy did not have asthma at age 10, while up to 40% of those with onset of wheezing and recurrent infections in infancy did have asthma.[55]

Blood Eosinophilia Test: A result of higher peripheral blood eosinophilia of ≥4% has been suggested as a weak predictor for asthma in school-age children.[56] The optimal cut-off for elevated blood eosinophils to support the diagnosis of asthma in preschool children is unclear.[57] Furthermore, changes of blood eosinophils through the preschool period and the potential role of food allergy, allergic rhinitis, and/or eczema is not fully clear.

Imaging Test: Imaging is rarely needed in diagnosing asthma. However, in cases of uncertainty with wheezing or coughing in children, a chest X-ray may be useful to rule out other medical conditions, for example atelectasis or pneumothorax. Advanced imaging such as chest CT or chest MRI may be performed after referral to a specialist for evaluating severe or difficult-to-treat asthma or ruling out other diagnoses.

6.4.2 Lung Function Testing in Preschool Children

The assessment of lung function could support the diagnosis of asthma in children with suggestive respiratory symptoms. Lung function testing may provide valuable insight into the presence and severity of airway obstruction but could also be used for monitoring disease progression and guiding treatment strategies. The most common lung function test in children older than five years to support the diagnosis of asthma is spirometry with additional bronchodilator reversibility testing. Spirometry testing in preschool children is challenging due to their limited ability to perform adequate breathing manoeuvres. Despite this, several other lung function techniques have been developed for this specific age group but may only be present in specialized clinics with moderate success rates or need of sedation.[58]

6.4.2.1 Impulse Oscillometry

The most common technique is impulse oscillometry (IOS), a non-invasive technique that measures airway resistance and reactance during normal breathing. Impulse oscillometry evaluates the resistance in the large airways (R5) and the small airways (R20), providing insight in airway obstruction and its location, after exercise, bronchodilator administration, and bronchial provocation tests. In wheezing children, IOS often shows elevated resistance, especially in the small airways, indicating an obstruction that may worsen during exacerbations or with recurrent wheezing.

6.4.2.2 Forced Oscillometry Technique

Forced oscillometry technique (FOT) measures airway resistance but using different frequencies than IOS to assess how easily air moves through the lungs. In preschool-age children with wheezing, FOT typically shows higher baseline resistance, especially in the lower airways, indicating obstruction, and possibly less after bronchodilator therapy.

6.4.2.3 Resistance Interrupter Technique

Resistance interrupter technique (Rint) is a technique used to measure airway resistance through a brief interruption of the airflow during normal breathing. Children with wheezing typically have elevated resistance values, suggesting airway narrowing or obstruction.

6.4.2.4 Multiple Breath Washout

Multiple breath washout (MBW) is used to assess the distribution of the air in the lungs, where it tries to detect inhomogeneity in the airways. Children inhale an inert gas and during normal breathing, the exhaled volume of this gas is measured. When children need more breaths to "wash out" the gas from the lungs, as in preschool-age children with wheezing, this suggests an increased lung clearance index (LCI), indicating abnormal ventilation distribution, particularly in the smaller airways.

6.4.2.5 Plethysmography

During plethysmography, the patient sits in a sealed chamber and small changes in pressure are measured as they breathe through a mouthpiece. When the patient inhales, the lung volume increases, causing a slight decrease in pressure in the chamber, and the reverse happens when they exhale. These changes of pressure allow for the calculation of lung volumes and airway resistance (sRaw). In children with wheezing, plethysmography often shows increased specific airway resistance (sRaw), indicating that their airways are more constricted. This higher resistance makes it harder for air to flow into and out of the lungs, a typical sign of airway obstruction in asthma.

6.4.2.6 Fractional Concentration of Exhaled Nitric Oxide (FeNO)

The FeNO test measures airway inflammation by the level of nitric oxide in parts per billion (PPB) in exhaled air. Various methods such as the offline and online methods have been used to measure FeNO in preschool children. Sedation is often needed in young preschool children due to the lack of subject cooperation. The standard method with exhalation flows at 50 ml/sec is successful in preschool children aged 4–6 years.[59, 60] FeNO cannot be used to diagnose asthma in preschool children because the limited standardization of measuring FeNO and high variability in the cut-offs for FeNO in this age group.

6.4.2.7 Trial Therapy

When lung function techniques are not available or if the preschool child is not able to adequately perform such tests, inhaled short-acting beta-agonists (SABAs) as a reliever and consideration of inhaled corticosteroids as maintenance therapy, both with a spacer, could be offered for children under five years.[8, 19] For preschool children who present with frequent asthma-related symptoms (such as symptoms occurring three times a week or more, or waking them at night), an eight-week trial of a moderate dose of inhaled corticosteroids could be considered. This trial therapy aims to assess whether maintenance therapy is needed. After the eight-week trial, the inhaled corticosteroids treatment could potentially be stopped, but reoccurrence of symptoms should be carefully monitored thereafter. If symptoms did not improve during the trial, an alternative diagnosis should be considered.

6.5 PREDICTION AND DIAGNOSING ASTHMA IN PRESCHOOL CHILDREN

Numerous prediction tools have been developed with the aim to predict asthma at school age in preschool children, of which a few have been externally validated.[61] The proposed tools that explored numerous risk factors and attempted to improve existing models with novel risk factors or measurements have limited predictive accuracy, with large variation in sensitivity and specificity, and have limited generalizability.[62] Nevertheless, all these models consistently identified wheezing during preschool age, eczema during preschool age, allergic sensitization (specific IgE in blood, skin prick test), and a parental history of asthma as key risk factors for developing asthma. A diagnosis of asthma in preschool children is therefore currently largely based on present history of recurrent respiratory symptoms combined with a careful history on risk factors related to respiratory symptoms, past history, and family history, and physical findings alongside careful consideration of the differential diagnostic possibilities. A positive family history of allergic disorders or the presence of eczema or allergic sensitization provide additional predictive support, as early allergic sensitization increases the likelihood that a wheezing child will develop persistent asthma.[32]

6.6 DIFFERENTIAL DIAGNOSIS OF ASTHMA IN PRESCHOOL-AGE CHILDREN

When evaluating a preschool child with suspected asthma, one must rule out other respiratory diseases that present with suggestive respiratory symptoms. The differential diagnosis of recurrent suggestive respiratory symptoms is quite extensive, but it can be narrowed down based on a thorough history and physical examination (Table 6.1). Atypical wheezing (Table 6.2) accompanied by warning signs such as persistent symptoms from birth, a productive wet cough as the primary symptom, the absence of symptom-free periods, failure to thrive, or recurrent pneumonia may indicate other underlying conditions. These conditions could include, for example, tracheobronchomalacia, primary ciliary dyskinesia (PCD), cystic fibrosis (CF), protracted bacterial bronchitis, immune deficiency, tuberculosis (TB), vascular ring, congenital lung malformations, bronchopulmonary dysplasia (BPD), or foreign body aspiration. One should focus first on common conditions such as gastro-oesophageal reflux disease (GERD) and upper airway diseases such as rhinitis and sinusitis, unless the evaluation supports pursuing more rare etiologies based on warning signs (Table 6.2).

Gastro-oesophageal reflux disease (GERD) is commonly diagnosed in young preschool children. Preschool children do not complain of the classic symptoms of heartburn or abdominal pain but rather present with excess burping or emesis, coughing after meals, or nocturnal cough or wheeze.[63] A diagnosis can be clinically suspected and confirmed with a positive response to an empiric therapy. Alternatively, a pH/impedance probe to document increased or prolonged events of acid and non-acid stomach contents in the oesophagus or radiographic studies such as a tailored barium swallow/upper gastrointestinal (GI) series may be utilized before treatment is started. Asthma and GERD symptoms may coexist and a diagnosis of one or the other is not mutually exclusive. There are conflicting studies regarding whether the treatment of GERD results in improved asthma symptoms and a decreased need for asthma medication.[64, 65]

Chronic sinusitis or rhinitis with associated postnasal drip may contribute to persistent cough in the preschool child patient. Typically, patients have evidence of persistent nasal congestion or drainage in association with the cough. The cough is more likely to be wet and/or productive and is worse at night or early morning. This type of cough will not improve with bronchodilator or inhaled corticosteroid therapy but often improves with the treatment of the underlying condition. The treatment can be started empirically, but a sinus CT may also be useful if considering a prolonged antibiotic course.[66]

Tracheo (broncho)malacia is a common anatomical defect seen in young children. Children with tracheomalacia often present with recurrent episodes of stridor, wheeze, or barky cough, which are worsened by crying, and a concurrent respiratory infection.[67, 68] The respiratory symptoms often subside while sleeping, in contrast to asthma symptoms that often worsen at night. In many patients, the symptoms are present between episodes of infection, but mild cases may be symptomatic only with infection or vigorous crying. Treatment with a bronchodilator result in no change or even worsens the symptoms because it results in diminished airway tone in the presence of malacia. Glucocorticoids, both systemic and inhaled, are also ineffective. For most patients, the symptoms associated with tracheomalacia resolve by age two, but more severe malacia may provide persistent symptoms. A bronchoscopy is the examination of choice in the diagnosis and assessment of tracheomalacia.

An evaluation for **less common aetiologies**, including a tracheoesophageal fistula (TEF), a vascular ring, or an underlying connective tissue disorder, should be pursued for severe or persistent presentations. Mechanical airway compression due to **congenital cardiac anomalies** should be considered in a patient with recurrent respiratory symptoms that have failed to improve with bronchodilator or corticosteroid therapy. Anatomic compression is obviously a less common etiology for recurrent wheeze compared with asthma, but it is often unrecognized in this age group. Compression can occur due to vascular rings or slings (right sided or double aortic arch, anomalous innominate artery, or pulmonary artery sling) or due to an enlargement of the cardiac and/or pulmonary vasculature (dilated pulmonary arteries, left atrial enlargement, or massive cardiomegaly). A classic presentation includes recurrent respiratory difficulties with wheezing and stridor. Many children have associated dysphagia or apnoea. The symptoms are usually aggravated by crying and concurrent respiratory viral infections. The severity of the symptoms is dependent on the location and the degree of the anomaly. When this diagnosis is suspected, a chest X-ray should be obtained with close attention to the side of the aortic arch, the size and shape of the cardiac silhouette, and for the presence of tracheal deviation or constriction. Esophagrams are sometimes used to evaluate for vascular rings and slings but are nonspecific and may be normal despite the presence of an anomaly if that anomaly does not compress the oesophagus. Of note, bronchoscopy is not diagnostic; rather, chest magnetic resonance imaging (MRI) of the chest or CT is employed to confirm the diagnosis.[69] Finally, congestive heart failure in young children rarely presents with wheezing, but it may present with a history of increased work of breathing.

The rare H-type **TEF** may need to be considered in a patient with recurrent respiratory symptoms, especially recurrent pneumonia or persistent infiltrates on a chest radiograph. These patients will not respond to conventional therapies, including bronchodilators and glucocorticoids. Most patients with TEF have additional birth anomalies. This type of TEF may be difficult to demonstrate by conventional radiographic studies, but a high-resolution CT is often used for the diagnosis. Bronchoscopy may also be useful.[70]

In a preschool child patient with an acute onset of wheeze, cough, or both, **foreign body aspiration** must be considered. On physical examination, the wheezing will often be unilateral or localized. A forced expiratory chest radiograph may demonstrate air trapping behind the foreign body (FB), but a normal image does not rule out a foreign body. The diagnosis is confirmed by bronchoscopy and removal of the FB. Typically, patients present with acute respiratory symptoms, but chronic symptoms or a history of infiltrate or pneumonia that fails to clear can also be presenting symptoms of a foreign body.[71]

Patients with **cystic fibrosis (CF)** classically present with a history of recurrent respiratory symptoms in association with systemic symptoms of failure to thrive, diarrhoea, and recurrent sinus and ear infections. Additionally, many more mild variants of classic CF may not have associated systemic symptoms. Therefore, in patients with recurrent pneumonia or those that have failed to respond to conventional therapies, one should consider CF in the differential diagnosis even when the heel prick screening was normal.[72]

Immunodeficiency disorders presenting with recurrent wheeze, cough, or both without superimposed infections, diarrhoea, rash, or failure to thrive is quite rare. Immunodeficiency should not be considered in the initial differential diagnosis of a young child with only recurrent wheeze, cough, or both.

TABLE 6.2
Atypical Wheeze: Warning Signs and Need for Further Investigation or Referral

Persistent symptoms from birth or very early onset
Productive wet cough as a main symptom
Never completely symptom free
Failure to thrive
Recurrent pneumonia
Failure to respond to asthma medications
Symptoms without typical triggers
Focal lung or cardiovascular signs, finger clubbing, or hypoxemia

6.7 CASE EVALUATION

Reviewing on the case of Noa in the beginning of this chapter, the information in this chapter may have helped to answer the questions of the parents.

1. **Does Noa have asthma?** Based on Noa's history of recurrent wheezing triggered by colds and pollens, along with nocturnal cough and his father's history of childhood asthma, and sensitization to cat dander and pollens, it is likely that Noa has asthma.
2. **"If so, will he 'grow out of it' or could we cure it?"** Approximately two-thirds of preschool children with asthma may no longer have asthma symptoms at older ages. Noa has risk factors, e.g. allergic sensitization, that put him at risk for persistent asthma. There is no cure for asthma. Parents are strongly advised to stop smoking, and depending on severity of uncontrolled symptoms, despite a trial period with inhalers and anti-allergic medication, are advised to remove the cats.
3. **"Is it necessary to start daily treatment?"** Noa could be treated with a short-acting beta-agonist (SABA) such as albuterol, administered via an inhaler with a spacer, to relieve his symptoms. An eight-week trial of inhaled corticosteroids (ICS) as maintenance treatment is advised when wheezing is present more than three times a week or is waking him up at night.

REFERENCES

1. L. B. Bacharier et al. *Journal of Allergy and Clinical Immunology: In Practice* (2021). DOI: S2213-2198(21)00250-6 [pii]. https://doi.org/10.1016/j.jaip.2021.02.045
2. Lara J. Akinbami et al. *NCHS Data Brief* (2012). PMID: 22617340
3. Dilini M. Kothalawala et al. *Pediatric Allergy and Immunology: Official Publication of the European Society of Pediatric Allergy and Immunology* (2020). https://doi.org/10.1111/pai.13247 PMID: 32181536

4. M. I. Asher et al. *The European Respiratory Journal* (1995). https://doi.org/10.1183/09031936.95.08030483 PMID: 7789502
5. Christian Rosas-Salazar et al. *The Lancet* (2023). https://doi.org/10.1016/S0140-6736(23)00811–5
6. M. Thompson et al. *BMJ* (2013). https://doi.org/10.1136/bmj.f7027
7. Heidi Makrinioti et al. *European Respiratory Journal* (2024). https://doi.org/10.1183/13993003.00624-2024
8. Global Initiative for Asthma. *Global Strategy for Asthma Management and Prevention* (2024). Available from: www.ginasthma.org
9. Terho Heikkinen. *Asko Järvinen Lancet* (2003). https://doi.org/10.1016/S0140-6736(03)12162-9 PMID: 12517470
10. Evelien R. van Meel et al. *Thorax* (2018). https://doi.org/10.1136/thoraxjnl-2017-210149 PMID: 29101282
11. Terho Heikkinen. *Asko Järvinen Lancet* (2003). https://doi.org/10.1016/S0140-6736(03)12162–9 PMID: 12517470
12. Christian Rosas-Salazar et al. *The Lancet* (2023). https://doi.org/10.1016/S0140-6736(23)00811-5
13. R. S.Cane Archives of Disease in Childhood (2000). https://doi.org/10.1136/adc.82.4.327
14. Craig Mellis Pediatric Clinics of North America (2009). https://doi.org/10.1016/j.pcl.2008.10.003
15. Georgios Liangas et al. *Pediatric Pulmonology* (2003). https://doi.org/10.1002/ppul.10313 PMID: 12833489
16. M. Thompson et al. *BMJ* (2013). https://doi.org/10.1136/bmj.f7027
17. Lara J. Akinbami et al. *NCHS Data Brief* (2012). PMID: 22617340
18. David M. Lang et al. *Pediatrics* (2004). https://doi.org/10.1542/peds.113.4.e341
19. NIH. *Asthma: Diagnosis, Monitoring and Chronic Asthma Management* (2021). London: National Institute for Health and Care Excellence (NICE). PMID: 32755129
20. E. Melén et al. *Clinical & Experimental Allergy* (2004). https://doi.org/10.1111/j.1365-2222.2004.01957.x
21. Piush J. Mandhane et al. *American Journal of Respiratory and Critical Care Medicine* (2005). https://doi.org/10.1164/rccm.200412-1738OC PMID: 15805179
22. Alet Wijga et al. *The Journal of Allergy and Clinical Immunology* (2011). https://doi.org/10.1016/j.jaci.2010.09.022 PMID: 21094994
23. Bénédicte Leynaert et al. *Thorax* (2012). https://doi.org/10.1136/thoraxjnl-2011-201249 PMID: 22334535
24. T. Keller et al. *Allergy* (2018). https://doi.org/10.1111/all.13312 PMID: 28960325
25. Hannah Burke et al. *Pediatrics* (2012). https://doi.org/10.1542/peds.2011-2196 PMID: 22430451
26. Michela Silvestri et al. *Pediatric Pulmonology* (2015). https://doi.org/10.1002/ppul.23037 PMID: 24648197
27. Kim F. E. van de Loo et al. *The European Respiratory Journal* (2016). https://doi.org/10.1183/13993003.00299-2015 PMID: 26541526
28. Weiwei Lin et al. *International Journal of Epidemiology* (2013). https://doi.org/10.1093/ije/dyt150 PMID: 23962958
29. Elaine Fuertes et al. *Environment International* (2020). https://doi.org/10.1016/j.envint.2020.105474 PMID: 31962272
30. Zhang Hehua et al. *Environmental Research* (2017). https://doi.org/10.1016/j.envres.2017.08.038 PMID: 28888196
31. Christina Tischer et al. *The European Respiratory Journal* (2017). https://doi.org/10.1183/13993003.02112-2015 PMID: 28642307
32. Sabina Illi et al. *The Lancet* (2006). https://doi.org/10.1016/S0140-6736(06)69286-6
33. Richard A. Sharpe et al. *The Journal of Allergy and Clinical Immunology* (2015). https://doi.org/10.1016/j.jaci.2014.07.002 PMID: 25159468
34. C. G. Tischer et al. *Allergy* (2011). https://doi.org/10.1111/j.1398-9995.2011.02712.x PMID: 21923669
35. Franca Rusconi et al. *American Journal of Epidemiology* (2017). https://doi.org/10.1093/aje/kwx021
36. Maria C. Magnus et al. *American Journal of Epidemiology* (2011). https://doi.org/10.1093/aje/kwr242 PMID: 22038100
37. Agnes M.M. Sonnenschein-van Der Voort et al. *Journal of Allergy and Clinical Immunology* (2014). https://doi.org/10.1016/j.jaci.2013.12.1082
38. James T.D. Gibbons et al. *ERJ Open Research* (2023). https://doi.org/10.1183/23120541.00046-2023
39. Agnes M. M. Sonnenschein-van der Voort et al. *The Journal of Allergy and Clinical Immunology* (2014). https://doi.org/10.1016/j.jaci.2013.12.1082 PMID: 24529685
40. Agnes M. M. Sonnenschein-van der Voort et al. *American Journal of Respiratory and Critical Care Medicine* (2012). https://doi.org/10.1164/rccm.201107-1266OC PMID: 22268138
41. HermanT.denDekkeretal.*TheJournalofAllergyandClinical Immunology* (2016). https://doi.org/10.1016/j.jaci.2015.08.050 PMID: 26548843
42. Sara M. Mensink-Bout et al. *American Journal of Respiratory and Critical Care Medicine* (2020). https://doi.org/10.1164/rccm.201905-0942OC PMID: 31597047
43. Ubong Peters et al. Chest (2018). https://doi.org/10.1016/j.chest.2017.07.010
44. Herman T. Den Dekker et al. *Journal of Allergy and Clinical Immunology* (2017). https://doi.org/10.1016/j.jaci.2016.06.022
45. Chen Hu et al. *Clinical and Translational Allergy* (2020). https://doi.org/10.1186/s13601-020-0310-7
46. J. A. Castro-Rodríguez et al. *American Journal of Respiratory and Critical Care Medicine* (2000). https://doi.org/10.1164/ajrccm.162.4.9912111 PMID: 11029352
47. Susan V. Lynch et al. *Journal of Allergy and Clinical Immunology* (2014). https://doi.org/10.1016/j.jaci.2014.04.018
48. Peter D. Sly et al. *Lancet* (2008). https://doi.org/10.1016/S0140-6736(08)61451-8 PMID: 18805338
49. L. J. Palmer et al. *The European Respiratory Journal* (2001). https://doi.org/10.1183/09031936.01.17406960 PMID: 11401066
50. Zaid W. El-Husseini et al. *The Lancet. Respiratory Medicine* (2020). https://doi.org/10.1016/S2213-2600(20)30363-5 PMID: 32910899
51. Cancan Qi et al. *Expert Review of Clinical Immunology* (2019).https://doi.org/10.1080/1744666X.2020.1686977PMID: 31674254
52. Bonnie R. Joubert et al. *Nature Communications* (2016). https://doi.org/10.1038/ncomms10577 PMID: 26861414
53. Bonnie R. Joubert et al. *American Journal of Human Genetics* (2016). https://doi.org/10.1016/j.ajhg.2016.02.019 PMID: 27040690
54. Herman T. den Dekker et al. *The European Respiratory Journal* (2019). https://doi.org/10.1183/13993003.01795-2018 PMID: 30765504
55. Suzanne Y. Ngo et al. *Pediatric Allergy and Immunology: Official Publication of the European Society of Pediatric Allergy and Immunology* (2023). https://doi.org/10.1111/pai.13999 PMID: 37492911
56. Dong Hyeon Lee et al. *Clinical and Experimental Pediatrics* (2020). https://doi.org/10.3345/kjp.2019.00640 PMID: 32024332
57. Sylvia Hartl et al. *The European Respiratory Journal* (2020). https://doi.org/10.1183/13993003.01874-2019 PMID: 32060069

58. Heidi Makrinioti et al. *European Respiratory Journal* (2024). https://doi.org/10.1183/13993003.00624-2024
59. Samatha Sonnappa et al. *The Journal of Allergy and Clinical Immunology* (2010). https://doi.org/10.1016/j.jaci.2010.04.018 PMID: 20579717
60. L. Pekka Malmberg et al. *Pediatric Allergy and Immunology: Official Publication of the European Society of Pediatric Allergy and Immunology* (2009). https://doi.org/10.1111/j.1399-3038.2009.00858.x PMID: 19496956
61. Dilini M. Kothalawala et al. *Pediatric Allergy and Immunology: Official Publication of the European Society of Pediatric Allergy and Immunology* (2020). https://doi.org/10.1111/pai.13247 PMID: 32181536
62. Silvia Colicino et al. *Clinical and Experimental Allergy: Journal of the British Society for Allergy and Clinical Immunology* (2019). https://doi.org/10.1111/cea.13336 PMID: 30657220
63. Osvaldo Borrelli et al. *Journal of Pediatric Gastroenterology and Nutrition* (2011). https://doi.org/10.1097/MPG.0b013e318216e1ad PMID: 21865976
64. Toni O. Kiljander et al. *American Journal of Respiratory and Critical Care Medicine* (2010). https://doi.org/10.1164/rccm.200910-1537OC PMID: 20110554
65. Writing Committee for the American Lung Association Asthma Clinical Research Centers et al. *JAMA* (2012). https://doi.org/10.1001/jama.2011.2035 PMID: 22274684
66. Ellen R. *Wald Clinical Reviews in Allergy & Immunology* (2006). https://doi.org/10.1385/CRIAI:30:3:143 PMID: 16785586
67. Jayna Doshi, Marzena E. Krawiec. *The Journal of Allergy and Clinical Immunology* (2007). https://doi.org/10.1016/j.jaci.2007.09.048 PMID: 18073123
68. Ruben Boogaard et al. *Chest* (2005). https://doi.org/10.1378/chest.128.5.3391 PMID: 16304290
69. Clare A. McLaren et al. *Paediatric Respiratory Reviews* (2008). https://doi.org/10.1016/j.prrv.2007.12.008 PMID: 18513668
70. Waseem M. Hajjar et al. *Annals of Thoracic Medicine* (2012). https://doi.org/10.4103/1817-1737.91553 PMID: 22347352
71. Joe Saliba et al. *Journal of Otolaryngology—Head & Neck Surgery = Le Journal D'oto-Rhino-Laryngologie Et De Chirurgie Cervico-Faciale* (2012). PMID: 22762702
72. Cystic Fibrosis Genotype-Phenotype Consortium. *The New England Journal of Medicine* (1993). https://doi.org/10.1056/NEJM199310283291804 PMID: 8166795

7 Diagnosis of Asthma in Older Children and Adults

Anchalee Senavonge and Paul M. O'Byrne

7.1 INTRODUCTION

Asthma is a chronic inflammatory disease of the airways that is characterized by recurrent respiratory symptoms of dyspnoea, wheezing, chest tightness, and/or cough, and that is associated with variable airflow obstruction [1]. Another characteristic feature of asthma is airway hyperresponsiveness, identified by an exaggerated response of the airways to a variety of stimuli [2]. Asthma usually begins in childhood, although sometimes the initial symptoms begin much later in life. Establishing the diagnosis can often be straightforward, particularly in older children; but in preschool children and older adults, the diagnosis can be difficult because of the difficulty in obtaining objective evidence of variable airflow obstruction in younger children and because of the possible presence of other diseases, which can present with symptoms similar to asthma, in older adults.

CASE PRESENTATION

A 52-year-old man presented with a one-year history of shortness of breath on exertion, being limited to less than two flights of stairs, chronic cough that was generally non-productive and was most troublesome at night, and intermittent chest tightness. He denied any wheezing or chest pain. His symptoms were worsened when exposed to extremes of temperature. He was a previous smoker, having smoked 25 pack-years, but had stopped smoking four years before, at which time he had presented to the Emergence Department with an acute myocardial infarction, which was managed with coronary angioplasty. His current medications were a beta-blocker, a statin, and daily low-dose aspirin. He had no history of atopic disease, nor any relevant family history. He had been told he had episodes of "bronchitis" as a young child but remembers very little detail about these episodes.

Initial investigations included a CXR, which was normal; spirometry, which showed a forced expired volume in one second (FEV$_1$) and forced vital capacity (FVC) of 1.9 L/4.4 L (ratio 43%) with normal values of 3.9 L/4.7 L. After short-acting inhaled β_2-agonist (SABA) treatment, the values were 2.0 L/4.5 L, showing no acute reversibility in airflow obstruction. Skin prick testing to common environmental allergens showed a positive response to house dust mite and grass pollen. Blood tests included a complete blood count and electrolytes, which were normal (no increase in blood eosinophils), and his total immunoglobulin E (IgE) was slightly elevated at 230. Thus, the patient presented with severe airflow obstruction and a long previous smoking history, atopy, and a history in childhood consistent with mild asthma.

A decision was made to begin treatment with a course of oral glucocorticoids (prednisolone 50 mg/day) for three weeks and a combination inhaler containing an inhaled corticosteroid (ICS), and a long-acting inhaled β_2-agonist (LABA) administered twice daily. At his return clinic visit, his symptoms had markedly improved; his cough was no longer troublesome at night, and his spirometry demonstrated values of 3.0 L/4.6 L (a 58% improvement in FEV$_1$). The diagnosis was established as asthma but with residual airflow obstruction, possibly related to his history of cigarette abuse. The prednisolone was discontinued, he was switched from a beta-blocker to an angiotensin receptor antagonist, and the combination inhaler was continued. He was left on low-dose aspirin, as he had no history of worsening symptoms with taking this medication. At the next follow-up visit, three months later, he remained largely symptom free, and his spirometry values were 2.9 L/4.4 L.

This case demonstrates a patient who was suspected of having chronic obstructive pulmonary disease (COPD) because of his long smoking history and who had no acute reversibility after inhaled β_2-agonists, but who demonstrated largely reversible airflow obstruction after treatment with glucocorticoids, confirming a diagnosis of asthma.

DOI: 10.1201/9781003287209-9

7.1.1 Role of Medical History in Establishing a Diagnosis

Patients with asthma seek medical attention because of respiratory symptoms. A cardinal feature of asthma symptoms is their variability. These symptoms are wheezing, chest tightness, episodic shortness of breath, and/or cough [1]. Importantly, none of these symptoms is diagnostic of asthma because similar symptoms can be present with other respiratory or even cardiac diseases (Table 7.1). It is important to elicit whether the symptoms are triggered or worsened by factors such as exercise, exposure to allergens, viral infections, and emotions, which would suggest a diagnosis of asthma. In some asthmatics (particularly children), wheezing and chest tightness are absent, and the only symptom the patient complains of is chronic cough. This has been labelled "cough-variant asthma" [3]; however, this terminology is not often used now, as with a careful history, other symptoms consistent with asthma are often elicited. Since the symptoms of asthma are nonspecific, the differential diagnosis is quite extensive, and the main goal for the physician is to consider and exclude other possible diagnoses (Table 7.1). The lack of specificity of the symptoms of asthma make it essential that the diagnosis is made demonstrating variable airflow obstruction, using objective measures of airflow obstruction.

Asthma clusters in families, and its genetic determinants appear to be linked to those of other allergic IgE-mediated diseases [4]. Thus, a personal or family history of asthma and/or allergic rhinitis, atopic dermatitis, or eczema increases the likelihood of a diagnosis of asthma.

Physical activity is an important cause of symptoms for most asthma patients, particularly in children, and for some it is the only cause. Exercise-induced bronchoconstriction does not usually develop during exercise, but 5–10 minutes afterward, and it resolves spontaneously within 30–45 minutes [5]. Prompt relief of symptoms after the use of inhaled β_2-agonist, or their prevention by pre-treatment with an inhaled β_2-agonist before exercise, supports a diagnosis of asthma.

Important aspects of personal history are exposure to agents known to worsen asthma in the home, such as dusty environments, forced air heating system, or exposure to allergens (e.g. pets or house dust mites, cockroaches) to which the patient is sensitized; workplace conditions, environmental tobacco smoke, or even the general environment (e.g. fumes from traffic).

In adult patients, a careful occupational history is essential to decide whether a possible workplace sensitizer is responsible for the onset of asthma. Several hundred different agents have been recognized as causing occupational asthma [6], only some of which are classical allergens, causing asthma through IgE-dependent mechanisms.

TABLE 7.1
Differential Diagnosis of Asthma

Pulmonary	COPD
	Sarcoidosis
	Eosinophilic bronchitis
	Pulmonary eosinophilia
	Cystic fibrosis
	Bronchiectasis
Neoplastic	Lung cancer
	Endobronchial tumours
	Lymphoma with hilar adenopathy
Cardiovascular	Left ventricular failure
	Pulmonary embolism
Other pathologies	Gastro-oesophageal reflux/aspiration
	Inhaled foreign body
	Vocal cord dysfunction
	Medication (e.g. ACE inhibitors)

7.1.2 Physical Examination

In mild asthma, the physical examination is usually not helpful, as it is normal under stable conditions but becomes characteristically abnormal during asthma exacerbations. Typical physical signs during an asthma exacerbation are wheezing on auscultation, cough, and signs of acute hyperinflation (e.g. poor diaphragmatic excursion at percussion, use of accessory muscles of respiration). In some asthmatics, wheezing may be detectable only on forced expiration or even be absent in the presence of very severe airflow obstruction. In these patients, however, the severity of asthma is mostly indicated by other signs, such as cyanosis, drowsiness, difficulty in speaking, tachycardia, hyperinflated chest, use of accessory muscles, and intercostal recession.

7.1.3 Lung Function Tests

While respiratory symptoms suggest asthma, the *sine qua non* for the diagnosis of asthma is the presence of reversible airflow obstruction, and/or airway hyperresponsiveness, or increased PEF variability, in subjects without airways obstruction [1].

7.1.3.1 Spirometry

Lung function tests play a critical role in both the diagnosis and follow-up of patients with asthma. Spirometric measurements, the forced expired volume in one second (FEV_1) and slow vital capacity (VC) or forced vital capacity (FVC), are the standard means for assessing airflow limitation (Figure 7.1). The FEV_1, the FVC, and the ratio of these two numbers are the measurements most widely used to document airflow obstruction. This is because these are the most reliable (reproducible and responsive) of all the measurements of lung function. Guidelines have been published by the American Thoracic Society and European Respiratory Society on the standardization of the measurement of spirometry and its interpretation [7]. The measurements, however, are mainly a reflection of larger airways obstruction.

Other measurements that can be obtained from a spirogram include flows at lower lung volumes, such as the FEF_{25-75}, which may better reflect smaller airways obstruction; however, these measurements are much less reliable than the FEV_1 and are not often used clinically for this reason. In addition, almost all studies that have related lung function measurements to other clinical outcomes, morbidity, quality of life, or even mortality in patients with airflow obstruction have used the FEV_1 as the reference measurement. Spirometry is recommended at the time of initial diagnosis and for the assessment of the severity of asthma [1]. It should be repeated to monitor the disease and when there is a need for reassessment, such as during exacerbations. Spirometry can usually be performed reliably in children as young as seven years and sometimes even younger [7].

Airflow limitation is usually defined by the reduction of post-bronchodilator FEV_1/FVC ratio <0.7. However, because this parameter decreases with aging, it should be confirmed by post-bronchodilator FEV_1/VC values below the lower limit of age-corrected normal values. Other pulmonary function measurements, such as measurements of lung volumes and gas transfer capacity, may be useful in determining the degree of hyperinflation and/or enlargement of airspaces, and these may help in the differential diagnosis with COPD but are not necessary for the diagnosis or for assessment of severity of asthma.

7.1.3.2 Peak Expiratory Flow (PEF)

If spirometry does not reveal airflow limitation at the time of the initial assessment of the patient, then home monitoring of PEF for two weeks may help to detect an increased variability of airway calibre and assist in making the diagnosis of asthma [8]. Daily monitoring of PEF (at a minimum in the morning upon awakening and in the evening hours, preferably both before and after bronchodilator inhalation) is also useful to assess the severity of asthma and its response to treatment, and it can help patients to detect early signs of asthma deterioration. Diurnal variability is calculated as follows:

$$\frac{PEF_{max} - PEF_{min}}{(PEF_{max} + PEF_{min})/2} \times 100$$

A diurnal variability of PEF of more than 20% is diagnostic of asthma, and the magnitude of the variability is broadly proportional to disease severity [9]. PEF monitoring may be of use not only in establishing a diagnosis of asthma and assessing its severity but also in uncovering an occupational cause for asthma [6]. When used in this way, PEF should be measured more frequently than twice daily, and special attention should be paid to changes occurring in and out of the workplace.

7.1.3.3 Reversibility to Bronchodilators

As already discussed, the demonstration of reversible airflow obstruction is required for a diagnosis of asthma and

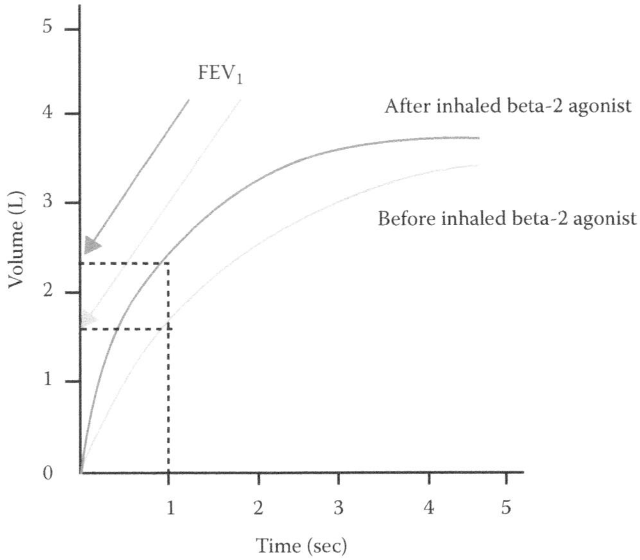

FIGURE 7.1 Measurements of FEV_1 before and 10 minutes after an inhaled β_2-agonist in an asthmatic patient. The FEV_1 value was 1.7 L before and 2.3 L after the inhaled β_2-agonist. This reversibility is consistent with a diagnosis of asthma.

a single demonstration of reversibility, defined as >12% reversibility and >200 mL in FEV_1 after bronchodilator can establish the diagnosis [1, 10] (Figure 7.1). However, reversibility is often not present, particularly in patients on treatment, and thus the absence of reversibility does not exclude the diagnosis. Repeated testing of reversibility of both clinical features and functional abnormalities may be useful in obtaining the best level of asthma control achievable and/or the best lung function for individual patients. Achieving and maintaining lung function at the best possible level is one of the objectives of asthma management [1].

7.1.3.4 Airway Hyperresponsiveness

Airway hyperresponsiveness consists of an increased sensitivity of the airways to constrictor agonists, as indicated by a smaller concentration of a constrictor agonist needed to initiate the bronchoconstrictor response, a steeper slope of the dose–response curve, and a greater maximal response to the agonist [2] (Figure 7.2). In asthmatic subjects, airway hyperresponsiveness is present to many chemical or physical stimuli, such as inhaled histamine [11] or the inhaled cholinergic agonist methacholine [12], as well as physical stimuli such as exercise [13], hyperventilation of cold dry air [14], and both hypotonic and hypertonic solutions, such as mannitol [15].

Methacholine inhalation challenge is the most widely used test to document airway hyperresponsiveness, and an abnormal methacholine challenge test can be demonstrated in almost all patients with current symptomatic asthma [2]. However, defining an exact level of airway responsiveness, which would distinguish asthmatic subjects from non-asthmatic subjects, is not possible because of a continuous distribution of airway responsiveness in the general

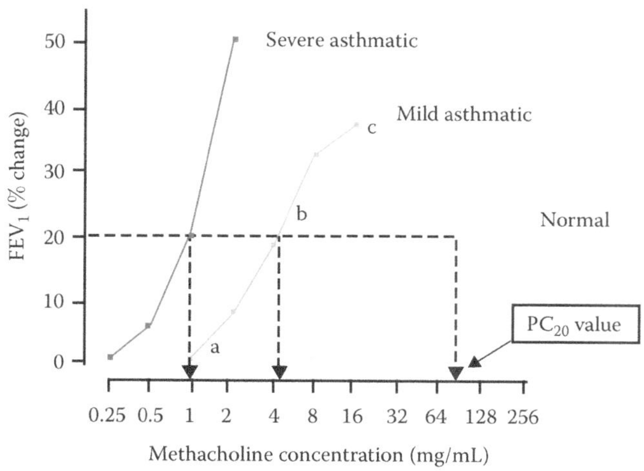

FIGURE 7.2 Dose–response curves obtained during inhalation challenges with methacholine in a severe asthmatic, a mild asthmatic, and a normal subject. The response to increasing inhaled doses of methacholine is measured by change in FEV_1 from baseline. Asthmatics have (a) a lower threshold (increased sensitivity); (b) a steeper slope of the dose–response curve (increased reactivity); (c) a greater maximal response to inhaled methacholine. The response is expressed as the provocative concentration of methacholine causing a 20% fall in FEV_1 (PC_{20}).

population, with asthmatic subjects in one tail of this distribution. In addition, even subjects with normal methacholine airway responsiveness can develop symptomatic asthma if exposed to specific stimuli to which they are sensitized, such as inhaled allergen [16]. The severity of airway hyperresponsiveness correlates with the severity of asthma, as determined by the amount of treatment needed to control asthma [12], with variability in PEF [17], and improvement in FEV_1 after inhaled bronchodilator [17].

Other challenge tests used clinically to document airway hyperresponsiveness include inhaled mannitol [18], exercise [13], and eucapnic voluntary hyperpnea [13], which are considered an "indirect" challenge procedure, causing bronchoconstriction by releasing bronchoconstrictor mediators from inflammatory cells in the airways.

Measurements of airway hyperresponsiveness are particularly useful in patients with normal airway calibre in whom a diagnosis of asthma is being considered; however, they are not useful in the presence of irreversible airflow limitation, thereby aiding in the differential diagnosis between asthma and COPD. Another important application of measuring airway responsiveness is the diagnosis of occupational asthma [6]. Lastly, measurement of airway responsiveness may be useful in determining the optimal treatment requirements in asthma [19].

7.1.4 Allergy Tests

The presence of allergic disorders in a patient's family history should be investigated in all patients with symptoms of asthma. A history provides important information about the patient's lifestyle and occupation, both of which influence exposure to allergens and the time, and factors possibly involved in onset and in exacerbations of asthma [20]. Skin tests with all relevant allergens present in the geographic area in which the patient lives are the primary diagnostic tool in determining allergic status. The main limitation of methods to assess allergic status is that a positive test does not necessarily mean that the disease is allergic in nature or that it is causing asthma, as some individuals have specific IgE antibodies without any symptoms, and it may not be causally involved. The relevant exposure and its relation to symptoms must be confirmed by patient history. Allergy tests should be considered especially in patients with complicated asthma, difficult to control or treat asthma, or those being considered for allergen immunotherapy (AIT), anti-IgE, or other biologic therapy.

7.2 ADDITIONAL TESTS

While the diagnosis and assessment of the severity of asthma can be fully established based on clinical history and lung function tests, additional tests are sometimes helpful to better characterize individual patients.

7.2.1 Imaging

While chest radiography may be useful to exclude diseases that may mimic asthma (Table 7.1), it is not required in the confirmation of the diagnosis of asthma. The utility of chest radiography is to exclude other conditions that may imitate or complicate asthma. Examples include pneumonia, cardiogenic pulmonary edema, pulmonary thromboembolism, tumours (especially those that result in airway obstruction with resulting peripheral atelectasis), and pneumothorax.

7.2.2 Assessment of Airway Inflammation

While airway biopsies and bronchoalveolar lavage may provide useful information in research protocols, they are considered too invasive for the diagnosis or staging of asthma. In contrast, non-invasive markers of airway inflammation have been increasingly used, particularly to differentiate asthma from COPD and to measure response to treatment. These non-invasive measurements include induced sputum and exhaled nitric oxide (FeNO). Induced sputum is not helpful in the diagnosis of asthma but can be very useful in the management of severe asthma [21]. In particular, induced sputum helps identify the persistence of airway eosinophilia or airway neutrophilia in patients with difficult-to-treat asthma, which can be useful in deciding on treatment strategies, particularly in the use of asthma biologics to reduce the risks of severe asthma exacerbations [22]. FeNO is increased in atopic asthma but less so in non-atopic asthma. A normal level of FeNO in a patient not using ICS may be helpful in excluding an asthma diagnosis [23]. FeNO measurements can also be helpful in monitoring adherence to inhaled corticosteroids [24], as it

TABLE 7.2
History, Symptoms, and Results of Pulmonary Function Tests in the Differential Diagnosis Between Asthma, ACO, and COPD

	Asthma	Asthma-COPD Overlap (ACO)	COPD
Onset	Often in childhood ≤ 20-year-old	Usually before 40 years old	Mid to late adult life ≥40-year-old
Smoking	Often non-smokers	Usually have history of smoking	Usually smokers
Daily cough and sputum	Often absent	Frequent	Frequent (chronic bronchitis)
Dyspnoea on effort	Variable and reversible to treatment	Constant in severe ACO	Constant, poorly reversible, and progressive
Nocturnal symptoms	Relatively common	Can occur	Relatively uncommon
Time course	Often improve with treatment or spontaneously	Partly improve with treatment	Slowly progressive over years
Airflow diurnal variability	Increased diurnal variability	n/a	Normal diurnal variability
Response to bronchodilator (FEV_1 ≥ 12% or ≥200 ml over baseline)	Good reversibility	Good reversibility	Poor reversibility
Airflow limitation Post-bronchodilator FEV_1/FVC <0.7	Usually not present (Variable airflow limitation)	Usually present (Persistent airflow limitation)	Present (Persistent airflow limitation)
FEV_1	≥80% good asthma control <80% poor asthma control	≥80% mild <80% severe	≥80% mild airflow limitation <80% severe airflow limitation
Lung function between symptoms	Usually normal	Frequently abnormal	Abnormal

is effectively reduced by inhaled corticosteroids but not by bronchodilators.

7.3 DIFFERENTIATING BETWEEN ASTHMA AND COPD

In adult patients, the most difficult diagnostic issue in patients with airflow obstruction, in past or current smokers, is differentiating between asthma and COPD. In most patients, the clinical presentation and the history provide the strongest diagnostic criteria to distinguish these conditions (Table 7.2). Results of pulmonary function tests, particularly spirometric measurements that show a nearly complete reversibility of airflow limitation, will confirm a diagnosis of asthma, and measurements that show poorly reversible airflow limitation may help to confirm the diagnosis of COPD (Table 7.2). Differential diagnosis between asthma and COPD becomes more difficult in elderly patients, in whom some features may overlap, such as smoking and atopy, and when the patient has airflow limitation that is poorly reversible after treatment. In these cases, symptoms, lung function, airway responsiveness, imaging, and even pathological findings may overlap and thus may not provide solid information to establish the diagnosis.

Asthma-COPD overlap (ACO) are those patients who have persistent airflow limitation together with clinical features that are consistent with both asthma and COPD [25]. The prevalence of asthma-COPD overlap is reported to range between 9% and 55%. The definition of ACO is not clear-cut, practically described as COPD patients with reversible lung function and/or aging asthmatic patients with incomplete reversible airway obstruction. Clinical characteristics and laboratory differentiating between asthma, ACO, and COPD are shown in Table 7.2 and Table 7.3.

Because an accurate diagnosis is needed to provide better treatment, it is important in these patients to undertake an individual approach and to perform additional tests. Reversibility to glucocorticoids alone or in combination with long-acting bronchodilators, measurements of lung volumes and diffusion capacity, analysis of sputum and FeNO, and imaging of the chest may demonstrate whether asthma or COPD is the predominant cause of airflow limitation (Table 7.3).

7.4 CONCLUSIONS

The diagnosis of asthma in older children and adults is made by the presence of symptoms consistent with asthma and the demonstration of variable airflow obstruction. The presence of the characteristic symptoms alone is not sufficient for an accurate diagnosis, as these are not specific for asthma. Variable airflow obstruction is usually documented by demonstrating changes in spirometry, particularly the FEV_1 and VC and the ratio of these numbers. The currently accepted definition of an improvement in FEV_1 that is consistent with asthma is >12% and >200 mL (most relevant when the FEV_1

TABLE 7.3
Ancillary Tests in the Differential Diagnosis Between Stable Asthma, ACOS, and COPD

Ancillary Test	Asthma	Asthma-COPD Overlap (ACO)	COPD
Airway hyperresponsiveness (AHR)	Increase in most patients, with or without airflow limitation	Increased if possible to measure	Usually not measurable due to airflow limitation
Lung volumes, residual volume, total lung capacity	Usually normal or, if increased, reversible	Usually irreversibly increased	Usually irreversibly increased
Diffusion capacity	Normal	Often decreased	Decreased
Allergy tests	Often positive	Often positive	Often negative
Imaging of the chest	Usually normal	Usually abnormal: hyperinflation	Usually abnormal: hyperinflation
Airway inflammation	Eosinophils and/or neutrophils	Eosinophils and/or neutrophils	Neutrophils ± eosinophils in sputum, lymphocytes in airways
Sputum	Eosinophilia	Eosinophilia	Neutrophilia
Exhaled NO	Increased	Increased	Usually normal Low in current smokers

is less than 1 L). This is often demonstrated within 10–30 minutes after the inhalation of a β_2-agonist, such as salbutamol. In some instances, however, the improvement in FEV_1 is only demonstrated after a more prolonged period of treatment with inhaled or oral glucocorticoids (as in the case presentation). In patients with mild asthma, or those on effective treatment, spirometry can be normal. In these situations, measurements of PEF over several weeks or the documentation of airway hyperresponsiveness to inhaled chemical mediators, such as methacholine or bronchoconstriction after exercise or inhaled mannitol, can establish the diagnosis.

Making the diagnosis of asthma can be challenging in patients (particularly younger children) who cannot reproducibly perform spirometry, and in adults with a smoking history and in whom there is fixed airflow obstruction (not reversible even after optimal treatment has been administered for a period of time). The presence of fixed airflow obstruction suggests a diagnosis of COPD, but this should be confirmed with ancillary testing, which may include measurements of lung volumes, diffusing capacity, and chest imaging. Measurements of inflammatory cells in blood or sputum or of FeNO are often not helpful in differentiating between asthma and COPD.

Making a diagnosis of asthma correctly is an essential step prior to the development of an asthma management plan. Unfortunately, this step is sometimes not completed, because either the managing healthcare professional is convinced by the history or the ability to document variable airflow obstruction is not readily available. This lack of precision in making the diagnosis is a common cause of patients being referred for specialist assessment because the asthma treatment recommended is ineffective.

REFERENCES

1. Global Initiative for Asthma: Global Strategy for Asthma Management and Prevention. 2023. www.ginasthma.org.
2. Nair, P., et al., Airway hyperresponsiveness in asthma: measurement and clinical relevance. *J Allergy Clin Immunol Pract* 2017; **5**:649–59.
3. Irwin, R.S., et al., Classification of cough as a symptom in adults and management algorithms: CHEST guideline and expert panel report. *Chest* 2018; **153**:196–209.
4. Bousquet, J., et al., Allergic Rhinitis and its Impact on Asthma (ARIA) Phase 4: Change management in allergic rhinitis and asthma multimorbidity using mobile technology. *J Allergy Clin Immunol* 2019; **143**:864–79.
5. Carlsen, K.H., et al., Exercise-induced asthma, respiratory and allergic disorders in elite athletes: epidemiology, mechanisms and diagnosis: part I of the report from the Joint Task Force of the European Respiratory Society (ERS) and the European Academy of Allergy and Clinical Immunology (EAACI) in cooperation with GA2LEN. *Allergy* 2008; **63**:387–403.
6. Tarlo, S.M. and C. Lemiere, Occupational asthma. *N Engl J Med* 2014; **370**:640–9.
7. Bhakta, N.R., et al., European respiratory society/American thoracic society technical statement: standardisation of the measurement of lung volumes, 2023 update. *Eur Respir J* 2023; **62**. https://doi.org/10.1183/13993003.01519-2022.
8. Reddel, H.K., G.B. Marks, and C.R. Jenkins, When can personal best peak flow be determined for asthma action plans? *Thorax* 2004; **59**:922–4.
9. Reddel, H.K., et al., Standardization of ambulatory peak flow monitoring: the importance of recent beta2-agonist inhalation. *Eur Respir J* 1998; **12**:9–14.
10. British Thoracic Society and Scottish Intercollegiate Guidelines Network. *British guideline on the management of asthma: a national clinical guideline*. British Thoracic Society and Scottish Intercollegiate Guidelines Network, 2019.
11. Cockcroft, D.W., et al., Bronchial reactivity to inhaled histamine: a method and clinical survey. *Clin. Allergy* 1977; **7**:235–43.
12. Juniper, E.F., P.A. Frith, and F.E. Hargreave, Airway responsiveness to histamine and methacholine: relationship to minimum treatment to control symptoms of asthma. *Thorax* 1981; **36**:575–9.
13. Anderson, S.D., Provocative challenges to help diagnose and monitor asthma: exercise, methacholine, adenosine, and mannitol. *Curr Opin Pulm Med* 2008; **14**:39–45.

14. O'Byrne, P.M., et al., Asthma induced by cold air and its relation to nonspecific bronchial responsiveness to methacholine. *Am Rev Respir Dis* 1982; **125**: 281–5.
15. Anderson, S.D., et al., Comparison of mannitol and methacholine to predict exercise-induced bronchoconstriction and a clinical diagnosis of asthma. *Respir Res* 2009; **10**:4–12.
16. Gauvreau, G.M., et al., Allergen provocation tests in respiratory research: building on 50 years of experience. *Eur Respir J* 2022; **60**. https://doi.org/10.1183/13993003.02782-2021.
17. Ryan, G., et al., Bronchial responsiveness to histamine: relationship to diurnal variation of peak flow rate, improvement after bronchodilator, and airway calibre. *Thorax* 1982; **37**:423–9.
18. Brannan, J.D., et al., The safety and efficacy of inhaled dry powder mannitol as a bronchial provocation test for airway hyperresponsiveness: a phase 3 comparison study with hypertonic (4.5%) saline. *Respir Res* 2005; **6**:144–52.
19. Sont, J.K., et al., Clinical control and histopathologic outcome of asthma when using airway hyperresponsiveness as an additional guide to long-term treatment. The AMPUL study group. *Am J Respir Crit Care Med* 1999; **159**:1043–51.
20. Bousquet, J., et al., The Allergic Rhinitis and Its Impact on Asthma (ARIA) approach of value-added medicines: as-needed treatment in allergic rhinitis. *J Allergy Clin Immunol Pract* 2022; **10**:2878–88.
21. Hargreave, F.E., Quantitative sputum cell counts as a marker of airway inflammation in clinical practice. *Curr Opin Allergy Clin Immunol* 2007; **7**: 102–6.
22. Brusselle, G.G. and G.H. Koppelman, Biologic therapies for severe asthma. *N Engl J Med* 2022; **386**:157–71.
23. Pedrosa, M., et al., Usefulness of exhaled nitric oxide for diagnosing asthma. *J Asthma* 2010; **47**:17–21.
24. Aung, H.W.W., et al., Assessing Inhaled corticosteroid adherence and responsiveness in severe asthma using beclometasone dipropionate/formoterol NEXThaler dose-counting and nitric oxide monitoring. *J Allergy Clin Immunol Pract* 2024; **12**:1539–46.
25. Postma, D.S. and K.F. Rabe, The Asthma-COPD overlap syndrome. *N Engl J Med* 2015; **373**:1241–9.

8 United Airways

Managing Patients with Allergic Rhinitis and Asthma

Glenis K. Scadding and Guy Scadding

CASE PRESENTATION

Stephen is 10 years old. He loves to play football. He suffers from hay fever in the summer, for which he takes an occasional antihistamine, but he still has an itchy, runny nose that blocks up and red, sore eyes. He often wheezes on running and is supposed to use salbutamol for this, but he usually forgets to take it. His legs become red and itchy when he walks through long grass.

One summer evening, Stephen is playing football in the park despite having a slight cold. He becomes wheezy, but he has no salbutamol, so he tries to play on. His asthma becomes much worse, and he collapses, almost unable to breathe. Fortunately, his friend gives him his own salbutamol and calls for an emergency ambulance on his cell phone, and Stephen is saved after rapid transfer to a nearby hospital.

Why Did Stephen Have Such a Bad Asthma Attack? Is This Unusual?

There are multiple potential causative factors (1):

- *Rhinitis that is uncontrolled.*
- *Exposure to a high allergen load . . .*
- *. . . at multiple sites—nose, eyes, chest, and skin.*
- *Undertreated asthma.*
- *Exercise.*
- *Intercurrent viral infection.*
- *Food-related, exercise-induced anaphylaxis. (This was discounted in Stephen's case, as he had not eaten for several hours prior to the attack.)*

Seasonal asthma exacerbations, which can be severe, are not uncommon. Unfortunately, asthma deaths include a proportion of people like Stephen whose asthma has previously been mild and largely ignored. This chapter explores the links between rhinitis and asthma.

Table 8.1 shows evidence for an association between rhinitis and asthma and the postulated mechanisms of their interaction.

As the majority of the literature related to rhinitis and asthma focuses on the allergic phenotype, the term "rhinitis" used in this chapter refers to "allergic rhinitis" unless stated otherwise.

8.1 ALLERGIC RHINITIS

Hay fever (seasonal allergic rhinitis [SAR] is a form of rhinitis that is frequently undiagnosed and undertreated) (2, 3). Seasonal allergen triggers vary geographically around the world, with grass pollen being the most common trigger in the United Kingdom. The highest grass pollen levels in the United Kingdom are at the end of June (early summer). As the air cools in the evening, pollen descends, and the levels inspired can be very high, particularly when exercising. Rhinitis is defined by the presence of two or more of the following nasal symptoms: rhinorrhoea, congestion, itching, and sneezing. It can be allergic, nonallergic, infective, or a combination of these (4). In children, allergy accounts for the majority of rhinitis cases, while in adults, allergy causes approximately one-third of cases. It is estimated that 25% of young people in the United Kingdom have rhinitis, which is similar to the prevalence of allergic rhinitis in other westernized countries.

Allergic rhinitis is associated with a biphasic immunologic response to an allergen, similar to that seen in allergic asthma. An early-phase reaction occurs almost immediately after an allergen exposure due to immunoglobulin E (IgE)-mediated mast cell degranulation and the release of chemical mediators such as histamine, leukotrienes, and prostaglandins. The late-phase reaction occurs several hours later, lasting for 12–24 hours and is associated with the activation of T cells and the recruitment, activation, and prolonged survival of eosinophils in the nasal mucosa (5). The resulting immediate symptoms in the nose are itching, sneezing, and rhinorrhoea. The late phase gives rise to nasal obstruction, a reduced sense of smell, and general hyperreactivity, which can extend throughout the respiratory tract (6, 7).

Asthma tends to be more severe in patients with perennial allergic rhinitis (8). Allergic-rhinitis-induced bronchial

DOI: 10.1201/9781003287209-10

TABLE 8.1
Evidence for a Link Between Rhinitis and Asthma and Postulated Mechanisms of Their Interaction

Evidence	References
Epidemiological	
Approximately 20–60% of patients with allergic rhinitis have clinical asthma, whereas >80% of patients with allergic asthma have concomitant rhinitis symptoms.	8, 14–16
The presence of rhinitis predicts the onset of asthma.	15
Worsening rhinitis negatively affects the course of asthma.	8, 11–13, 31
Treating rhinitis reduces the incidence of asthma exacerbations.	33–35
Pathological	
Allergic rhinitis patients have evidence of subclinical airways obstruction and inflammation even in the absence of overt asthma.	19, 20
Asthmatic patients have evidence of upper airway inflammation even in the absence of overt rhinitis.	22
Allergen challenge separately in the nasal or bronchial airways leads to marked inflammatory responses in the upper and lower airways, respectively.	6, 23–25
Allergens and aspirin can trigger exacerbations of both asthma and rhinitis and lead to inflammatory responses, involving increased expression of T2 cytokines.	5, 7, 26
Nasal allergen challenge leads to the production of circulating T2 effector cells responsible for promoting lower airways inflammation in mice.	7
Treating the upper airway with intranasal steroids reduces bronchial hyperresponsiveness.	9, 10
Possible Mechanisms of Upper and Lower Airway Interaction	
Absence of nasal functions—filtering, warming, and humidifying inspired air—allows direct contact of allergen and cold, polluted air with the lower airway epithelium.	
Spread of inflammation from one site to another via airways (airborne/droplet) or systemically (blood).	
Reflex activation of parasympathetic nerves by inflammation.	
Alteration of nitric oxide levels in nose may affect the larynx and bronchi.	
Postnasal "dripping" of infected material/cytokines passing to the lungs—implies microaspiration, mucous is reflexively swallowed.	

Source: Adapted from Scadding, G., Walker, S., *Prim. Care Respir.* J., 21, 222, 2012. 63

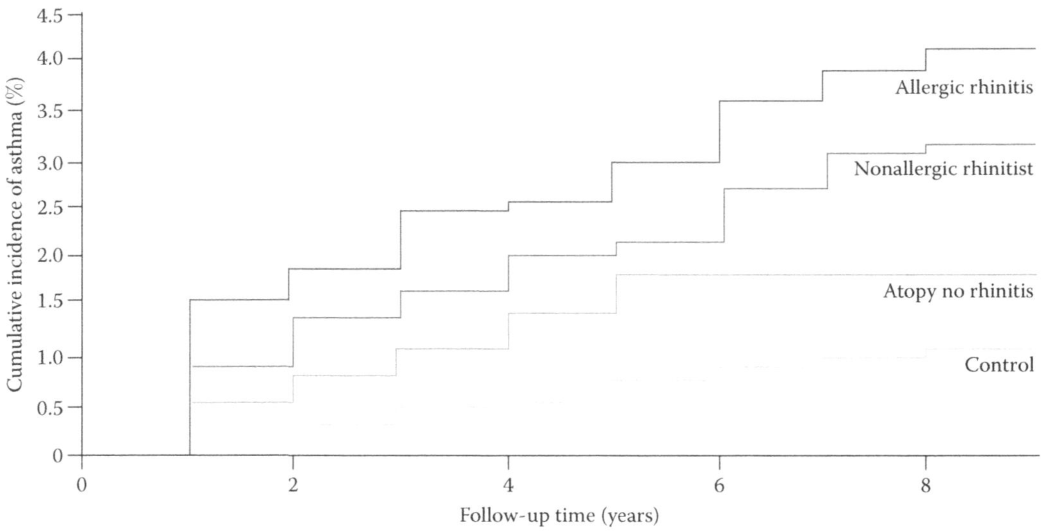

FIGURE 8.1 Association of rhinitis with the onset and incidence of asthma. (From Shaaban, R., Zureik, M., Soussan, D., et al., *Am. J. Respir. Crit. Care Med.*, 176, 659–666, 2007. With permission.)

hyperreactivity can be reduced by the use of nasal corticosteroids (9, 10). Concurrent rhinitis in asthma patients is associated with more asthma-related primary care visits and hospital referrals, as well as higher costs (11–13).

Epidemiological and pathophysiological studies show that rhinitis and asthma frequently coexist with over 80% of asthma patients having a coexisting upper airways disease (14, 15). Rhinitis, allergic or nonallergic, often precedes the development of asthma (See Figure 8.1) and is one of the strongest independent risk factors for asthma (14–17). This can be seen most clearly in the context of occupational asthma where the greatest risk for developing asthma is in the year after the onset of rhinitis (18). Many rhinitis patients without an overt diagnosis of asthma demonstrate subclinical changes such as inflammation in the lower airways and impaired lung function (19, 20). Equally, asthmatics may have upper airway inflammation, even in the absence of symptoms (21). There is proportionality between the extent of eosinophilia at both sites (22), probably explained by the fact that an allergen challenge at either site causes inflammation in both the upper and the lower airways (23–25). Rhinitis and asthma are thus considered by many as manifestations of the same "united" airway disease, interlinked by a common mucosa and nerve supply via systemic circulation (26, 27).

Most asthma exacerbations begin in the upper airway. Rhinovirus upper respiratory tract infections are the major precipitating factor for asthma exacerbations in both children and adults (28). Moreover, viral colds are more frequent and last longer in children and adults with allergic rhinitis (29, 30). As there is synergy between virus-induced and allergy-induced inflammations, not only is rhinovirus infection strongly associated with current wheezing, but also the greatest risk is seen in children who also have high levels of IgE antibodies to dust mites (31). In particular, asthmatic children who are sensitized to an allergen and then subsequently suffer combined exposure to that allergen and a naturally acquired viral upper respiratory tract infection are nearly 20 times more likely to be hospitalized for asthma (32).

Retrospective studies show that patients with asthma whose rhinitis is treated have fewer emergency visits and hospital admissions than those with untreated rhinitis, independent of asthma treatment (33–35). Chronic rhinitis is a high-risk comorbidity for 30-day hospital readmission of patients with asthma and chronic obstructive pulmonary disease (36).

The WHO Allergic Rhinitis and Its Impact on Asthma (ARIA) guidelines can be helpful in diagnosing and treating rhinitis (37). These guidelines recommend that people with asthma are assessed for rhinitis and vice versa so that they can be optimally managed. Additionally, useful pocket guides for rhinitis management are available at www.euforea.eu.

8.2 DIAGNOSIS OF RHINITIS

8.2.1 Taking a Specific History

Rhinitis can be broadly divided into three categories: allergic, infective, and non-allergic.

Mixed forms exist. Sneezing, an itchy nose and palate, and eye involvement suggest allergic rhinitis, although symptoms alone cannot reliably differentiate between allergic and non-allergic subtypes. The personal and family history of any allergic disease makes a diagnosis of allergic rhinitis more likely. The symptoms on exposure to relevant triggers such as pets, house dust, mould, and seasonal or occupational allergens may give a further indication of the probable causes. To guide subsequent treatment, it is important to ask whether the symptoms are intermittent or persistent and mild or moderate to severe (37) and to ask for an estimation of severity on a visual analogue scale. A previous study demonstrated that patients with rhinitis symptoms beginning later in life (age >35), no family history of allergies, no seasonality, and no symptoms around furry pets or odorants such as fragrances and perfumes had a greater than 98% likelihood of having non-allergic rhinitis before allergy skin and/or serology-specific IgE testing (38).

8.2.2 Physical Examination

Observation of the patient for signs of sniffing, nose rubbing, reduced nasal airflow, mouth breathing, and a transverse skin crease across the dorsum of the nose is helpful in determining the presence of rhinitis. Patients with allergic rhinitis may have erythematous eyes and "allergic shiners," which are a manifestation of chronic venous congestion. It is important to examine the nasal mucosa using a speculum and a head-mounted lamp, an endoscope if available, or simply use an otoscope with the largest earpiece. The nasal mucosa in allergic rhinitis is typically watery, swollen, and a slightly blue-grey shade of red. Additional features suggesting alternative diagnoses include the presence of nasal polyps (pale, shiny, white-grey, grapelike structures, often originating close to the middle turbinate), crusting, bleeding, septal perforation, mucopurulent discharge, and, from external observation, the presence of nasal bridge collapse or lupus pernio. The latter findings may warrant further assessment to rule out conditions such as vasculitis, sarcoidosis or relapsing polychrondritis, or other structural problems.

8.2.3 Allergen Identification: Skin Prick Tests/Serum IgE

A good medical history should include a thorough environmental history of the home and workplace to identify likely allergens and other non-allergic triggers that could be causing or aggravating the patient's symptoms. To assess the patient's atopic status, skin prick testing or serum-specific IgE testing to seasonal and perennial allergens should be performed. Patients with classical hay fever, with typical symptoms and seasonal timing, can often be diagnosed by their medical history alone. The British Society of Allergy and Clinical Immunology (BSACI) guidelines (4), recommend that skin prick tests are routinely used in secondary care in order to confirm or exclude underlying IgE sensitivity to common aeroallergens and to provide objective information to support the clinical history concerning an underlying allergic basis. In primary care, if skin prick tests are not available, serum-specific IgE tests may be requested. It should be kept in mind that both skin and serum tests alone identify allergic "sensitization"; however, a diagnosis of allergy requires positive tests to correlate with the patient's clinical history. Therefore, performing numerous screening tests in the absence of a compatible history is not recommended. A large, cross-sectional study used an irritant index questionnaire to reclassify patients with a physician diagnosis of allergic, non-allergic, or mixed rhinitis. The study found that both allergic and non-allergic rhinitis patients with a high-irritant burden had a significantly greater likelihood of having a diagnosis of asthma compared with allergic and non-allergic rhinitis patients with a low-irritant burden. This study indicates that quantifying the irritant burden in rhinitis patients results in distinct, "more severe" rhinitis phenotypes that may represent the difficult-to-treat rhinitis patient (39).

Additional investigations that may aid in the diagnosis and identification of the cause of rhinitis refractory to conventional treatment include:

- Complete blood count, erythrocyte sedimentation rate (ESR), and differential white cell count.
- C-reactive protein, if chronic infection is suspected.
- Thyroid function tests.
- Urine toxicology—if cocaine abuse is suspected.

Peak expiratory flow measurements and spirometry should be considered for all patients with anything more than mild, intermittent rhinitis to screen for an airway obstruction since allergic rhinitis is a risk factor for asthma. A diagnosis of asthma is more complicated and may be confused by symptoms of cough caused by rhinitis and postnasal drip, leading to either an inaccurate diagnosis or overtreatment of asthma. Few self-administered questionnaires are currently available for the assessment of both disorders (40). RHINASTHMA is a 30-item questionnaire, which differentiates between patients with rhinitis and patients with comorbid rhinitis and asthma, as well as controlled and uncontrolled asthma in asthmatic patients with symptomatic or nonsymptomatic rhinitis (41).

8.3 MANAGEMENT OF PATIENTS WITH COMORBID RHINITIS AND ASTHMA

Increasing evidence suggests that better management of rhinitis may result in decreased asthma comorbidity and an improved quality of life (33–35, 42).

This includes:

- Allergen and irritant identification and avoidance.
- Pharmacological treatment.
- Immunotherapy.
- Patient education.

8.3.1 Allergen Avoidance

To date, the results of meta-analyses of allergen avoidance studies, particularly for house-dust mites, have been disappointing (43). However, this may, in part, be due to methodological problems related to many of the published studies. If sufficient avoidance can be achieved, for example by relocating patients to a high altitude (44), improvements in symptoms, lung function, and allergen-induced bronchial hyperreactivity can be demonstrated. In real-life settings, allergen avoidance can be effective: one inner-city study of children with asthma, involving multiple intervention measures, proved effective (45), whereas another study utilizing a single intervention measure with allergen-impregnable bedcovers proved ineffective (46). There is evidence for a reduction of nose and eye symptoms by: nasal air filters compared with placebo filters in a pollen season study; (47) another placebo-controlled study demonstrated a reduction of both asthma and rhinitis symptoms using a nocturnal laminar airflow device, which removes particulate matter, including allergens, from the patients' breathing space; (48) and saline nasal douching, which reduces symptoms and inflammatory mediators simply by washing allergens out of the nose (49, 50).

8.3.2 Pharmacotherapy

8.3.2.1 Intranasal Corticosteroids

The EUFOREA guidelines recommend the treatment of allergic rhinitis according to an algorithm based on symptoms and their severity (Figure 8.2) (51). For any form of allergic rhinitis that is more than mild and intermittent, topical intranasal corticosteroids (INCS) are the first-line medication of choice. Meta-analyses have demonstrated these drugs to be more effective than H1-antihistamines (oral or topical), antileukotrienes, and the combination of H1-antihistamine plus antileukotriene (52–55). Topical corticosteroids reduce all nasal symptoms, including nasal obstruction, and they have also been shown to be beneficial for associated eye symptoms (56).

Systemic absorption is very low with nasal mometasone and fluticasone, with good long-term safety data in children and adults, but it is high for nasally administered betamethasone and dexamethasone (57). Although INCS may have a fast onset of action (within 6–8 hours), the maximal improvement in symptoms may not occur for at least two weeks. Minor nose bleeding may occur in 5–8% of patients and result in the need for discontinuation. This adverse effect can be reduced by judicious use of the spray, aiming the nozzle placed just inside the nose towards the lateral wall of the nasal cavity and spraying in two different directions: upwards and backwards. Sniffing should be avoided, as this pulls the spray straight back to the posterior pharynx and triggers swallowing. Very rarely, hypothalamic–pituitary axis suppression may occur with long-term use and guidelines advice monitoring growth in children.

8.3.2.2 H1-Antihistamines

H1-antihistamines are useful for mild symptoms, either intermittent or persistent. In the latter case, regular daily use is advisable because when they are withdrawn, the

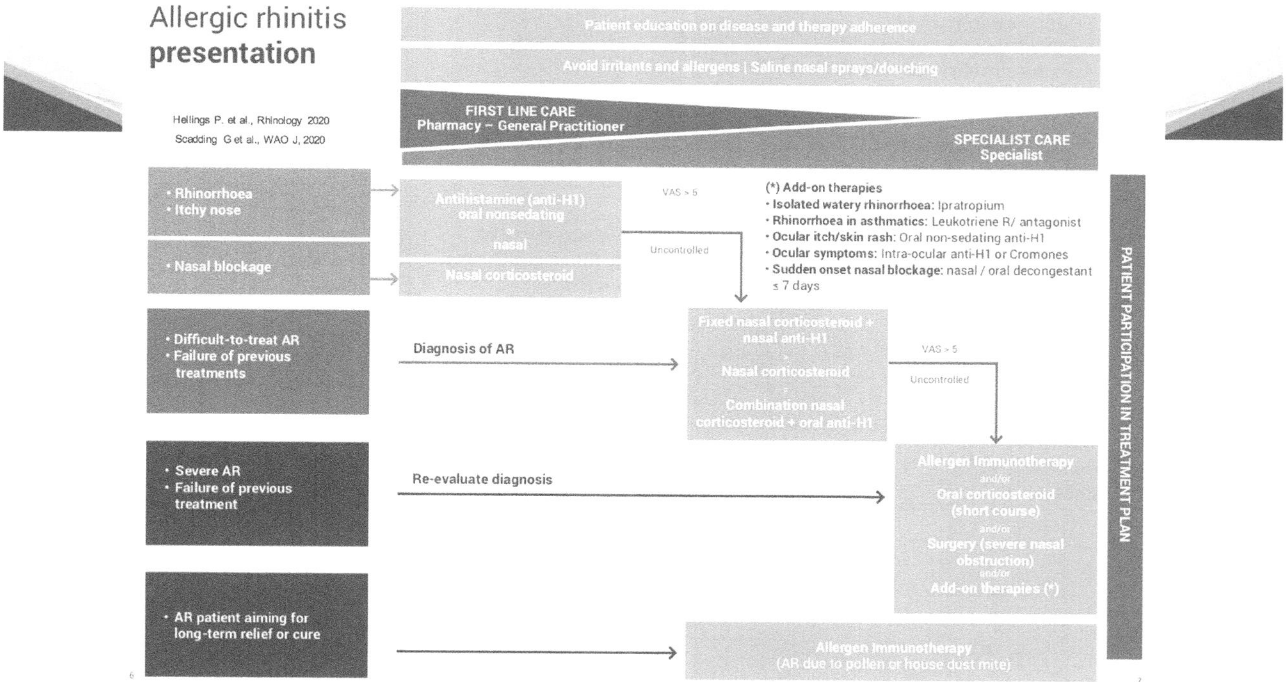

FIGURE 8.2 The EUFOREA guidelines for treatment of allergic rhinitis.

histamine receptor becomes more active and the symptoms can increase. H1-antihistamines are active against sneezing, rhinorrhea, and nasal itch, but are inferior to nasal corticosteroids in reducing nasal congestion. Most second-generation oral antihistamines (loratadine, cetirizine, fexofenadine, desloratidine, levocetirizine, misolastine, bilastine, rupatadine) reduce symptoms within one hour and are used once daily. Acrivastine is an exception to this rule; it has a rapid onset of action but lasts only eight hours. Availability of these second-generation antihistamines varies between countries. Topical nasal H1-antihistamines are available as azelastine and olopatadine, which have a 15-minute onset of action.

First-generation H1-antihistamines, such as chlorphenamine, may cause sedation with a resultant reduction in work and school performance; therefore, these should be avoided (58). Second-generation H1-antihistamines, especially fexofenadine, have a very low potential for sedation. All have few major drug interactions. Grapefruit impairs fexofenadine absorption and therefore should be avoided. The adverse effects of azelastine include local irritation and taste disturbance.

8.3.2.3 Combination Therapy

If the symptoms of rhinitis persist despite the use of antihistamines or topical INCS alone, it is important to review the diagnosis, check concordance with the treatment, and check the nasal spray technique. If the response remains poor, then most practitioners would recommend combined treatment with both a topical nasal corticosteroid and nasal H1-antihistamine (4). A combined spray containing both fluticasone propionate and azelastine is superior to either alone, another combination spray contains mometasone furoate and olopatadine.

8.3.3 Other Treatment Options (Figure 8.3)

- In cases of nasal blockage, the short-term use (i.e. <10 days) of an intranasal decongestant (e.g. ephedrine, xylometazoline, or oxymetazoline) may be beneficial. Regular prolonged use of topical decongestants leads to chronic nasal obstruction through tachyphylaxis and should therefore be avoided. However, recent studies have demonstrated that topical decongestants are well tolerated and do not cause rhinitis medicamentosa (nasal congestion rebound) when used in conjunction with an INCS. Oral decongestants, such as phenylephrine, show poor efficacy and cause adverse effects and therefore are not recommended for long-term use (59, 60).
- Oral leukotriene receptor antagonists (LTRAs) may be beneficial in patients with mild rhinitis, particularly in patients with comorbid asthma.
- Topical anticholinergic preparations such as ipratropium bromide may be beneficial in reducing rhinorrhea, particularly in the treatment of nonallergic (vasomotor) or allergic rhinitis.

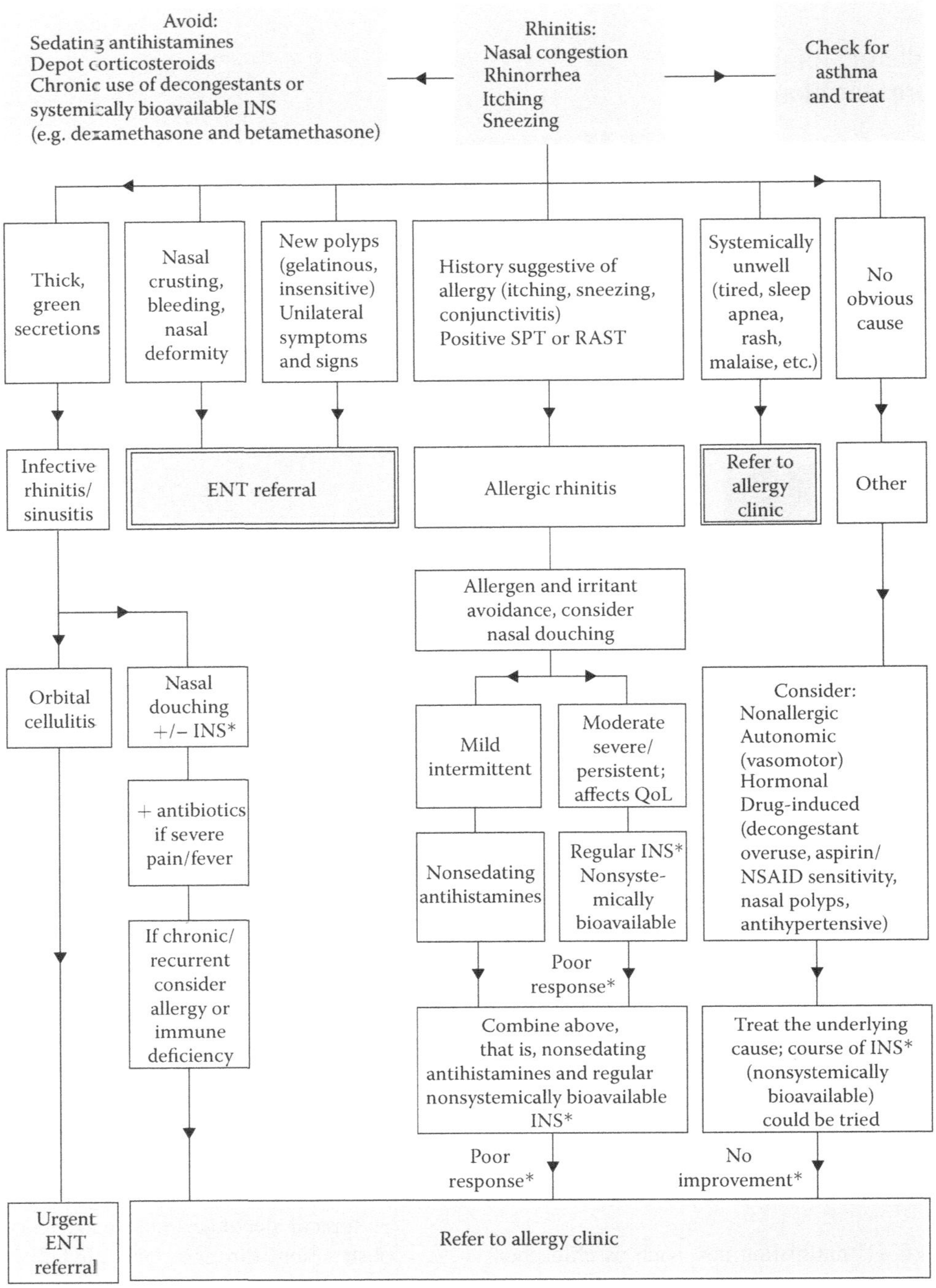

FIGURE 8.3 Other treatment options for allergic rhinitis.

Notes: **INS, intranasal corticosteroids; SPT, skin prick test; RAST, radioallergosorbent test; QoL, quality of life; NSAID, nonsteroidal anti-inflammatory drugs**

- Topical sodium cromoglicate is modestly effective, but it needs to be used 3–4 times a day. It is used by clinicians in the treatment of small children.
- Chromone and antihistamine-containing eye drops can be used alone or in combination with oral/topical nonsedating antihistamines and INCS for ocular symptoms if required.
- Systemic corticosteroids should rarely be used, but they have a role in severe nasal obstruction as a short-term rescue medication, particularly for important life events. The BSACI guideline recommends 0.5 mg/kg orally for five days in combination with a topical nasal corticosteroid, taken in the morning with food (4). Depot injections of corticosteroid are not recommended because risks of adverse events outweigh benefits (4).

Concordance with all treatments should be monitored regularly until patients reach a level of optimal symptom control.

8.3.3.1 Allergen Immunotherapy

Allergen immunotherapy is the only treatment that is able to alter the course of a disease, and it probably prevents progression from rhinitis to asthma (61). Previously performed only by subcutaneous injection, the recent confirmation of the efficacy and safety of sublingual immunotherapy (SLIT) has opened this avenue of therapy to a wider group of patients (62). Schedules for both approaches typically involve a three-year treatment programme and, depending on the allergen and formulation, use either weekly upwardly titrated dosing schedules, followed by maintenance injections every 4–6 weeks (4–9), pre-seasonal injections, or a daily sublingual tablet. Chronic, perennial uncontrolled asthma is a contraindication, and systemic reactions (particularly in patients with asthma), including urticaria, angioedema, bronchospasm, and anaphylaxis, can occur. For these reasons and also to ensure the appropriate targeting of the treatment to those patients most likely to benefit, immunotherapy is restricted to specialist allergy clinics. SLIT has the advantage of self-administration by the patient at home, following supervision of the first dose in the clinic. This route is currently underused in the United Kingdom; however, in the future, it should reduce overall treatment costs and environmental impact by reducing the need for the repeat clinic visits that are required for injection immunotherapy. Real-life studies from a very large database show that therapeutic responses with SLIT are as robust as with subcutaneous immunotherapy (SCIT) for grass pollen and house-dust mite (63).

8.3.3.2 Education and Prevention

The BSACI 4 and EUFOREA guidelines (51) emphasize the importance of education, particularly with regard to the negative effect that rhinitis may have on quality of life and the need for concordance. Relevant allergen avoidance should be discussed. The patient should be provided with information about the potential complications of rhinitis, such as asthma, sinusitis, and eustachian tube dysfunction. Information about therapy should be given, including a demonstration of the nasal spray technique where prescribed. Occupational rhinitis is considered a risk factor for occupational asthma and usually predates the onset of asthma. Of particular relevance to the workplace is primary prevention, particularly using non-powdered or non-latex gloves, and the avoidance of other occupational allergens known to cause sensitization (see Chapter 24). The superior efficacy and safety of the new-generation topical corticosteroids should be highlighted for those patients who are reluctant to use these drugs. Patients may be reluctant to use corticosteroids at more than one site, the nose as well as the lungs, but the contribution to the total corticosteroid load from INCS is minute compared with that from bronchial inhalers. Conversely, the contribution from untreated rhinitis to the overall disease burden can be considerable. In some asthmatic patients, the addition of nasal therapy allows a reduction in the inhaled dose.

8.4 SPECIAL CONSIDERATIONS

8.4.1 Treatment in Pregnancy

Pregnancy-associated rhinitis is self-limiting, and treatment should only be initiated if the benefit of the treatment outweighs the risk to the foetus (64). Saline nasal douching is safe and may help. For allergic rhinitis, INCS, such as budesonide, beclomethasone, triamcinolone, and fluticasone, have been widely used by pregnant women and are therefore considered safe. According to the American College of Obstetricians and Gynecologists (ACOG), (65) several over-the-counter (OTC) H1-antihistamines may be taken during pregnancy. Older, first-generation H1-antihistamines such as chlorphenamine and dexchlorpheniramine can be taken, but they may cause drowsiness. Newer, second-generation H1-antihistamines such as cetirizine and loratadine can also be taken with less risk of drowsiness.

Oral decongestant medication should be avoided in the first three months of pregnancy due to a possible risk of abdominal wall birth defects. Intranasal azelastine should also be avoided. Montelukast and zafirlukast are both considered safe to take during pregnancy.

Immunotherapy should not be initiated, but it can be continued during pregnancy (see Chapter 27).

8.4.2 Treatment in Children

EUFOREA also provides guidance for paediatric AR (66). AR therapy for children includes saline irrigation, H1-antihistamines, and nasal corticosteroids. Those with the lowest systemic bioavailability (budesonide, fluticasone, and mometasone) at the lowest dose for effective symptom control should be used, with monitoring of growth if the treatment is given long term.

HDM SLIT should be considered in children with early onset HDM-sensitive PAR, as evidence exists that earlier immunotherapy is associated with reduced progression to asthma and decreased healthcare costs in the long term (67).

8.5 REFERRAL

Treatment failure, which occurs in some 20% of rhinitis patients (68), should prompt a referral to either an allergist to assess whether the patient has allergic, nonallergic, or mixed rhinitis, and/or to an otolaryngologist to rule out structural abnormalities. The circumstances prompting referral to an allergist include:

- Inadequate control of symptoms.
- Recurrent nasal polyps.
- Patient systemically unwell as a result of rhinitis.
- Need for allergen or trigger identification or diagnosis.
- Consideration of immunotherapy.
- Presence of a multisystem allergy (e.g. rhinitis with asthma, eczema, or food allergy).

- Occupational rhinitis.

Referral to an ear, nose, and throat (ENT) clinic should be made if there is/are:

- Unilateral symptoms and signs, such as nasal obstruction (which may be due to a nasal tumour), nasal perforation, or ulceration.
- Thick, green nasal secretions, suggesting an acute or recurrent infective rhinosinusitis.
- Periorbital cellulitis (an emergency warranting an urgent ENT referral)
- New-onset nasal polyps.
- Significant nasal septal deviation or very enlarged turbinates in someone who is unresponsive to treatment; surgical management may be required to improve the nasal airway for access of topical medications.
- Evidence of persistent nasal crusting, nasal collapse, or bleeding from the nostrils, which may be signs of systemic disorders such as sarcoidosis or Wegener's granulomatosis.

8.6 CONCLUSIONS

Rhinitis and asthma frequently occur as comorbid conditions in adults and children as manifestations of the same inflammatory disease continuum. Rhinitis is a predictor of future asthma. It impacts negatively on asthma, leading to more severe disease, worse asthma control, and impaired quality of life, despite adherence to asthma treatment. Good treatment of rhinitis is likely to improve asthma control and outcomes. The WHO-ARIA recommendation is that patients with asthma and rhinitis should be treated for both conditions. Relevant allergens and triggers should be sought and excluded. The combination of intranasal and inhaled corticosteroids for persistent rhinitis and asthma should be considered, with the addition of other drugs including H1-antihistamines, chromones, and LTRAs as appropriate. The overall corticosteroid load should be reviewed on a regular basis to prevent unwanted side effects. Allergen-specific immunotherapy for allergic rhinitis has the potential to prevent the development of asthma in AR patients and to reduce exacerbations in asthmatics (69).

REFERENCES

1. Anagnostou K, Harrison B, Iles R, et al. Risk factors for childhood asthma deaths from the UK Eastern region confidential enquiry 2001–2006. *Prim Care Respir J* 2012;*21*(1):71–77.
2. Ryan D, Grant-Casey J, Scadding G, et al. Management of allergic rhinitis in UK primary care: Baseline audit. *Prim Care Respir J* 2005;*14*(4):204–209.
3. Maurer M, Zuberbier T. Under-treatment of rhinitis symptoms in Europe: Findings from a cross-sectional questionnaire survey. *Allergy* 2007;*62*(9):1057–1063.
4. Scadding GK, Durham S, Mirakian R, et al. BSACI guidelines for the management of allergic and non-allergic rhinitis. *Clin Exp Allergy* 2008;*38*(1):19–42.
5. Durham SR. Mechanisms of mucosal inflammation in the nose and lungs. *Clin Exp Allergy* 1998;*28*(Suppl 2):11–16.
6. Corren J, Adinoff AD, Irvin CG. Changes in bronchial responsiveness following nasal provocation with allergen. *J Allergy Clin Immunol* 1992;*89*:611–618.
7. KleinJan A, Willart M, van Nimwegen M, et al. United airways: Circulating Th2 effector cells in an AR model are responsible for promoting lower airways inflammation. *Clin Exp Allergy* 2010;*40*:494–504.
8. Magnan A, Meunier JP, Saugnac C, et al. Frequency and impact of AR in asthma patients in everyday general medical practice: A French observational cross-sectional study. *Allergy* 2008;*63*:292–298.
9. Agondi RC, Machado ML, Kalil J, et al. Intranasal corticosteroid administration reduces nonspecific bronchial hyperresponsiveness and improves asthma symptoms. *J Asthma* 2008;*45*(9):754–757.
10. Foresi A, Pelucchi A, Gherson G, et al. Once daily intranasal fluticasone propionate (200 micrograms) reduces nasal symptoms and inflammation but also attenuates the increase in bronchial responsiveness during the pollen season in allergic rhinitis. *J Allergy Clin Immunol* 1996;*98*(2):274–282.
11. Clatworthy J, Price D, Ryan D, et al. The value of self-report assessment of adherence, rhinitis and smoking in relation to asthma control. *Prim Care Respir J* 2009;*18*:300–305.
12. Brandão HV, Cruz CS, Pinheiro MC, et al. Risk factors for ER visits due to asthma exacerbations in patients enrolled in a program for the control of asthma and allergic rhinitis in Feira de Santana, Brazil. *J Bras Pneumol* 2009;*35*:1168–1173.
13. Price D, Zhang Q, Kocevar VS, et al. Effect of a concomitant diagnosis of AR on asthma-related health care use by adults. *Clin Exp Allergy* 2005;*35*:282–287.
14. Linneberg A, Henrik Nielsen N, Frolund L, et al. The link between AR and allergic asthma: A prospective population-based study. The Copenhagen allergy study. *Allergy* 2002;*57*:1048–1052.
15. Leynaert B, Neukirch F, Demoly P, et al. Epidemiologic evidence for asthma and rhinitis comorbidity. *J Allergy Clin Immunol* 2000;*106*(Suppl 5):S201–S205.
16. Shaaban R, Zureik M, Soussan D, et al. Allergic rhinitis and onset of bronchial hyperresponsiveness: A population-based study. *Am J Respir Crit Care Med* 2007;*176*(7):659–666.
17. Shaaban R, Zureik M, Soussan D, et al. Rhinitis and onset of asthma: A longitudinal population-based study. *Lancet* 2008;*372*:1049–1057.
18. Fishwick D, Barber CM, Bradshaw LM, et al. Standards of care for occupational asthma: An update. *Thorax* 2012;*67*(3):278–280.
19. Ciprandi G, Capasso M. Association of childhood perennial allergic rhinitis with subclinical airflow limitation. *Clin Exp Allergy* 2010;*40*(3):398–402.
20. Brown JL, Behndig AF, Sekerel BE, et al. Lower airways inflammation in allergic rhinitics: A comparison with asthmatics and normal controls. *Clin Exp Allergy* 2007;*37*(5):688–695.
21. Braunstahl G-J, Fokkens W. Nasal involvement in allergic asthma. *Allergy* 2003;*58*:1235–1243.
22. Gaga M, Lambrou P, Papageorgiou N, et al. Eosinophils are a feature of upper and lower airway pathology in non-atopic asthma, irrespective of the presence of rhinitis. *Clin Exp Allergy* 2000;*30*(5):663–669.

23. Inal A, Kendirli SG, Yilmaz M, et al. Indices of lower airway inflammation in children monosensitized to house dust mite after nasal allergen challenge. *Allergy* 2008;*63*(10):1345–1351.
24. Bonay M, Neukirch C, Grandsaigne M, et al. Changes in airway inflammation following nasal allergic challenge in patients with seasonal rhinitis. *Allergy* 2006;*61*:111–118.
25. Braunstahl GJ, Kleinjan A, Overbeek SE, et al. Segmental bronchial provocation induces nasal inflammation in AR patients. *Am J Respir Crit Care Med* 2000;*161*:2051–2057.
26. Simons FER. Allergic rhinobronchitis: The asthma-AR link. *J Allergy Clin Immunol* 1999;*104*:534–540.
27. Togias A. Mechanisms of nose-lung interaction. *Allergy* 1999;*54*(Suppl 57):94–105.
28. Busse WW, Lemanske RF Jr, Gern JE. Role of viral respiratory infections in asthma and asthma exacerbations. *Lancet.* 2010;*376*(9743):826–834.
29. Ciprandi G, Tosca MA, Fasce L. Allergic children have more numerous and severe respiratory infections than non-allergic children. *Pediatr Allergy Immunol* 2006;*17*(5):389–391.
30. Cirillo I, Marseglia G, Klersy C, et al. Allergic patients have more numerous and prolonged respiratory infections than non allergic subjects. *Allergy* 2007;*62*(9):1087–1090.
31. Soto-Quiros M, Avila L, Platts-Mills TA, et al. High titres of IgE antibodies to dust mite allergen and risk for wheezing among asthmatic children infected with rhinovirus. *J Allergy Clin Immunol* 2012;*129*:1499–1505.
32. Murray CS, Poletti G, Kebadze T, et al. Study of modifiable risk factors for asthma exacerbations: Virus infection and allergen exposure increase the risk of asthma hospital admissions in children. *Thorax* 2006;*61*(5):376–382.
33. Crystal-Peters J, Neslusan C, Crown WH, et al. Treating allergic rhinitis in patients with comorbid asthma: The risk of asthma-related hospitalizations and emergency department visits. *J Allergy Clin Immunol* 2002;*109*(1):57–62.
34. Adams RJ, Fuhlbrigge AL, Finkelstein JA, et al. Intranasal steroids and the risk of emergency department visits for asthma. *J Allergy Clin Immunol* 2002;*109*(4):636–642.
35. Corren J, Manning B, Thompson S, et al. Rhinitis therapy and the prevention of hospital care for asthma: A case-control study. *J Allergy Clin Immunol* 2004;*113*(3):415–419.
36. Singh U, Wangia-Anderson V, Bernstein JA. Chronic rhinitis is a high-risk comorbidity for 30-day hospital readmission of patients with asthma and chronic obstructive pulmonary disease. *J Allergy Clin Immunol Pract.* 2019 Jan;7(1):279–285.e6. https://doi.org/10.1016/j.jaip.2018.06.029. Epub July 25, 2018. PMID: 30053594.
37. Bousquet J, Khaltaev N, Cruz A, et al; World Health Organization; GA2(2) LEN; AllerGen. Allergic Rhinitis and its Impact on Asthma (ARIA) 2008 update (in collaboration with the World Health Organization, GA (2)LEN and AllerGen). *Allergy* 2008;*63*(Suppl 86):8–160.
38. Brandt D, Bernstein JA. Questionnaire evaluation and risk factor identification for nonallergic vasomotor rhinitis. *Ann Allergy Asthma Immunol* 2006;*96*(4):526–532.
39. Bernstein JA, Levin LS, Al-Shuik E, Martin VT. Clinical characteristics of chronic rhinitis patients with high vs low irritant trigger burdens. *Ann Allergy Asthma Immunol* 2012;*109*(3):173–178.
40. Demoly P, Bozonnat MC, Dacosta P, et al. The diagnosis of asthma using a self-questionnaire in those suffering from AR: A pharmaco-epidemiological survey in everyday practice in France. *Allergy* 2006;*61*:699–704.
41. Baiardini I, Pasquali M, Giardini A, et al. Rhinasthma: A new specific QoL questionnaire for patients with rhinitis and asthma. *Allergy* 2003;*58*(4):289–294.
42. Braido F, Baiardini I, Balestracci S, et al. Does asthma control correlate with quality of life related to upper and lower airways? A real life study. *Allergy* 2009;*64*:937–943.
43. Sheikh A, Hurwitz B, Nurmatov U, et al. House dust mite avoidance measures for perennial allergic rhinitis. *Cochrane Db Syst Rev* 2010;(7):CD001563.
44. Peroni DG, Boner AL, Vallone G, et al. Effective allergen avoidance at high altitude reduces allergen-induced bronchial hyperresponsiveness. *Am J Respir Crit Care Med* 1994;*149*(6):1442–1446.
45. Morgan WJ, Crain EF, Gruchalla RS, et al. Results of a home-based environmental intervention among urban children with asthma. *N Engl J Med* 2004;*351*(11):1068–1080.
46. Woodcock A, Forster L, Matthews E, et al. Control of exposure to mite allergen and allergen-impermeable bed covers for adults with asthma. *N Engl J Med* 2003;*349*(3):225–236.
47. O'Meara TJ, Sercombe JK, Morgan G, et al. The reduction of rhinitis symptoms by nasal filters during natural exposure to ragweed and grass pollen. *Allergy* 2005;*60*(4):529–532.
48. Boyle RJ, Pedroletti C, Wickman M, et al. Nocturnal temperature controlled laminar airflow for treating atopic asthma: A randomised controlled trial. *Thorax* 2012;*67*(3):215–221.
49. Garavello W, Romagnoli M, Sordo L, et al. Hypersaline nasal irrigation in children with symptomatic seasonal allergic rhinitis: A randomized study. *Pediatr Allergy Immunol* 2003;*14*(2):140–143.
50. Georgitis JW. Nasal hyperthermia and simple irrigation for perennial rhinitis. Changes in inflammatory mediators. *Chest* 1994;*106*(5):1487–1492.
51. Hellings PW, Scadding G, Bachert C et al. EUFOREA treatment algorithm for allergic rhinitis. *Rhinology* 2020 Dec 1;*58*(6):618–622.
52. Weiner JM, Abramson MJ, Puy RM. Intranasal corticosteroids versus oral H1 receptor antagonists in allergic rhinitis: Systematic review of randomised controlled trials. *BMJ* 1998;*317*(7173):1624–1629.
53. Yáñez A, Rodrigo GJ. Intranasal corticosteroids versus topical H1 receptor antagonists for the treatment of allergic rhinitis: A systematic review with meta-analysis. *Ann Allergy Asthma Immunol* 2002;*89*(5):479–484.
54. Di Lorenzo G, Pacor ML, Pellitteri ME, et al. Randomized placebo-controlled trial comparing fluticasone aqueous nasal spray in monotherapy, fluticasone plus cetirizine, fluticasone plus montelukast and cetirizine plus montelukast for seasonal allergic rhinitis. *Clin Exp Allergy* 2004;*34*(2):259–267.
55. Wilson AM, O'Byrne PM, Parameswaran K. Leukotriene receptor antagonists for allergic rhinitis: A systematic review and meta-analysis. *Am J Med* 2004;*116*(5):338–344.
56. Bernstein DI, Levy AL, Hampel FC, et al. Treatment with intranasal fluticasone propionate significantly improves ocular symptoms in patients with seasonal allergic rhinitis. *Clin Exp Allergy* 2004;*34*(6):952–957.
57. Demoly P. Safety of intranasal corticosteroids in acute rhinosinusitis. *Am J Otolaryngol* 2008;*29*(6):403–413.
58 Walker S, Khan-Wasti S, Fletcher M, et al. Seasonal allergic rhinitis is associated with a detrimental effect on examination performance in United Kingdom teenagers: Case-control study. *J Allergy Clin Immunol* 2007;*120*(2):381–387.
59. Vaidyanathan S, Williamson P, Clearie K, Khan F, Lipworth B. Fluticasone reverses oxymetazoline-induced tachyphylaxis of response and rebound congestion. *Am J Respir Crit Care Med* 2010;*182*(1):19–24.

60. Baroody FM, Brown D, Gavanescu L, DeTineo M, Naclerio RM. Oxymetazoline adds to the effectiveness of fluticasone furoate in the treatment of perennial allergic rhinitis. *J Allergy Clin Immunol* 2011;*127*(4):927–934.
61. Jacobsen L, Niggemann B, Dreborg S, et al. Specific immunotherapy has long-term preventive effect of seasonal and perennial asthma: 10-year follow-up on the PAT study. *Allergy* 2007;*62*(8):943–948.
62. Radulovic S, Wilson D, Calderon M, et al. Systematic reviews of sublingual immunotherapy (SLIT). *Allergy* 2011;*66*(6):740–752.
63. Contoli M, Porsbjerg C, Buchs S, Rask Larsen J, Freemantle N, Fritzsching B. Real-world, long-term effectiveness of allergy immunotherapy in allergic rhinitis: Subgroup analyses of the REACT study. *J. Allergy Clin Immunol* 2023;*152*(2):445–452.e4. ISSN 0091–6749. https://doi.org/10.1016/j.jaci.2023.02.024.
64. Demoly P, Piette V, Daures J-P. Treatment of allergic rhinitis during pregnancy. *Drugs* 2003;*63*(17):1813–1820.
65. https://www.acog.org/womens-health/experts-and-stories/ask-acog/what-medicine-can-i-take-for-allergies-while-im-pregnant#:~:text=Many%20people%20with%20allergies%20take,%2Dthe%2Dcounter%20allergy%20medication.
66. Scadding GK, Smith PK, Blaiss M et al. Allergic rhinitis in childhood and the new EUFOREA algorithm. *Front Allergy.* 2021 Jul 14;*2*:706589.
67. Hamelmann E, Hammerby E, Scharling KS, Pedersen M, Okkels A, Schmitt J. Quantifying the benefits of early sublingual allergen immunotherapy tablet initiation in children. *Allergy* 2024 Apr;*79*(4):1018–1027. https://doi.org/10.1111/all.15985. Epub December 26, 2023. PMID: 38146654
68. Bousquet J, Bachert C, Canonica GW, et al. Unmet needs in severe chronic upper airway disease (SCUAD). *J Allergy Clin Immunol* 2009;*124*(3):428–433.
69. Virchow JC, Backer V, Kuna P et al. Efficacy of a house dust mite sublingual allergen immunotherapy tablet in adults with allergic asthma: A randomized clinical trial. *JAMA*. 2016 Apr 26;*315*(16):1715–1725.

Section III

Asthma Triggers

9 Viral Infections in Asthma

René Lutter and Bart Hilvering

CASE REPORT

A 28-year-old female with a history of severe childhood onset eosinophilic asthma for which she receives monthly infusions with the biologic, anti-IL-5 (reslizumab), presented to the ER with an acute asthma attack. She suddenly became dyspneic at night with cough and midsternal thoracic pain radiating to her sides. Nebulization with salbutamol/ipratropium at home did not resolve her symptoms, prompting the decision to call an ambulance. In the ER, she appeared in acute respiratory distress with laboured breathing, increased respiratory rate (25/min), a rapid pulse of 110/min, BP of 127/86, and an oxygen saturation of 98%. Laboratory testing showed respiratory alkalosis and hypoxemia with an ABG: pH 7.50, pCO_2 of 3.6 kPa, O_2 of 8.9, BE 20.9 mmol/L, and a lactate of 1.9 mmol/L. Inflammatory parameters revealed a low CRP of 11 mg/L, leukocyte count of $5.0*10^9$/L, and eosinophil count $0.01*10^9$/L. The viral swab was positive for Influenza A by PCR testing. With oral glucocorticoids and ongoing salmeterol nebulization treatments, she initially improved and was admitted to the pulmonary ward. About 16 hours later, she suddenly deteriorated and was moved to the ICU for intubation and mechanical ventilation. Within 24 hours, she was able to be extubated and was started on non-invasive ventilation (CPAP). After a few hours, she was able to breath on her own with oxygen only. Three months later, after many hours of gradual training and physiotherapy, she was fully recovered.

This case emphasizes that patients with severe eosinophilic asthma who respond well to biologic treatment can still suffer from a severe exacerbation triggered by a viral infection. The nature and severity of the inflammatory response to viruses while on treatment with biologics is largely unknown. An example of a study that looked into this is the MEX study (1). Infectious triggers more often resulted in a non-eosinophilic inflammatory response in patients who were receiving treatment with mepolizumab (low FeNO and low sputum eosinophils), although when looking more carefully at the data, viral upper, and lower tract infections were divided fairly equally between groups (54% in the sputum eosinophil low group versus 40% in sputum eosinophil high group). To date, no other prospective studies looked into the nature of exacerbations while on biologics.

9.1 INTRODUCTION

Asthma is a chronic inflammatory airway disease that clinically manifests itself by periodic worsening of asthma symptoms, although some symptomology (e.g. difficulty in breathing, chest tightness, and daily coughing) may become persistent, certainly in more severe asthma. The acute worsening of asthma symptoms is associated with exposure to provoking factors that would normally not trigger a clinical response in healthy individuals. Therefore, from a biological perspective, asthma may be explained by exaggerated responses to provoking factors such as allergens in the case of allergic asthma, and, in non-allergic asthma, cold air, exercise, stress, smoke, odours, and respiratory viral infections. Allergens and respiratory viral infections are considered the main provoking factors, although each of the earlier mentioned factors, as well as poorly controlled disease, may be a synergistic factor in an asthma exacerbation. In this chapter, we will focus on respiratory viral infections, the acute worsening of asthma symptoms, the potential underlying causes, and the effect of therapeutic interventions. Many studies have addressed molecular pathways involved in anti-viral responses. Here, we have tried to bring together what we believe are the most relevant molecular pathways associated with respiratory viral infections associated with asthma (Figure 9.1).

9.2 RESPIRATORY VIRAL INFECTIONS

The COVID-19 pandemic and the societal responses have made us realize again that respiratory viruses can spread quickly and that behavioural changes such as coughing in your elbow pit, washing hands, and keeping distance can have a major effect on the spread of a virus. These behavioural changes reduced infections with SARS-CoV-2, the causative agent of COVID–19. However, the number of infections from RSV and influenza were also lower than one would typically expect during most of the COVID-19 pandemic (2). This in itself is a useful lesson that enables asthma patients to reduce exposure to respiratory viruses and reduce their risk of developing an exacerbation. This may be particularly effective during the seasonal viral peaks, which coincide with the start of the school during the fall season and in the winter during the holidays.

DOI: 10.1201/9781003287209-12

Infectivity/susceptibility:		
Docking sites affected	ACE2 expression (docking site for SARS) may be reduced by Th2 mediators, and CDHR expression (docking site for rhinovirus C) may be enhanced in—at risk—infants.	ICAM-1 expression (docking site for rhinovirus) is enhanced in asthma.
Defective innate defence	Formation of neutrophilic extracellular traps in asthma	Mucus over-production in asthma, enhanced numbers of eosinophils and cationic (positively charged) proteins in asthma.
Target cells for infection	Variable expression of ciliated epithelial cells targeted by rhinovirus type C.	
Viral replication and persistence		
Replicative phase and clearance of virus	Enhanced STING pathway activity in asthma, reduced viral clearance in some asthma patients.	
Host response to viral infection		
Response to viral infection	Reduced innate interferon production in asthma, synergy between allergic and viral responses, exaggerated epithelial responses in asthma.	

FIGURE 9.1 Overview of relevant mechanisms of viral infection in asthma patients: Responses to respiratory virus that may differ between asthma patients and healthy individuals. First column shows the various processes, second column shows differences that likely underlie heterogeneous responses to a respiratory viral infection in asthma, and third column shows differences without apparent effect.

Most respiratory viral infections are due to rhinovirus and less so by respiratory syncytial virus (RSV), coronavirus, and influenza, which may relate to the number of species within each viral genus and how well the virus spreads (2–4). For example, there now have been around 170 species of rhinovirus identified circulating worldwide (5), whereas there are only some genotypes of two subtypes of RSV, A and B (6). Apart from some coronaviruses such as SARS-CoV-2, SARS-CoV-1, and influenza, most respiratory viral infections cause relatively minor symptoms, and infections resolve quickly in individuals without asthma. Individuals with asthma frequently have acute worsening of asthma symptoms with a respiratory viral infection, which is associated with increased airway inflammation and enhanced airway hyperresponsiveness (7, 8). The impact of a respiratory viral infection depends on the severity and control of asthma. Whereas a respiratory viral infection in a well-controlled mild asthma patient may increase symptoms that merely require an adjustment of their maintenance and rescue medications, a poorly controlled asthma patient or a patient with severe asthma typically experiences an asthma exacerbation that requires oral corticosteroids and possibly hospitalization (7). The impact of a respiratory viral infection depends also on the virus type. Surprisingly, SARS-CoV-2 infections in asthma patients had relatively mild consequences, generally leading to slight variability in asthma symptoms (9). Rhinovirus that causes the common cold are the main inducers of an asthma exacerbation (10), emphasizing that the pathogenicity of a virus in healthy individuals does not directly relate to an exacerbation. So why does a respiratory viral infection in asthma patients have a very different effect from that in healthy individuals?

9.3 INFECTIVITY: ABILITY OF A VIRUS TO INFECT A CELL

Infectivity of a virus is determined by the nature of the virus and how well a virus transmits, i.e. survives its way from release by the spreading donor to the next host. "Survival" may not be the right term, as technically a virus is not a living organism. A virus can lose its capacity to infect and replicate in host cells. For example, rhinoviruses are acid and thermolabile (11). In virus challenge in man (CHIM) studies with rhinovirus 16 (RV16), it was observed that 20–30 minutes in solution without ice markedly reduced infectivity. Viruses can spread by aerosol and via surfaces, but not all viruses use both routes equally well. Once a viral particle enters the nasal compartment, it has to bind to a target cell and enter that cell to replicate. Viral species dock onto molecules that are expressed at the cell's surface, a so-called *porte d'entrée*, which facilitates infection of the cell. An overview of these cell surface molecules for the various viral species is provided in Table 9.1. The binding of the virus to these docking proteins is mediated by viral spike proteins. There is evidence suggesting a role for accessory molecules that promote binding of the spike proteins to docking proteins (12). At physiological pH, viral particles are negatively charged and thus may also interact with positively charged proteins at the cell surface, aiding binding to docking proteins.

TABLE 9.1
Respiratory Viruses and Their Docking Proteins

Viral species	Viral protein	Host protein
RV-A +-B (major group)	Capsid protein VP1	ICAM-1
Some RV-A (minor group)	Likely capsid protein VP2 (for RV2)	LDLR
RV-C	Likely and primarily capsid protein VP3	Co-receptor/CDHR3 (ciliated cells)
Coronavirus	Spike protein	CD13
SARS	Spike protein	ACE2
MERS	Spike protein	Dipeptidyl peptidase 4
Adenovirus	Penton base protein (RGD)	Coxsackievirus adenovirus receptor
Influenza	Hemagglutinin	*av* integrin
		sialic acid R
RSV	G protein (attachment)	Heparan sulphate
	F protein (fusion)	IGF1R/translocated nucleolin

Source: Overview of viral protein and their docking sites. An interesting paper showing efforts to interfere with viral attachment for influenza and coronavirus is that by Borisevich et al. Molecular Modelling of Viral Type I Fusion Proteins: Inhibitors of Influenza Virus Hemagglutinin and the Spike Protein of Coronavirus. *Viruses.* 2023 Mar 31;15 (4):902.

The expression of molecules that serve as docking sites differs between cell types, determining whether cells can be infected or not, and may differ for a cell type due to various conditions. For example, the expression of ACE2, the docking site for SARS viruses, on airway epithelial cells is reduced by Th2 mediators like IL-13 (9, 13). This may be an explanation for the minor effects of SARS viruses in asthma patients. ICAM1, which is the docking protein for most rhinoviruses, is a membrane-bound protein. Once ICAM1-expressing cells are exposed to interferon as part of the anti-viral response, the cell will start to generate an alternatively spliced form of ICAM1 that is soluble (14). This prevents more rhinovirus from infecting uninfected cells, as soluble ICAM1 has been found to be protective by its ability to bind unbound viral particles. Previously it has been shown that asthma patients were more susceptible to rhinovirus infection due to underlying airway inflammation consisting of cells that expressed more ICAM1 (14, 15). Interestingly, studies of cohabitating couples with similar infectious exposure risks where one spouse had asthma and the other did not found no differences between individuals for susceptibility to infection (16).

9.4 PREVENTING INFECTION

Both the innate and adaptive immune system influence the capacity of viruses to infect target cells. Because of their overall negative charge, viral particles have difficulty in passing the negatively charged mucus layer (17), unless the mucus layer is damaged, as seen with chronic respiratory diseases. However, studies on the prevalence of SARS-CoV-2 infections in patients with cystic fibrosis or primary ciliary dyskinesia have not revealed differences compared to the healthy population, but this may be different for other viruses.

Several innate immune cells have the capacity to engulf and inactivate (e.g. by reactive oxygen species) viruses, such as macrophages, which may be facilitated by opsonins like surfactant protein-A (18). Opsonins are extracellular proteins that can bind to pathogens such as viruses and particulate matter, promoting their phagocytosis. Eosinophilic granulocytes can bind and take up viruses by a major basic protein-mediated process (19). In addition, both neutrophilic and eosinophilic granulocytes have been shown to be able to release their nuclear DNA, forming extracellular traps (neutrophil and eosinophil extracellular traps [NETs and EETs]) that can capture viruses (20, 21). Finally, either due to vaccination or earlier similar or identical infections, protective antibodies may interfere with infection by blocking the interaction of viral spike proteins with target cell docking proteins. The predominant immunoglobulins at mucosal surfaces are IgA and IgM (22). These are typically produced by B cells under the epithelial layer in the lamina propria and can be transported to the apical side (i.e. the lumen) by the polymeric immunoglobulin receptor expressed at the basal side (23). This mechanism may facilitate removal of extra- and intracellular viruses (24), in which the apically released secretory IgA and IgM (sIgA, sIgM) have additional functions such as activating eosinophils via a receptor that binds free secretory component and sIgA (25). Most vaccinations are aimed at boosting an IgG response, but it should be realized that binding of viruses to their target cell is a rapid process, taking approximately an hour. Therefore, to be effective, antibodies have to be present in relatively high titers at the site of initial exposure. Once viral particles spread from the initially infected cells, the antibody titer may have increased, reducing further infection. Generally, it is difficult to prevent viral infections, but the course of the infection may be significantly attenuated by the presence of these protective antibodies.

9.5 INFECTION AND VIRAL REPLICATION

The major target cells in the nasal compartment are macrophages and nasal and subsequently bronchial epithelial cells, particularly ciliated epithelial cells. The epithelial cells are far more abundant than macrophages and therefore likely the predominant target cell. Bound viral particles either fuse with the cell membrane or are taken up and disassembled in the cytosol, where they release their viral genetic material in the host cell for replication. The processes leading to replication vary between viruses. However, coronavirus and rhinovirus, which are both single-stranded RNA viruses, follow a comparable path, which involves the formation of replication organelles (26). HRV-2B, which is a non-structural transmembrane protein of rhinoviruses, releases STING (stimulator of interferon genes) by interfering with the endoplasmic reticulum Ca2+ homeostasis (27). Among others, STING is a sensor of intracellular double-stranded (ds) DNA and via the cGAS-STING pathway will induce interferon production and an inflammatory response (28). However, the rhinovirus-induced release and activation of STING facilitates the binding of phosphatidylinositol-4-phosphate, which promotes transfer of STING to replicating organelles where STING will work as a scaffold (27). This trafficking occurred two to four hours post-viral exposure, again illustrating that infection is a rapid process. The replicative phase (in this study, six to eight hours after viral exposure) of rhinovirus occurs in these replication organelles.

In an earlier study with a GMP-prepared rhinovirus 16 (RV16UB), it was reported that varying doses did not affect the outcome of the infection, but the higher the dose, the earlier the viral peak was obtained (unpublished data). Studies looking into differences in viral load or between healthy individuals and asthma patients have been contradictory. In a prospective study (29) of natural infections, no differences were found over time in viral load between asthma patients and healthy individuals.

9.6 HOST RESPONSE TO VIRAL REPLICATION

During viral replication, viral dsRNA is generated, which triggers various anti-viral processes (30). Although endogenous dsRNA is produced, during normal cellular processes, the apparent abundancy of viral dsRNA will only trigger these responses. dsRNA is sensed by specific proteins such as RIG-I (retinoic acid-inducible gene-I), MDA5 (melanoma differentiation-associated protein 5), TLR-3 (toll-like receptor 3), and PKR (protein kinase R) (31–34). RIG-I, MDA5, and TLR-3 will induce an interferon response, which sets off the anti-viral response (33). PKR, when activated, will phosphorylate eukaryotic initiation factor 2 alpha, which will shut off protein synthesis (34). The enzyme OAS (2′-5′-oligoadenylate synthase) induced by interferon will promote RNA degradation by activating a latent ribonuclease (RNase-L) (35, 36). These and additional processes can lead to cell death (apoptosis), preventing further replication and spreading of virus. These dying cells will subsequently be phagocytosed to clear the infective virus.

Individuals respond to viral infections heterogeneously, and each virus type triggers a different response as they have evolved to manipulate or escape anti-viral responses. An example is the production of IL-10 by macrophages after exposure to the rhinovirus strain, RV14. Interestingly, a recently identified subpopulation of ciliated cells that are highly infectable due to their low interferon response suggests that local anti-viral responses can be determined by the presence of these distinct subsets of ciliated cells (37).

Individuals challenged with a fixed dose of virus, such as has been performed with RV16, has demonstrated that individual interferon responses and viral clearance differs between individuals (38). The regulation of interferon responses is highly complex, consisting of various interferon types (39).

9.7 DEFECTIVE INTERFERON RESPONSE IN ASTHMA

A similar variation of the interferon and anti-viral responses seen for healthy individuals is to be expected for asthma patients (40). It has been shown that the interferon responses to virus, in particular interferon-beta and -lambda, are impaired in the peripheral blood and airway mononuclear cells and epithelial cells for asthma patients (41–44). However, other studies have not been able to reproduce these findings (45–48). Possible explanations for these discrepant findings may be related to the severity and control of asthma and to experimental design. *In vivo* testing of mucosal epithelial cells may be influenced by other local effector cells, whereas *in vitro* these cellular interactions may be lost. Another interesting aspect of interferon-gamma production is that the mRNA encoding interferon-gamma can activate PKR via its pseudo-knot structure and down-regulate the interferon-gamma responses (49). This suggests that interferon production's profound impact on cell function is tailored by a negative feedback loop. Recently, another study reported that the viral infection of primary airway epithelial cells from asthma patients caused excessive RIG-I inflammasome activation, which impaired interferon production (50).

Although it would be expected that defective interferon production would affect viral load over time, studies have found no pronounced difference between viral loads in airway epithelial cells from asthma patients and healthy individuals. However, rhinovirus clearance from airway epithelial cells from some but not all asthma patients may be delayed (40, 50).

9.8 UNDERLYING CAUSES OF VIRUS-INDUCED EXACERBATIONS OF ASTHMA

The most obvious explanation for a viral-induced asthma exacerbation is the synergy between virus-induced and the allergen-induced immune responses, which is supported

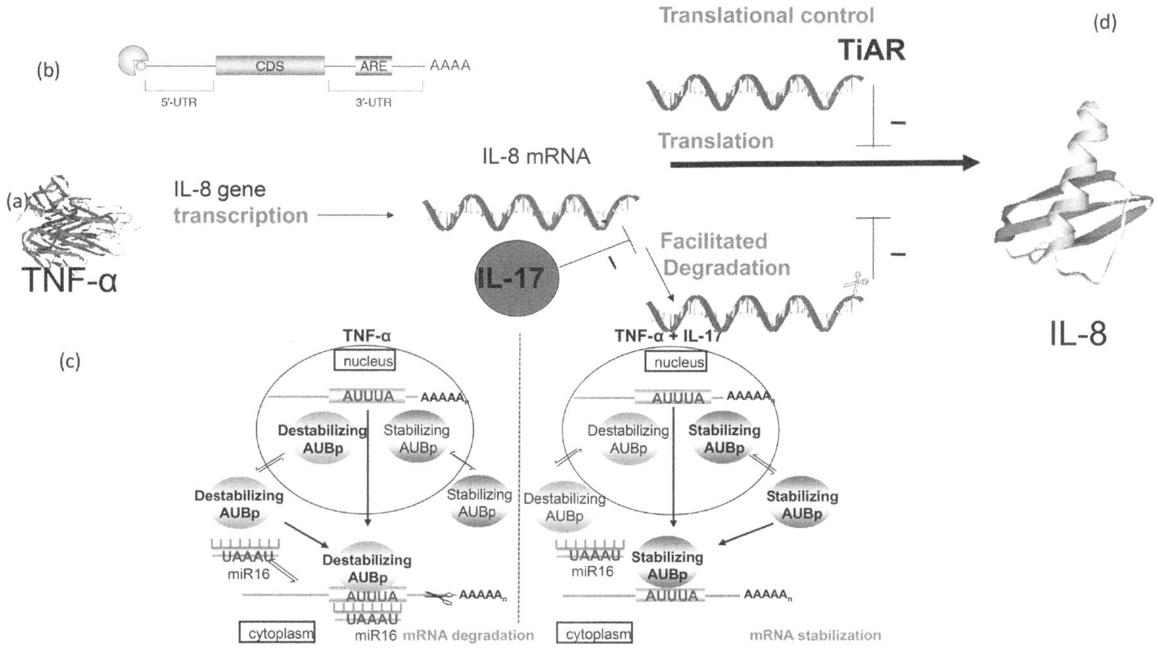

FIGURE 9.2 Defective translational control underlying exaggerated responses to a viral infection: Schematic presentation of how response gene expression is controlled, shown here for interleukin (IL)-8 (CXCL8). **(a)** Various stimuli can induce IL-8 gene transcription. There are around 800 response genes, many of which have been implicated in asthma, but only those that are transcribed at a certain stage are subjected to the subsequent processes. The transcript, mRNA **(b)**, consists of a coding sequence (CDS), encoding the protein, a 5′ - and 3′-untranslated region (UTR) and a poly A tail ($AAAAA_n$). These UTRs contain information for the cell, such as where to direct the transcript and how long before it should be degraded. Transcripts encoding a response protein typically are degraded rapidly (half-life ranges from minutes to an hour). AU-rich elements (ARE; also shown here as AUUUA) in the 3′-UTR have been particularly implicated in facilitating rapid mRNA degradation. Various mediators, some of which are generated during a viral infection, influence mRNA degradation. IL-17 (found in asthma) and IL-1β (generated during viral infection), for example, inhibit degradation of IL-8 mRNA, which leads to an exaggerated production of the encoded response gene, in this case IL–8. Degradation and stabilization are guided by AU-binding proteins (AUBp; **[c]**). In addition, there is regulation at the translational level by TiAR, a translational repressor that is translocated from the nucleus to the cytoplasm **(d)**, that limits the production of IL–8. It has been demonstrated that translocation of TiAR in bronchial epithelial cells from asthma patients is defective, leading to exaggerated IL-8 responses.

by several studies. For example, Spiteri *et al.* (51) demonstrated that nasal epithelial cells from sensitized asthma patients during a period of allergen exposure, express more ICAM-1, which may enable an infection with a higher viral load to occur. In a recent study, the exacerbation in allergen-sensitized mice was found to be induced by dsDNA and likely associated proteins in NETs but not EETs (52). Interestingly, breakdown of dsDNA by DNAses did substantially reduce the virus-induced exacerbation. Levels of IL-33, an alarmin released by airway epithelial cells in allergic asthma, were enhanced during a virus-induced exacerbation in a murine model of allergic asthma and inhibition of IL-33 attenuated this response (53). Others have shown that airway epithelial cells displayed exaggerated responses to stimuli manifesting as an enhanced production of various inflammatory and immune mediators (54). More recently, a defective translational control of response genes in bronchial epithelial cells from asthma patients has been reported that may explain these earlier findings (55). TIAR, which resides in the nucleus and controls the translation of hundreds of response genes, is translocated to the cytoplasm to halt the translation of response genes. This inhibitory mechanism limits responses, such as the production of inflammatory mediators (Figure 9.2). Defective control of response genes may lead to the exaggerated production of the proteins encoded by these response genes and underlie the enhanced responses by airway epithelial cells to a virus (56). Interestingly, bronchial epithelial cells collected a week after an *in vivo* rhinovirus challenge showed further enhanced responsiveness specifically involving endothelin-1, a potent bronchoconstrictor, compared to the primary bronchial epithelial cells collected prior to the viral challenge (57). This finding is consistent with the reported enhanced airway hyperresponsiveness in asthma patients post-viral challenge (8).

In infants, rhinoviruses type C and type A and RSV are the main inducers of bronchiolitis manifested as wheezing and have been linked to the subsequent development of childhood asthma (58). The epidemiological association of early-life respiratory viral infections with childhood asthma has led to the hypothesis that early-life viral infections may underlie the development of asthma (59).

Although not completely proven, the synergistic interaction of allergic and viral responses may lead to clinical asthma.

9.9 STRUCTURAL AND PHYSIOLOGICAL EFFECTS OF VIRAL INFECTION

Airway epithelial cells are polarized cells, which implies that cells can exercise distinct functions at their apical (luminal) and basolateral (site interacting with extracellular matrix) sides. A key characteristic of polarized cells are tight junctions, which may trigger polarization. Tight junctions interconnect neighbouring cells and limit paracellular movement of molecules and thus contribute to the physical barrier function of mucosal epithelial cells. Upon viral infection, epithelial cells will lose their polarized phenotype, and tight junctions are disrupted, leading to increased permeability across the mucosal barrier (60). This loss of tight junctions and polarization appears to recover after approximately seven days (unpublished data).

As a consequence of viral infection, anti-viral airway immune responses may be conditioned to respond differently. For example, the development of secondary bacterial infections (61) may occur due to induction of IDO1 (indoleamine 2,3-dioxygenase 1) by interferons (62). IDO1 oxidizes the essential amino acid tryptophan to formyl-L-kynurenine, which is degraded further by the kynurenine pathway to various metabolites, some of which are cytotoxic. Paradoxically, depletion of tryptophan interferes with viral replication, but viruses also require tryptophan for their synthesis (63). The formation of cytotoxic metabolites, as well the depletion of tryptophan, inhibit activation of immune cells, making the airway more vulnerable to bacterial infections (64). This pathway may be more particularly relevant for influenza infection than rhinovirus infections, which do not seem to lead to enhanced IDO1 expression (65). Interestingly, the IL-4 and IL-13 cytokines related to allergic inflammation, inhibit IDO1 expression (66), which may explain the reduced basal IDO1 activity in lung lumen of asthma patients (65).

9.10 EFFECTS OF INTERVENTIONS

There is a delay of a couple of days between infection and the worsening of symptoms in asthma, which is particularly clear from CHIM studies when the exact time of exposure to the virus is known. This makes development of an effective anti-viral treatment that can interfere with viral replication difficult to achieve for an infected asthma patient. Based on findings that interferon production is defective in asthma, trials with nebulized interferon type beta (67–69) were attempted but unfortunately met with futility.

Glucocorticoids, potent anti-inflammatory agents, are the cornerstone treatment for asthma exacerbations (70) and largely work by reducing viral-induced eosinophilic inflammation and interferon production and enhancing the production of CXCL-10, a strong pro-inflammatory stimulus (71–73). Despite the proposed effects of glucocorticoids on the anti-viral interferon response, there is no evidence that they affect viral load.

The initial case presented in this chapter of a severe asthma patient who developed a viral-induced asthma exacerbation despite being on reslizumab, an anti-IL-5 treatment (1) further emphasizes the complex host response to viral infections, which can also induce non-eosinophilic inflammation (74).

9.11 SUMMARY

In this chapter we aimed to provide an overview of the various molecular mechanisms implicated in respiratory viral infections, which focused on differences between asthma patients and healthy individuals. Although this overview is by no means complete, it provides an overall perspective of the intricate relationship between the host and virus, which also involves other effector cells such as B lymphocytes, regulatory T cells, and innate lymphoid cells (35). Understanding the nuances discussed about viral infectivity should help facilitate discussions between healthcare providers and their asthma patients about practical approaches to minimize the morbidity associated with acute viral infections and asthma exacerbations.

REFERENCES

1. McDowell PJ, Diver S, Yang F, Borg C, Busby J, Brown V, Shrimanker R, Cox C, Brightling CE, Chaudhuri R, Pavord ID, Heaney LG; Medical research council: Refractory asthma stratification programme (RASP-UK Consortium). The inflammatory profile of exacerbations in patients with severe refractory eosinophilic asthma receiving mepolizumab (the MEX study): a prospective observational study. *Lancet Respir Med.* 2021 Oct;9(10):1174–84
2. Principi N, Autore G, Ramundo G, Esposito S. Epidemiology of respiratory infections during the COVID-19 pandemic. *Viruses.* 2023 May 13;15(5):1160
3. Taylor S, Lopez P, Weckx L, Borja-Tabora C, Ulloa-Gutierrez R, Lazcano-Ponce E, Kerdpanich A, Angel Rodriguez Weber M, Mascareñas de Los Santos A, Tinoco JC, Safadi MA, Lim FS, Hernandez-de Mezerville M, Faingezicht I, Cruz-Valdez A, Feng Y, Li P, Durviaux S, Haars G, Roy-Ghanta S, Vaughn DW, Nolan T. Respiratory viruses and influenza-like illness: Epidemiology and outcomes in children aged 6 months to 10 years in a multi-country population sample. *J Infect.* 2017 Jan;74(1):29–41
4. Lam TT, Tang JW, Lai FY, Zaraket H, Dbaibo G, Bialasiewicz S, Tozer S, Heraud JM, Drews SJ, Hachette T, Chan PK, Koay ES, Lee HK, Tee KK, Liu Y, Fraaij P, Jennings L, Waris M, Krajden M, Corriveau A, Jalal H, Nishimura H, Nymadawa P, Badarch D, Watanabe A, Kabanda A, Sloots T, Kok J, Dwyer DE, Koopmans M; INSPIRE (International Network for the Sequencing of Respiratory Viruses). Comparative global epidemiology of influenza, respiratory syncytial and parainfluenza viruses, 2010–2015. *J Infect.* 2019 Oct;79(4):373–82
5. Esneau C, Duff AC, Bartlett NW. Understanding rhinovirus circulation and impact on illness. *Viruses.* 2022 Jan 13;14(1):141

6. Tabor DE, Fernandes F, Langedijk AC, Wilkins D, Lebbink RJ, Tovchigrechko A, Ruzin A, Kragten-Tabatabaie L, Jin H, Esser MT, Bont LJ, Abram ME; INFORM-RSV Study Group. Global molecular epidemiology of respiratory syncytial virus from the 2017–2018 INFORM-RSV study. *J Clin Microbiol.* 2020 Dec 17;59(1):e01828–20
7. https://ginasthma.org/wp-content/uploads/2024/05/GINA-2024-Strategy-Report-24_05_22_WMS.pdf (per October 2024)
8. Gern JE, Calhoun W, Swenson C, Shen G, Busse WW. Rhinovirus infection preferentially increases lower airway responsiveness in allergic subjects. *Am J Respir Crit Care Med.* 1997 Jun;155(6):1872–6
9. McPhee C, Yevdokimova K, Rogers L, Kraft M. The SARS-CoV-2 pandemic and asthma: What we have learned and what is still unknown. *J Allergy Clin Immunol.* 2023 Dec;152(6):1376–81
10. Jackson DJ, Gern JE. Rhinovirus infections and their roles in asthma: etiology and exacerbations. *J Allergy Clin Immunol Pract.* 2022 Mar;10(3):673–81
11. Hughes JH, Mitchell M, Hamparian VV. Rhinoviruses: kinetics of ultraviolet inactivation and effects of UV and heat on immunogenicity. *Arch Virol.* 1979;61(4):313–9
12. Everman JL, Sajuthi S, Saef B, Rios C, Stoner AM, Numata M, Hu D, Eng C, Oh S, Rodriguez-Santana J, Vladar EK, Voelker DR, Burchard EG, Seibold MA. Functional genomics of CDHR3 confirms its role in HRV-C infection and childhood asthma exacerbations. *J Allergy Clin Immunol.* 2019 Oct;144(4):962–71
13. Kimura H, Francisco D, Conway M, Martinez FD, Vercelli D, Polverino F, Billheimer D, Kraft M. Type 2 inflammation modulates ACE2 and TMPRSS2 in airway epithelial cells. *J Allergy Clin Immunol.* 2020 Jul;146(1):80–8
14. Whiteman SC, Spiteri MA. IFN-gamma regulation of ICAM-1 receptors in bronchial epithelial cells: soluble ICAM-1 release inhibits human rhinovirus infection. *J Inflamm.* 2008 Jun 5;5:8
15. Bianco A, Whiteman SC, Sethi SK, Allen JT, Knight RA, Spiteri MA. Expression of intercellular adhesion molecule-1 (ICAM-1) in nasal epithelial cells of atopic subjects: a mechanism for increased rhinovirus infection? *Clin Exp Immunol.* 2000 Aug;121(2):339–45
16. Corne JM, Marshall C, Smith S, Schreiber J, Sanderson G, Holgate ST, Johnston SL. Frequency, severity, and duration of rhinovirus infections in asthmatic and non-asthmatic individuals: a longitudinal cohort study. *Lancet.* 2002 Mar 9;359(9309):831–4
17. Kaler L, Iverson E, Bader S, Song D, Scull MA, Duncan GA. Influenza A virus diffusion through mucus gel networks. *Commun Biol.* 2022 Mar 22;5(1):249. https://doi.org/10.1038/s42003-022-03204-3. PMID: 35318436; PMCID: PMC8941132.
18. Barr FE, Pedigo H, Johnson TR, Shepherd VL. Surfactant protein-A enhances uptake of respiratory syncytial virus by monocytes and U937 macrophages. *Am J Respir Cell Mol Biol.* 2000 Nov;23(5):586–92
19. Sabogal Piñeros YS, Bal SM, Dijkhuis A, Majoor CJ, Dierdorp BS, Dekker T, Hoefsmit EP, Bonta PI, Picavet D, van der Wel NN, Koenderman L, Sterk PJ, Ravanetti L, Lutter R. Eosinophils capture viruses, a capacity that is defective in asthma. *Allergy.* 2019 Oct;74(10):1898–909
20. Jenne CN, Wong CH, Zemp FJ, McDonald B, Rahman MM, Forsyth PA, McFadden G, Kubes P. Neutrophils recruited to sites of infection protect from virus challenge by releasing neutrophil extracellular traps. *Cell Host Microbe.* 2013 Feb 13;13(2):169–80
21. Cortjens B, de Boer OJ, de Jong R, Antonis AF, Sabogal Piñeros YS, Lutter R, van Woensel JB, Bem RA. Neutrophil extracellular traps cause airway obstruction during respiratory syncytial virus disease. *J Pathol.* 2016 Feb;238(3):401–11
22. Matsumoto ML. Molecular mechanisms of multimeric assembly of IgM and IgA. *Annu Rev Immunol.* 2022 Apr 26;40:221–47. https://doi.org/10.1146/annurev-immunol-101320-123742
23. Norderhaug IN, Johansen FE, Schjerven H, Brandtzaeg P. Regulation of the formation and external transport of secretory immunoglobulins. *Crit Rev Immunol.* 1999;19(5–6):481–508
24. Schwartz-Cornil I, Benureau Y, Greenberg H, Hendrickson BA, Cohen J. Heterologous protection induced by the inner capsid proteins of rotavirus requires transcytosis of mucosal immunoglobulins. *J Virol.* 2002 Aug;76(16):8110–7
25. Lamkhioued B, Gounni AS, Gruart V, Pierce A, Capron A, Capron M. Human eosinophils express a receptor for secretory component. Role in secretory IgA-dependent activation. *Eur J Immunol.* 1995 Jan;25(1):117–25
26. den Boon JA, Nishikiori M, Zhan H, Ahlquist P. Positive-strand RNA virus genome replication organelles: structure, assembly, control. *Trends Genet.* 2024 Aug;40(8):681–93
27. Triantafilou M, Ramanjulu J, Booty LM, Jimenez-Duran G, Keles H, Saunders K, Nevins N, Koppe E, Modis LK, Pesiridis GS, Bertin J, Triantafilou K. Human rhinovirus promotes STING trafficking to replication organelles to promote viral replication. *Nat Commun.* 2022 Mar 17;13(1):1406
28. Zhang X, Bai XC, Chen ZJ. Structures and mechanisms in the cGAS-STING innate immunity pathway. *Immunity.* 2020 Jul 14;53(1):43–53
29. van Elden LJ, Sachs AP, van Loon AM, Haarman M, van de Vijver DA, Kimman TG, Zuithoff P, Schipper PJ, Verheij TJ, Nijhuis M. Enhanced severity of virus associated lower respiratory tract disease in asthma patients may not be associated with delayed viral clearance and increased viral load in the upper respiratory tract. *J Clin Virol.* 2008 Feb;41(2):116–21
30. Cottrell KA, Andrews RJ, Bass BL. The competitive landscape of the dsRNA world. *Mol Cell.* 2024 Jan 4;84(1):107–19
31. Thoresen D, Wang W, Galls D, Guo R, Xu L, Pyle AM. The molecular mechanism of RIG-I activation and signaling. *Immunol Rev.* 2021 Nov;304(1):154–68
32. Dias Junior AG, Sampaio NG, Rehwinkel J. A Balancing act: MDA5 in antiviral immunity and autoinflammation. *Trends Microbiol.* 2019 Jan;27(1):75–85
33. Li J, Yu J, Shen A, Lai S, Liu Z, He TS. The RNA-binding proteins regulate innate antiviral immune signaling by modulating pattern recognition receptors. *Virol J.* 2024 Sep 20;21(1):225
34. Hur S. Double-stranded RNA sensors and modulators in innate immunity. *Annu Rev Immunol.* 2019 Apr 26;37:349–75
35. Koul A, Hui LT, Lubna N, McKenna SA. Distinct domain organization and diversity of 2'-5'-oligoadenylate synthetases. *Biochem Cell Biol.* 2024 Aug 1;102(4):305–18.
36. Yang Z, Mitländer H, Vuorinen T, Finotto S. Mechanism of rhinovirus immunity and asthma. *Front Immunol.* 2021 Oct 6;12:731846. Erratum in: *Front Immunol.* 2021 Nov 16;12:800020
37. Basnet S, Mohanty C, Bochkov YA, Brockman-Schneider RA, Kendziorski C, Gern JE. Rhinovirus C causes

heterogeneous infection and gene expression in airway epithelial cell subsets. *Mucosal Immunol.* 2023 Aug;16(4):386–98.
38. Lutter R, Teitsma-Jansen A, Floris E, Lone-Latif S, Ravi A, Sabogal Pineros YS, Dekker T, Smids B, Khurshid R, Aparicio-Vergara M, Ruijschop R, Ravanetti L, Calame W, Kardinaal A, Albers R. The dietary intake of carrot-derived rhamnogalacturonan-I accelerates and augments the innate immune and anti-viral interferon response to rhinovirus infection and reduces duration and severity of symptoms in humans in a randomized trial. *Nutrients.* 2021 Dec 8;13(12):4395
39. Mesev EV, LeDesma RA, Ploss A. Decoding type I and III interferon signalling during viral infection. *Nat Microbiol.* 2019 Jun;4(6):914–24.
40. Ravi A, Chang M, van de Pol M, Yang S, Aliprantis A, Thornton B, Carayannopoulos LN, Bautmans A, Robberechts M, De Lepeleire I, Singh D, Hohlfeld JM, Sterk PJ, Krug N. Lutter R; U-BIOPRED study group. Rhinovirus-16 induced temporal interferon responses in nasal epithelium links with viral clearance and symptoms. *Clin Exp Allergy.* 2019 Dec;49(12):1587–97
41. Wark PA, Johnston SL, Bucchieri F, Powell R, Puddicombe S, Laza-Stanca V, Holgate ST, Davies DE. Asthmatic bronchial epithelial cells have a deficient innate immune response to infection with rhinovirus. *J Exp Med.* 2005;201:937–47
42. Gehlhar K, Bilitewski C, Reinitz-Rademacher K, Rohde G, Bufe A. Impaired virus-induced interferon-alpha2 release in adult asthmatic patients. *Clin Exp Allergy* 2006;36:331–7
43. Papadopoulos NG, Stanciu LA, Papi A, Holgate ST, Johnston SL. Rhinovirus-induced alterations on peripheral blood mononuclear cell phenotype and costimulatory molecule expression in normal and atopic asthmatic subjects. *Clin Exp Allergy* 2002;32:537–42
44. Contoli M, Message SD, Laza-Stanca V, Edwards MR, Wark PA, Bartlett NW, Kebadze T, Mallia P, Stanciu LA, Parker HL, et al. Role of deficient type III interferon-lambda production in asthma exacerbations. *Nat Med.* 2006;12:1023–6
45. Sykes A, Macintyre J, Edwards MR, Del Rosario A, Haas J, Gielen V, Kon OM, McHale M, Johnston SL. Rhinovirus-induced interferon production is not deficient in well controlled asthma. *Thorax* 2014;69: 240–6
46. DeMore JP, Weisshaar EH, Vrtis RF, Swenson CA, Evans MD, Morin A, Hazel E, Bork JA, Kakumanu S, Sorkness R, et al. Similar colds in subjects with allergic asthma and nonatopic subjects after inoculation with rhinovirus–16. *J Allergy Clin Immunol* 2009;124: 245–52.
47. Bochkov YA, Hanson KM, Keles S, Brockman-Schneider RA, Jarjour NN, Gern JE. Rhinovirus-induced modulation of gene expression in bronchial epithelial cells from subjects with asthma. *Mucosal Immunol.* 2010;3:69–80.
48. Kennedy JL, Shaker M, McMeen V, Gern J, Carper H, Murphy D, Lee WM, Bochkov YA, Vrtis RF, Platts-Mills T, et al. Comparison of viral load in individuals with and without asthma during infections with rhinovirus. *Am J Respir Crit Care Med* 2014;189:532–9
49. Kaempfer R. Interferon-gamma mRNA attenuates its own translation by activating PKR: a molecular basis for the therapeutic effect of interferon-beta in multiple sclerosis. *Cell Res.* 2006 Feb;16(2):148–53
50. Radzikowska U, Eljaszewicz A, Tan G, Stocker N, Heider A, Westermann P, Steiner S, Dreher A, Wawrzyniak P, Rückert B, Rodriguez-Coira J, Zhakparov D, Huang M, Jakiela B, Sanak M, Moniuszko M, O'Mahony L, Jutel M, Kebadze T, Jackson DJ, Edwards MR, Thiel V, Johnston SL, Akdis CA, Sokolowska M. Rhinovirus-induced epithelial RIG-I inflammasome suppresses antiviral immunity and promotes inflammation in asthma and COVID–19. *Nat Commun.* 2023 Apr 22;14(1):2329. Erratum in: *Nat Commun.* 2023 Jun 13;14(1):3493
51. Bianco A, Whiteman SC, Sethi SK, Allen JT, Knight RA, Spiteri MA. Expression of intercellular adhesion molecule-1 (ICAM-1) in nasal epithelial cells of atopic subjects: a mechanism for increased rhinovirus infection? *Clin Exp Immunol.* 2000 Aug;121(2):339–45
52. Toussaint M, Jackson DJ, Swieboda D, Guedán A, Tsourouktsoglou TD, Ching YM, Radermecker C, Makrinioti H, Aniscenko J, Bartlett NW, Edwards MR, Solari R, Farnir F, Papayannopoulos V, Bureau F, Marichal T, Johnston SL. Host DNA released by NETosis promotes rhinovirus-induced type-2 allergic asthma exacerbation. *Nat Med.* 2017 Jun;23(6):681–91. Erratum in: Nat Med. 2017 Nov 7;23(11):1384
53. Ravanetti L, Dijkhuis A, Dekker T, Sabogal Pineros YS, Ravi A, Dierdorp BS, Erjefält JS, Mori M, Pavlidis S, Adcock IM, Rao NL, Lutter R. IL-33 drives influenza-induced asthma exacerbations by halting innate and adaptive antiviral immunity. *J Allergy Clin Immunol.* 2019 Apr;143(4):1355–70.
54. Marini M, Vittori E, Hollemborg J, Mattoli S. Expression of the potent inflammatory cytokines, granulocyte-macrophage-colony-stimulating factor and interleukin-6 and interleukin-8, in bronchial epithelial cells of patients with asthma. *J Allergy Clin Immunol.* 1992 May;89(5):1001–9
55. Ravi A, Chowdhury S, Dijkhuis A, Bonta PI, Sterk PJ, Lutter R. Neutrophilic inflammation in asthma and defective epithelial translational control. *Eur Respir J.* 2019 Aug 15;54(2):1900547
56. Altman MC, Reeves SR, Parker AR, Whalen E, Misura KM, Barrow KA, James RG, Hallstrand TS, Ziegler SF, Debley JS. Interferon response to respiratory syncytial virus by bronchial epithelium from children with asthma is inversely correlated with pulmonary function. *J Allergy Clin Immunol.* 2018 Aug;142(2):451–9
57. Ravi A, Chowdhury S, Dijkhuis A, Dierdorp BS, Dekker T, Kruize R, Sabogal Piñeros YS, Majoor CJ, Sterk PJ, Lutter R. Imprinting of bronchial epithelial cells upon *in vivo* rhinovirus infection in people with asthma. *ERJ Open Res.* 2022 Apr 19;8(2):00522–2021
58. Hasegawa K, Mansbach JM, Bochkov YA, Gern JE, Piedra PA, Bauer CS, Teach SJ, Wu S, Sullivan AF, Camargo CA Jr. Association of rhinovirus c bronchiolitis and immunoglobulin e sensitization during infancy with development of recurrent wheeze. *JAMA Pediatr.* 2019 Jun 1;173(6):544–52
59. Sly PD, Kusel M, Holt PG. Do early-life viral infections cause asthma? *J Allergy Clin Immunol.* 2010 Jun;125(6):1202–5
60. Kast JI, McFarlane AJ, Głobińska A, Sokolowska M, Wawrzyniak P, Sanak M, Schwarze J, Akdis CA, Wanke K. Respiratory syncytial virus infection influences tight junction integrity. *Clin Exp Immunol.* 2017 Dec;190(3):351–9
61. Rynda-Apple A, Robinson KM, Alcorn JF. Influenza and bacterial superinfection: illuminating the immunologic mechanisms of disease. *Infect Immun.* 2015 Oct;83(10):3764–70
62. van der Sluijs KF, Nijhuis M, Levels JH, Florquin S, Mellor AL, Jansen HM, van der Poll T, Lutter R. Influenza-induced

expression of indoleamine 2,3-dioxygenase enhances interleukin-10 production and bacterial outgrowth during secondary pneumococcal pneumonia. *J Infect Dis.* 2006 Jan 15;193(2):214–22
63. Adams O, Besken K, Oberdörfer C, MacKenzie CR, Takikawa O, Däubener W. Role of indoleamine-2,3-dioxygenase in alpha/beta and gamma interferon-mediated antiviral effects against herpes simplex virus infections. *J Virol.* 2004 Mar;78(5):2632–6
64. Munn DH, Mellor AL. Indoleamine 2,3 dioxygenase and metabolic control of immune responses. *Trends Immunol.* 2013 Mar;34(3):137–43
65. van der Sluijs KF, van de Pol MA, Kulik W, Dijkhuis A, Smids BS, van Eijk HW, Karlas JA, Molenkamp R, Wolthers KC, Johnston SL, van der Zee JS, Sterk PJ, Lutter R; RESOLVE research team. Systemic tryptophan and kynurenine catabolite levels relate to severity of rhinovirus-induced asthma exacerbation: a prospective study with a parallel-group design. *Thorax.* 2013 Dec;68(12):1122–30
66. Yadav MC, Burudi EM, Alirezaei M, Flynn CC, Watry DD, Lanigan CM, Fox HS. IFN-gamma-induced IDO and WRS expression in microglia is differentially regulated by IL–4. *Glia.* 2007 Oct;55(13):1385–96
67. Djukanović R, Harrison T, Johnston SL, Gabbay F, Wark P, Thomson NC, Niven R, Singh D, Reddel HK, Davies DE, Marsden R, Boxall C, Dudley S, Plagnol V, Holgate ST, Monk P; INTERCIA study group. The effect of inhaled IFN-β on worsening of asthma symptoms caused by viral infections. A randomized trial. *Am J Respir Crit Care Med.* 2014 Jul 15;190(2):145–54
68. McCrae C, Olsson M, Gustafson P, Malmgren A, Aurell M, Fagerås M, Da Silva CA, Cavallin A, Paraskos J, Karlsson K, Wingren C, Monk P, Marsden R, Harrison T. INEXAS: A Phase 2 randomized trial of on-demand inhaled interferon beta-1a in severe asthmatics. *Clin Exp Allergy.* 2021 Feb;51(2):273–83
69. Watson A, Spalluto CM, McCrae C, Cellura D, Burke H, Cunoosamy D, Freeman A, Hicks A, Hühn M, Ostridge K, Staples KJ, Vaarala O, Wilkinson T. Dynamics of IFN-β responses during respiratory viral infection. Insights for therapeutic strategies. *Am J Respir Crit Care Med.* 2020 Jan 1;201(1):83–94
70. Sin DD, Man J, Sharpe H, Gan WQ, Man SF. Pharmacological management to reduce exacerbations in adults with asthma: a systematic review and meta-analysis. *JAMA.* 2004 Jul 21;292(3):367–76
71. Brightling CE, Green RH, Pavord ID. Biomarkers predicting response to corticosteroid therapy in asthma. *Treat Respir Med.* 2005;4(5):309–16
72. Singanayagam A, Glanville N, Girkin JL, Ching YM, Marcellini A, Porter JD, Toussaint M, Walton RP, Finney LJ, Aniscenko J, Zhu J, Trujillo-Torralbo MB, Calderazzo MA, Grainge C, Loo SL, Veerati PC, Pathinayake PS, Nichol KS, Reid AT, James PL, Solari R, Wark PAB, Knight DA, Moffatt MF, Cookson WO, Edwards MR, Mallia P, Bartlett NW, Johnston SL. Corticosteroid suppression of antiviral immunity increases bacterial loads and mucus production in COPD exacerbations. *Nat Commun.* 2018 Jun 8;9(1):2229
73. Gauthier M, Chakraborty K, Oriss TB, Raundhal M, Das S, Chen J, Huff R, Sinha A, Fajt M, Ray P, Wenzel SE, Ray A. Severe asthma in humans and mouse model suggests a CXCL10 signature underlies corticosteroid-resistant Th1 bias. *JCI Insight.* 2017 Jul 6;2(13):e94580
74. Sabogal Piñeros YS, Bal SM, van de Pol MA, Dierdorp BS, Dekker T, Dijkhuis A, Brinkman P, van der Sluijs KF, Zwinderman AH, Majoor CJ, Bonta PI, Ravanetti L, Sterk PJ, Lutter R. Anti-IL-5 in Mild asthma alters rhinovirus-induced macrophage, B-cell, and neutrophil responses (MATERIAL). A placebo-controlled, double-blind study. *Am J Respir Crit Care Med.* 2019 Feb 15;199(4):508–17

10 Asthma and Allergens

Anna Zhang, Sachin Baxi, and Wanda Phipatanakul

CASE

Kiara is a 10-year-old girl who was diagnosed with asthma at the age of three. She initially presented with multiple episodes of wheezing associated with viral upper respiratory infections in infancy. Around school age, she began to have more persistent symptoms of wheezing, necessitating frequent albuterol use. Despite the addition of daily maintenance with inhaled corticosteroid treatments, she continued to have difficulty with asthma exacerbations, especially during the winter and spring months. She was referred to an allergist for further evaluation. Further history was elicited including clear nasal discharge present on most days, and the development of itchy red eyes, clear nasal discharge, and frequent sneezing while at her grandmother's home, which has two cats. She had tried over-the-counter antihistamine therapy for these symptoms with limited results. She had no history of food allergies but did have eczema as an infant. Environmental history revealed the presence of mice and cockroaches in the home.

Physical exam showed injected conjunctivae and presence of Denny's lines. Nasal turbinates were edematous, pale, and boggy with clear rhinorrhea. There was a "cobblestone" appearance of her posterior pharynx. Cardiac, lung, and abdominal examinations were unremarkable. Skin exam showed scattered eczematous patches along the flexural areas of her upper and lower extremities.

Kiara underwent skin prick testing to an environmental allergen panel including common indoor and outdoor allergens with positive histamine and negative saline controls. Testing revealed sensitization to dust mite, cat, mouse, and cockroach, along with multiple tree and grass pollens. Testing was negative to dog, weeds, and molds.

Appropriate allergen avoidance and integrative pest management (IPM) strategies were discussed with Kiara's family. She was started on a leukotriene antagonist, a long-acting daily antihistamine, and a steroid nasal spray. The possibility of allergen immunotherapy was also discussed.

10.1 INTRODUCTION

Asthma is a heterogeneous disease that is influenced by multiple factors, including the environment, genetics, pollution, infection, and diet. Atopy, defined as a predisposition to developing allergic sensitization, is a strong predisposing factor for asthma development, and for over two decades, there has been increasing evidence that specific allergens can have a causative role in asthma development [1, 2]. Environmental allergen sensitivity can also play an important role in asthma disease severity and treatment. The percentage of patients with asthma sensitized to ≥1 environmental allergens approaches 80%, and atopy may be the causative factor in over 50% of asthma cases [3]. Increased exposure to allergens in sensitized individuals can lead to more asthma morbidity and increased healthcare utilization [4–6]. Amongst the many allergens found indoors, the primary aeroallergens to which asthmatics are sensitized include house dust mite, cat, dog, mouse, cockroach, and mold (Table 10.1). This chapter will describe specific indoor allergens, highlight their roles in asthma, and discuss strategies for avoidance and environmental remediation.

10.2 BRIEF IMMUNOLOGIC PRINCIPLES

In allergic asthma, individuals are sensitized to a variety of allergens. Upon re-exposure to an offending inhaled allergen, cross-linking of specific IgE occurs on the surface of mast cells and triggers a rapid release of inflammatory mediators from mast cells, including histamine, tryptase, and chymase. Within several hours, a late-phase reaction occurs that is characterized by release of leukotrienes, prostaglandins, and of CD4+ type 2 helper T cell cytokines such as IL-3, IL-4, IL-5, and IL–13. IL-4 is the major stimulus for IgE production, whereas IL-5 promotes eosinophil recruitment. The inflammatory mediator release causes increased vascular permeability, bronchial smooth muscle contraction, mucous secretion, and connective tissue matrix remodeling. The end result is chronic inflammation of the airways.

10.3 HOUSE DUST MITE

House dust mites are microscopic arachnids that thrive in warm, humid indoor environments. They are commonly found in bedding (mattresses and pillows) and other

DOI: 10.1201/9781003287209-13

TABLE 10.1
Indoor Allergen Classification

Common Name	Taxonomic Name	Major Allergen (s)	Molecular Weight(s) (kD)
House dust mite	*Dermatophagoides pteronyssinus, Dermatophagoides farinae*	Der p 1, Der f 1	24, 27
Cat	*Felis domesticus*	Fel d 1	17
Dog	*Canis familiaris*	Can f 1, Can f 2	23, 19
Cockroach	*Blatella germanica, Periplaneta americana*	Bla g 1, Bla g 2	46, 36
Mouse	*Mus musculus*	Mus m 1, Mus m 2	19,16

TABLE 10.2
Dust Mite Allergen Avoidance and Patient Education

Basic education principles	• Assess home environment. • Provide a general description of mites. • Avoid conditions for optimal dust mite growth (i.e. keep humidity <50%). • Identify local areas of dust mite growth (pillows, mattresses, box springs, carpet, upholstered furniture, draperies, stuffed animals).
Priorities for mites/allergens avoidance	**Bedroom** • Encase pillows (pore size <10 μm finely woven or vapor-permeable covers). • Encase mattress in vapor-permeable or plastic cover. • Encase box spring in vinyl or plastic. • Wash bedding weekly in hot water (>130° F). **Floor** • Vacuum weekly (wear mask; leave room 20 minutes after cleaning). • Ensure vacuum cleaner has good-quality bags (double thickness) and/or HEPA (high-efficiency particulate air) filter on air outlet. • Smooth floors cleaned by vacuuming plus damp mopping. • Loose rugs may be washed intermittently to remove allergens. **Furnishings** • If possible, replace with cleanable items that do not retain dust. • Possible compromise may be regularly washing loose covers of tightly woven cloth. **Long-term changes** • Reduce indoor relative humidity (A/C, dehumidifier, open windows). • Replace carpets with polished flooring (wood, vinyl, tile) if possible. • Replace upholstered furniture with leather, vinyl, or wood. • Replace draperies with shades or blinds that can be wiped down. • Avoid living in basements.

products with woven or stuffed material including stuffed animals. The most common species are *Dermatophagoides pteronyssinus* and *Dermatophagoides farinae*, and the primary allergens are Der p 1 and Der f 1. Proteases found in the dust mite's gut and fecal particles are potent inducers of allergic disease.

The association between house dust mite allergy and asthma has been well-characterized [1, 5]. In 1921, Kern first reported positive skin testing to house dust mites in asthmatics using dust from patients' homes [7]. House dust mite sensitization is present in over 50% of asthmatics and is a known risk factor for development of childhood asthma [8]. A study by Sporik et al. showed a relative risk of asthma development approximately five times greater in subjects with high levels of dust mite allergen exposure (>10 μg/g) [2]. Celedon et al. demonstrated that early exposure to house dust mite was associated with increased risk of asthma and late-onset wheezing [9].

There are several approaches to house dust mite remediation (Table 10.2), and experts agree that a comprehensive strategy is best. This would include the use of dust mite encasings or fabrics with pore size diameters less than 6–10 μm for bedding [10, 11], washing linens weekly in hot water greater than 130° F, removal of carpeting and upholstery especially in the bedroom, keeping humidity levels in the home less than 50%, and using a HEPA (high-efficiency particulate air) filter vacuum weekly. Hardwood or linoleum floors are preferred over carpeted floors. If carpeting is unable to be removed, steam vapor treatments of carpeting has been found to be more effective in dust mite removal compared to vacuuming [12]. Platts-Mills et al. looked at long-term effects of avoiding house dust mite allergen in nine asthmatics. Clinical symptoms and morning peak flow measurements improved in all subjects, and five subjects tolerated significant increases in the concentration of histamine necessary to provoke a 30% fall in FEV_1 (forced expiratory volume in one second) [13]. Recently, Murray et al. sought to elucidate the effectiveness of dust-mite-impermeable encasings on reducing asthma symptoms in children. They enrolled over 400 mite-sensitized children with asthma in a randomized control trial. Over an intervention period lasting one year, Murray et al. demonstrated that dust-mite-impermeable covers reduced dust mite levels on children's mattresses by 84% and that the subsequent risk of going to the emergency department for an asthma exacerbation was 45% less. However, there was no difference found in the risk of prednisolone use. Nonetheless, this study highlighted the potential for dust-mite-impermeable covers to improve asthma control in mite-sensitized children [14].

10.4 CAT AND DOG

Domestic animal allergies are common in people with asthma. The primary cat allergen is Fel d 1, which is found in saliva, dander, and hair, and is produced in sebaceous, salivary, and anal glands. Cat allergen can take several months to degrade once the primary source is removed from an indoor environment. This allergen has been found in dust samples taken from environments without cat exposure including schools and day cares [15, 16]. The major dog allergen is Can f 1, which is also found in hair, saliva, and dander. Both cat and dog allergens consist of small particles capable of rapid aerosolization.

The role of pet allergen exposure and sensitization is unclear, as there is controversy over whether early, frequent exposure to pets will lead to sensitization or induce tolerance. Several recent studies suggest protective effects in reducing allergic sensitization in infants exposed to pet allergens [17–19]. Ingram et al., however, reported a strong correlation between asthma and children sensitized and exposed to increased levels of cat and dog allergen [20]. Overall, there is general agreement that cat and dog allergens in sensitized asthmatic individuals can be problematic. Cat allergen exposure in sensitized individuals is also associated with decreased lung function in young children [21].

Individuals with dog allergies who desire a dog are commonly recommended to seek hypoallergenic ones. However, there is a lack of evidence to describe any dog breed as truly "hypoallergenic." Vredegoor et al. compared Can f 1 levels from hair and coat samples of commonly touted hypoallergic dogs (Labradoodle, poodle, Spanish waterdog, and Airedale terrier) and non-hypoallergenic dogs. They found that there were significantly higher Can f 1 levels in the samples from hypoallergenic dogs compared to non-hypoallergenic dogs. Moreover, there was minimal variability of Can f 1 levels between breeds and essentially no difference in airborne Can f 1 levels between breeds [22].

TABLE 10.3
Avoidance Measures for Pet Allergens

Basic principles	• Emphasis on control using allergy-proof encasings, furnishings (cleanable), carpets (removal/cleanable surfaces), and clothing (change if contaminated, wash regularly). • Low confidence on methods relying on chemicals. • Focus on air filtration as pet allergen is airborne for prolonged periods of time.
Control of source	• Encourage eviction of animal, particularly where clinical effects are obvious and sensitization is present. • If not possible, limit animal's territory to indoor cleanable areas (kitchen) and confine outdoors at other times. • Note that allergens can be persistent and last many months, and control may require aggressive cleaning and removal of heavily contaminated items.
Additional comments	• Measures may be required to prevent significant transport of allergen to houses without pets from houses with furry pets and from public buildings. • Production varies widely between animals and, over time, is not well-understood, and it is unlikely that truly allergen-free breeds of cats or dogs exist.

Avoidance measures for pet allergens are summarized in Table 10.3. While the best method is to remove the pet from the home, this is often difficult for families. If the pet remains, it is generally recommended to remove the pet from the bedroom and confine it to one area of the home as much as possible. Other effective strategies include regular bathing of the pet, removal of carpeting, use of allergy-proof encasings for bedding, and use of HEPA filters. Recently, Satyaraj et al. demonstrated a novel approach by which anti-Fel d 1 IgY was safely added to cat food and, once ingested, not only reduced Fel d 1 levels in cat saliva, hair, and dander but also improved allergic symptoms in individuals with a known cat allergy [23]. However, individuals with asthma were excluded from this pilot study. Future research is needed to investigate the impact of anti-Fel d 1 IgY on cat-allergic pet owners with asthma. If shown to reduce asthma symptoms, this approach may offer a promising alternative for cat owners unwilling or unable to relinquish their pet or employ other allergen reduction strategies.

10.5 COCKROACH

The primary indoor species of cockroach are *Blattella germanica* (German cockroach) and *Periplaneta americana*

(American cockroach). The major allergens are Bla g 1 and Bla g 2, which are found in fecal material, saliva, secretions, and debris. Cockroaches thrive in warm, humid environments. Infestation is associated with inner-city environments, high population density, and low socioeconomic status. Exposure to cockroach allergen in the home has also been associated with incident doctor-diagnosed asthma and recurrent wheezing [24]. Using the National Cooperative Inner-City Asthma Study (NCICAS) cohort, Rosenstreich et al. demonstrated that children who were sensitized to cockroach and had evidence of elevated cockroach antigen levels in their homes had significantly higher rates of asthma-related hospitalization and more days of wheezing [25]. Cockroach allergen is also prevalent in schools. Over 66% of collected dust samples from urban Baltimore elementary schools had detectable levels of cockroach allergen [15]. A similar study found detectable levels in 77% of 11 urban high schools in the Northeastern US [26]. Research is ongoing regarding the association of cockroach allergen and asthma morbidity in the school setting.

Eliminating and preventing cockroach infestations are best accomplished with IPM, as summarized in Table 10.4. This would include the removal of potential food sources, the use of insecticides, pesticides, and bait traps, and the sealing of holes or cracks in the home. However, several home-based interventions have yielded mixed results on the effectiveness of cockroach abatement in reducing asthma morbidity. Rabito et al. showed that insecticidal baiting reduced cockroach exposures in homes and was associated with improved asthma symptoms in children [27]. Morgan et al. demonstrated similar results but using allergen impermeable covers, HEPA filters, and professional pest control in inner-city homes [28]. Although DiMango et al. reduced cockroach allergen levels in the home using a multifaceted approach, there was no reduction in asthma pharmacologic therapy [29].

TABLE 10.4
Cockroach Management and Control Procedures

Perform careful inspection to detect insect hiding places and travel routes, and to identify food sources (grease, cooking debris).

Remove sources of food and household food wastes (do not keep garbage cans inside, avoid exposed pet food and snack food containers).

Remove or repair leaking faucets or condensation on pipes.

Before applying insecticide, perform a good general cleaning so that the insects are more likely to eat the gels or baits.

Apply insecticides using gels or baits in selected areas. In the kitchen, apply gel spots to cracks, crevices, the junctures of cupboards or walls with floors, and counters. Bait traps are just as effective as the gel baits if used properly.

Perform a section treatment after one or two weeks.

After one week following application of insecticide, perform thorough house cleaning, removing grease and other food debris.

Wash bedding, curtains, and clothing.

Consider same principles for rodent or other pest management.

10.6 MOUSE

The major mouse allergens are Mus m 1 and Mus m 2, which are found in mouse urine, dander, and hair follicles [30]. Similar to cockroach, mouse infestations are more prevalent in urban and high population density environments [31]. Phipatanakul et al. sought to identify predictors of significant indoor mouse allergen exposure in metropolitan Boston homes of infants at risk for developing allergic diseases, due to parental histories of asthma or allergies. The authors identified visible mouse droppings and the spring as predictors of higher mouse allergen levels and suggested IPM strategies may need to be more intensely applied in the spring, although yearlong strategies are likely necessary to tackle this potential public health problem in the school environment [32].

Both homes and schools have been identified as sites for significant mouse allergen exposure, which can lead to sensitization and worsening asthma morbidity in children [33–36]. Phipatanakul et al. detected mouse allergen in 95% of homes from the National Cooperative Inner-City Asthma Study, and also demonstrated that higher mouse allergen levels led to significantly higher rates of mouse sensitization [37]. Several studies, including the first School Inner-City Asthma Study (SICAS-1) and second School Inner-City Asthma Intervention Study (SICAS-2), have detected mouse allergens in 98–99.5% of dust samples in Northeastern urban schools [35, 36]. SICAS-1 evaluated several hundred students with asthma from 37 inner-city elementary schools in the Northeast. This study found that increased school exposure to mouse allergens was linked with increased odds of having an asthma symptom-day and lower FEV_1 independent of sensitization [35]. Similarly, Matsui et al. found that mouse-sensitized inner-city children who were exposed to greater levels of Mus m 1 had 50% more days of symptoms and 80% more days of beta-agonist use compared to other children [34].

Mitigation strategies for mouse infestations include removing food and water sources, sealing known entryways, and using traps or rodenticides [12]. There have been a number of home and school-based studies evaluating the effects of mouse allergen reduction on asthma morbidity. While SICAS-2 overall found no significant difference in the number of symptom-days students with asthma experienced after implementation of either school-wide IPM or classroom HEPA filter purifiers, school-wide IPM reduced asthma symptoms by 63% during the fall/winter exacerbation season, although not sustained, and secondarily reduced missed school days due to asthma [36].

The Mouse Allergen and Asthma Intervention Trial (MAAIT) found no significant difference in the number of symptom-days between children with asthma who received IPM and pest management or pest management alone at home for mouse allergen reduction [38]. However, it was noted that those who experienced ≥75% reduction in mouse allergen exposure had greater increases in pre-bronchodilator FEV_1 and pre- and post-bronchodilator FEF_{25-75} over one year, indicating the possibility of improved lung function growth and outcomes long term [39]. Further analysis of the MAAIT identified several predictors of successful reduction in mouse allergen levels. These predictors were characteristics of the homes studied, including higher baseline levels of mouse allergen, presence of exposed holes in the living room, and greater percentage of clear bedroom flooring [40].

10.7 POLLEN AND MOLD

Detailed descriptions of the complexities involved in pollen and mold species are beyond the scope of this review, which will provide an introduction into these allergens and how exposures can trigger asthma exacerbations or worsen symptoms in sensitized individuals.

Pollen's role in nature is to transport the male gamete to the female part of a flower through wind, animal, or insect dispersal. In most parts of the US, trees pollinate in the spring, grass pollinates from late spring to early summer, and weeds pollinate in late summer through the fall. The National Allergy Bureau (NAB) is part of the American Academy of Allergy, Asthma and Immunology and supplies the public with estimates of pollen and spore counts (https://pollen.aaaai.org). Trees are either seed bearing (gymnosperms) or flowering (angiosperms), and most allergenic trees are in the flowering group [41]. Birch, oak, elm, and maple trees are common in the Northeast and less prevalent in the Southwest [42]. A single birch tree flower cluster can produce 6 million pollen grains. Species like ragweed, lamb's quarter, and plantain are found throughout the US. A single ragweed plant can expel a million pollen grains in a day. Grass pollen is a common cause of springtime allergies. Northern grasses in the US include timothy, orchard, meadow, rye, Kentucky, redtop, and vernal, while southern grasses include Bermuda, Bahia, and Johnson.

Fungal spores are responsible for both seasonal and perennial allergy symptoms. Outdoor spores peak in the midsummer and diminish with the first hard frost in regions that experience cold winter seasons. *Alternaria* is the most prevalent mold in dry, warm climates and is commonly found in soil, seeds, and plants. *Cladosporium* is the most prevalent spore in temperate regions and is the most commonly identified outdoor fungus. It is found on dead plants or vegetable matter. *Aspergillus* is often found in house dust, compost heaps, and dead vegetation. *Penicillium* is found in soil, food and grains, and house dust. It grows in water-damaged buildings, wallpaper, and decaying fabrics. All of these molds induce allergic rhinitis, asthma, and hypersensitivity pneumonitis.

Intact pollens range from 10 to 100 μm, though most have diameters between 20 and 35 μm, while fungal spores range from 2 to 50 μm [43]. Large particles are removed by the nasal mucosa and upper tracheobronchial passages. However, particles <5 μm generally reach the alveoli of the lungs [44]. An intact pollen is too large to reach the alveoli, but studies have shown that submicronic pollen-derived bioaerosols can reach the alveoli. For example, ryegrass pollen ruptures on contact with water and releases microscopic starch particles (0.5–2.5 μm) containing major grass allergen [45]. Such bioaerosols have been shown to be expulsed from pollens and mold spores [46–49]. While rain can wash pollen grains or spores from the air, the expulsed bioaerosols can trigger asthma exacerbations. Bioaerosols are thought to be associated with thunderstorm asthma epidemics [44, 46–49]. In Melbourne, in 1987, there was a fivefold increase in asthma ED visits in a 24-hour period after a thunderstorm. In 1989, there was a tenfold increase with 277 ED visits [44, 50]. In 1994, in London, 40 patients presented with asthma flares within 24 hours of a storm [51, 52].

There are a number of studies describing asthma morbidity secondary to fungal exposure. *Alternaria* sensitivity has been found to be a risk factor for severe asthma attacks and epidemic asthma [53, 54]. Targonski et al. demonstrated that Chicago asthma deaths were more than two times higher on days when there were 1000 spores/m^3 [55]. Baxi et al. studied the effects of fungal exposures on students with asthma using the SICAS cohort. Fungal spores were detected in all classroom samples. They found that students sensitized and exposed to *Alternaria* had 3.2 more symptom-days per two-week period as compared to students sensitized but not exposed to *Alternaria*. That difference would extrapolate to almost six more asthma symptom-days per month and roughly 50 more asthma symptom-days per school year [56].

The Environmental Relative Moldiness Index (ERMI) scale can be used to compare mold contamination in homes across the United States. This metric was created in collaboration with the US Environmental Protection Agency and the Department of Housing and Urban Development. To generate this scale, 1083 homes underwent PCR quantification of 36 mold species, which were categorized into two groups. Group 1 contained 26 molds commonly associated with water damage in the home. Group 2 contained 10 molds commonly found outdoors. A numerical ERMI value was determined by calculating the difference between the sum of the logs of group 1's mold concentrations and the sum of the logs of group 2's mold concentrations. These ERMI values were plotted to generate a standardized scale.

One review of six epidemiological studies spanning six US cities demonstrated that children and adults with asthma lived in homes with significantly higher ERMI values than comparison homes [57]. Another prospective study found that, in a group of 176 infants, those who lived in homes with ERMI values >5.2 had more than twice the risk of developing asthma than those who lived in homes with lower ERMI values [58]. With the later addition of 116 more infants to this cohort, Reponen et al. demonstrated that each increase in the ERMI value by 10 was associated with a 1.8 times greater risk of developing asthma at age seven [59].

Howard et al. assessed ERMI values in homes and schools in the Northeast US and found that group 1 mold

TABLE 10.5
Mold Management and Control Measures

Locate mold-contaminated items and remove them.
Clean moist areas, as these are prone to mold growth.
Repair leaks.
Reduce humidity to <50%.

levels were similar in homes and schools, but group 2 mold levels were significantly higher in schools, indicating the need for interventions to target those outdoor-sourced molds [60]. Vesper et al. conducted a *post hoc* analysis of SICAS-2 that investigated the effect of school-wide HEPA filtration on ERMI values and students' FEV_1. The authors concluded that HEPA filtration significantly reduced group 1 mold levels and ERMI values. Moreover, students in classrooms with HEPA filters experienced a significant, average increase of 4.22% in their FEV_1 compared to students in classrooms without HEPA filtration [61].

It is not possible to control the pollen or mold spore level outside the home, but one can control the amount of allergen that gets inside. Two major components of control are keeping windows and doors closed during high counts and bathing to remove allergens from the hair and body (Table 10.5). HEPA filters can reduce pollen in the home [62]. A number of trials have shown that immunotherapy is beneficial in treating allergen-induced asthma [63–68]. Abramson et al. conducted a meta-analysis for the Cochrane Database of 20 prospective, randomized, placebo-controlled trials of immunotherapy for asthma between 1960 and 1990 and concluded that immunotherapy reduces asthma symptoms and use of asthma medications and improves bronchial hyperreactivity [67].

10.8 CLIMATE CHANGE

Human industrialization and air pollution have contributed immensely to global climate change and the accelerated rise in temperatures worldwide. Rising temperatures have been associated with increases in natural disasters such as thunderstorms, forest fires, floods, and droughts. Natural disasters themselves have been associated with worsening asthma symptoms. As discussed previously, thunderstorms have been theorized to induce asthma exacerbations via aerosolization of pollen grains [69]. Wildfire smoke has been thought to trigger asthma attacks via disruption of the respiratory epithelial barrier and shifting of T cell to T helper 2 cells. Air pollutants can cause inflammatory reactions in the respiratory tract and predispose individuals to asthma exacerbations [70].

Rising temperatures have contributed to warmer, more humid conditions, which are conductive to the growth of many indoor and outdoor allergens, including pollen and mold. The shift in outdoor temperatures affects the timing, quantity, and dispersion of pollen, which in turn, can affect the prevalence, severity, and duration of allergy symptoms [70]. Since 1990, pollen seasons in North America have lengthened by 20 days and contained 21% more pollen [71]. Further research is needed to examine the effects of climate change on the allergenicity of outdoor environmental allergens, as this dynamic may carry serious implications for those afflicted by allergy-induced asthma.

10.9 CURRENT AND FUTURE RESEARCH

In recent years, research has greatly expanded to examine the role of indoor allergens both in the home and school [72]. The identification of urban exposures such as cockroach and mouse, along with their associations with allergen sensitization and asthma morbidity, have naturally led to ongoing research focused on methods for allergen reduction, notably IPM. This comprehensive approach involves education, extermination, maintaining proper food storage, use of air filters, and sealing of holes and cracks in the home. Allergen reduction has been shown to improve asthma symptoms in individuals in environments with significant levels of mouse and dust mite allergens but has yielded mixed results for cockroach allergens [13, 14, 27–29, 39]. In one promising pilot study, anti-Fel d 1 IgY was added to cat food and, once ingested, was associated with decreased levels of detectable Fel d 1 allergen level and reduced allergic symptoms in cat-allergic owners without asthma [23]. If translational to pet owners with asthma and to other domestic animals, this approach may offer an enticing solution to sensitized pet owners. Ongoing studies are also attempting to understand the role of single versus multifaceted interventions to a variety of allergen exposures in homes and schools. These results may prove to be important targets for effective and efficient intervention strategies to reduce allergenic triggers. Furthermore, there remains a growing need for climate change research to investigate whether and how the allergenicities of environmental allergens are evolving worldwide.

10.10 CONCLUSION

In atopic individuals, indoor and outdoor environmental allergens can play a significant role in asthma development and asthma morbidity. Patients with asthma, as in our patient case, can benefit from skin testing to identify common environmental inhalant allergens, including dust mite, cat, dog, cockroach, mouse, pollen, and mold. Once culprit allergens are identified, the focus should shift to appropriate environmental remediation strategies, including education, avoidance, carpet removal, allergy-proof encasings, air filtration, HEPA filtered vacuums, and IPM. The results thus far are promising, but ongoing research is needed to further discern whether and by what methods early reduction of indoor allergen exposures can alleviate asthma morbidity. At the same time, we must renew our efforts to combat global climate change, as it may carry serious implications for the allergenicity of outdoor environmental allergens.

REFERENCES

1. Sears, M. R., et al., *Clinical and Experimental Allergy* (1989).
2. Sporik, R., et al., *N Engl J Med* (1990).
3. Arbes, S. J., Jr., et al., *J Allergy Clin Immunol* (2007). PMID 17889931.
4. Platts-Mills, T. A., et al., *J Allergy Clin Immunol* (1997).
5. Squillace, S. P., et al., *Am J Respir Crit Care Med* (1997).
6. Platts-Mills, T., et al., *Am Fam Physician* (2007). PMID 17894137.
7. Kern, R. A., *J Immunol* (1921).
8. Peat, J. K., et al., *Am J Respir Crit Care Med* (1996).
9. Celedon, J. C., et al., *J Allergy Clin Immunol* (2007). PMID 17507083.
10. Halken, S., et al., *J Allergy Clin Immunol* (2003). P
11. Baxi, S. N. and W. Phipatanakul, *Adolesc Med State Art Rev* (2010). PMID 20568555.
12. Maciag, M. C. and W. Phipatanakul, *Ann Allergy Asthma Immunol* (2022). PMID 35227902.
13. Platts-Mills, T. A., et al., *Lancet* (1982).
14. Murray, C. S., et al., *Am J Respir Crit Care Med* (2017). PMID 28282501.
15. Amr, S., et al., *Ann Allergy Asthma Immunol* (2003). PMID 12546335.
16. Instanes, C., et al., *Indoor Air* (2005). PMID 16108908.
17. Ownby, D. R., et al., *JAMA* (2002). PMID 12190366.
18. Ownby, D. R. and C. C. Johnson, *Curr Opin Allergy Clin Immunol* (2003). PMID 14612678.
19. Perzanowski, M. S., et al., *J Allergy Clin Immunol* (2008). PMID 18395554.
20. Ingram, J. M., et al., *J Allergy Clin Immunol* (1995).
21. Lowe, L. A., et al., *Arch Pediatr Adolesc Med* (2004). PMID 15466689.
22. Vredegoor, D. W., et al., *J Allergy Clin Immunol* (2012). PMID 22728082.
23. Satyaraj, E., et al., *Allergy* (2019). PMID 31498459.
24. Litonjua, A. A., et al., *J Allergy Clin Immunol* (2001).
25. Rosenstreich, D. L., et al., *N Engl J Med* (1997). PMID 9134876.
26. Chew, G. L., et al., *Indoor Air* (2005). PMID 15982269.
27. Rabito, F. A., et al., *J Allergy Clin Immunol* (2017). PMID 28108117.
28. Morgan, W. J., et al., *N Engl J Med* (2004). PMID 15356304.
29. DiMango, E., et al., *J Allergy Clin Immunol Pract* (2016). PMID 27025297.
30. Mortelliti, C. L., et al., *Immunol Allergy Clin North Am* (2022). PMID 36265973.
31. Permaul, P., et al., *Pediatr Allergy Immunol* (2012). PMID 22672325.
32. Permaul, P., et al., *Ann Allergy Asthma Immunol* (2013). PMID 24054369.
33. Phipatanakul, W., et al., *J Allergy Clin Immunol* (2000). PMID 11112889.
34. Matsui, E. C., et al., *Ann Allergy Asthma Immunol* (2006). PMID 17069107.
35. Sheehan, W. J., et al., *JAMA Pediatr* (2017). PMID 27893060.
36. Phipatanakul, W., et al., *JAMA* (2021). PMID 34547084.
37. Phipatanakul, W., et al., *J Allergy Clin Immunol* (2000). PMID 11112889.
38. Matsui, E. C., et al., *JAMA* (2017). PMID 28264080.
39. Grant, T., et al., *J Allergy Clin Immunol* (2020). PMID 31866099.
40. Akar-Ghibril, N., et al., *J Allergy Clin Immunol Pract* (2021). PMID 34265449.
41. Esch, R. and Bush, RK, Aerobiology of Outdoor Allergens. In: Adkinson NF, Yunginger, JW, Busse WW, eds., *Middleton's Allergy Principles & Practice* (2009). Elsevier.
42. Kagen, S., et al., *Aeroallergen PhotoLibrary of North America* (2004).
43. Portnoy, J. and C. Barnes, *Immunol Allergy Clin North Am* (2003). PMID 14524382.
44. Suphioglu, C., *Int Arch Allergy Immunol* (1998). PMID 9693274.
45. Suphioglu, C., *Int Arch Allergy Immunol* (1998).
46. Grote, M., et al., *J Allergy Clin Immunol* (2000). PMID 10856148.
47. Taylor, P. E., et al., *J Allergy Clin Immunol* (2002). PMID 11799365.
48. Taylor, P. E., et al., *Clin Exp Allergy* (2004). PMID 15479275.
49. Taylor, P. E. and H. Jonsson, *Curr Allergy Asthma Rep* (2004). PMID 15283882.
50. Bellomo, R., et al., *Med J Aust* (1992). PMID 1603007.
51. Celenza, A., et al., *BMJ* (1996). PMID 8595333.
52. Davidson, A. C., et al., *BMJ* (1996). PMID 8595332.
53. O'Hollaren, M. T., et al., *N Engl J Med* (1991). PMID 1987459.
54. Pulimood, T. B., et al., *J Allergy Clin Immunol* (2007). PMID 17624415.
55. Targonski, P. V., et al., *J Allergy Clin Immunol* (1995). PMID 7751516.
56. Baxi, S. N., et al., *Ann Allergy Asthma Immunol* (2019). PMID 30904580.
57. Vesper, S. and L. Wymer, *Int J Hyg Environ Health* (2016). PMID 26861576.
58. Reponen, T., et al., *Ann Allergy Asthma Immunol* (2011). PMID 21802019.
59. Reponen, T., et al., *J Allergy Clin Immunol* (2012). PMID 22789397.
60. Howard, E. J., et al., *J Allergy Clin Immunol Pract* (2021). PMID 33091637.
61. Vesper, S. J., et al., *J Asthma* (2022). PMID 35341426.
62. Sublett, J. L., et al., *J Allergy Clin Immunol* (2009). PMID 19910039.
63. Walker, S. M., et al., *Allergy* (1995). PMID 7573829.
64. Durham, S. R., et al., *N Engl J Med* (1999). PMID 10441602.
65. Walker, S. M., et al., *J Allergy Clin Immunol* (2001). PMID 11149996.
66. Moller, C., et al., *J Allergy Clin Immunol* (2002). PMID 11842293.
67. Abramson, M. J., et al., *Cochrane Database Syst Rev* (2003). PMID 14583928.
68. *J Allergy Clin Immunol* (2007). PMID 17765078.
69. Luschkova, D., et al., *Allergo J Int* (2022). PMID 35693463.
70. al., Z. C. S. e., *Front Allergy* (2022).
71. Anderegg, W. R. L., et al., *Proc Natl Acad Sci U S A* (2021). PMID 33558232.
72. Salo, P. M., et al., *J Allergy Clin Immunol* (2009). PMID 19577284.

11 Air Pollutants

Meghan E. Rebuli, Chris Carlsten, and Neil E. Alexis

CASE PRESENTATION

A 56-year-old grocery store clerk with well-controlled asthma moved from the Southeastern US to the Pacific Northwest to be closer to family. She found a new family physician to care for her and her family, and no changes were deemed necessary in her medical regimen. However, within approximately 10 months of settling into her new environment, the summer fire season erupted, and she noted a marked increase in wheezing. Her new physician recommended that she increase the as-needed use of her LABA/ICS inhaler and doing so helped somewhat but did not allow her return to wheeze-free baseline. Frustrated, she reached out for further solutions.

Her care provider had seen recommendations in a family practice journal regarding portable HEPA filters to reduce particulate matter from wildfire smoke. The patient obtained one and noted her wheezing to be further reduced but still slightly above baseline. She searched for further solutions and ultimately saw an allergist in consultation. The allergist performed skin prick testing and revealed clear positivity to local tree species, noting that his colleagues' recent study documented a rapid increase in pollen concentrations over the past two decades. Interestingly, the pattern of increased pollen correlated strongly with increased temperatures in the region. The patient began routine nasal saline rinses, with which her wheezing resolved completely.

11.1 INTRODUCTION

Asthma is a disease characterized by intermittent bronchoconstriction due to increased airway responsiveness to both allergic and nonallergic stimuli. Airways inflammation is a key underlying feature of this disease. Epidemiological evidence from the last two decades has shown that exposure to inhaled environmental pollutants such as ozone, particulate matter (PM), diesel exhaust (DE), and biological/microbial agents contribute significantly to the morbidity associated with asthma, including increasing exacerbation frequency [1–4]. Evidence also suggests that some causal relationships exist with new onset asthma in children, namely with nitrogen dioxide (NO_2) and black carbon, and less clearly with ozone and traffic-related PM [5]. More recently, as climate change is on the rise, other sources of air pollution, such as wildfire smoke, has been investigated as a potential exacerbation risk for individuals with asthma [6–8]. Further, personal product use has also been reported as a potential risk for individuals with asthma, such as increased exposure to phthalates from hair care and cosmetic products [9], as well as harmful components of cigarettes, e-cigarettes, and marijuana smoking, but detailed contributions from these personal use agents are beyond the scope of this chapter [10–15]. As noted in the preceding case study, exposure to wildfire smoke in combination with exposure to high levels of a local allergen, was the likely cause of enhanced wheeze in a patient who, prior to this new routine exposure, was symptomatically quiescent. This case study draws our attention to the potential role climate change plays in increasing inhaled exposures to both pollutants and allergens that can enhance asthma exacerbation rates, as increasing global temperatures are predicted to contribute to elevated and prolonged allergen and wildfire seasons. Prior studies have also suggested that air pollutant exposures can enhance the bioavailability of allergens, resulting in an interactive effect [16–18].

The public health concern regarding the effect of air pollution on asthma is valid and supported by science. It is estimated that over 137 million people in the United States live in areas that are not in compliance with current air pollutant standards [19]. Therefore, poor air quality in many places remains a significant problem for susceptible individuals, such as those with asthma. This chapter will review our current understanding of the link between asthma and air pollution and factors that impact this relationship, by examining association-based evidence from epidemiological and cohort studies, as well as effects-based evidence generated from controlled chamber exposure studies.

11.2 MODIFYING FACTORS

At the outset, it is prudent to recognize that a myriad of factors must be considered when discussing the impact of air pollution on asthma. These factors can all contribute to the heterogeneity in the results often observed across studies when examining this complex area. These factors are typically related to (a) subject phenotype such as age (childhood vs. adult asthma), race, sex and gender, body mass index (BMI), clinical phenotype, inflammatory endotype (Th2-high/Th2-low), and genotype; (b) differences in study design and analysis techniques, that is, the proximity to exposure versus the estimation of exposure by using land-use regression modelling; (c) implementation of different exposure matrices; and

DOI: 10.1201/9781003287209-14

(d) use of a range of methods to measure clinical and biological outcomes. For example, studying asthma exacerbation in existing asthmatics is quite different from assessing whether a pollutant is causing new-onset asthma. Likewise, the measurement and sampling techniques for inflammatory biomarkers in patients are not necessarily interchangeable or comparable; for example, the use of induced sputum examines the surfaces of the central airways compared with bronchoalveolar lavage, which reflects events in the more distal airways [20]. Therefore, caution must be used when making direct study comparisons or including studies in meta-analyses where different measurement and analysis methodologies have been used.

It is important to highlight a few modifying factors that have garnered significant attention in recent studies investigating the effects of inhaled exposures on asthmatics, namely sex, genotype, and sputum neutrophil response. Studies investigating tobacco smoke exposure have identified increased incidence of asthma attacks in males compared to females [21]. Prenatal exposure to ambient ultrafine particles alters the risk of incident asthma in a sex-dependent manner based on exposure window, particularly females exposed in late pregnancy [22]. However, it should be noted that evidence of sex differences in response to inhaled exposures in individuals with asthma is limited, as many studies control or adjust for sex rather than factor sex into analyses as a biological variable. As researchers comply with the National Institutes of Health's Sex as a Biological Variable Policy, evidence may continue to emerge [23]. Further complicating this analysis is asthma incidence and is known to be differentially sex-specific by life stage. Asthma is known to be more prevalent in male children than female children, switching in prevalence to a majority in females at puberty, and again back to increased prevalence in males at perimenopause and periandropause [24], which may complicate the understanding of the role of pollutants on asthma incidence.

In terms of genotype, a recent pilot study showed that individuals who were null for the glutathione-S-transferase Mu1 (GSTM1) gene were more likely to have a robust inflammatory response in the airways following wood smoke exposure [25]. Studies have also pointed to a neutrophil response phenotype whereby a subset of individuals have an increased sputum percentage neutrophil response over baseline (>10% points) following exposure to ozone, endotoxin, and wood smoke particles [26, 27]. Other factors including diet and microbiome, that may play a role in altered incidence or exacerbation of asthma in response to air pollution, are under investigation [28–30]. Future studies must consider the role of effect modifiers, such as sex, genotype, inflammatory endotype, and other factors in the analyses.

11.3 AIR POLLUTION AND ASTHMA EXACERBATION

It is widely accepted that air pollution can exacerbate asthma in those individuals who already have the condition. Many studies from the past several years have reported significant associations between exposure to air pollution (ozone, PM, diesel exhaust particles [DEPs], mould/fungal spores) and asthma exacerbations, and in the case of certain pollutants such as ozone, a lag time of 1–2 days following exposure is correlated with increased admissions to emergency departments (ED) for respiratory complaints [31–36]. Air pollution is thought to influence frequency of asthma exacerbation in a myriad of ways [37] and can impair lung development in the perinatal period and childhood. Reported mechanisms include augmentation of allergen sensitization, increased airway inflammation [38], impaired immune host-defence against pathogens [39, 40], and induction of bronchospasm.

Recent studies continue to support the association between air pollution and asthma. For example, a study examined rates of asthma exacerbation in 54,632 children in the Philadelphia metropolitan region and found positive associations between $PM_{2.5}$ during both warm and cold months (OR:1.03, 95% CI: 0.98–1.08 and 1.05, 95% CI: 1.02–1.07) and ozone only during cold months (OR: 1.08, 95% CI: 1.02–1.14) [41]. A meta-analysis of case-crossover studies examining emergency department visits and/or hospital admissions (common surrogates for asthma exacerbation) found 22 studies over a 16-year period and NO2, PM2.5, CO, and ozone showed a significant association (OR: 1.02, 95% CI: 1.01,1.04; OR: 1.03: 1.01,1.05; OR: 1.05, 1.01,1.09, and OR: 1.03: 1.01,1.06, respectively) [42]. A more comprehensive meta-analysis of 84 studies analysed similar surrogates for asthma exacerbation, along with symptoms, lung function changes, and medication use in time-series or case-crossover studies using same-day (lag 0) or prior day (lag 1) pollutant exposure [43]. Similar to the previous meta-analysis, they found in both lag models, when effects of all pollutants except SO_2 were included (air quality index [AQI]), PM2.5, PM10, NO_2, CO, ozone), larger effects were seen in children and in metrics of asthma exacerbation including symptoms, lung function changes, and medication use, rather than emergency department visits or hospital admissions [43]. These more current epidemiological data in the form of aggregated meta-analyses strengthen the long-held view that there is a clear association between air pollution and asthma exacerbation.

Not only can air pollution exposure exacerbate existing asthma, but there are also areas of active research exploring whether air pollution is a risk factor for progression from asthma to chronic obstructive lung disease [37, 44]. For example, in a 2016 study, it was found that increased air pollution exposure resulted in threefold greater odds of developing asthma-chronic obstructive pulmonary disease (COPD) overlap syndrome (ACOS) [44].

11.4 AIR POLLUTION AND NEW-ONSET ASTHMA

A recent report evaluated available evidence on the role of traffic-related air pollutants (TRAPs) in new-onset asthma [5]. The workshop was conducted to evaluate all the current available evidence on the link between TRAPs and new onset asthma from the conglomeration of studies in the fields of epidemiology, clinical research, and basic mechanistic science. The authors found that there is sufficient evidence of a causal relationship between new onset childhood asthma and long-term exposure to outdoor air pollution. Strong evidence from a number of studies from the Southern California Children's Health Study that identified increased risk of new-onset childhood asthma from TRAP exposure [45–47] and a meta-analysis of prenatal air pollution exposure studies that identified associations for NO_2 and PM10 [48]. Results from adult studies were more inconclusive, but while positive associations have been identified between TRAP and asthma onset in adults, including increased hazard ratios for NO_2, a causal relationship cannot yet be established [5]. Thus the evidence suggests that in addition to air pollution acting as an exacerbating agent, air pollutants, particularly traffic-related ones, may be contributing to the development of new-onset asthma, particularly in children.

11.5 INTERVENTIONS

To combat the effects of air pollution on asthma exacerbation, clinical interventions can be utilized, such as medication optimization, informed usage of air pollution monitoring to avoid exposure to "bad air" days [49], use of high-efficiency particulate air (HEPA) filtration indoors (Figure 11.1) to reduce particle load, and advocacy for increased air quality regulation stringency. Medication optimization and management, along with personal air pollution monitoring through mobile health (mHealth) applications, has been shown to reduce severe asthma exacerbation, enhancing patient self-management of their asthma [50]. In a study of HEPA filters on childhood asthma control, indoor HEPA filter usage reduced TRAP particulate concentration and improved asthma control and quality of life in children with poorly controlled asthma [51]. Other strategies that are also currently under investigation to reduce risk of the effects of air pollution include ingestion of antioxidant supplements [52], but these investigations are in early stages and need further confirmation [53].

While a large number of epidemiological and cohort studies can highlight the association between disease and exposure and provide weight of evidence for causality, they are quite limited in ability to assess how individual pollutants affect the biology and physiology of asthma. Better suited to address these questions, controlled chamber exposure studies are used in which individuals (asthmatics and non-asthmatics) are exposed to selected pollutants under carefully controlled conditions, such as exposure duration, pollutant concentration, and ventilation or breathing rate. Clinical and biological outcome measures are obtained both before and after exposure. Much evidence has been acquired from these types of controlled exposure studies to further our understanding of how pollutants are exerting their effects on the biology and physiology of asthma and may set the stage for broader epidemiologic investigations [45].

11.6 EFFECT OF AIR POLLUTANTS ON ASTHMA BIOLOGY

To understand how oxidant pollutants such as ozone, or organism-derived pollutants such as endotoxin, affect the biology of asthma, it is important to appreciate the constitutive state of the asthmatic airway prior to exposure in terms of inflammation, immunology, and physiology. This will allow a better appreciation of how the asthmatic airway is predisposed to respond to a particular air pollutant, especially since pollutants differ in their mechanisms of action. For example, pollutants such as ozone or PM [46, 47] will induce oxidative stress responses, whereas pollutants with biological components adhered to their surface, such as bacterial endotoxin on coarse size PM (PM2.5–10), peptidoglycan/gram-positive bacteria on swine dust, or allergens may exert their effects primarily or initially through innate immune mechanisms [48, 54–56].

In terms of airways inflammation, there are different inflammatory cell endotypes to be recognized (eosinophilic, neutrophilic, paucigranulocytic), and these differ according to the stability of the disease (stable vs. acute) and whether it is present in children or adults. For acute asthma, the eosinophilic phenotype predominates in children (50%), while in adults, the neutrophilic phenotype predominates (82%) and is negatively correlated with lung function and airflow obstruction [57–59]. For stable asthma, the paucigranulocytic phenotype appears to be the most common in both children and adults. In terms of microbial presence, evidence is emerging that respiratory microbiome dysbiosis may play a role in asthma [60, 61]. Dysbiosis refers to an imbalance of the microbes present in the lung compared to the healthy microbiome. Multiple bacterial taxa have been implicated in asthma incidence in children, even predictive of future asthma diagnosis when detected in the upper airway (*Streptococcus pneumoniae*, *Haemophilus influenzae*, and *Moraxella catarrhalis*) [61]. In the lower airway, dysbiosis has been associated with distinct asthma phenotype, such as Proteobacteria being associated with neutrophilic asthma. In contrast, members of the Bacteroidetes phyla, such as *Prevotella*, were more commonly found in control patients without asthma, identifying a potential beneficial microbe [60]. In general, asthmatic patients have increased lower respiratory tract symptoms, greater impairment of their lung function, and increased bronchial hyperresponsiveness. However, pertinent to how they may respond to inhaled pollutants, asthmatics have a diminished innate immune response capability and depleted levels of antioxidants [62–66]. For example, modified immune capability includes altered cell surface marker expression and decreased phagocytosis, where the latter effect was positively correlated with markers of asthma severity and would be expected to lead to reduced clearance of cellular debris, PM, or pathogens [67]. Similarly, muted interferon gamma (IFNγ) and interleukin (IL)-10 responses following a challenge with an experimental rhinovirus infection, have been observed in individuals with asthma [68]. Together, these pieces of evidence suggest reduced host-defence capacity, making individuals with asthma more susceptible to the deleterious effects of inhaled pollutants.

As evidence of the role of antioxidants in asthma, a nested-control study found that plasma α-tocopherol and platelet-activating factor acetylhydrolase (PAF-AH) were associated with decreased risk of incident asthma (OR: 0.52, 95% CI: 0.32–.084, OR: 0.63; 95% CI: 0.42–0.93, respectively) [65]. Further, patients with asthma have been shown to be deficient in levels of the potent antioxidant, ascorbic acid, in their airways, reducing their ability to neutralize endogenously derived free radicals produced from activated inflammatory cells and contributing to increased susceptibility to inhaled environmental oxidants, such as ozone [66].

11.7 OZONE

Asthmatics have been studied for several years following controlled inhalation challenges with pollutants such as ozone, endotoxin, PM, and DEPs. Among these pollutants, ozone has been the most extensively examined. Following a controlled exposure to ozone, the most noted and consistent effects observed in both asthmatics and non-asthmatics are symptoms such as pain on deep inspiration, decrements in lung function (FEV_1 and FVC), increased neutrophil levels, and elevated pro-inflammatory cytokines (IL-8, IL-6) in the airways [69, 70]. Other less consistent effects that have been reported include increased airway reactivity and increased airway eosinophil levels in atopic individuals [71]. Several studies have attempted to distinguish effects of ozone between individuals with and without asthma, these reports similarly implicate increased inflammatory signalling, both through gene expression and protein analyses in individuals with asthma as compared to controls [72, 73]. For example, Hernandez et al. examined spirometric and inflammatory responses to two hours of 0.4 ppm ozone exposure in individuals with allergic asthma and healthy volunteers. They observed that individuals with asthma had significantly increased expression of CD23,

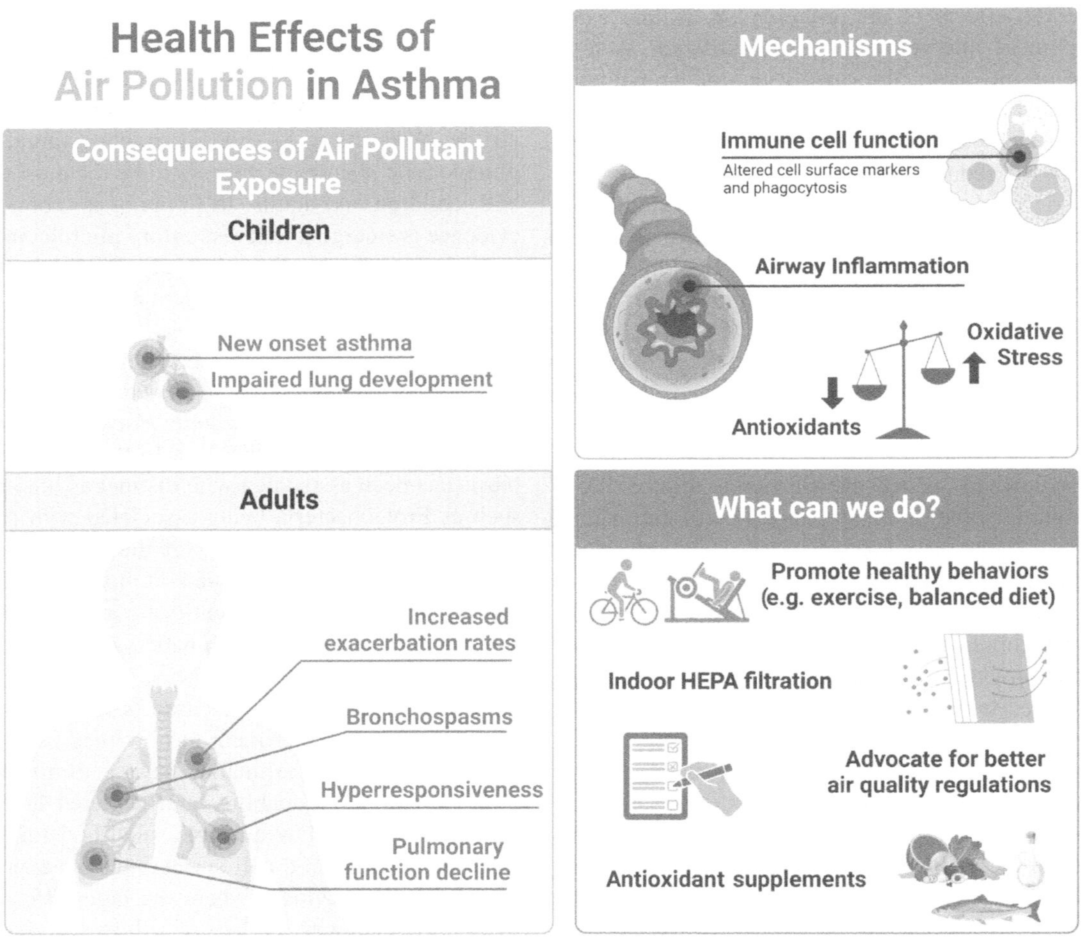

FIGURE 11.1 Health effects of air pollution in asthma: The schematic summarizes the consequences of air pollutant exposure in both children and adults (left), mechanisms of action (top right), and potential ways to mitigate effects of air pollution exposure in asthma (bottom right). Abbreviations: HEPA = high efficiency particulate air. Note: Physiological effects in left panel are not denoted in anatomically accurate locations. (Figure created with BioRender.)

FcεRI, and TLR4 on sputum macrophages and increased levels of pro-inflammatory cytokines [74]. Similarly, Leroy et al. [72] found increased expression of genes associated with inflammation and remodelling in the bronchoalveolar lavage (BAL) of asthmatics following ozone, particularly the gene for osteopontin (OPN), secreted phosphoprotein 1 (*SPP1*). In that study, expression increased 2.1 and sixfold with 100 ppb and 200 ppb levels of ozone for four hours. Interestingly, Gomez et al. [75] demonstrated the existence of microRNA networks and genes in asthmatics that are associated with features of asthma severity, including hsa-miR-223–3p, a neutrophil-derived microRNA that is significantly increased following ozone exposure.

Together, the data suggests that, following acute ozone exposure, asthmatics may be primed for enhanced immune responses to subsequently inhaled pollutants. Potentially, biomarkers may be useful in predicting which individual asthmatics may have an exaggerated inflammatory response to ozone, thereby making them more susceptible to subsequently inhaled allergenic stimuli. Thus far, potential biomarkers on circulating monocytes (CD11b) and neutrophils (CD14) have been associated with response to pollutant exposure in asthma [76, 77]. Other markers, such as malondialdehyde levels in exhaled breath condensate, have also been proposed [71]. However, a definitive and validated biomarker of response to ozone in people with asthma in a large clinical study has not yet been identified.

11.8 ENDOTOXIN

Although perhaps not generally considered an air pollutant by classic definition, endotoxin or lipopolysaccharide (LPS) is ubiquitous in nature, an active component of PM-induced airway cell toxicity [78], an active component of both house dust and occupational dust [79–81], and more recently has been found to be capable of biocorona formation on engineered nanoparticles [82]. Endotoxin is a known enhancing factor for asthma severity [83] and can act as an adjuvant for the subsequent response to inhaled allergens in the nasal [84] and lower airways [85]. These data suggest that atopy plays an important role in how endotoxin exerts its effect in asthma. Newton et al. tested this hypothesis in an occupational cohort and identified that atopic workers may be more susceptible to endotoxin-associated respiratory symptoms [86]. Further supporting this idea, significant associations have been reported between the magnitude of the LPS-induced polymorphonuclear neutrophil (PMN) response and baseline levels of eosinophils, suggesting that atopy plays an important role in the sensitivity of asthmatics to LPS [87].

Epidemiological studies have also indicated an association between emergency room visits for asthma and co-exposures to residential endotoxin and ambient PM2.5 in adults and children (OR 5.01; 95% CI 2.54–9.87), as well as NO_2 in children (OR 5.01, 95% CI 1.65–7.18) [88]. Further, each log10-unit increase in endotoxin levels has been associated with increased odds of severe asthma exacerbation in children living near roadways (OR 4.21; 95% CI 1.5–12) [89]. A study out of Japan has also identified that high household endotoxin exposure may be involved in the development of incident asthma, increasing the odds ratio for wheeze and asthma from 24–36 months of age [88]. Thus, in addition to acting as an allergen adjuvant, endotoxin may also function as an independent air pollutant.

It is important to note that effects of endotoxin in asthmatics may differ by dose, relatively high (>30,000 EU) or low (10,000 EU). At high doses (>30,000 EU), endotoxin will induce lung function decline, symptoms such as malaise, fever, chills, and neutrophil influx to the airways with blunted phagocytic capacity, as measured by an increase in the percentage of neutrophils in the sputum [76, 90–93]. In contrast, at low LPS levels (10,000 EU), asthmatics demonstrated significant upregulation of the cell-surface markers associated with innate immunity and antigen presentation (CD14, CD11b, CD16, HLA-DR, CD86, FceR1), and an increased expression of the genes that modulate antigen presentation (HLA-DR, MCP1), immune activation (CD14, IL-1β), and inflammation (ICAM1, iκBα) [94]. *In vitro* evidence also shows that small concentrations of endotoxin (<1 ng/mL) activate alveolar macrophages, causing the release of several pro-inflammatory mediators [95], again suggesting that low-dose endotoxin is an innate immune stimulant or primer. Although the dose–response effect of endotoxin is also present in non-asthmatics, it may be more significant in susceptible populations such as asthmatics. For example, it has been established that asthmatics require a lower dose of LPS to elicit bronchoconstriction and inflammation than that required by non-asthmatics [94, 96]. Overall, the evidence suggests that the effect of dose is clearly important when describing the toxic effects of endotoxin on asthma.

To combat the effects of endotoxin on the airway, several clinical trials have been conducted using pharmaceutical drugs and dietary supplements, evaluating their effects on response to endotoxin exposure. Two have successfully demonstrated reduction in endotoxin effects—gamma tocopherol isoform of vitamin E reduced sputum eosinophilia and endotoxin-induced sputum neutrophilia in individuals with asthma, while IL-1 receptor antagonist, anakinra, reduced endotoxin-induced airway inflammation in healthy controls [97, 98]. Further work is needed to validate these findings in larger cohorts, but these studies provide promising evidence of potential preventative measures that can be utilized to reduce the effects of endotoxin.

11.9 DIESEL EXHAUST AND DIESEL EXHAUST PARTICLES

As discussed earlier in the chapter, epidemiological evidence supports the role of TRAP, which includes diesel exhaust (DE), in new onset asthma, particularly in children, with some evidence of association, also in adults. To strengthen causal evidence of effects of components of TRAP that can be more easily regulated, such as diesel exhaust, controlled exposure studies of the effects of diesel exhaust have been conducted. Results from 19 diesel-exhaust-controlled exposure studies on individuals with asthma prior to 2020 were recently reviewed where methods as well as results were described in detail [99, 100]. Multiple studies, primarily at DE exposure levels of 300 $\mu g/m^3$ PM10, reported airway hyperreactivity (1.7–4.8 mg/mL decrease in PC_{20} compared to filtered air exposure), increased obstruction (6.4% decrease FEV_1% compared to 24 hours post filtered air exposure), and increased airway resistance (6.5% increase compared to filtered air). Increased airway resistance was also found as an effect in a study using a lower dose (100 $\mu g/m^3$ PM10). Airway inflammation findings, however, were inconsistent across studies in individuals with asthma, which contrasts with healthy subjects [38]. A few studies have also explored mechanisms of action, finding evidence of a role of increased oxidative stress, epigenetic marks, neurogenic inflammation, and adipokines in DE-based health effect mechanisms. The role of oxidative stress was based on increased nitrite as measured through exhaled breath condensate and reductions in airway hyperresponsiveness following antioxidant supplementation. However, despite some insights into potential mechanisms, more research is needed to elucidate this fully. In addition to the identified effects of DE alone, multiple controlled exposure studies have also included co-exposures, which better mimics TRAP as a complex inhaled exposure mixture. Co-exposures including allergens, ozone, and pathogens have induced synergistic effects with DE; however, the majority of these studies have been conducted only in healthy subjects [99, 100].

11.9.1 Biomass Fuels

About 2.4 billion persons live in households in which biomass fuels (BMFs) are the primary fuel for cooking, heating, or both [101, 102], with more than 90% of subjects in rural areas in less-developed countries (LDCs) using BMFs. BMFs for indoor cooking stoves include wood, charcoal, dung, and crop residues. Biomass emissions, however, can also technically include cigarette smoke, and most studies on this topic have not previously controlled for tobacco smoke exposure [103]. All of these are important sources of indoor air pollution, particularly in developing countries and LDCs. Epidemiologic studies have reported associations between BMF and asthma. A study in Ethiopia found that, in a hospital-based matched case-control study of 483 participants, tobacco smoking, use of solid fuels for cooking, including wood and agriculture residues, were associated with development of asthma [104]. Similarly, in Sri Lanka a study of 262 children, incidence of infection-induced asthma was higher in female children where households used biomass fuel and kerosene versus petroleum gas or electricity for cooking (RR 1.77, 95% CI 1.098–2.949) [105]. Data also suggest that children with wheeze may experience more severe asthma symptoms with exposure to biomass fuels [106]. Other studies have demonstrated increase in respiratory symptoms [107]. However, field-wide results are mixed, and none have demonstrated a causal link [103]. The success of the measures to reduce exposure to BMF has begun to be assessed for their effect on respiratory health outcomes; however, currently these results are also mixed. Recent studies in Guatemala and Bolivia suggest that use of more efficient cookstoves may reduce risk of allergic asthma and rhinitis in children exposed before six months of age [108] and improve respiratory health-related quality of life metrics with use of ventilated cookstoves to reduce household air pollution exposure [109]. However, a study in Peru did not find differences in lung function or respiratory symptoms in 180 women randomized to a petroleum gas intervention stove when compared to use of biomass [110, 111]. Whether interventions, such as replacement of cookstoves with more efficient methods, are sustainable without sociological and economic intervention is also currently up for debate [112].

11.10 WILDFIRE SMOKE

Wildfire smoke exposures are a growing concern, as climate change is linked to increasing land being burned each decade [113]. Studies have found associations between wildfire smoke and cardiopulmonary outcomes that are similar to the literature on PM2.5, of which wildfire smoke particulate is a substantial component [114]. Respiratory health effects appear to be substantial in those with existing respiratory disease, such as asthma and COPD. Wildfire smoke days has been shown to increase asthma exacerbations [115], first use of respiratory medications in early life exposure [116], asthma-related hospital visits [117], and, with prolonged exposure, persistent symptoms [7]. In a meta-analysis of children 0–18 years of age, there was a consistent increase in asthma-related hospital visits within the first three days of exposure [118], affirming strong associations of wildfire smoke on asthma outcomes. Firefighters are also particularly at risk, with recent studies identifying that firefighters have an increased risk of asthma consultations post fire (measure of new onset asthma; OR 2.56; 95% CI 1.75–3.74) [119]. While epidemiological evidence of associations between asthma and wildfire smoke exposure are strong, controlled exposure studies have been conducted to provide potential causal evidence. Most controlled exposures used wood smoke as a model for more complex wildfires. Reviewed in Schwartz et al., 12 human controlled exposure studies had been undertaken as of 2020, with a large variation in study design that limited strong conclusions on effects [120]. These studies did consistently find effects on the airways, including airway function, with more limited evidence of effects on systemic inflammation, cardiovascular function, and oxidative stress. The most recent report on a controlled exposure study, not included in the previous review, has found evidence of increased airway inflammation in individuals with asthma at 24 hours following wood smoke exposure [25]. Thus, while overall evidence of adverse health associations is strong, there is an intriguing pattern of respiratory greater than cardiovascular

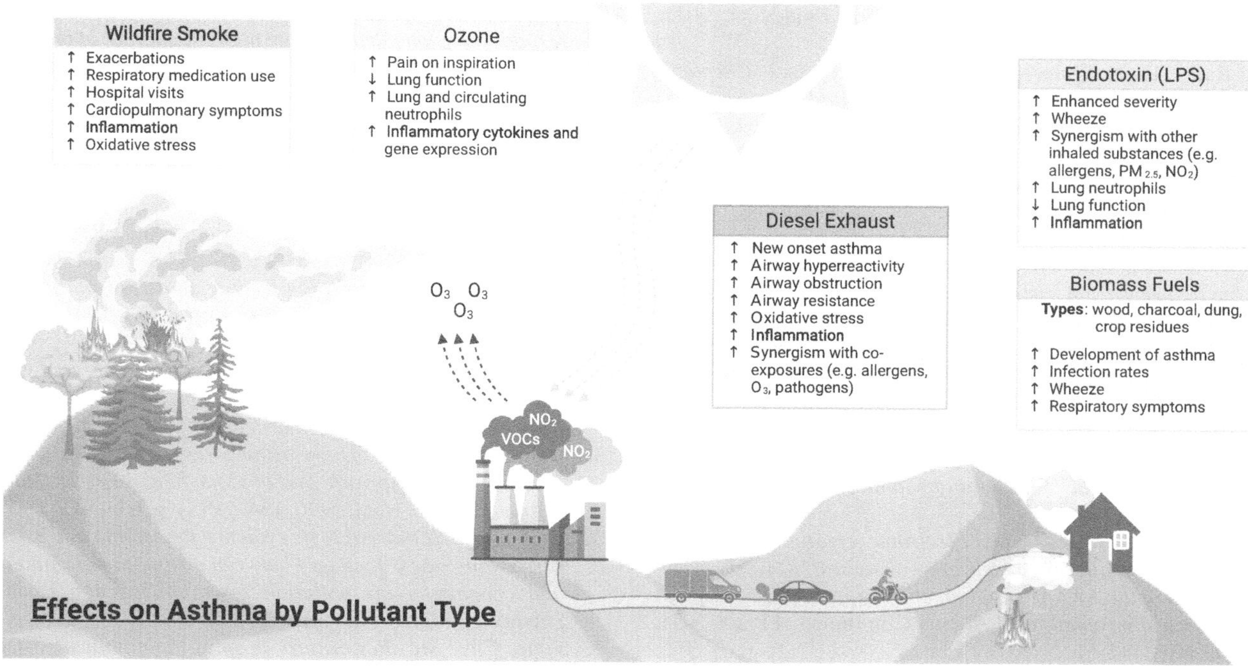

FIGURE 11.2 Effects on asthma by pollutant type: The schematic summarizes the effects of individual pollutant types on asthma. From left to right: wildfire smoke, ozone, diesel exhaust, endotoxin, and biomass fuels. Depictions of each pollutant source are accompanied by a summary box with asthma effects above each source. Abbreviations: O_3 = ozone, VOCs = volatile organic compounds, NO_2 = nitrogen dioxide, LPS = lipopolysaccharide, PM2.5 = particulate matter 2.5 μm or smaller in size. (Figure created with BioRender.)

decrements (in contrast to the pattern observed for the effect of TRAP), and an associated dearth of detailed understanding of causality of effects due to wildfire smoke (Figure 11.2).

11.11 SUMMARY AND FUTURE DIRECTION

Evidence from epidemiology and cohort-based studies establishes a clear link between exposure to air pollution and asthma exacerbation. Further, traffic-related air pollution has newly been established as a causal agent for new-onset asthma in children. However, evidence for new and emerging exposures like wildfire smoke is only beginning to emerge. Controlled exposure and *in vitro* studies have provided evidence that pollutants such as ozone, PM, or endotoxin affect the biology of asthma by increasing inflammation in the airways and modifying the innate immune capability of the airways. The constitutive state of the asthmatic airway in terms of inflammation, innate immune responsiveness, and antioxidant defence capability are all important factors to consider when analysing how a particular pollutant may be exerting its effect on the biology of asthma. Additional modifying factors, specifically sex, genotype, inflammatory endotype, neutrophil response in the airways, and diet, among others, require careful attention as to their role in the effect of air pollution on asthma. Additionally, as exposure to air pollution may be growing, especially in light of climate change, more attention is needed in areas of exposure prevention, mitigation, and treatment. Future studies will have to include these factors in an already complex equation as we move forward with emerging evidence.

REFERENCES

1. Peden, D.B., *Air pollution in asthma: effect of pollutants on airway inflammation*. Ann Allergy Asthma Immunol, 2001. **87**(6 Suppl 3): p. 12–7. doi: 10.1016/s1081-1206(10)62334-4. PMID: 11770676.
2. McDonnell, W.F., et al., *Long-term ambient ozone concentration and the incidence of asthma in nonsmoking adults: The AHSMOG study*. Environ Res, 1999. **80**(2 Pt 1): p. 110–21.
3. Bates, D.V., *Observations on asthma*. Environ Health Perspect, 1995. **103** (Suppl 6): p. 243–7.
4. Thurston, G.D., et al., *Respiratory hospital admissions and summertime haze air pollution in Toronto, Ontario: Consideration of the role of acid aerosols*. Environ Res, 1994. **65**(2): p. 271–90.
5. Thurston, G.D., et al., *Outdoor air pollution and new-onset airway disease. An official American thoracic society workshop report*. Ann Am Thorac Soc, 2020. **17**(4): p. 387–98.
6. Reid, C.E. and M.M. Maestas, *Wildfire smoke exposure under climate change: Impact on respiratory health of affected communities*. Curr Opin Pulm Med, 2019. **25**(2): p. 179–87.
7. Beyene, T., et al., *'Breathing fire': Impact of prolonged bushfire smoke exposure in people with severe asthma*. Int J Environ Res Public Health, 2022. **19**(12).
8. Holm, S.M., M.D. Miller, and J.R. Balmes, *Health effects of wildfire smoke in children and public health tools: A*

narrative review. J Expo Sci Environ Epidemiol, 2021. **31**(1): p. 1–20.
9. Raley, E., L. Quirós-Alcalá, and E.C. Matsui, *Chemical exposures via personal care products and the disproportionate asthma burden among the U.S. Black population.* J Allergy Clin Immunol Pract, 2021. **9**(9): p. 3290–2.
10. Hickman, E. and I. Jaspers, *Current E-cigarette research in the context of asthma.* Curr Allergy Asthma Rep, 2020. **20**(10): p. 62.
11. Li, X., et al., *Association between E-cigarettes and asthma in adolescents: A systematic review and meta-analysis.* Am J Prev Med, 2022. **62**(6): p. 953–60.
12. Chand, B.R. and H. Hosseinzadeh, *Association between e-cigarette use and asthma: A systematic review and meta-analysis.* J Asthma, 2022. **59**(9): p. 1722–31.
13. Wills, T.A., et al., *E-cigarette use and respiratory disorders: An integrative review of converging evidence from epidemiological and laboratory studies.* Eur Respir J, 2021. **57**(1).
14. Hernandez, M.L., et al., *Electronic cigarettes and their impact on allergic respiratory diseases: A work group report of the AAAAI environmental exposures and respiratory health committee.* J Allergy Clin Immunol Pract, 2021. **9**(3): p. 1142–51.
15. Rebuli, M.E., et al., *The E-cigarette or vaping product use-associated lung injury epidemic: Pathogenesis, management, and future directions: An official american thoracic society workshop report.* Ann Am Thorac Soc, 2023. **20**(1): p. 1–17.
16. Carlsen, H.K., et al., *Birch pollen, air pollution and their interactive effects on airway symptoms and peak expiratory flow in allergic asthma during pollen season—a panel study in Northern and Southern Sweden.* Environ Health, 2022. **21**(1): p. 63.
17. Eckl-Dorna, J., et al., *Exposure of rye (Secale cereale) cultivars to elevated ozone levels increases the allergen content in pollen.* J Allergy Clin Immunol, 2010. **126**(6): p. 1315–7.
18. Stawoska, I., et al., *Air pollution in the places of Betula pendula growth and development changes the physicochemical properties and the main allergen content of its pollen.* PLOS ONE, 2023. **18**(1): p. e0279826.
19. American Lung Association. *State of the Air.* 2022; Available from: https://www.lung.org/getmedia/74b3d3d3-88d1-4335-95d8-c4e47d0282c1/SOTA-2022.pdf.
20. Alexis, N.E., et al., *Induced sputum derives from the central airways: Confirmation using a radiolabeled aerosol bolus delivery technique.* Am J Respir Crit Care Med, 2001. **164**(10 Pt 1): p. 1964–70.
21. Becerra, B.J., D. Arias, and M.B. Becerra, *Sex-specific association between environmental tobacco smoke exposure and asthma severity among adults with current asthma.* Int J Environ Res Public Health, 2022. **19**(9).
22. Wright, R.J., et al., *Prenatal ambient ultrafine particle exposure and childhood asthma in the Northeastern United States.* Am J Respir Crit Care Med, 2021. **204**(7): p. 788–96.
23. Clayton, J.A., *Applying the new SABV (sex as a biological variable) policy to research and clinical care.* Physiol Behav, 2018. **187**: p. 2–5.
24. Pignataro, F.S., et al., *Asthma and gender: The female lung.* Pharmacol Res, 2017. **119**: p. 384–90.
25. Alexis, N.E., et al., *Development of a screening protocol to identify persons who are responsive to wood smoke particle-induced airway inflammation with pilot assessment of GSTM1 genotype and asthma status as response modifiers.* Inhal Toxicol, 2022. **34**(11–12): p. 329–39.
26. Fry, R.C., et al., *Individuals with increased inflammatory response to ozone demonstrate muted signaling of immune cell trafficking pathways.* Respir Res, 2012. **13**(1): p. 89.
27. Hernandez, M.L., et al., *Atopic asthmatic patients have reduced airway inflammatory cell recruitment after inhaled endotoxin challenge compared with healthy volunteers.* J Allergy Clin Immunol, 2012. **130**(4): p. 869–76 e2.
28. Tashiro, H., et al., *Sex differences in the impact of dietary fiber on pulmonary responses to ozone.* Am J Respir Cell Mol Biol, 2020. **62**(4): p. 503–12.
29. Brigham, E.P., et al., *A pilot feeding study for adults with asthma: The healthy eating better breathing trial.* PLOS ONE, 2017. **12**(7): p. e0180068.
30. Hosseini, B., et al., *The effects of increasing fruit and vegetable intake in children with asthma on the modulation of innate immune responses.* Nutrients, 2022. **14**(15).
31. Delfino, R.J., et al., *Daily asthma severity in relation to personal ozone exposure and outdoor fungal spores.* Am J Respir Crit Care Med, 1996. **154**(3 Pt 1): p. 633–41.
32. Delfino, R.J., *Epidemiologic evidence for asthma and exposure to air toxics: Linkages between occupational, indoor, and community air pollution research.* Environ Health Perspect, 2002. **110** (Suppl 4): p. 573–89.
33. Pope, C.A., 3rd, *Respiratory hospital admissions associated with PM10 pollution in Utah, Salt Lake, and Cache Valleys.* Arch Environ Health, 1991. **46**(2): p. 90–7.
34. Schwartz, J., et al., *Particulate air pollution and hospital emergency room visits for asthma in Seattle.* Am Rev Respir Dis, 1993. **147**(4): p. 826–31.
35. Peters, A., et al., *Short-term effects of particulate air pollution on respiratory morbidity in asthmatic children.* Eur Respir J, 1997. **10**(4): p. 872–9.
36. Mortimer, K.M., et al., *The effect of air pollution on inner-city children with asthma.* Eur Respir J, 2002. **19**(4): p. 699–705.
37. Pfeffer, P.E., I.S. Mudway, and J. Grigg, *Air pollution and asthma: Mechanisms of harm and considerations for clinical interventions.* Chest, 2021. **159**(4): p. 1346–55.
38. Orach, J., C.F. Rider, A.C.Y. Yuen, C. Schwartz, N. Mookherjee, C. Carlsten, *Controlled diesel exhaust exposure induces a concentration-dependent increase in airway inflammation: A clinical trial.* Ann Am Thorac Soc, 2023. **20**(6): p. 834–42. doi: 10.1513/AnnalsATS.202209-762OC. PMID: 36930796.
39. Rebuli, M.E., et al., *Electronic-cigarette use alters nasal mucosal immune response to live-attenuated influenza virus. a clinical trial.* Am J Respir Cell Mol Biol, 2021. **64**(1): p. 126–37.
40. Rebuli, M.E., A.M. Speen, E.M. Martin, K.A. Addo, E.A. Pawlak, E. Glista-Baker, C. Robinette, H. Zhou, T.L. Noah, I. Jaspers, *Wood smoke exposure alters human inflammatory responses to viral infection in a sex-specific manner. A randomized, placebo-controlled study.* Am J Respir Crit Care Med, 2019. **199**(8): p. 996–1007. doi: 10.1164/rccm.201807-1287OC. PMID: 30360637; PMCID: PMC6467301.
41. Huang, W., et al., *Effects of ambient air pollution on childhood asthma exacerbation in the Philadelphia metropolitan Region, 2011–2014.* Environ Res, 2021. **197**: p. 110955.
42. Orellano, P., et al., *Effect of outdoor air pollution on asthma exacerbations in children and adults: Systematic review and multilevel meta-analysis.* PLOS ONE, 2017. **12**(3): p. e0174050.
43. Huang, J., et al., *Outdoor air pollution and the risk of asthma exacerbations in single lag0 and lag1 exposure patterns: A systematic review and meta-analysis.* J Asthma, 2022. **59**(11): p. 2322–39.

44. To, T., et al., *Progression from asthma to chronic obstructive pulmonary disease. is air pollution a risk factor?* Am J Respir Crit Care Med, 2016. **194**(4): p. 429–38.
45. Park, Y., C. Lee, and J.Y. Jung, *Digital healthcare for airway diseases from personal environmental exposure.* Yonsei Med J, 2022. **63**(Suppl): p. S1–13.
46. Khusial, R.J., et al., *Effectiveness of myaircoach: A mhealth self-management system in asthma.* J Allergy Clin Immunol Pract, 2020. **8**(6): p. 1972–9.e8.
47. James, C., et al., *HEPA filtration improves asthma control in children exposed to traffic-related airborne particles.* Indoor Air, 2020. **30**(2): p. 235–43.
48. Bolcas, P.E., et al., *Vitamin D supplementation attenuates asthma development following traffic-related particulate matter exposure.* J Allergy Clin Immunol, 2019. **143**(1): p. 386–94.e3.
49. Moreno-Macias, H. and I. Romieu, *Effects of antioxidant supplements and nutrients on patients with asthma and allergies.* J Allergy Clin Immunol, 2014. **133**(5): p. 1237–44; quiz 1245.
50. Alexis, N.E., *Controlled chamber studies showed protective effect of nonsteroidal antiinflammatory drugs against ozone exposure: The stage was set for broader epidemiologic investigation.* Am J Respir Crit Care Med, 2020. **201**(12): p. 1583.
51. Michaeloudes, C., et al., *Molecular mechanisms of oxidative stress in asthma.* Mol Aspects Med, 2022. **85**: p. 101026.
52. Enweasor, C., C.H. Flayer, and A. Haczku, *Ozone-induced oxidative stress, neutrophilic airway inflammation, and glucocorticoid resistance in asthma.* Front Immunol, 2021. **12**: p. 631092.
53. Biddle, T.A., et al., *Aerosolized aqueous dust extracts collected near a drying lake trigger acute neutrophilic pulmonary inflammation reminiscent of microbial innate immune ligands.* Sci Total Environ, 2023. **858**(Pt 3): p. 159882.
54. Poole, J.A., et al., *Repetitive organic dust exposure in vitro impairs macrophage differentiation and function.* J Allergy Clin Immunol, 2008. **122**(2): p. 375–82, 382.e1–4.
55. Yurakova, T.R., et al., *HDM induces distinct immunometabolic phenotype in macrophages in TLR4-dependent manner.* Biochim Biophys Acta Mol Basis Dis, 2022. **1868**(12): p. 166531.
56. Thorne, P.S., *Environmental endotoxin exposure and asthma.* J Allergy Clin Immunol, 2021. **148**(1): p. 61–63.
57. Tliba, O. and R.A. Panettieri, Jr., *Paucigranulocytic asthma: Uncoupling of airway obstruction from inflammation.* J Allergy Clin Immunol, 2019. **143**(4): p. 1287–94.
58. Kuruvilla, M.E., F.E. Lee, and G.B. Lee, *Understanding asthma phenotypes, endotypes, and mechanisms of disease.* Clin Rev Allergy Immunol, 2019. **56**(2): p. 219–33.
59. Carr, T.F., A.A. Zeki, and M. Kraft, *Eosinophilic and noneosinophilic asthma.* Am J Respir Crit Care Med, 2018. **197**(1): p. 22–37.
60. Hilty, M., et al., *Disordered microbial communities in asthmatic airways.* Plos One, 2010. **5**(1): p. e8578.
61. Wilson, N.G., A. Hernandez-Leyva, and A.L. Kau, *The ABCs of wheeze: Asthma and bacterial communities.* PLOS Pathog, 2019. **15**(4): p. e1007645.
62. Hosseini, B., et al., *Children with asthma have impaired innate immunity and increased numbers of type 2 innate lymphoid cells compared with healthy controls.* Front Immunol, 2021. **12**.
63. Barnig, C. and B.D. Levy, *Innate immunity is a key factor for the resolution of inflammation in asthma.* Eur Respir Rev, 2015. **24**(135): p. 141.
64. Quon, B.S. and C.H. Goss, *Adult-onset asthma prevention. Should we be investing in antioxidant defense?* Am J Respir Crit Care Med, 2014. **191**(1): p. 4–5.
65. Larkin, E.K., et al., *New risk factors for adult-onset incident asthma. A nested case–control study of host antioxidant defense.* Am J Respir Crit Care Med, 2014. **191**(1): p. 45–53.
66. Kongerud, J., et al., *Ascorbic acid is decreased in induced sputum of mild asthmatics.* Inhal Toxicol, 2003. **15**(2): p. 101–9.
67. Alexis, N.E., et al., *Association between airway hyperreactivity and bronchial macrophage dysfunction in individuals with mild asthma.* Am J Physiol Lung Cell Mol Physiol, 2001. **280**(2): p. L369–75.
68. Newcomb, D.C. and R.S. Peebles, Jr., *Bugs and asthma: A different disease?* Proc Am Thorac Soc, 2009. **6**(3): p. 266–71.
69. Goodman, J.E., et al., *Short-term ozone exposure and asthma severity: Weight-of-evidence analysis.* Environ Res, 2018. **160**: p. 391–7.
70. Balmes, J., *Effect of GSTM1 Genotype on Ozone-Induced Allergic Airway Inflammation*, M. Arjomandi, H. Wong, and N. Holland, Editors. 2012. Prepared for the California Air Resources Board and the California Environmental Protection Agency.
71. Vagaggini, B., et al., *Increase in markers of airway inflammation after ozone exposure can be observed also in stable treated asthmatics with minimal functional response to ozone.* Respir Res, 2010. **11**(1): p. 5.
72. Leroy, P., et al., *Inflammatory and repair pathways induced in human bronchoalveolar lavage cells with ozone inhalation.* PLOS ONE, 2015. **10**(6): p. e0127283.
73. Hernandez, M., et al., *Airway cells from atopic asthmatic patients exposed to ozone display an enhanced innate immune gene profile.* J Allergy Clin Immunol, 2012. **129**(1): p. 259–61.e1–2.
74. Hernandez, M.L., et al., *Atopic asthmatic subjects but not atopic subjects without asthma have enhanced inflammatory response to ozone.* J Allergy Clin Immunol, 2010. **126**(3): p. 537–44.e1.
75. Gomez, J.L., et al., *A network of sputum MicroRNAs is associated with neutrophilic airway inflammation in asthma.* Am J Respir Crit Care Med, 2020. **202**(1): p. 51–64.
76. Alexis, N.E., M.W. Eldridge, and D.B. Peden, *Effect of inhaled endotoxin on airway and circulating inflammatory cell phagocytosis and CD11b expression in atopic asthmatic subjects.* J Allergy Clin Immunol, 2003. **112**(2): p. 353–61.
77. Svendsen, E.R., et al., *Circulating neutrophil CD14 expression and the inverse association of ambient particulate matter on lung function in asthmatic children.* Ann Allergy Asthma Immunol, 2007. **99**(3): p. 244–53.
78. Soukup, J.M. and S. Becker, *Human alveolar macrophage responses to air pollution particulates are associated with insoluble components of coarse material, including particulate endotoxin.* Toxicol Appl Pharmacol, 2001. **171**(1): p. 20–6.
79. Liebers, V., T. Brüning, and M. Raulf, *Occupational endotoxin exposure and health effects.* Arch Toxicol, 2020. **94**(11): p. 3629–44.
80. Carnes, M.U., et al., *House dust endotoxin levels are associated with adult asthma in a U.S. Farming population.* Ann Am Thorac Soc, 2017. **14**(3): p. 324–31.
81. Mendy, A., et al., *Endotoxin clustering with allergens in house dust and asthma outcomes in a U.S. National study.* Environ Health, 2020. **19**(1): p. 35.

82. Li, Y., et al., *Bacterial endotoxin (lipopolysaccharide) binds to the surface of gold nanoparticles, interferes with biocorona formation and induces human monocyte inflammatory activation*. Nanotoxicology, 2017. **11**(9–10): p. 1157–75.
83. Ishida, T., et al., *Association of protein and endotoxin in outdoor air with emergency department visits for children and adults with asthma in Fukuoka, Japan*. Biol Pharm Bull, 2020. **43**(9): p. 1361–6.
84. Eldridge, M.W. and D.B. Peden, *Airway response to concomitant exposure with endotoxin and allergen in atopic asthmatics*. J Toxicol Environ Health A, 2000. **61**(1): p. 27–37.
85. Berger, M., et al., *Lipopolysaccharide amplifies eosinophilic inflammation after segmental challenge with house dust mite in asthmatics*. Allergy, 2015. **70**(3): p. 257–64.
86. Newton, A.N., et al., *Atopy as a modifier of the relationships between endotoxin exposure and symptoms among laboratory animal workers*. Ann Work Expo Health, 2017. **61**(8): p. 1024–8.
87. Alexis, N., et al., *CD14-dependent airway neutrophil response to inhaled LPS: Role of atopy*. J Allergy Clin Immunol, 2001. **107**(1): p. 31–5.
88. Mendy, A., et al., *Synergistic association of house endotoxin exposure and ambient air pollution with asthma outcomes*. Am J Respir Crit Care Med, 2019. **200**(6): p. 712–20.
89. Hasunuma, H., et al., *Effects of early-life exposure to dust mite allergen and endotoxin on the development of asthma and wheezing: The Japan environment and children's study*. Clin Transl Allergy, 2021. **11**(8): p. e12071.
90. Rylander, R., et al., *Pulmonary function and symptoms after inhalation of endotoxin*. Am Rev Respir Dis, 1989. **140**(4): p. 981–6.
91. Michel, O., et al., *Inflammatory response to acute inhalation of endotoxin in asthmatic patients*. Am Rev Respir Dis, 1992. **146**(2): p. 352–7.
92. Michel, O., et al., *Dose-response relationship to inhaled endotoxin in normal subjects*. Am J Respir Crit Care Med, 1997. **156**(4 Pt 1): p. 1157–64.
93. Michel, O., *Role of house-dust endotoxin exposure in aetiology of allergy and asthma*. Mediat Inflamm, 2001. **10**(6): p. 301–4.
94. Alexis, N.E., et al., *Development of an inhaled endotoxin challenge protocol for characterizing evoked cell surface phenotype and genomic responses of airway cells in allergic individuals* Ann Allergy Asthma Immunol, 2008. **100**(3): p. 206–15.
95. Dubin, W., et al., *Asthma and endotoxin: Lipopolysaccharide-binding protein and soluble CD14 in bronchoalveolar compartment*. Am J Physiol, 1996. **270**(5 Pt 1): p. L736–L744.
96. Kline, J.N., et al., *Variable airway responsiveness to inhaled lipopolysaccharide*. Am J Respir Crit Care Med, 1999. **160**(1): p. 297–303.
97. Hernandez, M.L., et al., *IL-1 receptor antagonist reduces endotoxin-induced airway inflammation in healthy volunteers*. J Allergy Clin Immunol, 2015. **135**(2): p. 379–85.
98. Burbank, A.J., et al., *Gamma tocopherol-enriched supplement reduces sputum eosinophilia and endotoxin-induced sputum neutrophilia in volunteers with asthma*. J Allergy Clin Immunol, 2018. **141**(4): p. 1231–8.e1.
99. Long, E. and C. Carlsten, *Controlled human exposure to diesel exhaust: Results illuminate health effects of traffic-related air pollution and inform future directions*. Part Fibre Toxicol, 2022. **19**(1): p. 11.
100. Long, E., C. Schwartz, and C. Carlsten, *Controlled human exposure to diesel exhaust: A method for understanding health effects of traffic-related air pollution*. Part Fibre Toxicol, 2022. **19**(1): p. 15.
101. Noonan, C.W. and J.R. Balmes, *Biomass smoke exposures: Health outcomes measures and study design*. Inhal Toxicol, 2010. **22**(2): p. 108–12.
102. Reddy, A.K., R.H. Williams, and T.B. Johansson, *Energy after Rio: Prospects and challenges*. UNDP: New York, 1997.
103. Simkovich, S.M., et al., *The health and social implications of household air pollution and respiratory diseases*. NPJ Prim Care Respir Med, 2019. **29**(1): p. 12.
104. Abebe, Y., et al., *Determinants of asthma in Ethiopia: Age and sex matched case-control study with special reference to household fuel exposure and housing characteristics*. Asthma Res Pract, 2021. **7**(1): p. 14.
105. Ranathunga, N., et al., *Effect of household air pollution due to solid fuel combustion on childhood respiratory diseases in a semi urban population in Sri Lanka*. BMC Pediatr, 2019. **19**(1): p. 306.
106. Oluwole, O., et al., *Household biomass fuel use, asthma symptoms severity, and asthma underdiagnosis in rural schoolchildren in Nigeria: A cross-sectional observational study*. BMC Pulm Med, 2017. **17**(1): p. 3.
107. Regalado, J., et al., *The effect of biomass burning on respiratory symptoms and lung function in rural Mexican women*. Am J Respir Crit Care Med, 2006. **174**(8): p. 901–5.
108. Lu, W., et al., *Biomass smoke exposure and atopy among young children in the Western highlands of Guatemala: A prospective cohort study*. Int J Environ Res Public Health, 2022. **19**(21).
109. Alexander, D., et al., *Ventilated cookstoves associated with improvements in respiratory health-related quality of life in rural Bolivia*. J Public Health (Oxf), 2014. **36**(3): p. 460–6.
110. Kaali, S., D. Jack, and A.G. Lee, *The conundrum of cleaner cookstove interventions: Necessary but insufficient?* Am J Respir Crit Care Med, 2020. **203**(11): p. 1336–8.
111. Checkley, W., et al., *Effects of a household air pollution intervention with liquefied petroleum gas on cardiopulmonary outcomes in Peru: A randomized controlled trial*. Am J Respir Crit Care Med, 2020. **203**(11): p. 1386–97.
112. Schilmann, A., et al., *A follow-up study after an improved cookstove intervention in rural Mexico: Estimation of household energy use and chronic PM2.5 exposure*. Environment International, 2019. **131**: p. 105013.
113. Liu, J.C., et al., *Particulate air pollution from wildfires in the Western US under climate change*. Climatic Change, 2016. **138**(3): p. 655–66.
114. Rice, M.B., et al., *Respiratory impacts of wildland fire smoke: Future challenges and policy opportunities. an official american thoracic society workshop report*. Ann Am Thorac Soc, 2021. **18**(6): p. 921–30.
115. Moore, L.E., et al., *Impacts of wildfire smoke and air pollution on a pediatric population with asthma: A population-based study*. Int J Environ Res Public Health, 2023. **20**(3).
116. Dhingra, R., C. Keeler, B.S. Staley, et al., *Wildfire smoke exposure and early childhood respiratory health: a study of prescription claims data*. Environmental Health. 2023. **22**(1): p. 48.

117. Heaney, A., et al., *Impacts of fine particulate matter from wildfire smoke on respiratory and cardiovascular health in California*. Geohealth, 2022. **6**(6): p. e2021GH000578.
118. Henry, S., et al., *Assessing the risk of respiratory-related healthcare visits associated with wildfire smoke exposure in children 0–18 years old: A systematic review*. Int J Environ Res Public Health, 2021. **18**(16).
119. Cherry, N., et al., *Respiratory outcomes of firefighter exposures in the Fort McMurray fire: A cohort study from Alberta Canada*. J Occup Environ Med, 2021. **63**(9): p. 779–86.
120. Schwartz, C., A.K. Bølling, and C. Carlsten, *Controlled human exposures to wood smoke: A synthesis of the evidence*. Part Fibre Toxicol, 2020. **17**(1): p. 49.

12 Exercise-Induced Bronchoconstriction

Justin Greiwe, Anil Nanda, and Sharmilee M. Nyenhuis

CASE PRESENTATION

A 24-year-old female presents to the office with shortness of breath and severe nasal congestion after strenuous exercise sessions that increasingly seem to be affecting her athletic performance. She is a professional soccer player currently on the roster for the US women's national team preparing for the Olympic Games. Dyspnea occurs after several minutes of exercise and is associated with wheezing, chest tightness, and a non-productive cough. The patient also notes increased nasal congestion, postnasal drainage, sneezing, and rhinorrhea during the spring and fall months. Symptoms have been bothersome for years, but she has learned to push through the symptoms. She has no other significant past medical history and denies any history of asthma but has been hesitant to discuss her symptoms with the training staff for fear of losing playing time. Physical examination is unremarkable, and pulmonary function testing revealed a forced vital capacity (FVC) of 1.75 (119% predicted), a forced expiratory volume in 1 sec (FEV_1) of 1.47 (113% predicted), and a forced expiratory flow at 25%–75% (FEF_{25-75}) of 1.65 (100% predicted) without response to a beta-2 agonist bronchodilator. Given the concerning history and her status as an Olympic athlete, indirect provocation with eucapnic voluntary hyperpnea (EVH) was completed, and she was found to have a 14% pre-/post-challenge reduction in FEV_1, confirming the diagnosis of exercise-induced bronchoconstriction (EIB). Skin prick testing (SPT) to inhalants indicated sensitization to trees, grass, ragweed pollens, and Alternaria mold spores. A fractional exhaled nitric oxide (FeNO) test was 12 ppb, indicating no evidence of eosinophilic airway inflammation. Based on the patient's tests, she was started on a nasal corticosteroid to reduce nasal congestion during exercise to better control her underlying seasonal allergic rhinitis. She was also instructed to use a short-acting beta-2 adrenergic agonist 15 minutes before all exercise activity along with a standard pre-competition warm-up. A follow-up visit six weeks later revealed that she was now able to complete all of her training workouts and that her performance on the field significantly improved. Her nasal congestion dramatically improved as well, allowing her to breathe through her nose while running. A six-month follow-up evaluation was recommended.

12.1 INTRODUCTION

Exercise-induced bronchospasm (EIB) is defined as a transient narrowing of the lower airway with an associated increase in airway resistance during or following exercise.[1–3] EIB is a more accurate descriptor of this condition than is exercise-induced asthma (EIA) because exercise induces bronchoconstriction, not asthma, and not all EIB is associated with chronic asthma.[4] Indeed, the term "exercise-induced asthma" should be abandoned.[3]

This chapter addresses the two forms of EIB: EIB in patients who do not have evidence of chronic asthma (called EIB alone); and EIB in patients who also have chronic asthma (called EIB with asthma). EIB alone, which is less common, occurs with strenuous exercise, and it has been studied in schoolchildren, armed-forces recruits, and highly competitive and elite athletes.[1, 5–8] EIB alone may be considered a form of injury-related lung disease. The more common condition, EIB with asthma, is seen in as many as 90% of asthmatic patients.[1–3] In contrast, EIB alone without known asthma is seen in 40–50% of patients who have allergic rhinitis, 10% of the general population, and as many as 60% of elite or highly competitive athletes.[1–3] The prevalence of EIB in athletes who do not otherwise have asthma depends on the intensity and the duration of exercise and is particularly prevalent in the most strenuous endurance sports, with the highest degree of ventilation injuring the airway in conjunction with environmental irritants such as cold air. Thus, ice hockey, cross-country skiing, skating, cycling, mountain biking, swimming, rowing, and track and field ("athletics") have the highest prevalence of EIB alone without known asthma (ranging up to 60%). Less strenuous sports, such as badminton, baseball, and diving, have a lesser prevalence of EIB.[9, 10]

EIB with asthma may represent the earliest sign of asthma in childhood and may be the last sign to resolve after an exacerbation.[1] The prevalence of EIB in patients who have underlying chronic asthma depends on the sport or activity, the environment, and the degree of control of the underlying asthma.[1–4] EIB reflects the control (or lack of control) of asthma and the evidence of airway bronchial hyperreactivity. The more severe the EIB is, the more poorly controlled the chronic asthma will be.[2, 4] In the Expert Panel Report (EPR) of the National Asthma Education and Prevention Program (NAEPP-3), EIB is listed as an important indicator of the impairment of pulmonary function.[11] In the most up-to-date 2020 Focused Updates to the Asthma Management

DOI: 10.1201/9781003287209-15

Guidelines, EIB was not mentioned.[12] EIB exacerbations suggest the need to increase controller therapy for underlying asthma.[1–4]

A history of respiratory symptoms alone, during, or following exercise, is not reliable for the diagnosis of EIB.[1–4, 13, 14] EIB is identified by establishing objective evidence for a fall in post-exercise FEV_1 of at least 10% from its pre-exercise value, after eight minutes of strenuous aerobic exercise. Exercise is conducted to achieve at least 80–95% of the maximum heart rate as a surrogate for a maximum voluntary ventilation (MVV) of 40–80% of the predicted maximum.[1–3, 15] In children aged 3–6 years, a fall in FEV in one-half second (FEV0.5) may be used to define EIB.[16] The fall in FEV_1 may begin during exercise; in 80% of patients, the fall in FEV_1 occurs between 5 and 12 minutes and rarely as late as 30 minutes post exercise.[17] Recovery from the bronchoconstriction occurs within 30–60 minutes after exercise is completed.[18] Repeated exercise within 2–4 hours may lead to a refractory period in 50% of individuals, in which exercise does not induce additional bronchoconstriction [18].

This chapter describes the epidemiology, pathogenesis, presentation, diagnosis, and management (both pharmaceutical and nonpharmaceutical) of EIB alone and EIB with asthma. The appropriate management of EIB should allow patients, whether recreational or elite athletes or nonathletic patients with activity-induced symptoms, to have a healthy lifestyle, with the ability to participate in physical activity, including their selected sports activities.[1–4]

12.2 EPIDEMIOLOGY

The prevalence of EIB varies with the population being studied, including age, sex, ethnicity, urbanization, exercise level of intensity, type of exercise challenge, criteria for a positive test, the presence or absence of chronic asthma, and environmental conditions, including the season in which the challenge is being performed.[3, 19] A recent systematic review and meta-analysis estimated the global prevalence of EIB among children and adolescents at 9% (IC95%: 8–10%), with a higher rate (12%) in Asia-Pacific and America.[20] The review included 66 studies with 55,696 participants and 5670 cases of EIB. The prevalence of EIB was higher among child/adolescent athletes (15%; 95% CI: 9–21%) and children/adolescents with asthma (46%; 95% CI: 39–53%). A study published in 2020 found an estimated prevalence of EIB to be 23.1% (95% confidence interval [CI]: 14.5–33.8) among adolescent athletes.[21] This study diagnosed EIB using exercise treadmill test (EIB was defined as a decrease of $FEV_1 \geq 10\%$ from baseline).[21] Other reports using free-running exercise in adolescent athletes reported a prevalence of 9.4%. The range in prevalence among adolescent athletes is 9–38% and appears to depend on testing used to screen from free-running exercise to eucapnic voluntary hyperventilation (EVH).[20, 21]

The socioeconomic and environmental impact of EIB was demonstrated in two surveys in Ghana performed 10 years apart (1993 and 2003) using a six-minute free-running test among children aged 9–13 years. The urban rich children demonstrated an increased prevalence of EIB from 4.2% to 8.3%, whereas the urban poor children had an increased prevalence from 1.4% to 3.0%, and the rural poor prevalence increased from 2.2% to 3.9%.[22, 23]

Prevalence is affected by gender and urbanization, with girls (8.5%) more likely than boys (6.4%), and an urban setting (8.9%) more likely than a rural setting (7%) to have a positive challenge with a six-minute run using a 15% fall in PEF.[24] Ethnic and racial differences are also noted, with African Americans having a higher prevalence of EIB (13%) than European Americans (2%) using a free-running test with PEF monitoring.[25]

A British study used cycle ergometry in nine-year-old Asian children from the Indian subcontinent and found a 3.6 times higher prevalence of EIB than in White urban children when EIB was defined as at least a 15% fall in PEF within 10 minutes of the end of the exercise.[26]

In elite athletes, the prevalence of EIB has been reported to be 18–50% in winter Olympians following an exercise challenge; the prevalence was 50% in skiers with a field exercise and 30–35% in figure skaters with an exercise challenge.[27, 28] In summer athletes, using EVH to screen, the prevalence of EIB was 50%; with the same technique in winter Olympians, the prevalence was 45%.[29, 30] In asymptomatic individuals with a history of EIB only but no history of asthma, the prevalence of EIB was 12%, and EIB was predictive of adult asthma.[31] As previously described, sex-related differences in the prevalence of EIB in athletes have been identified. A systematic literature review identified 60 studies evaluating EIB and/or atopy in post-pubertal adult athletes ($n = 7501$). These studies reported a higher prevalence of atopy in male versus female athletes and a significantly higher rate of atopic EIB in male versus female athletes. This suggests an interaction between male sex, exercise, and atopic status in the course of EIB among adult athletes.[32]

In Olympic athletes, the prevalence of EIB was highest in athletes participating in the most strenuous endurance sports, ranging from winter sports with 17.6% in cross-country skiing and 16.2% in speed skating, to summer sports with 15.3% in cycling, 11.3% in swimming, and 10.1% in the modern pentathlon.[33] In another study, scuba divers had a 17% prevalence of EIB defined as a 15% fall in FEV_1 from baseline secondary to the use of inhaled hypertonic saline (4.5%), a surrogate for an exercise challenge.[34]

Elite athletes have a higher prevalence of EIB related to certain atmospheric conditions such as high pollen levels, high pollution, chemical exposure, and cold air.[3] EIB can be present with or without symptoms, but symptoms alone are not a sensitive index for the diagnosis of EIB. Thus the prevalence varies not only with the form of the exercise but also with the type of challenge that is used to elicit EIB (surrogate or exercise).[3] Other factors related to the presence of EIB include environmental factors such as chlorinated pools, ice hockey rinks surfaced with fossil fuel, a family history of atopy, uncontrolled asthma, lower respiratory illness, a personal history of atopy, and urbanization.[4]

EIB has an impact on physical functioning including school activities and emotional functioning in quality of life. This impact was demonstrated in studies in high school athletes and in children in Tokyo with EIB with and without asthma, and in telephone surveys of parents of 4- to 17-year-old children with current asthma and adults aged 18 years and older.[35–38]

Children with EIB were profoundly impacted, with lower scores in the areas of physical functioning, emotional functioning, and school activities compared with those without EIB.[37] In the telephone survey, the most frequently reported symptoms of EIB were cough, wheezing, and shortness of breath. In a large survey of EIB, more than one in five (22.2%) of 4- to 12-year-old children with EIB avoided selected activities and almost one in three (31.8%) of 13- to 18-year-old adolescents with EIB reported avoidance of activities related to EIB.[36, 38] Parents reported that asthma impacted their children "a lot or some" in 30% of sports or recreation activities, in 30.9% of normal non-sports-related activities, and in 26% of other outdoor activities. Despite the frequency of EIB, only 23% stated that they used bronchodilators always or most of the time, and 43.4% reported that they "never" used bronchodilators.[36] Parents frequently express worries that asthma may limit exercise in their children; however, if they were properly educated and their children's EIB was better managed, these concerns could be resolved in most cases.[39]

12.3 PATHOGENESIS (TABLE 12.1)

The physiological determinant for EIB is the transfer or loss of water from the airway surface in response to the inspiration and conditioning of large amounts of dry air in a short period of time.[1–3] There are two theories for the evolution of EIB: the more widely accepted osmolar theory and the possibly contributory thermal theory. The osmolar theory postulates that mediator release follows degranulation of the mast cells caused by a hyperosmolar environment created by dehydration.[1–3, 22, 40] The thermal theory suggests that EIB is a vascular event with vasoconstriction as a result of airway cooling and reactive hyperemia following rewarming (Table 12.1).[1–3]

The evaporation of water results in the cooling and dehydration of the airway. Dehydration creates a hyperosmolar environment that leads to degranulation of the mast cells with a mediator release, including histamine, tryptase, leukotrienes, and prostaglandins, as well as chemotactic factors leading to the recruitment of inflammatory cells, most notably eosinophils but also lymphocytes and neutrophils. This response is also associated with reverse axonal sensory nerve mediator release. This orchestrated release of mediators, cytokines, and chemokines contributes to bronchial smooth muscle constriction, airway inflammation characterized by dense infiltrates of inflammatory cells (lymphocytes and eosinophils) and increased inspissated mucus secretions and cellular debris due to the denudation of the bronchial epithelial cells. Epithelial cell injury leads to an increase in transglutaminase 2, which regulates phospholipases and the leukotriene pathway. Leukotrienes are more predominant than prostaglandins in the airways of patients with EIB, and they play a significant role in inducing bronchoconstriction mediated by the sensory nerves and the release of mucus from goblet cells (MUCSAC).[22] Thus EIB is the outcome of the dehydration of the airway leading to a hyperosmolar environment. Extensive studies of the airway cells, mucosa, epithelium, exhaled breath condensate, proteomics, the genetics of the airway mucosa, sputum, and bronchoalveolar lavage support the osmolar mechanism of action for EIB.[22]

EIB alone without known asthma in the competitive or elite athlete is postulated to be due to an overuse injury to the airway. Hyperventilation, often of cold and dry air, results in compensation by the airway down to the smaller airways, where there is an enhanced risk of injury to the epithelium.[1–3, 22, 41] Plasma exudation occurs in the repair process so that repeated exposure leads to smooth muscle hyperresponsiveness and EIB.[40, 41] This is seen in endurance athletes, particularly those exercising in cold climates and swimmers.[40, 42–45]

Another contributing factor to the pathogenesis of EIB may be environmental exposures to fine ($PM_{2.5}$) and nano-/ultra-fine particulate matter ($PM_{0.1}$; <0.1 mm diameter). The main source of $PM_{2.5}$ and $PM_{0.1}$ is from fossil fuel combustion emissions. These small particles can have alveolar deposition, which may be exacerbated by high ventilations of exercise.[46, 47] High levels of $PM_{0.1}$ have been identified at indoor ice rinks where a fossil-fueled Zamboni is used for ice resurfacing[29, 48, 49] and at athletic fields located close to major roadways.[50] Exposure to high levels of nano-/ultra-fine particulate matter along with high ventilation exercise and a genetic susceptibility may explain the high reported prevalence of asthma and EIB in ice rink athletes.[27–29, 48, 51]

TABLE 12.1
Pathogenesis 1–3, 25

EIB alone	Syndrome of overuse injury in competitive or elite athletes
EIB with asthma	Osmolar theory with contributory thermal theory peripherally with cold air

Note: Pronounced leukotriene production is regulated by epithelial injury via transglutaminase (TGM2) and phospholipase A2.

12.4 CLINICAL PRESENTATION OF EIB

The symptoms of EIB include cough, wheeze, chest tightness (or chest pain in children), shortness of breath, dyspnea, excessive mucus production, and "feeling out of shape" even though the individual is really in an acceptable physical condition.[3, 14, 52–58] The signs and symptoms may also be vague, including poor performance, heavy legs, muscle cramps, sore throat, and stomachache.[3, 14, 30, 52, 53] Post-race cough is the most commonly reported symptom in elite athletes. Nevertheless, a sensitivity/specificity analysis did not demonstrate the effectiveness of self-reported symptoms as a negative or positive predictor of changes in the pulmonary function after exercise.[3, 14, 53]

Rundell noted that in elite cold-weather athletes, 91% of EIB-positive athletes had at least one symptom, whereas 48% of EIB-negative athletes also had at least one symptom.[3, 14] Parsons et al. reported similar findings in collegiate athletes, with both EIB-positive and EIB-negative athletes having a similar prevalence of symptoms.[55] This is consistent with other studies that show that the percentage change in FEV_1 from pre- to post-challenge follows a normal distribution, suggesting that there is no specific cut-off point for a fall in FEV_1 that distinguishes between those individuals with or without EIB.[52]

Additionally, exercise-induced dyspnea is one of the most common symptoms of EIB. It has been demonstrated that many individuals who are thought to have EIB have other conditions that contribute to or precipitate their symptoms, including exercise-induced hyperventilation, exercise-related laryngomalacia, exercise-precipitated vocal cord dysfunction, nasal congestion, gastroesophageal reflux disease (GERD), cardiac abnormalities, and poor conditioning.[59, 60] In one study, only 8% of children presenting with exercise-induced dyspnea had EIB; the remaining 92% had another diagnosis that manifested as EIB [60].

12.5 DIAGNOSIS OF EIB (TABLE 12.2)

A self-reported history alone does not predict who will have a positive exercise challenge, and therefore it is not reliable for the diagnosis of EIB. The outcome of a challenge may also be modified by the training environmental conditions and the level of competition, particularly in competitive or elite athletes.[3, 13–15, 24, 56, 61–64] Therefore, an evaluation of EIB mandates objective pulmonary function monitoring with exercise at 85%–90% of the maximum heart rate (40%–80% of MVV). This level of exercise may be achieved by exercising for six minutes (in children) and eight minutes (in adults) at a minute ventilation of at least 17.5–21 times FEV_1 and up to 30 times FEV_1 for EVH. The latter two ventilation rates equal 60%–85% of MVV.[3, 15, 56, 64] Interestingly, when exercise is performed in a laboratory (e.g. on a treadmill) rather than in the venue in which an athlete participates, there may be a high rate of false-negative results for EIB. This may be due to the natural variability of EIB, but it is likely to be impacted more by factors that affect the airway response, including type, duration, and intensity of exercise, temperature and humidity of the inspired air, pollutants in the air, time since the last episode of EIB, and the duration of medication withholding (Table 12.2).[15, 56]

The most commonly used and effective procedure for the diagnosis of EIB is a laboratory exercise treadmill challenge, which uses a protocol that incrementally increases the exercise intensity rapidly over 2–4 minutes followed by 6–8 minutes of strenuous exercise for a total of 10 minutes. The ventilation for athletes should be more than 21 times the FEV_1 during the final eight minutes. Protocols generally encourage that patients breathe medical-grade dry air with a nose clip while running or cycling at a level sufficient to increase the heart rate to 80%–95% of the maximum heart rate (max HR = 220−age in years).[15, 56]

Free running or running on a treadmill may be preferable to cycling because ventilation increases more rapidly when running. Again, as noted, the patient should breathe dry air to ensure a low water content of inspired air. The apparatus to produce cool air is considerably more complex, and few laboratories provide both dry and cool air. If available, cool air may be preferable in skiers to simulate the natural environment in which they participate.[1–3]

There is a natural variation in the airway reactivity to exercise so that a single negative test may not be sufficient to rule out EIB.[15, 56] As many as 25% of individuals without known asthma but with exercise-induced symptoms may have one positive test and one negative test when an exercise is repeated under the same conditions over a short span of days.[15] A natural variation can also occur with known asthmatic patients in whom exposure to allergens or irritants can temporarily increase the severity of EIB, and the elimination of these factors will diminish the severity of EIB.[64]

Generally, elite athletes should be evaluated using a sports-specific exercise that reproduces the symptoms in the laboratory that occur "on the field."[3, 24, 29] The environmental conditions, including temperature, humidity, pollen level, and pollution index, may impact the response on the field and are difficult to replicate in the laboratory.

Measurements of FEV_1 are made in duplicate at 0, 3, 5, 10, 15, 20, and 30 minutes after exercise, and the highest (best) value at each post-exercise stage is used in the calculations. Full FVC maneuvers should not be performed post-exercise; an FEV_1 lasting at least two seconds but no more than three seconds leads to less fatigue than a full FVC maneuver.[1–3, 56]

The percentage fall in FEV_1 is:

$$100 \times \frac{(\text{Best pre-challenge } FEV_1 - \text{lowest best post-challenge } FEV_1)}{\text{Best pre-challenge } FEV_1}$$

where the lowest FEV_1 post-challenge is the best (highest) FEV_1 at the stage with the largest fall in FEV_1.

The diagnosis of EIB requires at least a 10% fall in FEV_1, preferably at two or more time points post-challenge. The severity of EIB may be rated based on the fall in FEV_1 as mild (>10% but <25%), moderate (>25% but <50%), and severe (>50%), from pre-challenge.[1–3] Other end points are time to recovery to 95% of baseline FEV_1 and area under the curve (AUC) until 30 minutes post-exercise. Flow rates (FEF25–75) and PEF are rarely useful.

Given the variability in the performance of exercise challenges, surrogate challenges have been developed to assess EIB.[29] These include inhaling dry powder mannitol (Aridol)

TABLE 12.2
Diagnostic Tests (1–3): Challenges to Perform When Response to Bronchodilator Shows <12% and 200 mL Increase in FEV_1 3

	Advantage	Disadvantage	Diagnostic Cutoff
Indirect challenge	Specificity	Sensitivity less than with methacholine	At least a 10% fall in FEV_1 from baseline
Exercise: cycle, treadmill, run, sport	Specificity	Requires facilities to perform challenge (e.g., laboratory equipped with treadmill and crash cart)	At least a 10% fall in FEV_1 from baseline
Surrogate challenges	Specificity; requires no exercise equipment	Sensitivity less than with methacholine	At least a 10% fall in FEV_1 from baseline
Mannitol	Specificity; requires no exercise equipment; commercially available; relatively inexpensive; produces a response–dose ratio	May not diagnose mild asthma	PD_{15}: at least a 15% fall in FEV_1 from baseline or 10% fall in FEV_1 between stages
EVH	Standard for evaluating Olympic athletes to confirm EIB	May be more sensitive than mannitol for EIB	At least a 10% fall in FEV_1 from baseline
Hypertonic saline	Specificity (88%)	Sensitivity (46%); not standardized	At least a 15% fall in FEV_1 from baseline
Adenosine monophosphate 151	Sensitivity (70%); specificity (94%)	Sputum eosinophilia; not approved by the FDA; limited publications support its use in this setting	At least a 10% fall in FEV_1 from baseline
Direct challenge	Sensitivity	May lack specificity	PC_{20}: at least a 20% fall in FEV_1 from baseline
Methacholine	Sensitivity	May lack specificity	PC_{20}: at least a 20% fall in FEV_1 from baseline

and EVH. EVH is the recommended test for Olympic athletes. Mannitol is a graduated dose–response test, which has intrinsic safety and may provide the level of sensitivity (e.g. using the response–dose ratio [RDR]). In contrast to other challenges, patients undergoing EVH may be more susceptible to severe reactions with extreme falls in FEV_1.[1–3]

EVH was developed in the 1980s to evaluate armed forces personnel for EIB. The EVH test requires inhalation of a fixed dry gas mixture containing 4.9–5% carbon dioxide, 21% oxygen, and the remaining balance of nitrogen.[65] The procedure necessitates hyperventilation of the dry gas mixture for six minutes at 30 times FEV_1 to reach about 85% of MVV. The higher ventilation achieved (vs. 17–21 times FEV_1 with exercise) and the use of dry air result in a low rate of false-negative outcomes for EIB. However, EVH is a challenge without a standardized dose response and is very potent with the potential for a larger fall in FEV_1 than that with a graduated test such as the inhalation of mannitol (or methacholine). EVH should probably not be the first challenge performed for individuals with a documented diagnosis of asthma.[65] However, EVH has been useful in the diagnosis of previously undiagnosed elite athletes and in excluding asthma in others previously clinically diagnosed as having EIB.[66–68] The disadvantages of EVH are a sore throat from breathing dry air, the need for a very low-resistance breathing circuit, and, as noted, severe falls in FEV_1.[1–3] Following the EVH challenge, FEV_1 is evaluated for about 30 minutes. A sustained fall in FEV_1 of at least 10% following EVH is consistent with EIB;[67, 69, 70] EVH is considered the gold standard for the diagnosis of asthma in Olympic athletes who are being screened for EIB. Nevertheless, general screening of all elite athletes for EIB with EVH is not recommended, as there is a relatively low prevalence of EIB among these athletes, suggesting that a history of EIB is unreliable.[13]

For individuals with known asthma, a mannitol dry powder challenge could be the initial procedure to evaluate the potential for EIB. This challenge test is standardized, and patients rarely have large falls in FEV_1, as may be seen with the exercise challenge or EVH; moreover, exercise and EVH do not provide an RDR.[1–3]

Mannitol creates a hyperosmolar environment, which causes a mediator release similar to exercise and EVH. The challenge involves the inhalation of progressively increasing doses of mannitol powder to a cumulative dose of 635 mg, with determinations of FEV_1 60 seconds after each dose. The mannitol kit is commercially available in many countries, with prepackaged capsules containing 5, 10, 30, or 40 mg of mannitol and an Osmohaler device to deliver the drug.[71, 72] The FEV_1 is determined in duplicate. A fall of 15% from baseline in FEV_1 (or a fall of 10% between doses) at a cumulative dose of no more than 635 mg is considered a positive test. The test has a repeatability of about one doubling dose. Spontaneous recovery usually occurs rapidly after a mannitol challenge;[71–73] in those with known asthma who are not receiving ICS (inhaled corticosteroids), there is a consistent relationship between mannitol PD15 and the percentage fall in FEV_1 after exercise and EVH. This relationship is not as consistent in patients using ICS or in those without a defined asthma diagnosis.[74] A mannitol challenge completed in less than 35 minutes demonstrated sensitivities of 64%, 75%, and 83% to characterize exercise-associated FEV_1 falls of 10%, 15%, and 20%, respectively.[72]

Hypertonic saline (4.5%) is not commercially available for challenge testing, but it has been used for the diagnosis of EIB and airway hyperresponsiveness in individuals with known asthma.[75] During a saline challenge, the nebulizer output is kept unchanged, and the dose of saline is increased consecutively by doubling the inhalation time beginning with 0.5 minutes, then one, two, four, and eight minutes, with subjects inhaling at tidal volumes. FEV_1 is determined in duplicate one minute after each challenge step, and the best (highest) of the duplicate readings at each stage is used. The challenge is terminated when FEV_1 falls ≥15% or more from baseline or the cumulative inhalation time of 15.5 minutes is achieved.[76] The level of aerosol delivered is determined by the alteration in the weight of the nebulizer. A 15% fall in FEV_1 in response to an inhalation of 23 g of saline or less is considered a positive result.[76] The sensitivity of a 4.5% saline provocative dose to diagnose EIB (with a fall in FEV_1 of at least 10%) was 53.9% with a specificity of 84.7% in a pediatric population.[77] Adenosine monophosphate is another investigational surrogate diagnostic test that creates a hyperosmolar environment.[3, 75]

In a review of 20 relevant studies of diagnostic tests versus exercise challenge tests, the sensitivity and specificity for each test were as follows:[78]

- Self-report of symptoms to detect EIB (two studies): sensitivity 36.8%, specificity 85–86%
- Sports-specific challenge for exercise bronchoprovocation to detect EIB (five studies): sensitivity 0–100%, specificity 0–100%
- EVH (seven studies) to detect EIB: sensitivity 25–90%, specificity 0–71%
- Free-running test (three studies) to detect EIB: sensitivity 60–67%, specificity 47–67%
- Mannitol (three studies) to detect EIB: sensitivity 58–96%, specificity 65–78%

These studies reflect small numbers and heterogeneity, with different study populations of adult and pediatric patients, elite and professional athletes, and different methods to induce EIB. This demonstrates that there is no consensus on a gold standard that replaces the standard exercise challenge to diagnose EIB.[78]

Direct challenges with pharmaceutical agents such as methacholine (which is available commercially) and histamine (which is investigational) are not recommended for the diagnosis of EIB because they are not specific for EIB. Although methacholine may be used to exclude reactive airway disease, winter athletes who had a positive methacholine challenge did not demonstrate bronchoconstriction when evaluated with exercise, EVH, or mannitol.[8] A positive methacholine challenge in cold-weather athletes may reflect airway injury with bronchial hyperresponsiveness secondary to the hyperventilation of cold and dry air. Athletes performing in cold and dry environments, in swimming pools, or on ice rinks with air polluted with irritants may have airway hyperresponsiveness secondary to injury. In these patients, a methacholine challenge is not recommended for the diagnosis of EIB because a positive methacholine challenge merely reflects nonspecific airway injury. Individuals with "ski asthma," with airway hyperresponsiveness to methacholine and symptoms simulating asthma, fail to respond to ICS. This finding corroborates the contention that ski asthma with a positive methacholine challenge represents nonspecific airway injury with hyperresponsiveness and not the characteristic airway inflammation seen with chronic asthma.[79]

Comparative studies of EVH and methacholine in swimmers showed that the majority of swimmers who have positive EVH challenges also have positive methacholine challenges.[43] However, discrepancies exist because it is not uncommon to see a patient who has a positive EVH challenge and a negative methacholine challenge.[4, 80]

The differential diagnosis of EIB should include vocal cord dysfunction, cardiac and/or pulmonary abnormalities, and poor exercise conditioning, which all mimic EIB. Vocal cord dysfunction usually presents with inspiratory stridor with flattening and/or premature closure of the inspiratory loop on pulmonary function testing.[3] Dyspnea alone usually suggests poor physical conditioning and, less frequently, exercise-induced hyperventilation or other pulmonary conditions such as chronic obstructive pulmonary disease (COPD) or restrictive lung conditions (e.g. obesity).[60] Patients with dyspnea may rarely have cardiac disorders (including arrhythmias, congestive heart failure, structural disease such as myopathies or idiopathic hypertrophic subaortic stenosis, or mitochondrial defects), gastrointestinal diseases (such as GERD), or skeletal abnormalities such as scoliosis. Cardiopulmonary exercise testing may be needed to determine whether symptoms are resulting from exercise-induced dyspnea and hyperventilation, particularly in children and adolescents.[81]

Rarely, if pruritus and urticaria are coexistent with symptoms suggesting EIB, then exercise-induced anaphylaxis syndromes with or without food dependence should be considered. With the proper use of diagnostic exercise challenge testing and rhinolaryngoscopy to visualize vocal cord adduction for vocal cord dysfunction, these other conditions can be ruled in or out.[1–3, 59, 60]

12.6 MANAGEMENT; PHARMACEUTICAL AND NONPHARMACEUTICAL AGENTS (TABLES 12.3 AND 12.4)

Treatment goals of EIB management include minimizing and preventing symptoms with exercise, achieving and maintaining therapeutic control with minimal side effects, and maximizing lung function to achieve peak performance.[82] An emphasis should be placed on education of appropriate inhaler technique, medication adherence, and environmental controls. Any comorbid conditions, including rhinitis, sinusitis, gastroesophageal reflux disease (GERD), anxiety, depression, obstructive sleep apnea, and viral infections, including COVID-19, should be treated.[81,82] The treatment of individuals who have EIB requires an awareness of the variability of patient responses and regular follow-up to establish an effective treatment plan. The environmental conditions, the type of activity, and the underlying asthma must all be carefully evaluated when initiating and adjusting therapies.[33]

As noted earlier, EIB is triggered by inhaling dry air, leading to a hyperosmolar airway, resulting in airway inflammation and bronchoconstriction. The severity of EIB may be diminished in some patients by inspiring warm and humid air during exercise.[84] Nevertheless, severe EIB can still develop in patients inhaling hot dry air.[85] Thus it is important to recognize that the principal stimulus for EIB is loss of water rather than airway rewarming. Medications that are effective in blocking the physiological effects of the bioactive mediators released from inflammatory cells as a result of this hyperosmolar state in the airway are useful in preventing EIB.[86–91]

12.7 BETA-AGONISTS

To prevent EIB, either inhaled short-acting beta-agonists (SABAs) or long-acting beta-agonists (LABAs) can be administered 15–30 minutes prior to exercise on an intermittent basis in the majority of individuals.[92–94] SABAs have an onset of action within 5–20 minutes with a duration of activity of about 2–4 hours.[92, 95, 96] Inhaled beta-agonists inhibit EIB by activating two sites of beta-2 receptors on the mast cells to inhibit mediator release and on the bronchial smooth muscle to block contraction in response to mediators including histamine, leukotrienes, and prostaglandin D2.[1]

Beta-agonists alone are able to treat the bronchoconstrictive component of EIB, but they have no impact on inflammation.[96, 97] A tolerance to beta-agonist therapy develops with daily administration at the level of both the mast cell and the airway smooth muscle within a week of regular use, and this tachyphylaxis is not impacted by simultaneous therapy with ICS.[1–3]

Tolerance is reflected first by shortening the duration of protection to 2 hours with SABAs and to 4–6 hours with LABAs.[96, 98–103] Additionally, the time to recovery to baseline FEV_1 following exercise may be extended after prolonged use of beta-agonists. The dose of inhaled beta-agonists needed to achieve protection may be higher if a daily beta-agonist is administered.[104, 105] The EIB episode may be more severe with daily administration of a beta-agonist.[105] The likely mechanism of tolerance is a decreased number or a downregulation of beta-2 adrenergic receptors on the mast cells.[98, 106] Tachyphylaxis is often managed by increasing the dose of the beta-agonist prior to exercise, making the problem even worse. Intermittent use of a beta-agonist, no more than three times a week, for prophylaxis or treatment, is most effective in preventing tachyphylaxis.[107] The discontinuation of a beta-agonist for three days will generally lead to a return of responsiveness to beta-agonists.[102]

12.8 ANTICHOLINERGIC AGENTS

Anticholinergic agents, such as ipratropium bromide, have been inconsistent in attenuating EIB; however, it is clear that some patients do respond to this therapy. This agent has bronchodilator activity by inhibiting vagally mediated bronchomotor tone. Ipratropium has been used alone and in conjunction with SABAs for acute exacerbations of asthma, but it has not been consistent in double-blind, placebo-controlled investigations, and intrapatient variability has been reported.[108–111]

12.9 CHROMONES AND NONSTEROIDAL ANTI-INFLAMMATORY AGENTS

Chromones are mast cell stabilizing medications that block EIB.[112] These agents, including sodium cromoglycate and nedocromil sodium, are administered by inhalation, immediately prior to exercise, to provide up to 60% inhibition of EIB; but they are no longer available in the United States.[112] Complete inhibition of EIB is defined as a fall in FEV_1 post-exercise of no more than 10%.[1, 2] The duration of these agents' protection is usually less than four hours, but their onset of action is immediate so they can be inhaled just prior to exercise on an as-needed basis.[2, 113] Tolerance has not been reported to the recurrent administration of these drugs. These agents reportedly work by inhibiting the release of prostaglandin D2 and leukotrienes.[113] Unfortunately, the armamentarium of medications to treat EIB has been significantly weakened since these agents are no longer available.

12.10 LEUKOTRIENE ANTAGONISTS

Leukotriene receptor antagonists (LTRAs) such as montelukast and zafirlukast and 5-lipoxygenase inhibitors such as zileuton provide approximately 60% protection against EIB. Montelukast is the most commonly used agent. It is administered as a tablet and should be taken about two hours prior to the activity so that it can be fully effective.[114] Although it is not effective for all asthmatic patients, it can provide protection for as long as 24 hours.[115, 116] Unlike beta-agonists, montelukast can be taken continuously, daily, prophylactically, and without tolerance developing.[116] Montelukast promotes the recovery of FEV_1 to baseline by decreasing the time to recovery, and it diminishes the duration and severity of the asthma episode following exercise.[1–3] Combination therapy with loratadine may provide effective attenuation of EIB with a decreased mediator release.[117–119] Zafirlukast, a second leukotriene antagonist, has a duration of action of about eight hours.[118, 119] Zileuton, a 5-lipoxygenase inhibitor, has a duration of prophylaxis for EIB of four hours, equivalent to zafirlukast, but it is less efficacious by eight hours than zafirlukast, montelukast, and salmeterol, and there is no difference between it and placebo by 12 hours.[119–121]

12.11 NONPHARMACEUTICAL MANEUVERS

Nonpharmacologic management strategies of EIB include wearing a face mask, avoiding cold air, and warming up

TABLE 12.3
Nonpharmacological Therapy 1–3, 127–132, 147–150

Breathing through mouth/face mask
Warm-up refractory period
Vitamin C
Fish oil
Low-salt diet
Aerobic conditioning

TABLE 12.4
Pharmacological Therapy 109, 111, 112, 121, 124

Beta-agonists: long acting and short acting (LABA, SABA)
Anticholinergic agents
Montelukast
Nonsteroidal agents
Inhaled corticosteroids (ICS)
Combination therapy (such as ICS plus LABA or ICS plus SABA)

prior to exercise.[122] In addition, a low sodium diet, intake of omega-3 polyunsaturated fatty acids and ascorbic acid, as well as weight loss have been demonstrated to attenuate EIB in small, placebo-controlled trials.[122–125] Further maneuvers that can attenuate or provide prophylaxis against EIB include hydration and inspiring air conditioned to the physiological temperature and humidity, which may provide 80% or more protection, similar to medications (Table 12.3).[111, 115, 116, 126–130]

Recurrent exercise repeated within a limited period of time from the first exercise (e.g. about two hours) will lead to a refractory period of tolerance to further bronchoconstriction.[127] A pre-exercise intense warm-up approximately equivalent to maximal heart rate or peak oxygen consumption has been associated with a 10% improvement in the reduction of FEV_1 after exercise.[131] One potential mechanism is an intense pre-exercise warm-up induces a refractory period in which exercise does not cause EIB for about four hours.[131] Respiratory warm-ups consisting of normocapnic hyperpnea have also been shown to diminish the post-exercise fall in FEV_1 after exercise.[131] Respiratory muscle training can also improve EIB.[131]

The use of face masks utilizing a heat and moisture exchange can reduce EIB in colder and dryer environments by the retention of water vapor, allowing rebreathing. This may decrease the number of airway generations required for adjusting the inspired air to the physiological conditions.[1–3] Face masks can also potentially reduce the detrimental effects of air pollution on asthma.[131]

12.12 APPROACH TO TREATMENT OF EIB WITH ASTHMA

As described earlier, SABA or LABA may be administered up to 30 minutes prior to exercise, as many as three times a week, to prevent mild intermittent episodes of EIB. Tolerance to SABA and LABA occurs after only a few doses and is indicated by decreased bronchodilation when these drugs are given for an asthma exacerbation, even with concomitant ICS therapy.[99, 102, 132–134] This tolerance may lead the patient or healthcare provider to further increase the use of beta-agonists with a greater chance of adverse events and no increase in efficacy. However, despite the concern regarding the daily use of beta-agonists leading to tolerance and impairing the response to emergency therapy for asthma, there are limited data to support that this tolerance is clinically important in the elite athlete.[61] With competitive and elite athletes who exercise daily or even more frequently, the use of beta-agonists for prophylaxis during or following exercise could theoretically lead to exceeding the optimal guidelines for beta-agonist monotherapy stated in the National Heart, Lung, and Blood Institute (NHLBI) and the Global Initiative for Asthma (GINA) guidelines, and tolerance could then potentially be of clinical importance.[1–3, 61]

If asthma is more persistent and not well-controlled, then either montelukast or ICS may be started. Montelukast is administered once a day at night, with onset within about two hours and a duration of about 24 hours. Montelukast is effective in at least one-half of asthmatic patients, but the other half will have no improvement with this drug. No tolerance develops to montelukast, as occurs with beta-agonists. ICS therapy is indicated for persistent asthma that is mild to severe and that does not respond to beta-agonists or montelukast (Table 12.4).[1, 2]

Nonsteroidal medications, such as mast cell stabilizers (MCS), cromolyn (cromoglycate), or nedocromil, are also deemed effective for chronic mild persistent asthma, as stated in previous NHLBI guidelines. Cromolyn has been demonstrated to be effective versus a placebo in decreasing the fall in FEV_1 after a EVH challenge in the most competitive or elite athletes with EIB.[113] These findings support the importance of the mast cell mediator release in EIB severity. The limitation of the study is that cromoglycate was compared in a single dose with a placebo, not with an active comparator.[61, 113] In a Cochrane analysis of 20 randomized, controlled trials, nedocromil (4 mg inhaled 15–60 minutes prior to exercise) significantly diminished the severity and the duration of EIB in both adults and children.[112] A Cochrane analysis of eight studies demonstrated no significant difference between cromolyn and nedocromil in the maximum decrease in FEV_1, complete protection (defined as the maximum percentage fall in FEV_1 less than 10% from baseline), clinical protection (defined as 50% improvement over a placebo), or side effects.[135] Unfortunately, as noted earlier, neither agent is marketed or sold in the United States, the United Kingdom, or Europe.

ICS therapy is indicated in both adults and children who have chronic persistent asthma not responsive to beta-agonist and montelukast. When administered on a daily basis, these agents have been demonstrated to be effective in decreasing the severity of EIB.[1–3] The dose and the duration of the therapy are dependent on the various preparations.[1–3, 126] ICS therapy is the most widely utilized and the most effective inhaled anti-inflammatory therapy preferred in both the NHLBI and GINA guidelines.[1–3] ICS therapy prevents asthma episodes and enhances quality of life and pulmonary functions while diminishing airway inflammation and hyperresponsiveness as well as the severity and frequency of exacerbations and mortality.[136, 137] Used in the recommended doses, ICS therapy requires days to weeks to become fully effective. The onset of the effects of ICS therapy usually requires 7–14 days and is most efficacious after eight weeks of treatment.[64] ICS may be administered in very high doses a few hours prior to exercise for EIB alone in competitive athletes, but this is not recommended as an ongoing clinical practice.[138]

Our understanding of the efficacy of ICS therapy is derived from similar studies lasting from three weeks to two years in children and adults. In a study with budesonide (800 µg bid) versus a placebo, in which adults were randomized to treatment for six weeks of therapy, there was a post-exercise fall in FEV_1 of 7% in the budesonide cohort and 22% in the placebo cohort with similar outcomes in pediatric studies.[61, 139] When combination therapy was examined, the ICS component remained effective in controlling the severity of EIB when the beta-agonist was withdrawn from the combination therapy.[140] ICS, including budesonide, ciclesonide, and fluticasone, have been demonstrated to be efficacious in decreasing the severity of EIB within 3–12 weeks of the initiation of ICS therapy.[128, 129, 141, 142] The time to onset of protection is quicker with higher doses of ICS than with lower doses.[126] ICS alone, used daily, are effective, as the majority of individuals with EIB have normal spirometry and require a beta-agonist only prior to exercise. However, in individuals with an abnormal baseline spirometry, the combination of ICS with LABAs has been demonstrated to be effective in decreasing the severity of EIB.[141, 142] Combination therapy with LABAs, including salmeterol and formoterol, is often used in the management of asthma that is not controlled with ICS therapy alone. The combinations (of ICS with LABA) are usually prescribed in fixed combinations but may be administered as separate inhalers. The use of monotherapy with LABAs for chronic or persistent asthma is never recommended on a continuous basis because of the danger of adverse outcomes with therapeutic failure and the danger of asthma exacerbation.[143] However, a review of the literature indicates that combined fluticasone and salmeterol was more effective than fluticasone alone for the prophylaxis of EIB with asthma.[144] Similarly, in a randomized, double-blind investigation, combination therapy with budesonide and formoterol was more effective in improving asthma control and symptoms compared with budesonide alone.[145] As noted earlier, a pilot study in children with clinically stable asthma, who were being treated with a combination therapy (ICS and LABA), demonstrated that the removal of the LABA reduced the severity of EIB and may even have eliminated it.[140] This observation suggests that ICS alone may be more effective over time than the combination of ICS and LABA for EIB. Indeed, patients should attempt to discontinue the inhaled beta-agonist prior to exercise to determine whether EIB is still present. This policy will avoid administering inhaled beta-agonists when these agents are unnecessary.[1]

An evidence-based review of the literature reveals that SABA provided greater protection than MCS in 12 studies.[78] However, combining SABAs and MCS provided no further benefits in five studies. LTRAs, MCS, ipratropium bromide, and interval warm-up routines demonstrated a statistically significant reduction in EIB with asthma, measured as the mean difference in the percentage fall in FEV_1 and 95% confidence intervals when compared with a placebo. Nine studies demonstrated the efficacy of single-dose interventions with LTRA (8.9% mean difference); 17 studies with nedocromil sodium (15.6% mean difference); four studies with interval warm-up (10.6% mean difference); four studies with ICS (5% mean difference); two studies with continuous high-intensity warm-up (9.8% mean difference); and three studies with continuous low-intensity warm-up versus no warm-up (12.6% mean difference).[78] Notably, after daily LABA use for 3–4 weeks in four studies, the percentage fall in FEV_1 following an exercise challenge at two and four weeks was greater than at day one, presumably related to tachyphylaxis. Interestingly, both SABA and LABA continue to lessen EIB in patients with known asthma when given prophylactically, even though the effect of these drugs is diminished by tachyphylaxis with a prolonged time to recovery.[78, 96, 98–104]

Supplements to the diet such as fish oil and vitamin C as well as a low-salt diet have been demonstrated to be effective for protection against EIB.[146, 147] However, these studies, while often placebo controlled, were performed in individuals with mild EIB and do not apply to the more severe forms of EIB.[146, 147] Agents such as heparin, theophylline, furosemide, and calcium channel blockers have also been evaluated as therapy for EIB, but there is insufficient evidence to recommend their routine use.[1–3]

Maintaining physical conditioning may raise the threshold for EIB.[148, 149] For the elite athlete, national and global guidelines and standards as well as regulations must be followed. For the elite athlete with EIB alone, the use of ICS in large doses (i.e. beclomethasone at 1500 µg given four hours prior to exercise) or cromolyn sodium or beta-agonists given prior to exercise have some demonstrated efficacy,[113, 138] but a reduction in prolonged training and the avoidance of triggers in the environment may be the only effective management of EIB.[1–3] Chronic use of ICS is less effective in the setting of neutrophil predominance with EIB alone.[1, 2, 61, 80]

12.13 SPECIAL CONSIDERATIONS

12.13.1 Athletes

Cardiovascular fitness should be emphasized in athletes at all levels, including beginners. For high school and college athletes, identifiable and individualized asthma and EIB action plans are essential.[82] Governing body regulations exist regarding athletes at all levels, and these athletes should be aware of the most current rules.[82] National

Collegiate Athletic Association (NCAA) allows B2-agonist therapy, with medical documentation.[82] Similarly, the World Anti-Doping Agency generally permits the use of B2-agonists and ICS by athletes with appropriate medical justification.[82] Psychological factors, including measured mental toughness (MT) scores, can also impact EIB.[150]

12.13.2 Children

Children may avoid exercise-related activities due to fear of symptoms. Addressing both caregiver and patient concerns regarding exercise and treatment options is vital. Aerobic conditioning and improved physical fitness can also be helpful in children.[151]

12.13.3 Older Adults

There are few studies specifically on older adults with EIB. Exercise has been shown to be beneficial in older adults with asthma.[152] Older adults frequently have associated comorbid conditions, such as cardiovascular disease and depression, that should also be addressed.[153]

12.14 CONCLUSION

EIB occurs in approximately up to 20% of the general population, including up to 90% of people with asthma.[154] EIB has bronchoconstrictive and inflammatory components. Proposed mechanisms include increases in osmolarity, thermal gradient changes, and cooling of the airway. Objective tools that can aid in the diagnosis include spirometry with bronchodilator reversibility testing and bronchoprovocation testing. Nonpharmacologic therapies include avoiding cold air, use of facial masks, and pre-exercise warm-ups, as well as certain diets. Pharmacologic treatments may include SABA, ICS, and leukotriene inhibitors. Any comorbidities, such as rhinitis, sinusitis, GERD, obstructive sleep apnea, anxiety, and depression, should also be evaluated for and appropriately treated. Special populations, including children, older adults, and athletes, may need to have more specific interventions. Additional research will be helpful in assessing, monitoring, and treating EIB in the future.

12.15 DECLARATION OF INTEREST

SN receives funding from the National Institutes of Health. The authors alone are responsible for the content, preparation, and writing of this chapter.

REFERENCES

1. Anderson SD. Exercise-induced bronchoconstriction in the 21st century. *J Am Osteopath Assoc.* 2011 Nov;111(11 Suppl 7):S3–10.
2. Anderson SD, Kippelen P. Assessment and prevention of exercise-induced bronchoconstriction. *Br J Sports Med.* 2012 May;46(6):391–6.
3. Weiler JM, Anderson SD, Randolph C, Bonini S, Craig TJ, Pearlman DS, et al; American Academy of Allergy, Asthma and Immunology; American College of Allergy, Asthma and Immunology; Joint Council of Allergy, Asthma and Immunology. Pathogenesis, prevalence, diagnosis, and management of exercise-induced bronchoconstriction: a practice parameter. *Ann Allergy Asthma Immunol.* 2010 Dec;105(6 Suppl):S1–47.
4. Khan DA. Exercise-induced bronchoconstriction: burden and prevalence. *Allergy Asthma Proc.* 2012 Jan–Feb;33(1):1–6.
5. Bougault V, Turmel J, Boulet LP. Bronchial challenges and respiratory symptoms in elite swimmers and winter sport athletes: Airway hyperresponsiveness in asthma: its measurement and clinical significance. *Chest.* 2010 Aug;138(2 Suppl):31S–37S.
6. Langdeau JB, Boulet LP. Is asthma over- or under-diagnosed in athletes? *Respir Med.* 2003 Feb;97(2):109–14.
7. Lund TK, Pedersen L, Anderson SD, Sverrild A, Backer V. Are asthma-like symptoms in elite athletes associated with classical features of asthma? *Br J Sports Med.* 2009 Dec;43(14):1131–5.
8. Sue-Chu M, Brannan JD, Anderson SD, Chew N, Bjermer L. Airway hyperresponsiveness to methacholine, adenosine 5-monophosphate, mannitol, eucapnic voluntary hyperpnoea and field exercise challenge in elite cross-country skiers. *Br J Sports Med.* 2010 Sep;44(11):827–32.
9. Weiler JM, Layton T, Hunt M. Asthma in United States Olympic athletes who participated in the 1996 Summer Games. *J Allergy Clin Immunol.* 1998 Nov;102(5):722–6.
10. Weiler, J.M. and E.J. Ryan, 3rd, Asthma in United States Olympic athletes who participated in the 1998 Olympic winter games. *J Allergy Clin Immunol*, 2000. 106(2): 267–71.
11. National Asthma Education and Prevention Program. Expert panel report 3 (EPR-3): Guidelines for the diagnosis and management of asthma-summary report 2007. *J Allergy Clin Immunol.* 2007 Nov;120(5 Suppl):S94–138.
12. Expert Panel Working Group of the National Heart, Lung, and Blood Institute (NHLBI) administered and coordinated National Asthma Education and Prevention Program Coordinating Committee (NAEPPCC), Cloutier MM, Baptist AP, Blake KV, Brooks EG, Bryant-Stephens T, DiMango E, et al. 2020 Focused updates to the asthma management guidelines: a report from the national asthma education and prevention program coordinating committee expert panel working group. *J Allergy Clin Immunol.* 2020 Dec;146(6):1217–70.
13. Parsons JP, Cosmar D, Phillips G, Kaeding C, Best TM, Mastronarde JG. Screening for exercise-induced bronchoconstriction in college athletes. *J Asthma.* 2012 Mar;49(2):153–7.
14. Rundell KW, Im J, Mayers LB, Wilber RL, Szmedra L, Schmitz HR. Self-reported symptoms and exercise-induced asthma in the elite athlete. *Med Sci Sports Exerc.* 2001 Feb;33(2):208–13.
15. Anderson SD, Pearlman DS, Rundell KW, Perry CP, Boushey H, Sorkness CA, et al. Reproducibility of the airway response to an exercise protocol standardized for intensity, duration, and inspired air conditions, in subjects with symptoms suggestive of asthma. *Respir Res.* 2010 Sep 1;11(1):120.
16. Vilozni D, Bentur L, Efrati O, Barak A, Szeinberg A, Shoseyov D, et al. Exercise challenge test in 3- to 6-year-old asthmatic children. *Chest.* 2007 Aug;132(2):497–503.
17. van Leeuwen JC, Driessen JM, de Jongh FH, van Aalderen WM, Thio BJ. Monitoring pulmonary function during exercise in children with asthma. *Arch Dis Child.* 2011 Jul;96(7):664–8.

18. Freed AN, Anderson SD. Exercise induced bronchoconstriction: Human models. In: Kay, A.B., J. Bousquet, P.G. Holt, and A.P. Daplan (eds.), *Allergy and Allergic Diseases*, pp. 808–822. Oxford: Blackwell Scientific Publications, 2009.
19. Goldberg S, Mimouni F, Joseph L, Izbicki G, Picard E. Seasonal effect on exercise challenge tests for the diagnosis of exercise-induced bronchoconstriction. *Allergy Asthma Proc.* 2012 Sep–Oct:33(5):416–20.
20. de Aguiar KB, Anzolin M, Zhang L. Global prevalence of exercise-induced bronchoconstriction in childhood: A meta-analysis. *Pediatr Pulmonol.* 2018 Apr;53(4):412–25.
21. Ersson K, Mallmin E, Malinovschi A, Norlander K, Johansson H, Nordang L. Prevalence of exercise-induced bronchoconstriction and laryngeal obstruction in adolescent athletes. *Pediatr Pulmonol.* 2020 Dec;55(12):3509–16.
22. Hallstrand TS. New insights into pathogenesis of exercise-induced bronchoconstriction. *Curr Opin Allergy Clin Immunol.* 2012 Feb;12(1):42–8.
23. Addo-Yobo EO, Woodcock A, Allotey A, Baffoe-Bonnie B, Strachan D, Custovic A. Exercise-induced bronchospasm and atopy in Ghana: two surveys ten years apart. *PLOS Med.* 2007 Feb;4(2):e70.
24. De Baets F, Bodart E, Dramaix-Wilmet M, Van Daele S, de Bilderling G, Masset S, et al. Exercise-induced respiratory symptoms are poor predictors of bronchoconstriction. *Pediatr Pulmonol.* 2005 Apr;39(4):301–5.
25. Kukafka DS, Lang DM, Porter S, Rogers J, Ciccolella D, Polansky M, et al. Exercise-induced bronchospasm in high school athletes via a free running test: incidence and epidemiology. *Chest.* 1998 Dec;114(6):1613–22.
26. Jones CO, Qureshi S, Rona RJ, Chinn S. Exercise-induced bronchoconstriction by ethnicity and presence of asthma in British nine year olds. *Thorax.* 1996 Nov;51(11):1134–6.
27. Wilber RL, Rundell KW, Szmedra L, Jenkinson DM, Im J, Drake SD. Incidence of exercise-induced bronchospasm in Olympic winter sport athletes. *Med Sci Sports Exerc.* 2000 Apr;32(4):732–7.
28. Mannix ET, Farber MO, Palange P, Galassetti P, Manfredi F. Exercise-induced asthma in figure skaters. *Chest.* 1996 Feb;109(2):312–5.
29. Rundell KW, Anderson SD, Spiering BA, Judelson DA. Field exercise vs laboratory eucapnic voluntary hyperventilation to identify airway hyperresponsiveness in elite cold weather athletes. *Chest.* 2004 Mar;125(3):909–15.
30. Holzer K, Anderson SD, Douglass J. Exercise in elite summer athletes: challenges for diagnosis. *J Allergy Clin Immunol.* 2002 Sep;110(3):374–80.
31. Porsbjerg C, von Linstow ML, Ulrik CS, Nepper-Christensen SC, Backer V. Outcome in adulthood of asymptomatic airway hyperresponsiveness to histamine and exercise-induced bronchospasm in childhood. *Ann Allergy Asthma Immunol.* 2005 Aug;95(2):137–42.
32. Rodriguez Bauza DE, Silveyra P. Sex differences in exercise-induced bronchoconstriction in athletes: a systematic review and meta-analysis. *Int J Environ Res Public Health.* 2020 Oct 5;17(19):7270.
33. Carlsen KH, Anderson SD, Bjermer L, Bonini S, Brusasco V, Canonica W, et al; European Respiratory Society; European Academy of Allergy and Clinical Immunology. Exercise-induced asthma, respiratory and allergic disorders in elite athletes: epidemiology, mechanisms and diagnosis: part I of the report from the Joint Task Force of the European Respiratory Society (ERS) and the European Academy of Allergy and Clinical Immunology (EAACI) in cooperation with GA2LEN. *Allergy.* 2008 Apr;63(4):387–403.
34. Anderson SD, Wong R, Bennett M, et al. Summary of the knowledge and thinking about asthma and diving since 1993. *Diving Hyperb Med.* 1993;36:12–22.
35. Parsons JP, Craig TJ, Stoloff SW, Hayden ML, Ostrom NK, Eid NS, et al. Impact of exercise-related respiratory symptoms in adults with asthma: exercise-induced bronchospasm landmark national survey. *Allergy Asthma Proc.* 2011 Nov–Dec;32(6):431–7.
36. Ostrom NK, Eid NS, Craig TJ, Colice GL, Hayden ML, Parsons JP, et al. Exercise-induced bronchospasm in children with asthma in the United States: results from the exercise-induced bronchospasm landmark survey. *Allergy Asthma Proc.* 2011 Nov–Dec;32(6):425–30.
37. Kojima N, Ohya Y, Futamura M, Akashi M, Odajima H, Adachi Y, et al. Exercise-induced asthma is associated with impaired quality of life among children with asthma in Japan. *Allergol Int.* 2009 Jun;58(2):187–92.
38. Hallstrand TS, Curtis JR, Aitken ML, Sullivan SD. Quality of life in adolescents with mild asthma. *Pediatr Pulmonol.* 2003 Dec;36(6):536–43.
39. Correia MA Jr, Rizzo JA, Sarinho SW, Cavalcanti Sarinho ES, Medeiros D, Assis F. Effect of exercise-induced bronchospasm and parental beliefs on physical activity of asthmatic adolescents from a tropical region. *Ann Allergy Asthma Immunol.* 2012 Apr;108(4):249–53.
40. Anderson SD, Kippelen P. Airway injury as a mechanism for exercise-induced bronchoconstriction in elite athletes. *J Allergy Clin Immunol.* 2008 Aug;122(2):225–35; quiz 236–7.
41. Anderson SD, Kippelen P. Exercise-induced bronchoconstriction: pathogenesis. *Curr Allergy Asthma Rep.* 2005 Mar;5(2):116–22.
42. Stensrud T, Mykland KV, Gabrielsen K, Carlsen KH. Bronchial hyperresponsiveness in skiers: field test versus methacholine provocation? *Med Sci Sports Exerc.* 2007 Oct;39(10):1681–6.
43. Stadelmann K, Stensrud T, Carlsen KH. Respiratory symptoms and bronchial responsiveness in competitive swimmers. *Med Sci Sports Exerc.* 2011 Mar;43(3):375–81.
44. Bougault V, Turmel J, St-Laurent J, Bertrand M, Boulet LP. Asthma, airway inflammation and epithelial damage in swimmers and cold-air athletes. *Eur Respir J.* 2009 Apr;33(4):740–6.
45. Rundell KW, Spiering BA, Evans TM, Baumann JM. Baseline lung function, exercise-induced bronchoconstriction, and asthma-like symptoms in elite women ice hockey players. *Med Sci Sports Exerc.* 2004 Mar;36(3):405–10.
46. Daigle CC, Chalupa DC, Gibb FR, Morrow PE, Oberdörster G, Utell MJ, et al. Ultrafine particle deposition in humans during rest and exercise. *Inhal Toxicol.* 2003 May;15(6):539–52.
47. Chalupa DC, Morrow PE, Oberdörster G, Utell MJ, Frampton MW. Ultrafine particle deposition in subjects with asthma. *Environ Health Perspect.* 2004 Jun;112(8):879–82.
48. Rundell KW. Pulmonary function decay in women ice hockey players: is there a relationship to ice rink air quality? *Inhal Toxicol.* 2004 Mar;16(3):117–23.
49. Rundell KW. High levels of airborne ultrafine and fine particulate matter in indoor ice arenas. *Inhal Toxicol.* 2003 Mar;15(3):237–50.
50. Rundell KW, Caviston R, Hollenbach AM, Murphy K. Vehicular air pollution, playgrounds, and youth athletic fields. *Inhal Toxicol.* 2006 Jul;18(8):541–7.
51. Provost-Craig MA, Arbour KS, Sestili DC, Chabalko JJ, Ekinci E. The incidence of exercise-induced bronchospasm in competitive figure skaters. *J Asthma.* 1996;33(1):67–71.

52. Weiler JM, Bonini S, Coifman R, Craig T, Delgado L, Capão-Filipe M, Passali D, Randolph C, Storms W; Ad Hoc Committee of Sports Medicine Committee of American Academy of Allergy, Asthma & Immunology. American academy of allergy, asthma & immunology work group report: exercise-induced asthma. *J Allergy Clin Immunol.* 2007 Jun;119(6):1349–58.
53. Rundell KW, Wilber RL, Szmedra L, Jenkinson DM, Mayers LB, Im J. Exercise-induced asthma screening of elite athletes: field versus laboratory exercise challenge. *Med Sci Sports Exerc.* 2000 Feb;32(2):309–16.
54. Rundell KW, Slee JB. Exercise and other indirect challenges to demonstrate asthma or exercise-induced bronchoconstriction in athletes. *J Allergy Clin Immunol.* 2008 Aug;122(2):238–46; quiz 247–8.
55. Parsons JP, Kaeding C, Phillips G, Jarjoura D, Wadley G, Mastronarde JG. Prevalence of exercise-induced bronchospasm in a cohort of varsity college athletes. *Med Sci Sports Exerc.* 2007 Sep;39(9):1487–92.
56. Crapo RO, Casaburi R, Coates AL, Enright PL, Hankinson JL, Irvin CG, et al. Guidelines for methacholine and exercise challenge testing–1999. This official statement of the American thoracic society was adopted by the ATS board of directors, July 1999. *Am J Respir Crit Care Med.* 2000 Jan;161(1):309–29.
57. Cockcroft D, Davis B. Direct and indirect challenges in the clinical assessment of asthma. *Ann Allergy Asthma Immunol.* 2009 Nov;103(5):363–9; quiz 369–72, 400.
58. Carlsen KH, Engh G, Mørk M. Exercise-induced bronchoconstriction depends on exercise load. *Respir Med.* 2000 Aug;94(8):750–5.
59. Vasudev M. Evaluation of paradoxical vocal fold motion. *Ann Allergy Asthma Immunol.* 2012 Oct;109(4):233–6.
60. Abu-Hasan M, Tannous B, Weinberger M. Exercise-induced dyspnea in children and adolescents: if not asthma then what? *Ann Allergy Asthma Immunol.* 2005 Mar;94(3):366–71.
61. Pedersen L, Elers J, Backer V. Asthma in elite athletes: pathogenesis, diagnosis, differential diagnoses, and treatment. *Phys Sportsmed.* 2011 Sep;39(3):163–71.
62. McKenzie DC, Boulet LP. Asthma, outdoor air quality and the Olympic Games. *CMAJ.* 2008 Sep 9;179(6):543–8.
63. Fitch KD, Sue-Chu M, Anderson SD, Boulet LP, Hancox RJ, McKenzie DC, et al. Asthma and the elite athlete: summary of the international Olympic committee's consensus conference, Lausanne, Switzerland, January 22–24, 2008. *J Allergy Clin Immunol.* 2008 Aug;122(2):254–60, 260.e1–7.
64. Anderson SD, Lambert S, Brannan JD, Wood RJ, Koskela H, Morton AR, et al. Laboratory protocol for exercise asthma to evaluate salbutamol given by two devices. *Med Sci Sports Exerc.* 2001 Jun;33(6):893–900.
65. Anderson SD, Argyros GJ, Magnussen H, Holzer K. Provocation by eucapnic voluntary hyperpnoea to identify exercise induced bronchoconstriction. *Br J Sports Med.* 2001 Oct;35(5):344–7.
66. Dickinson J, McConnell A, Whyte G. Diagnosis of exercise-induced bronchoconstriction: eucapnic voluntary hyperpnoea challenges identify previously undiagnosed elite athletes with exercise-induced bronchoconstriction. *Br J Sports Med.* 2011 Nov;45(14):1126–31.
67. Argyros GJ, Roach JM, Hurwitz KM, Eliasson AH, Phillips YY. Eucapnic voluntary hyperventilation as a bronchoprovocation technique: development of a standardized dosing schedule in asthmatics. *Chest.* 1996 Jun;109(6):1520–4.
68. Ansley L, Kippelen P, Dickinson J, Hull JH. Misdiagnosis of exercise-induced bronchoconstriction in professional soccer players. *Allergy.* 2012 Mar;67(3):390–5.
69. Spiering BA, Judelson DA, Rundell KW. An evaluation of standardizing target ventilation for eucapnic voluntary hyperventilation using FEV1. *J Asthma.* 2004 Oct;41(7):745–9.
70. Brummel NE, Mastronarde JG, Rittinger D, Philips G, Parsons JP. The clinical utility of eucapnic voluntary hyperventilation testing for the diagnosis of exercise-induced bronchospasm. *J Asthma.* 2009 Sep;46(7):683–6.
71. Brannan JD, Anderson SD, Perry CP, Freed-Martens R, Lassig AR, Charlton B; Aridol Study Group. The safety and efficacy of inhaled dry powder mannitol as a bronchial provocation test for airway hyperresponsiveness: a phase 3 comparison study with hypertonic (4.5%) saline. *Respir Res.* 2005 Dec 9;6(1):144.
72. Anderson SD, Charlton B, Weiler JM, Nichols S, Spector SL, Pearlman DS; A305 Study Group. Comparison of mannitol and methacholine to predict exercise-induced bronchoconstriction and a clinical diagnosis of asthma. *Respir Res.* 2009 Jan 23;10(1):4.
73. Holzer K, Anderson SD, Chan HK, Douglass J. Mannitol as a challenge test to identify exercise-induced bronchoconstriction in elite athletes. *Am J Respir Crit Care Med.* 2003 Feb 15;167(4):534–7.
74. Brannan JD, Koskela H, Anderson SD, Chew N. Responsiveness to mannitol in asthmatic subjects with exercise- and hyperventilation-induced asthma. *Am J Respir Crit Care Med.* 1998 Oct;158(4):1120–6.
75. Anderson SD. Indirect challenge tests: Airway hyperresponsiveness in asthma: its measurement and clinical significance. *Chest.* 2010 Aug;138(2 Suppl):25S–30S.
76. Anderson SD, Brannan JD. Methods for "indirect" challenge tests including exercise, eucapnic voluntary hyperpnea, and hypertonic aerosols. *Clin Rev Allergy Immunol.* 2003 Feb;24(1):27–54.
77. Riedler J, Reade T, Dalton M, Holst D, Robertson C. Hypertonic saline challenge in an epidemiologic survey of asthma in children. *Am J Respir Crit Care Med.* 1994 Dec;150(6 Pt 1):1632–9.
78. Dryden DM, Spooner CH, Stickland MK, Vandermeer B, Tjosvold L, Bialy L, Wong K, Rowe BH. Exercise-induced bronchoconstriction and asthma. *Evid Rep Technol Assess (Full Rep).* 2010 Jan;(189):1–154, v–vi.
79. Sue-Chu M, Karjalainen EM, Laitinen A, Larsson L, Laitinen LA, Bjermer L. Placebo-controlled study of inhaled budesonide on indices of airway inflammation in bronchoalveolar lavage fluid and bronchial biopsies in cross-country skiers. *Respiration.* 2000;67(4):417–25.
80. Pedersen L, Winther S, Backer V, Anderson SD, Larsen KR. Airway responses to eucapnic hyperpnea, exercise, and methacholine in elite swimmers. *Med Sci Sports Exerc.* 2008 Sep;40(9):1567–72.
81. Weiler JM, Brannan JD, Randolph CC, Hallstrand TS, Parsons J, Silvers W, et al. Exercise-induced bronchoconstriction update–2016. *J Allergy Clin Immunol.* 2016 Nov;138(5):1292–5.e36.
82. Greiwe J, Cooke A, Nanda A, Epstein SZ, Wasan AN, Shepard KV 2nd, et al. Work group report: perspectives in diagnosis and management of exercise-induced bronchoconstriction in athletes. *J Allergy Clin Immunol Pract.* 2020 Sep;8(8):2542–55.
83. Spector S, Tan R. Exercise-induced bronchoconstriction update: therapeutic management. *Allergy Asthma Proc.* 2012 Jan–Feb;33(1):7–12.
84. Anderson SD, Schoeffel RE, Follet R, Perry CP, Daviskas E, Kendall M. Sensitivity to heat and water loss at rest and during exercise in asthmatic patients. *Eur J Respir Dis.* 1982 Sep;63(5):459–71.

85. Anderson SD, Schoeffel RE, Black JL, Daviskas E. Airway cooling as the stimulus to exercise-induced asthma—a re-evaluation. *Eur J Respir Dis*. 1985 Jul;67(1):20–30.
86. Reiss TF, Hill JB, Harman E, Zhang J, Tanaka WK, Bronsky E, et al. Increased urinary excretion of LTE4 after exercise and attenuation of exercise-induced bronchospasm by montelukast, a cysteinyl leukotriene receptor antagonist. *Thorax*. 1997 Dec;52(12):1030–5.
87. O'Sullivan S, Roquet A, Dahlén B, Larsen F, Eklund A, Kumlin M, et al. Evidence for mast cell activation during exercise-induced bronchoconstriction. *Eur Respir J*. 1998 Aug;12(2):345–50.
88. Leff JA, Busse WW, Pearlman D, Bronsky EA, Kemp J, Hendeles L, et al. Montelukast, a leukotriene-receptor antagonist, for the treatment of mild asthma and exercise-induced bronchoconstriction. *N Engl J Med*. 1998 Jul 16;339(3):147–52.
89. Brannan JD, Gulliksson M, Anderson SD, Chew N, Seale JP, Kumlin M. Inhibition of mast cell PGD2 release protects against mannitol-induced airway narrowing. *Eur Respir J*. 2006 May;27(5):944–50.
90. Brannan JD, Gulliksson M, Anderson SD, Chew N, Kumlin M. Evidence of mast cell activation and leukotriene release after mannitol inhalation. *Eur Respir J*. 2003 Sep;22(3):491–6.
91. Brannan JD, Anderson SD, Gomes K, King GG, Chan HK, Seale JP. Fexofenadine decreases sensitivity to and montelukast improves recovery from inhaled mannitol. *Am J Respir Crit Care Med*. 2001 May;163(6):1420–5.
92. Pearlman DS, Rees W, Schaefer K, Huang H, Andrews WT. An evaluation of levalbuterol HFA in the prevention of exercise-induced bronchospasm. *J Asthma*. 2007 Nov;44(9):729–33.
93. Larsson K, Carlsen KH, Bonini S. Anti-asthmatic drugs: treatment of athletes and exercise induced bronchoconstriction. *Eur Respir Mon*, 2005;33:73–88.
94. Anderson SD. Single-dose agents in the prevention of exercise-induced asthma: a descriptive review. *Treat Respir Med*. 2004;3(6):365–79.
95. Anderson SD, Seale JP, Rozea P, Bandler L, Theobald G, Lindsay DA. Inhaled and oral salbutamol in exercise-induced asthma. *Am Rev Respir Dis*. 1976 Sep;114(3):493–500.
96. Anderson SD, Caillaud C, Brannan JD. Beta2-agonists and exercise-induced asthma. *Clin Rev Allergy Immunol*. 2006 Oct–Dec;31(2–3):163–80.
97. Bisgaard H. Long-acting beta (2)-agonists in management of childhood asthma: A critical review of the literature. *Pediatr Pulmonol*. 2000 Mar;29(3):221–34.
98. Scola AM, Chong LK, Suvarna SK, Chess-Williams R, Peachell PT. Desensitisation of mast cell beta2-adrenoceptor-mediated responses by salmeterol and formoterol. *Br J Pharmacol*. 2004 Jan;141(1):163–71.
99. Nelson JA, Strauss L, Skowronski M, Ciufo R, Novak R, McFadden ER Jr. Effect of long-term salmeterol treatment on exercise-induced asthma. *N Engl J Med*. 1998 Jul 16;339(3):141–6.
100. Johnson M. Molecular mechanisms of beta (2)-adrenergic receptor function, response, and regulation. *J Allergy Clin Immunol*. 2006 Jan;117(1):18–24; quiz 25.
101. Haney S, Hancox RJ. Recovery from bronchoconstriction and bronchodilator tolerance. *Clin Rev Allergy Immunol*. 2006 Oct–Dec;31(2–3):181–96.
102. *Haney S, Hancox RJ. Rapid onset of tolerance to beta-agonist bronchodilation. Respir Med. 2005 May;99(5):566–71.*
103. Drotar DE, Davis BE, Cockcroft DW. Tolerance to the bronchoprotective effect of salmeterol 12 hours after starting twice daily treatment. *Ann Allergy Asthma Immunol*. 1998 Jan;80(1):31–4.
104. Storms W, Chervinsky P, Ghannam AF, Bird S, Hustad CM, Edelman JM; Challenge-rescue study group. A comparison of the effects of oral montelukast and inhaled salmeterol on response to rescue bronchodilation after challenge. *Respir Med*. 2004 Nov;98(11):1051–62.
105. Hancox RJ, Subbarao P, Kamada D, Watson RM, Hargreave FE, Inman MD. Beta2-agonist tolerance and exercise-induced bronchospasm. *Am J Respir Crit Care Med*. 2002 Apr 15;165(8):1068–70.
106. Peachell P. Regulation of mast cells by beta-agonists. *Clin Rev Allergy Immunol*. 2006 Oct–Dec;31(2–3):131–42.
107. Davis BE, Reid JK, Cockcroft DW. Formoterol thrice weekly does not result in the development of tolerance to bronchoprotection. *Can Respir J*. 2003 Jan–Feb;10(1):23–6.
108. Knöpfli BH, Bar-Or O, Araújo CG. Effect of ipratropium bromide on EIB in children depends on vagal activity. *Med Sci Sports Exerc*. 2005 Mar;37(3):354–9.
109. Boulet LP, Turcotte H, Tennina S. Comparative efficacy of salbutamol, ipratropium, and cromoglycate in the prevention of bronchospasm induced by exercise and hyperosmolar challenges. *J Allergy Clin Immunol*. 1989 May;83(5):882–7.
110. Boner AL, Vallone G, De Stefano G. Effect of inhaled ipratropium bromide on methacholine and exercise provocation in asthmatic children. *Pediatr Pulmonol*. 1989;6(2):81–5.
111. Blake K. Review of guidelines and the literature in the treatment of acute bronchospasm in asthma. *Pharmacotherapy*. 2006 Sep;26(9 Pt 2):148S–55S.
112. Spooner CH, Spooner GR, Rowe BH. Mast-cell stabilising agents to prevent exercise-induced bronchoconstriction. *Cochrane Database Syst Rev*. 2003;2003(4):CD002307.
113. Kippelen P, Larsson J, Anderson SD, Brannan JD, Dahlén B, Dahlén SE. Effect of sodium cromoglycate on mast cell mediators during hyperpnea in athletes. *Med Sci Sports Exerc*. 2010 Oct;42(10):1853–60.
114. Pearlman DS, van Adelsberg J, Philip G, Tilles SA, Busse W, Hendeles L, et al. Onset and duration of protection against exercise-induced bronchoconstriction by a single oral dose of montelukast. *Ann Allergy Asthma Immunol*. 2006 Jul;97(1):98–104.
115. Philip G, Pearlman DS, Villarán C, Legrand C, Loeys T, Langdon RB, Reiss TF. Single-dose montelukast or salmeterol as protection against exercise-induced bronchoconstriction. *Chest*. 2007 Sep;132(3):875–83.
116. Edelman JM, Turpin JA, Bronsky EA, Grossman J, Kemp JP, Ghannam AF, et al. Oral montelukast compared with inhaled salmeterol to prevent exercise-induced bronchoconstriction. A randomized, double-blind trial. Exercise Study Group. *Ann Intern Med*. 2000 Jan 18;132(2):97–104.
117. Hallstrand TS, Moody MW, Wurfel MM, Schwartz LB, Henderson WR Jr, Aitken ML. Inflammatory basis of exercise-induced bronchoconstriction. *Am J Respir Crit Care Med*. 2005 Sep 15;172(6):679–86.
118. Dahlén B, Roquet A, Inman MD, Karlsson O, Naya I, Anstrén G, et al. Influence of zafirlukast and loratadine on exercise-induced bronchoconstriction. *J Allergy Clin Immunol*. 2002 May;109(5):789–93.
119. Coreno A, Skowronski M, Kotaru C, McFadden ER Jr. Comparative effects of long-acting beta2-agonists, leukotriene receptor antagonists, and a 5-lipoxygenase inhibitor on exercise-induced asthma. *J Allergy Clin Immunol*. 2000 Sep;106(3):500–6.
120. Krawiec ME, Wenzel SE. Leukotriene inhibitors and nonsteroidal therapies in the treatment of asthma. *Expert Opin Pharmacother*. 2001 Jan;2(1):47–65.

121. Kraft M. LTRA inhibition of exercise-induced bronchoconstriction. *Postgrad Med.* 2000 Sep 15;108(4 Suppl):32–9.
122. Koya T, Ueno H, Hasegawa T, Arakawa M, Kikuchi T. Management of Exercise-Induced Bronchoconstriction in Athletes. *J Allergy Clin Immunol Pract.* 2020 Jul-Aug;8(7):2183–92.
123. Tecklenburg SL, Mickleborough TD, Fly AD, Bai Y, Stager JM. Ascorbic acid supplementation attenuates exercise-induced bronchoconstriction in patients with asthma. *Respir Med.* 2007 Aug;101(8):1770–8.
124. Mickleborough TD, Lindley MR, Montgomery GS. Effect of fish oil-derived omega-3 polyunsaturated Fatty Acid supplementation on exercise-induced bronchoconstriction and immune function in athletes. *Phys Sportsmed.* 2008 Dec;36(1):11–7.
125. Mickleborough TD, Fogarty A. Dietary sodium intake and asthma: an epidemiological and clinical review. *Int J Clin Pract.* 2006 Dec;60(12):1616–24.
126. Subbarao P, Duong M, Adelroth E, Otis J, Obminski G, Inman M, et al. Effect of ciclesonide dose and duration of therapy on exercise-induced bronchoconstriction in patients with asthma. *J Allergy Clin Immunol.* 2006 May;117(5):1008–13.
127. Larsson J, Perry CP, Anderson SD, Brannan JD, Dahlén SE, Dahlén B. The occurrence of refractoriness and mast cell mediator release following mannitol-induced bronchoconstriction. *J Appl Physiol* (1985). 2011 Apr;110(4):1029–35.
128. Jónasson G, Carlsen KH, Hultquist C. Low-dose budesonide improves exercise-induced bronchospasm in schoolchildren. *Pediatr Allergy Immunol.* 2000 May;11(2):120–5.
129. Hofstra WB, Neijens HJ, Duiverman EJ, Kouwenberg JM, Mulder PG, Kuethe MC, Sterk PJ. Dose-responses over time to inhaled fluticasone propionate treatment of exercise- and methacholine-induced bronchoconstriction in children with asthma. *Pediatr Pulmonol.* 2000 Jun;29(6):415–23.
130. Hermansen MN, Nielsen KG, Buchvald F, Jespersen JJ, Bengtsson T, Bisgaard H. Acute relief of exercise-induced bronchoconstriction by inhaled formoterol in children with persistent asthma. *Chest.* 2006 May;129(5):1203–9.
131. Dickinson J, Amirav I, Hostrup M. Nonpharmacologic strategies to manage exercise-induced bronchoconstriction. *Immunol Allergy Clin North Am.* 2018 May;38(2):245–58.
132. Pauwels RA, Löfdahl CG, Postma DS, Tattersfield AE, O'Byrne P, Barnes PJ, et al. Effect of inhaled formoterol and budesonide on exacerbations of asthma. Formoterol and Corticosteroids Establishing Therapy (FACET) International Study Group. *N Engl J Med.* 1997 Nov 13;337(20):1405–11.
133. Hancox RJ, Taylor DR. Long-acting beta-agonist treatment in patients with persistent asthma already receiving inhaled corticosteroids. *BioDrugs.* 2001;15(1):11–24.
134. Elers J, Strandbygaard U, Pedersen L, Backer V. Daily use of salmeterol causes tolerance to bronchodilation with terbutaline in asthmatic subjects. *Open Respir Med J.* 2010 Apr 21;4:48–50.
135. Kelly KD, Spooner CH, Rowe BH. Nedocromil sodium versus cromoglycate for the pre-treatment of exercise induced bronchoconstriction in asthma. *Cochrane Database Syst Rev.* 2000;(2):CD002169.
136. Suissa S, Ernst P, Benayoun S, Baltzan M, Cai B. Low-dose inhaled corticosteroids and the prevention of death from asthma. *N Engl J Med.* 2000 Aug 3;343(5):332–6.
137. Jeffery PK, Godfrey RW, Adelroth E, Nelson F, Rogers A, Johansson SA. Effects of treatment on airway inflammation and thickening of basement membrane reticular collagen in asthma. A quantitative light and electron microscopic study. *Am Rev Respir Dis.* 1992 Apr;145(4 Pt 1):890–9.
138. Kippelen P, Larsson J, Anderson SD, Brannan JD, Delin I, Dahlen B, Dahlen SE. Acute effects of beclomethasone on hyperpnea-induced bronchoconstriction. *Med Sci Sports Exerc.* 2010 Feb;42(2):273–80.
139. Vathenen AS, Knox AJ, Wisniewski A, Tattersfield AE. Effect of inhaled budesonide on bronchial reactivity to histamine, exercise, and eucapnic dry air hyperventilation in patients with asthma. *Thorax.* 1991 Nov;46(11):811–6.
140. Kersten ET, Driessen JM, van Leeuwen JC, Thio BJ. Pilot study: The effect of reducing treatment on exercise induced bronchoconstriction. *Pediatr Pulmonol.* 2010 Sep;45(9):927–33.
141. Weiler JM, Nathan RA, Rupp NT, Kalberg CJ, Emmett A, Dorinsky PM. Effect of fluticasone/salmeterol administered via a single device on exercise-induced bronchospasm in patients with persistent asthma. *Ann Allergy Asthma Immunol.* 2005 Jan;94(1):65–72.
142. Pearlman D, Qaqundah P, Matz J, Yancey SW, Stempel DA, Ortega HG. Fluticasone propionate/salmeterol and exercise-induced asthma in children with persistent asthma. *Pediatr Pulmonol.* 2009 May;44(5):429–35.
143. Lazarus SC, Boushey HA, Fahy JV, Chinchilli VM, Lemanske RF Jr, Sorkness CA, et al; Asthma Clinical Research Network for the National Heart, Lung, and Blood Institute. Long-acting beta2-agonist monotherapy vs continued therapy with inhaled corticosteroids in patients with persistent asthma: a randomized controlled trial. *JAMA.* 2001 May 23–30;285(20):2583–93.
144. Reynolds NA, Lyseng-Williamson KA, Wiseman LR. Inhaled salmeterol/fluticasone propionate: a review of its use in asthma. *Drugs.* 2005;65(12):1715–34.
145. Noonan M, Rosenwasser LJ, Martin P, O'Brien CD, O'Dowd L. Efficacy and safety of budesonide and formoterol in one pressurised metered-dose inhaler in adults and adolescents with moderate to severe asthma: a randomised clinical trial. *Drugs.* 2006;66(17):2235–54.
146. Mickleborough TD, Murray RL, Ionescu AA, Lindley MR. Fish oil supplementation reduces severity of exercise-induced bronchoconstriction in elite athletes. *Am J Respir Crit Care Med.* 2003 Nov 15;168(10):1181–9.
147. Mickleborough TD, Lindley MR, Ionescu AA, Fly AD. Protective effect of fish oil supplementation on exercise-induced bronchoconstriction in asthma. *Chest.* 2006 Jan;129(1):39–49.
148. Ram FS, Robinson SM, Black PN, Picot J. Physical training for asthma. *Cochrane Database Syst Rev.* 2005 Oct 19;(4):CD001116.
149. Hallstrand TS, Bates PW, Schoene RB. Aerobic conditioning in mild asthma decreases the hyperpnea of exercise and improves exercise and ventilatory capacity. *Chest.* 2000 Nov;118(5):1460–9.
150. Zeiger JS, Weiler JM. Special considerations and perspectives for exercise-induced bronchoconstriction (EIB) in Olympic and other elite athletes. *J Allergy Clin Immunol Pract.* 2020 Jul–Aug;8(7):2194–201.
151. Milgrom H, Taussig LM. Keeping children with exercise-induced asthma active. *Pediatrics.* 1999 Sep;104(3):e38.
152. Turner S, Eastwood P, Cook A, Jenkins S. Improvements in symptoms and quality of life following exercise training in older adults with moderate/severe persistent asthma. *Respiration.* 2011;81(4):302–10.
153. Baptist AP, Busse PJ. Asthma over the age of 65: all's well that ends well. *J Allergy Clin Immunol Pract.* 2018 May–Jun;6(3):764–73.
154. Pongdee T, Li JT. Exercise-induced bronchoconstriction. *Ann Allergy Asthma Immunol.* 2013 May;110(5):311–5.

Section IV

Asthma Education and Outcomes

13 Asthma Education

Vanessa M. McDonald, Kirsten R. Murray, and Peter G. Gibson

CASE STUDY

Lucy is a 42-year-old female non-smoker who presented to the ambulatory care asthma clinic of a tertiary care hospital for clinical review following an admission to hospital with an acute exacerbation of her asthma. She is a non-smoker with a history of asthma since childhood. This is her first hospital presentation since childhood. Her main exacerbation trigger is respiratory tract infections. Her body mass index (BMI) is 31.6 kg/m^2, and she is atopic, with no avoidable allergen exposures.

Asthma Control

Lucy said that her asthma was fine now. However, when asked specifically about her asthma symptoms, she said that she had woken from her sleep with a cough and wheeze on three or four nights over the past week, she had symptoms of asthma each morning on waking, and, when probed, she stated that her activity was somewhat limited during moderate exercise but that this was normal. She was using inhaled short-acting beta-2 adrenergic agonists three times per day for the relief of her symptoms. Her forced expiratory volume in 1 sec (FEV_1) was 2.10 L (72% predicted), her forced vital capacity (FVC) was 3.25 L (90% predicted), and her FEV_1/FVC (forced expiratory ratio [FER]) was 0.65. Her best peak flow reading was 400 L/min. T2 biomarkers were positive with a peripheral blood eosinophil count of 0.5 ×10 L9 and a fractional exhaled nitric oxide (FENO) measure of 89 ppb. Her assessment indicated that her asthma was uncontrolled, with active T2 inflammation.

Current Prescribed Treatment

- Fluticasone propionate/salmeterol xinafoate 250/25 µg, 1 inhalation bd via a pressurized metered-dose inhaler (pMDI) and a valved holding chamber (spacer)
- Terbutaline 500 µg via a Turbuhaler as needed

Asthma Management Skills and Knowledge

Adherence

Lucy said that she was adherent to her prescribed treatment. However, she said that she had missed two doses of her combination inhaled corticosteroid/long-acting beta-2 adrenergic agonist (ICS/LABA) in the past week.

Asthma Knowledge and Symptom Perception

Lucy had a lifelong history of asthma. While she was aware of the role of her inhaled therapies, she had never undergone an asthma education and self-management programme. Her symptom perception was poor.

Inhaler Technique

Lucy's inhaler technique with both her pMDl and spacer was optimal. Her technique using the Turbuhaler was inadequate; she held it horizontally (instead of vertically) during activation and did not inhale rapidly or deeply. Inhaler device polypharmacy was also evident with this regimen.

Self-Monitoring

Lucy was not monitoring her symptoms or her peak flow readings. She did not own a peak flow meter and was not familiar with self-monitoring diaries.

Exacerbation Management

Lucy had a written action plan that was prescribed by her general practitioner (GP) 20 years ago. The maintenance therapy and escalation plan were not reflective of her current treatment regimen.

DOI: 10.1201/9781003287209-17

Biomarkers

Lucy's FeNO and peripheral blood eosinophils are elevated, indicating the presence of T2 high inflammation that should be responsive to inhaled corticosteroid treatment. Of interest, Lucy's FeNO is raised even in the presence of an elevated BMI. Whether higher BMI is associated with lower FeNO in adults with asthma remains debatable, with studies reporting conflicting data).[1]

Case Summary

Lucy has uncontrolled asthma with T2 inflammation and poor symptom perception. Her treatment knowledge is adequate, but she is not aware of the severity of her asthma, the level of poor control, how to recognize exacerbations, or how to escalate treatment. Her current treatment plan does not reflect guideline-based management, and she would benefit from a change to maintenance and reliever therapy (MART). The number of devices she uses could be minimized, and a change to MART with a pMDI and spacer would achieve this. While she reports adherence to her treatment of greater than 80%, this may not be an accurate reflection of what is actually occurring.

Lucy would benefit from education to improve her knowledge of the desired level of asthma control, the role of T2 inflammation, and the impact of treatment, symptom recognition, and new treatment recommendations. She will start self-monitoring her symptoms and/or her peak flow, and she will need a personalized written action plan for exacerbation management. An extra pulmonary trait that could impact her asthma is her obesity, and person-centred education of the impact of obesity on asthma and potential treatment options would be beneficial. Regular follow-up will be required.

13.1 INTRODUCTION

We have presented Lucy, a 42-year-old female with asthma, who was recently admitted to hospital with an acute exacerbation of her asthma. Currently, she has ongoing poor symptom control despite being prescribed a combination high-dose ICS/LABA. An assessment of her asthma management skills and knowledge indicates that several areas require addressing. Asthma education will be integral to Lucy's management of her asthma.

Asthma education not only involves the transfer of information and knowledge, but it also incorporates strategies to improve skills and change attitudes, ultimately leading to behavioural change.[2, 3] This approach is termed *asthma self-management education.*

In this chapter, we will describe the essential components of effective education and discuss best-practice recommendations. We will also present evidence supporting asthma self-management education in a number of different patient populations and settings.

13.2 ASTHMA EDUCATION

Three decades of unequivocal evidence supports asthma self-management education and its ability to improve the morbidity of this disease in both children and adults.[4–6] As such, asthma self-management education is fundamental to optimal asthma management.

Self-management support is defined as

> the systematic provision of education and supportive interventions by health-care staff to increase patients' skills and confidence in managing their health problems, including regular assessment of progress and problems, goal setting, and problem-solving support. Self-management is defined as the tasks that individuals must undertake to live well with one or more chronic conditions. These tasks include having the confidence to deal with medical management, role management, and emotional management of their conditions.[7]

Meta-analyses of randomized controlled trials (RCT) have identified the essential components of asthma self-management education.[8, 9] The most effective programmes include the transfer of information, skills training, behavioural support, regular medical follow-up, the delivery of written asthma action plans (WAAPs), and regular monitoring of symptoms or lung function by the patient. These are achieved through effective therapeutic patient–clinician partnerships using a person-centred approach (Figure 13.1).[10] While successful asthma self-management programmes have considerable variability, they remain a multifaceted intervention and are most effective when their components are delivered in combination rather than as individual aspects.[9, 11]

Asthma self-management education can be delivered in a variety of settings. Improvements in asthma knowledge and control have been demonstrated in programmes delivered in the primary care outpatient, hospital, and emergency department settings.[11, 12] The advancement of electronic and mobile health (eHealth and mHealth) interventions and telehealth platforms has exploded the potential for patients to access asthma education and self-management help outside the clinic. Common digital health interventions for asthma education and self-management include mobile applications, text messaging services, telehealth platforms, wearables/monitoring devices, and Smartinhalers. The use of digital health platforms has been generally well-accepted, especially in an adolescent population. A systematic review has shown that adolescents were more comfortable using digital asthma action plans over traditional written ones

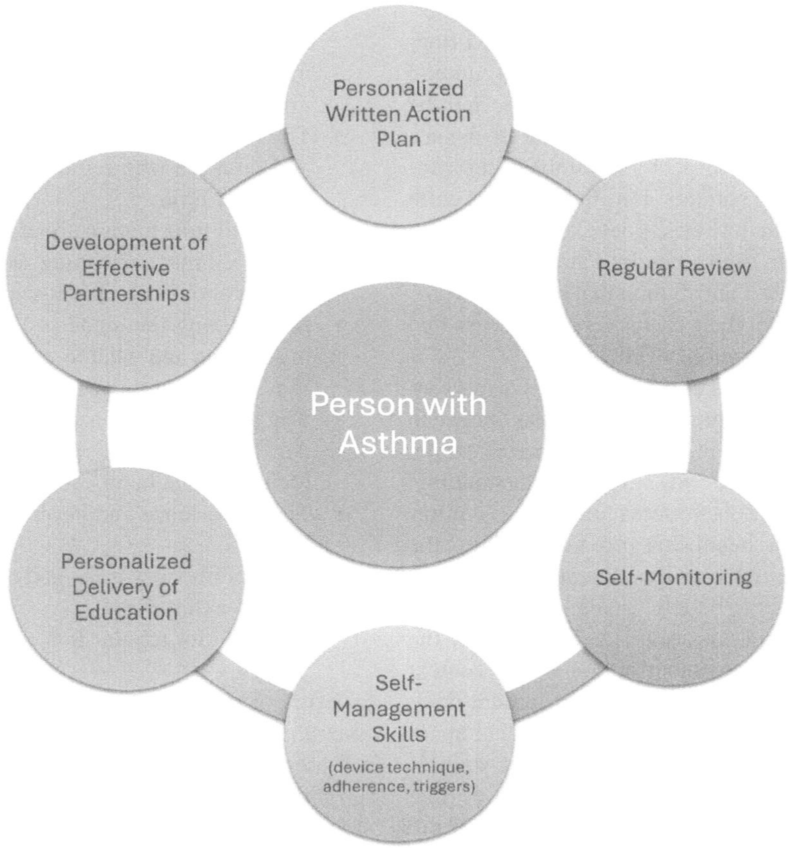
Personalized
Written Action
Plan
Regular Review
Self-Monitoring
Self-
Management
Skills
(device technique,
adherence, triggers)
Personalized
Delivery of
Education
Development of
Effective
Partnerships
Person with
Asthma

FIGURE 13.1 Key components of effective asthma education, placing the patient at the centre of the educative process. (Diagram created by the authors.)

and found e- and mHealth interventions helpful and convenient for asthma advice, information about asthma, self-monitoring, reminders, motivational messages, and to share information with others.[13] Digital health platforms that are personalized and interactive have also shown promise in improving medication adherence and asthma outcomes such as asthma control, and quality of life.[14] However, when choosing a digital platform for asthma education and self-management, care must be taken to ensure the quality and reliability of the resource. The landscape of asthma self-management platforms is currently unregulated, and the first evaluations of their content and functionality against best practice guidelines are only just underway.

Models of care that have reported the best outcomes are those that are implemented in secondary care settings[2] or that transcend multiple care settings for patients with moderate to severe asthma.[15] Personalization of asthma self-management education is essential for maintaining patient engagement and ensuring patient motivation to optimize implementation of asthma self-management strategies. The treatable traits model of care is one approach that has been effective in personalizing patient education, treatment, and self-management for people with severe asthma.[15] Using a multidimensional assessment, comorbidities, risk factors, and self-management skills specific to the individual are identified. These phenotypic and endotypic traits are targeted to deliver personalized treatment and self-management education for the individual.[16]

13.3 ESSENTIAL COMPONENTS OF ASTHMA EDUCATION

13.3.1 Developing Effective Patient–Clinician Partnerships

The development of effective patient–clinician partnerships is an important aspect of asthma self-management. One model that facilitates effective partnerships is patient-centred care. The concept of "patient centeredness" was first presented in medical literature in the mid-1950s by Balint,[17] who contrasted this concept with illness-centred medicine. The paradigm of person-centred care relates to holism, suggesting that patients be treated from a biopsychosocial perspective, placing the person at the centre of their own care[18] (Figure 13.1).

The hallmark features of patient-centred care concern the creation and maintenance of respectful and collaborative relationships between patients, their families, and healthcare staff, and the recognition of individuality.[10] Patient-centred care requires the clinician to have an appreciation of the patient's expectations, beliefs, and concerns; an understanding of the patient's personal circumstances; a willingness and motivation to provide information surrounding the diagnosis, pathology, treatment, and prognosis; and the knowledge to inform evidence-based treatment decisions. Healthcare providers should respect and establish the contribution of the patient and patients' families to their health decisions, recognizing their values, goals, experience, and knowledge of their own health needs. Patients and their families should respect the contribution that healthcare providers can make, including their professional expertise and their knowledge about the options available.[19]

Shared patient–clinician decision-making is a person-centred, collaborative communication process between healthcare professionals and patients to optimize asthma management decisions based on mutual understanding, respect, and agreement. This process involves (1) information sharing where the healthcare provider explains the management options available to the patient; (2) a discussion of patient preferences, beliefs, goals, and values in relation to the management options; (3) a discussion of the pros and cons of each management option in the context of the patient's specific circumstances; (4) a mutual decision that is agreed upon by the patient and clinician about the best asthma management plan for the patient; and (5) the asthma management plan, which is reviewed over time as the patient's asthma and circumstances change. There is evidence that shared decision-making with people with asthma improves medication and management adherence and patient (and parent) satisfaction.[20] Shared decision-making has been incorporated into the Global Initiative for Asthma (GINA) clinical best practice guidelines for choice of inhaler device, medication, and dose choice, which have been proved to lead to improved adherence and asthma outcomes.[2, 21]

13.3.2 Assessment of Knowledge and Skills and Provision of Information

The content and style of the information transfer and skills training will somewhat depend on the specific needs of the patient, taking into consideration the patient's age, level of health literacy, disease severity, and environmental factors such as the patient's social and emotional status and family support.[2] There are, however, core information and skills that must be included, and these are illustrated in the suggested content checklist for asthma education consultations (Table 13.1). These content areas can be addressed during the initial consultation, and they can be reinforced and reviewed during follow-up consultations.

With respect to the transfer of information, asthma education should include:

- The provision of information relating to the nature of asthma and its mechanisms, including the concept of different asthma subtypes;
- Asthma treatment, including the concept of different classes of asthma medication, when to use medications, possible side effects, and ways to minimize these side effects;
- The concept that asthma is a long-term condition, and, as such, the requirements for treatment are also long term;
- Practical information about how to use the inhaled therapy, inhaler cleaning instructions, and information about knowing when the device is empty;
- Recognizing the signs and symptoms of worsening asthma and what to do if they occur;
- Ways of preventing exacerbations;
- Trigger identification, avoidance, and management;
- An assessment of adherence and discussions focusing on adherence-aiding strategies;
- The importance and benefits of self-monitoring;
- WAAPs;
- Extra pulmonary traits and comorbidities that may impact asthma; and
- The need for regular follow-up.

In terms of asthma management skills, inhaler technique assessment and correction are vital, as are the initiation of self-monitoring of the symptoms and/or peak flows, the prescription, and an agreement on a written action plan that includes the course of action to take following an increase in asthma signs and symptoms.[2, 12]

13.3.3 Inhaler Technique

Adequate skill in the use of inhaler devices is integral to achieving good asthma outcomes. The majority of asthma medications are delivered via the inhaled route, as this offers the best balance between efficacy and safety.[22] Unfortunately, as many as 90% of patients have poor inhalation technique.[23] This is an ongoing problem. A systematic review reporting direct observation of inhaler technique in people with asthma and COPD, covering the period from 1975 to 2014, alarmingly reported that rates of correct technique did not improve over a 40-year period.[24] This is important, as inadequate inhaler technique is associated with poor asthma outcomes including increased risk asthma attacks.[25] The assessment and correction of inhaler technique are therefore essential features of asthma education and can effectively overcome errors and improve outcomes.[4] A number of known factors can increase the error rate for inhalation devices, and these factors need to be considered when educating patients and choosing the inhaled therapy. Both older people and people with more severe airflow limitation are at greatest risk of poor inhaler technique, which is related to decreased cognitive function and manual dexterity in older people and reduced peak inspiratory flow rates in both older people and those with severe airflow obstruction.[23, 24, 26] Furthermore, data suggests that there is a lack of education and instruction on inhalation technique among patients who are prescribed treatment; as

TABLE 13.1
Content of Asthma Education Consultations

	Case Study "Lucy"
Nature of Disease	
Provide basic patient-centred review of respiratory anatomy and asthma physiology, including the concept of asthma as an inflammatory disease and the concept of airway narrowing. Include discussion on the type of asthma the individual has.	
Asthma Treatment	
Concept of asthma medication classes	
Actions—relievers for bronchoconstriction; preventers for airway inflammation, and the benefit of combination maintenance and reliever therapy	
When to use medication	
Possible side effects and ways to minimize	
Inhaler Technique	
Assess inhaler technique.	Needs correction
Correct inhaler technique.	Minimize the number
Continually reassess and correct inhaler technique at follow-up.	
Assess and, when possible, correct inhaler device polypharmacy.	
Self-Monitoring	
Establish patient preference for self-monitoring.	Commenced on peak flow and symptom monitoring
Have the patient understand the rationale for self-monitoring.	
Commence either peak flow or symptom monitoring based on the patient's ability and preference.	
Continually review self-monitoring at follow-up.	
Asthma Control	
Ensure the patient understands the concept of good asthma control.	Poor control
Ensure the patient is able to recognize the signs and symptoms of worsening asthma and knows the actions to take.	Poor recognition Given a written action plan
Written Action Plan	
Prescribe a written action plan.	Plan developed
Include the patient in the decision-making process.	Treatment changed
Ensure the patient understands and accepts the treatment recommendations.	Knowledge and agreement of plan
Provide the patient with prescriptions for the recommended treatments.	Assessed
Reinforce the plan at follow-up.	
Review the plan following each exacerbation or every six months.	
Adherence	
Assess adherence to treatment.	Requires ongoing assessment and review
Establish reason for nonadherence in a supportive and nonjudgmental way.	
Discuss ways to implement adherence-aiding strategies.	
Triggers	
Identify relevant trigger factor with the patient.	
Provide advice on trigger factor management.	
Review regularly.	
Smoking	N/A
Establish smoking status.	
Engage in discussions about smoking cessation.	
Individual Patients' Needs	
Establish what is important to each patient.	
Ensure patients' needs are addressed.	
Allow time to explore patients' questions and concerns.	
Review extra-pulmonary traits and provide targeted education on the impacts on asthma and treatment options.	Person-centred discussion and education about obesity and asthma
Follow-up/review	

N/A, not applicable.
Source: Adapted from McDonald, V.M. and Gibson, P.G., *Allergy Frontiers: Diagnosis and Health Economics*, Springer Publishing, Japan, 2009. With permission.

many as 25% of asthma or chronic obstructive pulmonary disease (COPD) patients have never been provided with inhaler device instruction.[27] This may be related to clinicians' confidence to educate patients, as other data suggests that up to 89.2% of health professionals are unable to demonstrate adequate inhaler technique.[28] The document "Inhaler Technique" (https://assets-stage.nationalasthma.org.au/resources/Inhaler-technique-checklist_NPS-Medicinewise_2020.pdf) details the essential steps that are required to develop an adequate technique for each of the most common inhaler devices used in asthma treatment. The following is a TEACHER mnemonic to aid in the vital steps for inhaler technique education.

Tailor: Individualize the device to the patient's needs.
Educate: Educate and demonstrate the correct technique.
Assess: Assess the patient's ability for using the device.
Correct: Correct the technique.
Have Another Go: After correction, reassess.
Evaluate: Is this the correct device for this patient?
Reduce: Minimize the number of devices prescribed.

These include the need to individualize the choice of inhaler to the individual patient's skill and preference; the need to explain and demonstrate to the patient how to use the device, and why an effective technique is important; the need to assess the patient's technique and to correct the essential steps when necessary; and the continued evaluation of the patient's technique as his or her proficiency may decrease over time, therefore reassessment every 2–3 months is recommended.[26] Finally, we advise minimizing the number of different devices prescribed to avoid inhaler device polypharmacy.[29, 30]

Over time, there has been a progressive increase in the types of inhalation devices used in the management of asthma and other obstructive airway diseases; this has led to the frequent problem of inhaler device polypharmacy, which is the use of multiple types of inhalation devices by one individual.[29, 30] We have previously demonstrated that this is a common problem among adults with asthma and that an inadequate inhalation device technique is most common among patients using three or more delivery devices.[29] As the array of devices continues to increase, this is becoming a very important issue to address.

Figure 13.2 provides guidance for the selection of inhaler devices, taking into consideration the potential errors. Regardless of the device selected, the practitioner must demonstrate the technique and provide regular reassessment and instruction.[2]

13.3.4 Self-Monitoring

Self-monitoring is the regular self-recording of symptoms and/or peak expiratory flow (PEF) measurements that patients perform in their homes and work or school environments. Self-monitoring is useful, as it provides patients with a tool for assessing their level of asthma control and aids in the recognition of the early signs of an exacerbation.

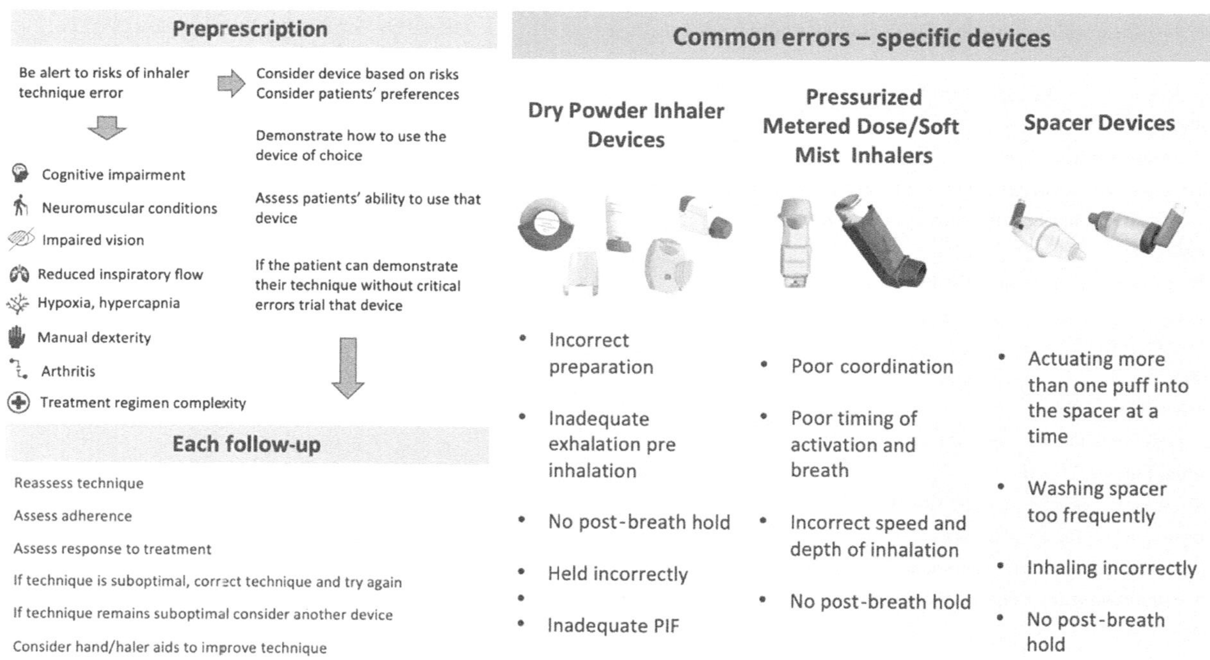

FIGURE 13.2 Guide to inhaler device selection recognizing the potential problems associated with the optimal technique. (Content has been reproduced with permission from the Centre of Excellence in Treatable Traits, originally developed as part of the Centre of Excellence in Treatable Traits [https://treatabletraits.org.au].)

When compared to environmental data and other comorbidities, self-monitoring can provide indications of what may trigger a patient's asthma symptoms. Self-monitoring also assists clinicians in reviewing the level of asthma control over time, and the results provide clinicians with data to determine the action to be taken at certain points of the early exacerbation written action plan and monitor new treatment behaviours. Self-monitoring has traditionally been performed using handwritten symptom diaries. However, this method is inefficient and can take time to identify, communicate, and compare symptom trends over time. Digital applications provide a unique opportunity to not only record symptom trends over time but efficiently and meaningfully represent and compare self-monitoring data.[2, 31] They also present the opportunity to better embed self-monitoring behaviours into daily routines, using mobile notifications, prompts, reminders, and alarms.[32]

In children, it appears that symptom-based action plans are superior to peak-flow-based plans, but it is not known if this is related to differences in adherence for either option.[33] In adult patients, a number of studies have compared the two forms of monitoring, and a meta-analysis concluded that, when self-monitoring is coupled with a written action plan, the results from symptom or peak flow monitoring are equivalent.[34] One study did, however, show that patients preferred symptom monitoring over the use of peak flow[35] and that, while adherence to self-monitoring can be poor, the notion of establishing individual patient preferences is important in determining the approach each patient might take.

While the effects of peak flow or symptom monitoring are equivalent, each has its pros and cons. Peak flows provide more objective data and may be more useful in patients (such as in the earlier "Lucy" case study) who have a poor perception of their symptoms;[36] however, they may be considered by patients as less practical and an unnecessary financial burden. Conversely, symptom monitoring provides less objective data, but it is less costly and more practical. In some patients, symptoms may deteriorate before a fall in the peak flow is evident; in this group of patients, symptom monitoring is preferred.

Several other factors should also be considered when establishing and reviewing self-monitoring practices with patients. Factors such as health literacy, cognition, and the ability to record symptoms or peak flow are important. Additionally, patients should be provided with information or examples about the rationale and the benefits of self-monitoring, including the interpretation and the relevance of the results on asthma control. A chart display also influences the ability to recognize deteriorating asthma.[37]

13.3.5 Regular Review

A regular medical review is another key element contributing to the success of asthma self-management education.[2] The review provides practitioners with the opportunity to assess asthma control, measure lung function, review treatment response, reinforce asthma knowledge and skills, and maintain an effective partnership with the patient.

The key questions to assess during the review are the frequency of symptoms, including nocturnal awakening and symptoms on waking up in the morning. The degree of activity limitation and the frequency of short-acting beta-2 adrenergic agonist use should also be elicited, as should the exacerbation history.

Due to the time pressures faced by medical practitioners, asthma education opportunities may be limited during both the initial consultation and at follow-up review. Working in partnership with asthma educators, specialist nurses, and allied health professionals will increase the asthma education opportunities for patients.

Follow-ups after acute attacks of asthma are particularly important, as these are the best predictors of a future attack.[38, 39] These attacks put people with asthma at high risk of adverse outcomes, including death. The UK's National Review of Asthma Deaths (NRAD)[40] alarmingly reported that 10% of the confirmed deaths from asthma occurred within four weeks of discharge from hospital for treatment of an acute attack, and over one-fifth occurred in people who had attended an emergency department in the past year. It is therefore of utmost importance that people receive follow-up with their primary care practitioner promptly following an attack. The NRAD and society guidelines recommend that this occurs within two working days of an acute attack, and during the follow-up, the diagnosis should be confirmed, treatment and skills optimized, a written action plan discussed, adherence addressed, and future risk assessed. Levy et al. suggest that this can be operationalized by leaving one appointment available each day for acute asthma follow-ups. If not needed, the day can be easily used by other patients.[39]

13.3.6 Written Asthma Action Plans

Exacerbations are a common feature in asthma, putting the patient at immediate risk for distress, hospitalization, and even death. Acute exacerbations represent a significant contribution to healthcare costs.[41] Exacerbations may occur over days or weeks and, as such, patients frequently have an opportunity to recognize their deterioration and escalate their treatment to reduce both the severity of the exacerbation and the recovery time. Written asthma action plans (WAAPs) are used to facilitate asthma management, particularly exacerbation management.[2, 42]

WAAPs are developed by a medical practitioner or an accredited nurse practitioner to provide patients with written instructions, either in the form of printed, digital, or pictorial information. WAAPs include instructions about a patient's maintenance treatment and how to escalate treatment during both moderate and severe asthma exacerbations.[2] They are an essential component in the effective self-management of asthma[43] and are a key recommendation of international clinical practice asthma guidelines.[2]

When written action plans are coupled with self-management education there is irrefutable evidence to support their effect on reducing asthma morbidity.[42] Unfortunately, the uptake of WAAPs in practice remains poor. A population survey in South Australia demonstrated that the proportion of people who stated that they had a WAAP was 42% in 1995, which fell to 20.8% in 2003.[44] Since then, there has been a slight improvement with 28% of people who reported having asthma as a long-term condition, indicating they have a written asthma action plan—an increase from 21% in 2007–2008.[45]

The reasons for the low-level uptake of WAAPs by healthcare professionals are likely to be multifactorial; they may reflect the poor training of doctors and other health professionals in creating and delivering negotiated action plans in partnership with people with asthma,[46] suggesting a need for additional training in self-management plans among health professionals. It may also be related to the time required for medical practitioners to develop and effectively convey the plan to the patient. This can be overcome by developing asthma management programmes in partnership with asthma educators, specialist nurses, and other allied healthcare professionals. Finally, the poor uptake could be related to the attitudes of clinicians and patients regarding the importance of such plans. In a study published by the present authors, the importance of the clinical problems experienced by older people with asthma and COPD was rated by both patients and their physicians. The problems related to self-management, including WAAPs,[47] received the lowest rating of importance from patients and doctors. This suggests a need to improve clinicians' and patients' knowledge of the efficacy and benefits of written action plans.

Many different written action plan templates are available to aid both clinicians and patients in completing these agreed treatment plans. Examples may be found at the following websites: https://www.nationalasthma.org.au/health-professionals/asthma-action-plans/asthma-action-plan-library (accessed 11/07/2024), http://www.aaaai.org/Aaaai/media/MediaLibrary/PDF%20Documents/Libraries/NEW-WEBSITE-LOGO-asthma-action-plan_HI.pdf (accessed 11/07/2024), and https://asthma.ca/wp-content/uploads/2020/06/Asthma-Action-Plan_optimized.pdf (accessed 11/07/2024).

Gibson and Powell[42] undertook a study to review the evidence supporting WAAPs, and they recommended that the key components of WAAPs include detail describing:

- When to increase treatment (action point);
- How to increase treatment;
- For how long; and
- When to seek medical help.

An example of a WAAP incorporating these components for the "Lucy" case study is presented in Figure 13.3. In addition to the written component, engagement with the patient is also essential to ensure that he or she understands the plan, agrees to the treatment recommendations, and has the capacity to implement all elements of the plan.

13.3.7 Adherence

Adherence to medical advice is a well-known problem in people with asthma,[48] and as health professionals, we need to recognize and expect nonadherence. The reality that patients do not always follow the prescribed treatment advice has been evident for thousands of years. As Hippocrates said:

> [B]e alert to the faults of the patients which make them lie about their taking of the medicines prescribed and when things go wrong, refuse to confess that they have not been taking their medicine.[49]

He was referring to health behaviour that is now referred to as nonadherence. There are now several terms used in the medical literature to describe a patient's health behaviour regarding treatment. These include *compliance*, *adherence*, and *concordance*. While these terms are frequently used interchangeably, their different meanings must be recognized.

The now largely outmoded term "compliance" refers to the extent to which the patient's behaviour matches the prescriber's advice.[50] Compliance is associated with negative connotations, as it infers that the role of the prescriber is to issue treatment and the role of the patient is to follow orders.[50, 51] This term inadequately captures the collaboration that is essential to effective, best-practice patient–clinician partnerships.[2]

> The preferred term "adherence" refers to the extent to which a patient's behaviour with respect to their medication, diet or lifestyle is consistent or matches the recommendations of the prescriber.[50, 51]

In contrast with the term "compliance," adherence is intended to be nonjudgmental. Adherence alludes to the process of deciding appropriate treatment after proper discussion between the clinician and patient. It implies that the patient is not obliged to accept a particular treatment if it does not appeal to them and the patient is not held solely responsible for nonadherence.[51]

Concordance is a more complex notion that relates to the relationship between the patient and the prescriber. Concordance fits the model of person-centred care as it recognizes the need for patients and clinicians to work in partnership to reach agreement around treatment decisions and that patients and clinicians may have opposing views.[50, 51] Concordance can be thought of as the process required for achieving adherence.

It is well-known that adherence in chronic disease can be poor, and this is particularly true in chronic respiratory conditions. In a meta-analysis of 569 studies, adherence to therapy in respiratory diseases ranked poorly, with a mean adherence rate of 68.8%, which was 15th out of 17

My Symbicort (budesonide/formoterol) Rapihaler 100/3 Asthma Action Plan

Anti-inflammatory Reliever With or without Maintenance

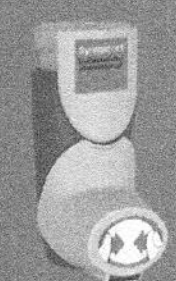

Name: Lucy Chapter

Date: 01-Jul-2024

Plan discussed with: (name of health care professional) Dr A Asthma

My usual best peak flow (if used): 400 l/min

National Asthma Council AUSTRALIA

Usual Medical Contact: Name and telephone number

NORMAL MODE

MY SYMBICORT ASTHMA TREATMENT IS:

☑ Symbicort Rapihaler 100/3 mcg

☑ Use with a spacer

RELIEVER

I should take 2 separate puffs (1 at a time) of my Symbicort whenever needed for relief of my asthma symptoms

I should always carry my Symbicort with me to use as a reliever when needed

MY REGULAR MAINTENANCE TREATMENT EVERY DAY IS : *(enter number of puffs or 0 if no regular daily treatment prescribed)*

2 Puffs in the morning (0, 2, 4)

2 Puffs in the evening (0, 2, 4)

MY ASTHMA IS STABLE IF:

- I do not wake up at night or in the morning because of asthma
- My asthma has not interfered with my usual activities (e.g housework, school, exercise)

OTHER INSTRUCTIONS
(e.g. what to do before exercise, when to see my doctor)

Have your asthma reviewed every six months or after any asthma worsening (attack)

Use one puff of Symbicort with your spacer 10 minutes prior to exercise.

ASTHMA FLARE UP

IF OVER A PERIOD OF 2–3 DAYS:

- My asthma symptoms are getting worse or not improving

OR

- I am using more than to 12 Symbicort reliever puffs a day

OR

- Peak flow below: 320 (delete if not used)

I SHOULD:

✓ **Continue to use my Symbicort to relieve my symptoms and my regular daily Symbicort (if prescribed) (up to a total maximum of 24 puffs in a day)**

☑ Contact my doctor

☐ Start a course of prednisolone

COURSE OF PREDNISOLONE TABLETS:

Take ____ mg prednisolone tablets each morning for ____ days; OR

IF I NEED MORE THAN 24 SYMBICORT PUFFS (TOTAL) IN ANY DAY,

- I must see my doctor or go to hospital the same day

ASTHMA EMERGENCY

SIGNS OF AN ASTHMA EMERGENCY

- My asthma symptoms are getting worse quickly
- I am finding it very hard to breathe or speak
- My Symbicort is not helping

IF I HAVE ANY OF THE ABOVE DANGER SIGNS, I SHOULD DIAL 000 FOR AN AMBULANCE AND SAY I AM HAVING A SEVERE ASTHMA ATTACK.

WHILE I AM WAITING FOR THE AMBULANCE:

- Sit upright and keep calm
- I should keep taking my Symbicort as needed
- If only Ventolin® is available, take 4 puffs as often as needed until help arrives
- Even if my symptoms appear to settle quickly I should seek medical advice right away
- ☐ Use my adrenaline autoinjector

OTHER INSTRUCTIONS

FIGURE 13.3 Example of a written asthma action plan. (Adapted from the Symbicort Asthma Action Plan, National Asthma Council Australia, found at https://assets-stage.nationalasthma.org.au/resources/Symbicort_Asthma_Action_Plan_Rapihaler_01.06.2020.pdf, with permission)

Note: Trade names have been used to represent the language used in patient communication.

different diseases.[52] A prospective study of asthma found that 24% of severe exacerbations were attributable to nonadherence.[53]

Two distinct patterns of behaviour are associated with nonadherence: intentional and unintentional nonadherence.[14, 54, 55] Factors that can influence adherence can be assigned to three domains—the physician, the patient, and the healthcare system—and are summarized in Figure 13.4. Understanding the behaviour patterns and views contributing to nonadherence in individuals should guide education content and delivery and help develop personalized adherence-aiding strategies.

Intentional nonadherence occurs when patients make purposeful decisions to take and perform treatments in a way other than that prescribed. This often refers to the self-adjustment or titration of treatment according to the patient's symptoms or beliefs or to the cessation of treatment earlier than prescribed.[50] Intentional nonadherence usually results when the patient weighs the risks against the benefits of taking medication and makes a decision based on their reasoning.[56] While intentional nonadherence may result from a balance of reasoning, the decision could result from poor knowledge about the treatment or from an erroneous understanding regarding the nature or consequence of the problem, the prescribed therapy, and the potential benefit of treatment. Therefore, this form of nonadherence can often be addressed through strategies that improve patients' knowledge and influence their health beliefs and concerns.[57]

Unintentional nonadherence occurs when patients do not adhere to treatment advice due to reasons out of their control.[50] These are often related to cognitive impairments, language barriers, and physical disabilities. In the case of an older person with asthma, this could relate to impaired vision or musculoskeletal problems affecting his or her ability to use inhaled medications. Further unintentional nonadherence could also result from ineffective communication or inaccurate recollection of the prescribed treatment prescription.[55, 57] Studies of how well patients retain health information suggest that less than 50% of the information conveyed by the physician is recalled immediately after an office visit.[58]

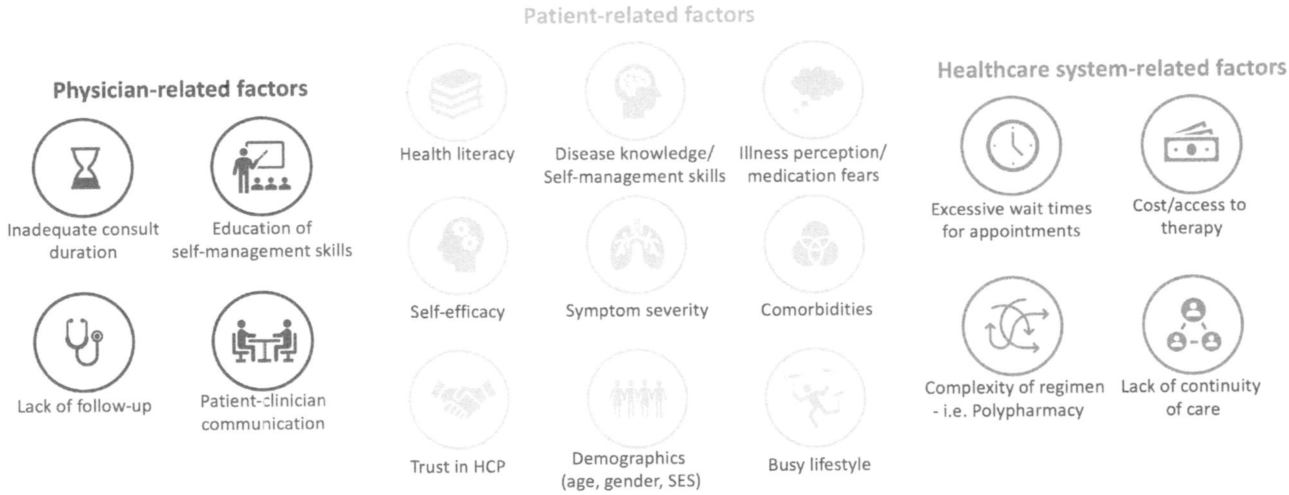
Patient-related factors
Physician-related factors
Inadequate consult duration
Education of self-management skills
Lack of follow-up
Patient-clinician communication
Health literacy
Disease knowledge/ Self-management skills
Illness perception/ medication fears
Self-efficacy
Symptom severity
Comorbidities
Trust in HCP
Demographics (age, gender, SES)
Busy lifestyle
Healthcare system-related factors
Excessive wait times for appointments
Cost/access to therapy
Complexity of regimen - i.e. Polypharmacy
Lack of continuity of care

FIGURE 13.4 Factors influencing adherence.[59, 60]

Recognizing nonadherence, establishing the reasons for nonadherence (Figure 13.4), and working with patients to improve their adherence are essential elements of asthma education.

13.4 ASTHMA EDUCATION IN DIFFERENT POPULATIONS

Asthma self-management education has been tested in many different patient groups, including adults, children and adolescents, elderly people, pregnant women, and culturally and linguistically diverse populations. Evidence supports asthma self-management education in these populations and recognizes that the education should be tailored to the specific needs of the population.[5, 59]

13.4.1 Adults

Many RCTs of asthma education have been conducted in adults with asthma, and the results of these trials have been summarized in Cochrane systematic reviews.[34, 61] One review examined limited education that included the provision of information only. The review included 12 RCTs, and the results indicated that the provision of information alone was effective in terms of improving knowledge, but it did not reduce asthma morbidity, hospital admissions, or unscheduled doctors' visits for asthma. Furthermore, these studies showed that the provision of information alone did not improve lung function or reduce medication use. From this analysis, it can be concluded that limited education involving the transfer of information alone improves knowledge but not asthma health outcomes.[62] A second systematic review evaluated 36 RCTs comparing self-management education with usual medical care. This analysis demonstrated that self-management education is effective in reducing hospitalizations, emergency department and unscheduled physician office visits, as well as reducing days off work or school, reducing nocturnal asthma, and improving patients' quality of life. The estimated number needed to treat (NNT) with asthma self-management education in order to prevent one asthma hospitalization is 20 and to prevent one emergency department visit the NNT is eight.[2] The authors conclude that asthma self-management education that includes the provision of information, self-monitoring by either PEF or symptoms, regular medical review, and a WAAP improves the health outcomes for adults with asthma.[63]

13.4.2 Older People

Older people with asthma are an important population, as the morbidity and mortality from asthma in this population is high.[64] The optimal self-management education for older people with asthma is still unclear. In the majority of the studies included in the previously described systematic review, the participants were a mean age of less than 52 years, and older people were excluded in some of the trials.[63] While asthma deaths have fallen in younger populations over the last few decades, Australia, for example, has witnessed a rise in mortality in older adults.[65] While advances in pharmacotherapy and self-management education policy initiatives have led to positive outcomes in younger people with asthma, the same has not been seen in older people, suggesting that the results of these RCTs cannot be extrapolated or applied to older populations who remain at risk.[66]

While less data exists in relation to self-management techniques in older people, some trials have examined interventions in this population. Huang et al. also conducted a RCT in older people with moderate to severe asthma involving telephone interventions. This trial had three arms: usual care, individualized education with weekly telephone consults, and the former plus peak flow monitoring. Written information was provided in large fonts and used pictures with few words. Participants in the two intervention arms demonstrated significant improvements in their asthma knowledge and skills, self-care behaviours and self-efficacy, and prebronchodilator FEV_1 compared with a control group.[67] In an RCT of 172 people with asthma over the age of 55, participants received a six-session asthma self-management intervention delivered via group sessions and telephone calling compared to the control (30-minute asthma education session). The intervention led to significant reductions in asthma exacerbations and improved asthma control and self-management score.[68]

These studies suggest that older people with asthma can be instructed in an effective self-management programme and achieve improvements in self-management efficacy,[67, 68] quality of life,[69] lung function,[67] asthma control, and exacerbations.[68] The benefits of asthma self-management education come from integrated programmes with active involvement by the participant.

13.4.3 Pregnant Women

Irrespective of the level of asthma severity, exacerbations of asthma in pregnant women are common. Achieving good control in this population is vital, as uncontrolled asthma during pregnancy is associated with adverse maternal and foetal outcomes.[70] Asthma self-management education in this population has been shown to improve asthma knowledge and skills. Murphy et al.[71] conducted a study in which pregnant women were recruited from the antenatal clinic of a tertiary hospital. The women were interviewed by an asthma educator at 20 and 33 weeks' gestation. Their asthma knowledge and skills were poor at the baseline visit but improved significantly following education by the asthma educator, suggesting that asthma self-management education should be integrated into standard antenatal care.[71]

A RCT of a virtual model of asthma care compared to a face-to-face model was conducted by Thomas et al. in 200 pregnant women with asthma. The primary outcome was uptake, and the secondary outcome was asthma control. Both groups received a consult with a respiratory physician and an asthma educator, and auxiliary digital support including text messages, written education materials, and a smartphone application. While uptake was better in the virtual care model, asthma control improved significantly in both groups.[72, 73]

An important aspect of asthma education for pregnant women is to ensure that they understand the importance of good asthma control to avoid poor maternal and foetal outcomes. The safety of asthma treatment during pregnancy must also be stressed, as pregnant women may have concerns about using their treatment and a misconstrued understanding of the risk of taking medications during pregnancy may lead to poor adherence and adverse outcomes. An online toolkit for managing asthma during pregnancy, including information for families and health professionals, is available at https://asthmapregnancytoolkit.org.au.

13.4.4 Children

A number of systematic reviews have demonstrated the value of asthma self-management education in paediatric and adolescent populations.[6, 68] While the setting and the type of intervention varies, the reviews are supportive of educational intervention for children with asthma. In the review by Wolf et al., the effects of self-management education in children were evaluated. Thirty-two RCTs were included, and the results of the analysis indicated that self-management education by children was associated with improvements in airflow obstruction and self-efficacy. Furthermore, education was also associated with a reduction in emergency department presentations and reduced absenteeism from school.[74] Asthma self-management education is recognized as standard practice in children and adolescents with asthma.[2]

Kneale et al. reported a systematic review of school-based self-management interventions compared to control. These interventions reduced hospital admission and emergency department visits. Studies that engaged parents were conducted outside of children's free time and used a theoretical framework that was more likely to be implemented successfully.[6]

13.5 SUMMARY

Asthma self-management education is an effective and integral part of asthma management in both adults and children. It can be successfully delivered in a variety of settings and platforms. The key components of asthma self-management education involve the transfer of information to improve knowledge, skills training, self-monitoring, the prescription of WAAPs, and regular medical review. These components of asthma education are best delivered in a model of person-centred care where the needs of the individual patient are understood and effective clinician–patient partnerships are developed.

REFERENCES

1. H. Zhang, et al., *Front Physiol* (2023). https://doi.org/10.3389/fphys.2023.1019123
2. Global Initiative for Asthma, GINA (2024). www.ginasthma.org
3. V. M. McDonald, et al., Springer (2009). https://doi.org/10.1007/978-4-431-98349-1_26
4. R. Fortescue, et al., *Cochrane Database Syst Rev* (2017). https://doi.org/10.1002/14651858.CD012286.pub2
5. G. B. McCallum, et al., *Cochrane Database Syst Rev* (2017). https://doi.org/10.1002/14651858.CD006580.pub5
6. K. Harris, et al., *Cochrane Database Syst Rev* (2019). https://doi.org/10.1002/14651858.CD011651.pub2
7. K. Adams, et al., The National Academies Press. (2004). https://doi.org/10.17226/11085
8. H. Pinnock, et al., *BMC Med* (2017). https://doi.org/10.1186/s12916-017-0823-7
9. T. Dhippayom, et al., *J Allergy Clin Immunol Pract* (2022). https://doi.org/10.1016/j.jaip.2021.09.049

10. V. M. McDonald, et al., *Respirology* (2024). https://doi.org/10.1111/resp.14644
11. M. N. Eakin, et al., *JAMA Pediatrics* (2020). https://doi.org/10.1001/jamapediatrics.2020.3375
12. B. Murray, et al., *Br J Nurs* (Mark Allen Publishing) (2018). https://doi.org/10.12968/bjon.2018.27.7.396
13. A. R. van Buul, et al., *Clin Ehealth* (2020). https://doi.org/10.1016/j.ceh.2020.06.001
14. A. Chan, et al., *Cochrane Database Syst Rev* (2022). https://doi.org/10.1002/14651858.CD013030.pub2
15. V. M. McDonald, et al., *Eur Respir J* (2020). https://doi.org/10.1183/13993003.01509–2019
16. V. M. McDonald, et al., *Med J Aust* (2022). https://doi.org/10.5694/mja2.51464
17. M. Balint, *Lancet* (1955). https://doi.org/10.1016/s0140-6736(55)91061-8
18. A. Coulter, et al., *Future Hosp J* (2016). https://doi.org/10.7861/futurehosp.3-2-114
19. B. Dow, et al., *The Victorian Government Department of Human Services* (2006).
20. D. A. Bukstein, et al., *Ann Allergy Asthma Immunol* (2020). https://doi.org/10.1016/j.anai.2020.06.030
21. Y. J. Taylor, et al., *J Asthma* (2018). https://doi.org/10.1080/02770903.2017.1362423
22. S. Anderson, et al., *Pharmacol Rev* (2022). https://doi.org/10.1124/pharmrev.120.000108
23. A. S. Melani, et al., *Respir Med* (2011). https://doi.org/10.1016/j.rmed.2011.01.005
24. J. Sanchis, et al., *Chest* (2016). https://doi.org/10.1016/j.chest.2016.03.041
25. O. S. Usmani, et al., *Respir Res* (2018). https://doi.org/10.1186/s12931-017-0710-y
26. S. Bosnic-Anticevich, et al., *J Allergy Clin Immunol Pract* (2023). https://doi.org/10.1016/j.jaip.2023.04.031
27. F. Lavorini, et al., *Respir Med* (2008). https://doi.org/10.1016/j.rmed.2007.11.003
28. V. Plaza, et al., *J Allergy Clin Immunol Pract* (2018). https://doi.org/10.1016/j.jaip.2017.12.032
29. McDonald VM, et al., *Med J Aust* (2005). https://doi.org/10.5694/j.1326-5377.2005.tb06680.x
30. S. Bosnic-Anticevich, et al., *Int J Chron Obstruct Pulmon Dis* (2017). https://doi.org/10.2147/copd.S117196
31. S. McLean, et al., *Cochrane Database Syst Rev* (2010). https://doi.org/10.1002/14651858.CD007717.pub2
32. A. Kaplan, et al., *Ther Adv Chronic Dis* (2023). https://doi.org/10.1177/20406223231209329
33. S. K. Bhogal, et al., *Cochrane Database Syst Rev* (2006). https://doi.org/10.1002/14651858.CD005306.pub2
34. H. Powell, et al., *Cochrane Database Syst Rev* (2002). https://doi.org/10.1002/14651858.CD004107
35. A. Harver, et al., *J Asthma* (2009). https://doi.org/10.3109/02770900903274475
36. P. G. Gibson, *J Allergy Clin Immunol* (2000). https://doi.org/10.1067/mai.2000.108307
37. R. M. Turner, et al., *J Clin Epidemiol* (2012). https://doi.org/10.1016/j.jclinepi.2011.04.012
38. V. M. McDonald, et al., *Respirology* (2019). https://doi.org/10.1111/resp.13389
39. M. L. Levy, et al., *NPJ Prim Care Respir Med* (2018). https://doi.org/10.1038/s41533-018-0087-5
40. M. L. Levy, Asthma still kills: Little change over five decades. *NPJ Prim Care Respir Med*. 2014;24(1):14029. https://doi.org/10.1038/npjpcrm.2014.29
41. J. G. Zein, et al., *PLOS ONE* (2016). https://doi.org/10.1371/journal.pone.0157301
42. P. G. Gibson, et al., *Thorax* (2004). https://doi.org/10.1136/thorax.2003.011858
43. H. Pinnock, *Breathe* (Lausanne, Switzerland) (2015). https://doi.org/10.1183/20734735.015614
44. D. H. Wilson, et al., *Med J Aust* (2006). https://doi.org/10.5694/j.1326-5377.2006.tb00207.x
45. Australian Institute of Health and Welfare. 2018. Australia's Health 2018: In Brief. https://www.aihw.gov.au/reports/australias-health/australias-health-2018/contents/overview
46. N. Ring, et al., *Patient Educ Couns* (2011). https://doi.org/10.1016/j.pec.2011.01.025
47. V. M. McDonald, et al., *Prim Care Respir J* (2011). https://doi.org/10.4104/pcrj.2011.00025
48. J. Murphy, et al., *J Asthma* (2021). https://doi.org/10.1080/02770903.2020.1711916
49. Hippocrates, (200 BC).
50. R. Horne, *Chest* (2006). https://doi.org/10.1378/chest.130.1_suppl.65S
51. S. Chakrabarti, *World J Psychiatry* (2014). https://doi.org/10.5498/wjp.v4.i2.30
52. L. K. Williams, et al., *J Allergy Clin Immunol* (2011). https://doi.org/10.1016/j.jaci.2011.09.011
53. M. Banning, *Int J Nurs Stud* (2008). https://doi.org/10.1016/j.ijnurstu.2008.02.009
54. R. F. McLoughlin, et al., (2022). https://doi.org/10.1183/2312508X.erm9722
55. A. L. Wroe, *J Behav Med* (2002). https://doi.org/10.1023/A:1015866415552
56. J. Holmes, et al., *Breathe* (2021). https://doi.org/10.1183/20734735.0037–2021
57. J. T. Lindsay, et al., *Patient Prefer Adherence* (2013). https://doi.org/10.2147/ppa.S38208
58. R. P. Kessels, *J R Soc Med* (2003). https://doi.org/10.1177/014107680309600504
59. E. L. McQuaid, *Ann Allergy Asthma Immunol* (2018). https://doi.org/10.1016/j.anai.2018.03.024
60. S. Amin, et al., *Patient Prefer Adherence* (2020). https://doi.org/10.2147/ppa.S234651
61. S. Tapp, et al., *Cochrane Database Syst Rev* (2007). https://doi.org/10.1002/14651858.CD003000.pub2
62. P. G. Gibson, et al., *Cochrane Database Syst Rev* (2002). https://doi.org/10.1002/14651858.CD001005
63. P. G. Gibson, et al., *Cochrane Database Syst Rev* (2002). https://doi.org/10.1002/14651858.CD001117
64. J. K. Khosa, et al., *J Asthma Allergy* (2023). https://doi.org/10.2147/jaa.S293081
65. V. M. McDonald, et al., *Australia's J Ageing* (2008). https://doi.org/10.1111/j.1741-6612.2008.00322.x
66. S. Battaglia, et al., *Breathe* (2016). https://doi.org/10.1183/20734735.002816
67. T. T. Huang, et al., *J Adv Nurs* (2009). https://doi.org/10.1111/j.1365-2648.2008.04874.x
68. A. P. Baptist, et al., *Ann Allergy Asthma Immunol* (2020). https://doi.org/10.1016/j.anai.2019.12.015
69. A. S. Buist, et al., *Am J Respir Crit Care Med* (2006). https://doi.org/10.1164/rccm.200510-1606OC
70. V. E. Murphy, *Breathe* (Sheffield, England) (2015). https://doi.org/10.1183/20734735.007915
71. V. E. Murphy, et al., *Eur Respir J* (2005). https://doi.org/10.1183/09031936.05.00135604
72. D. Thomas, et al., *Eur Respir J* (Under Review) (2024).
73. D. Thomas, et al., *Lancet Respir Med* (2024). https://doi.org/10.1016/s2213-2600(24)00080-8
74. F. M. Wolf, et al., *Cochrane Database Syst Rev* (2003). https://doi.org/10.1002/14651858.Cd000326

14 Adherence and Outcomes

Andrew Bush

CASE STUDY

The patient is a 13-year-old girl who was referred after having five admissions to hospital in the previous year, three requiring intravenous glucocorticoid therapy. She had been prescribed a fluticasone/salmeterol Accuhaler 500/50 strength, Montelukast 5 mg daily, and uniphyllin 400 mg twice daily. She uses salbutamol several times a day most days. Her total IgE is 2081, with raised specific IgE to house dust mite, tree and grass pollen, and cat and dog. Her peripheral blood eosinophil count is 0.9 cells/μλ, and she is referred for either omalizuab (for which she is ineligible due to the high IgE level), mepolizuab or dupilumab, for which she meets criteria. The first step was a protocolized, multidisciplinary team assessment [1–3] including assessment of adherence:

- *On history taking and using the MARS-5 questionnaire, she reports >95% adherence [4], confirmed by her mother (who actually does not witness the medication being taken).*
- *Theophylline is undetectable in blood testing despite her stating she had taken her morning dose.*
- *GP prescription records are accessed and show she has filled prescriptions for only two fluticasone/salmeterol accuhalers in the previous 18 months but fills prescriptions for two salbutamol cannisters a month. The hospital to which she has been admitted five times confirms they have not dispensed any fluticasone/salmeterol.*
- *She is unable to locate her fluticasone/salmeterol during a nurse-led home visit.*

The conclusion was that poor adherence was a major contributory factor, and she was given a Smartinhaler® to electronically monitor activation of the device. At the start of monitoring, her first second forced expired volume (FEV_1) was 76% predicted, and her fractional exhaled nitric oxide (FeNO) was elevated at 113 ppb. She achieves 89% adherence during three months' monitoring, her FEV_1 rose to 109%, and her FeNO normalized at 18 ppb. She had no asthma attacks, and she rarely used her salbutamol. The team is now able to simplify her medication regime, including reduction in her daily inhaled corticosteroid dose in support of her ongoing efforts to adhere.

14.1 DEFINITION AND INTRODUCTION TO THE PROBLEM

According to the World Health Organization (WHO), adherence is defined as "the extent to which a person's behaviour-taking medication, following a diet, and/or executing lifestyle changes corresponds with agreed recommendations from a healthcare provider" [5]. Agreed in this context means "agreed between the patient and the physician." However, in all sorts of contexts, people "agree" for many reasons, often to terminate a conversation! It may be difficult to be sure whether the patient really agrees and that that agreement stands the test of time. The term "recommendations" is also contentious. If the recommendation is solidly evidence-based, such as treatment of a patient with fully sensitive tuberculosis where the outcome is predictable, failure to adhere is illogical. However, if my recommendations as a healthcare professional are opinion and not evidence-based, is the imperative to adhere the same?

There are three components of adherence [6]: (1) initiation of therapy (primary adherence, was the prescription ever filled?), (2) implementation of therapy (did the patient use the treatment as recommended?), and (3) persistence with the regime. Primary nonadherence has been less studied and presumably indicates that any agreement between physician and patient was spurious. In one study of nearly 200,000 e-prescriptions in several conditions across the developmental spectrum, less than 80% were ever filled; this figure was 72% for new medications. Primary adherence rates were higher (87%) for primary care and for children and adolescents 18 years and younger. Nonadherence was most common for newly prescribed medications treating chronic conditions.

Children referred to tertiary care for assessment for biologic therapy for severe asthma most frequently have suboptimal basic management [7], and if this can be optimized, asthma outcomes have been demonstrated to improve [8]. The commonest reason why asthma outcomes are poor is low adherence to prescribed medications. In a seminal study [9], 80 of 292 (27%) severe asthmatics who were being considered for a randomized controlled trial of azithromycin as an add-on therapy were nonadherent

DOI: 10.1201/9781003287209-18

and were not recruited. Poor adherence is the major contributory factor to poor asthma outcomes, including severe attacks and death [10–14].

14.2 IS ADHERENCE EVEN POSSIBLE?

The acronym KISS stands for "Keep It Simple, Silly," and adherence may be impossible if the regime is too complex (discussed in more detail later in the chapter) or the patient is provided with a medication delivery device that is hard to use. Thus the first step is an assessment of how the child uses the device. Regardless of what any theoretical laboratory constructs may suggest, the optimal device for young persons is the one they can and will use. The importance of checking technique is often overlooked not merely clinically but also in research studies [15].

14.3 PARADOXICAL NONADHERENCE: TAKING TOO MUCH TREATMENT

Most adherence interventions aim to increase the amount of medication that the patient uses. There is increasing interest in the use of biomarkers to titrate treatment. This specifically may lead to a proposed dose reduction, but, interestingly, patients and families may be reluctant to do this and, seemingly paradoxically, continue to take more treatment than they need [16, 17]. The reasons are not well explored but may include a reluctance to change what appears to be a winning formula and the fact that physicians have in the past stressed the importance of absolutely regular, twice daily therapy. The result is adherence leading to overtreatment.

14.4 RATIONAL NONADHERENCE

If the prescribed treatment is not working because the actual diagnosis is an endobronchial foreign body, then not taking treatment is rational and wrong diagnosis of paediatric asthma is all too common [18, 19]. Also, respiratory symptoms in a known asthma patient may not be due to asthma. For example, exercise-induced dyspnea may be due to deconditioning (very commonly) or a breathing pattern disorder including exercise-induced laryngeal obstruction [20, 21], neither of which responds to escalating asthma therapy. These possibilities should always be considered before trying to improve adherence. Likewise, the child has poor adherence, but good asthma control is probably being prescribed too high a level of medication, and reducing the dose may be rational. Therefore, there is an important caveat to studies that provide figures such as "at least 80% adherence is needed for benefit from inhaled corticosteroids (ICS)" [11, 22] because this is predicated on the assumption that the dose is appropriate for the young person.

Conversely, if the child is persistently documented as being nonadherent (below) and has poor asthma outcomes, the next step is to see whether outcomes improve with directly observed therapy. If they do not, then either the diagnosis is wrong or the child has genuine severe, therapy-resistant asthma, and deployment of biologicals (omalizumab, mepolizumab, dupilumab) may be appropriate.

Physicians need also to acknowledge that we have sometimes in the past insisted on adherence to an unnecessarily rigorous regime. Early asthma guidelines propagated the mantra that asthma is a disease of airway inflammation and that it was essential to use ICS every day irrespective of symptoms to suppress this underlying inflammation or airway scarring (remodelling). It is now clear that for many with mild, intermittent asthma, outcomes are at least as good with less use of medication using inhaled corticosteroids only intermittently [23]. This is another example of rational nonadherence! Of course, this is not true for those with more severe asthma, and, at least in adults, there is evidence that uncontrolled Type 2 inflammation is a marker of future risk of an asthma exacerbation [24]. However, the wrong advice given (in good faith) to asthma patients previously and criticism for not following it should induce a degree of humility into ongoing discussions regarding adherence!

Another variant of "rational" nonadherence may be hidden gain. Uncontrolled asthma may be used by the child as an excuse to avoid disagreeable activities such as cross-country running on a cold winter day. The family may benefit from financial support such as (in the UK) a disability living allowance because the child has "bad asthma." These sorts of motives may mean that there is no incentive to improve adherence and outcomes, which may be particularly difficult to address [25]. Potential strategies are discussed in Section 14.10.

14.5 METHODS OF ASSESSING ADHERENCE

These are summarized in Table 14.1.

In order to show that adherence issues are contributing to poor asthma outcomes, it is necessary to demonstrate that (1) adherence as well as asthma outcomes are poor at baseline and (2) improved adherence leads to better outcomes. Assessment of outcomes can be in several domains. Although spirometry may improve, it is generally a less important asthma outcome measure in children than in adults. Relevant outcomes to patients include asthma attacks, short-acting bronchodilator therapy use, and quality of life. Generally, asking the family about adherence is always done but generally not helpful. However, GINA guidelines have provided a useful framework that may increase success by using a nonjudgemental approach [26]. Questions we have found useful are shown in the text box "Non-Threatening Questions That May Be Useful When Discussing Adherence." I also stress that only two types of people come to my clinic: those who swear they never miss a dose of their inhaler but are not being truthful and those who are honestly taking their medication about the failings that we all share.

TABLE 14.1
Methods of Assessing Adherence

Adherence Tool	Comment	Baseline or Response (see text)
Asking the child and family	Nonjudgemental questions assuming that nonadherence is normal may help, but this is generally unreliable.	Baseline adherence and at follow-up, whether adherence has improved, dubious clinical utility
Questionnaires	These seem to work better in a research context. In our hands have never been useful in the clinic; children and families tell us what they think we want to hear.	Baseline adherence and at follow-up, whether adherence has improved, dubious clinical utility
Prescription records	Picking up a prescription does not mean the medication has been utilized, but failure to access a prescription means the medication cannot be being used. May need to access several sources, e.g. primary care, urgent care facility.	Baseline adherence and also risk if there is a combination of poor uptake of inhaled corticosteroids and accessing three or more short-acting β2-agonist cannisters. One caveat is that, since in the UK asthma medications are free for children but there is a prescription charge for adults, some carers with asthma may access their own reliever therapy on their child's prescription. Can be used as a surrogate of response to improved adherence.
Home visit (face-to-face or virtual)	If the medication cannot be located or is out of date, good adherence is very unlikely. Also, medications are sometimes also found stockpiled and/or never removed from their original boxes, again pointing to nonadherence.	Baseline adherence
Monitoring of medication blood levels	Applicable in clinical practice if the child is prescribed daily theophylline or prednisolone and has taken the morning dose. Neither medication is commonly used for maintenance therapy. Blood levels of inhaled medications are a research tool only. A high plasma cortisol in a child prescribed maintenance oral steroids is strongly suggestive of poor adherence.	Baseline adherence, can be repeated to demonstrate response to improved adherence.
Electronic activation monitor, e.g. Smartinhaler®	Can only say if and when the device has been activated, not whether used correctly. Can be combined with automated alerts to take medication and/or feedback as to adherence.	Baseline adherence and response to improved adherence
Electronic devices with inspiratory flow sensor	Not yet widely available, and usually measures only peak inspiratory flow, not inspired volume. Can be combined with automatic feedback as to adherence. Can be combined with automated alerts to take medication.	Baseline adherence and response to improved adherence
Response to directly observed therapy by mobile phone	Very labour-intensive	Response to improved adherence
Directly observed therapy at school	Does not work if child does not go to school. School must engage in close observation. Cannot be done on weekends or on school holidays.	Response to improved adherence
Response to admission for directly observed therapy	Resource-intensive	Response to improved adherence
Response to a single dose of intramuscular triamcinolone	Guarantees adherence and determines whether the child is steroid-sensitive; response highly suggestive of previous poor adherence.	Response to improved adherence
Breathomics: Volatile organic compounds	Futuristic and only in the research domain currently.	Potentially could be used to determine baseline adherence and response to improved adherence

EXAMPLES OF NON-THREATENING QUESTIONS THAT MAY BE USEFUL WHEN DISCUSSING ADHERENCE

These questions can be adapted for the parents of younger children to determine also whether the child is supervised when taking medication:

- Do you know who are the worst people for remembering to take medications? A clue is that there is one in the room and it's not you. (Answer: Doctors. If a doctor tells you they have finished a course of antibiotics, they are often not telling the truth.)
- A lot of people find it is difficult to remember inhalers in the morning in the rush to get to school on time. Is this a time that is difficult for you as well?
- People like you work a lot harder at school than I ever did, and you must get a ton of homework to do. Does all that stuff mean it is difficult to remember your evening inhaler dose?
- Weekends are a time when there is less routine compared to during the week, and many people find they forget medications on the weekend because of the lack of routine. Do you think you may also have this problem?

Sometimes poor adherence comes as a genuine surprise to the families, who believe they have been supervising their child's use of inhaler medications. However, in sensitive and skilled discussions with a respiratory nurse, they come to realize that they have not actually witnessed a child (especially a younger child) taking the medication but have merely asked if it has been taken as they leave the house to go to school. Once identified, that problem is often readily rectified.

Exhaled nitric oxide (FeNO) is a marker of airway type 2 inflammation, especially interleukin-(IL)4 and IL-13 driven [27]. This has been suggested to be an objective marker of adherence [28]; however, interpretation needs to be cautious. A raised FeNO is a pointer to the diagnosis of asthma but is also seen in atopic children with no airway disease [29]. Some children continue with a raised FeNO despite adherence being assured by using intramuscular triamcinolone, so a raised FeNO may not necessarily be due to poor adherence [30]. However, if the FeNO is high in a child with poorly controlled asthma and falls during any form of directly observed therapy (FeNO suppression test), then this is suggestive of previous poor adherence [31].

Increasingly, electronic monitoring devices are being used clinically, and many are currently available or in development [32]. A device is attached to the inhaler, which records the timing of any activation; this precludes deception by dose dumping (activating multiple times while awaiting a consultation). Furthermore, adherence is capped at 100% morning and evening after the prescribed number of activations. Some devices are Bluetooth-enabled and can be linked to an app. These devices are currently considered the gold standard, and although they are much more useful than merely asking questions, they are not without problems. In our clinic, up to 30% of monitors are lost, a considerable financial outlay, and the suspicion is always that a lost device is a ruse to prevent detection of poor adherence. Popular reasons for poor recorded adherence include temporary loss of the device, or it was left behind during time away, or the device was not working, which is the only excuse that can be verified. A recent study using electronic monitoring demonstrated four patterns of adherence and outcomes (Table 14.2). Notably, even though the children knew they were being monitored, more than half were

TABLE 14.2
Findings During Electronic Inhaler Monitoring and Their Interpretation

Findings	Interpretation
Adherence good, ACT & FEV_1 improve, FeNO falls	Previously poorly adherent, becomes adherent during monitoring, and medications work when taken
Adherence poor, no improvement in asthma outcomes	Differential is wrong diagnosis, refractory nonadherence or STRA tired of taking medications which do not work Determine what happens with DOT
Adherence good, continued poor asthma control or recurrent asthma attacks	Either true STRA, or inhaler being activated but used incorrectly, check technique and see what happens with DOT ensuring correct inhaler technique
Adherence poor, but asthma outcomes good	Likely overtreated, rational poor adherence Reduce prescribed medications

Abbreviations: ACT, Asthma Control Test; DOT, directly observed therapy; FeNO, fractional exhaled nitric oxide; FEV_1, first second forced expired volume; STRA, severe therapy resistant asthma nonadherent [33]. Patients have expressed concerns about data security and feeling "big brother is watching you" [32]. Despite all these caveats, these devices are the current best option in clinical practice. Monitoring is usually for three months, and we have shown that the benefits of increased adherence during this period are maintained over a subsequent three-month period [34].

Electronic monitoring devices have been taken to the next level by monitoring inhalation as well as activation. Unsurprisingly, these have shown that merely measuring activation over-estimates adherence [35]. However, there are two components of effective inhalation—peak inspiratory flow and total inspired volume—and both need to be correct if the medication is to be maximally useful. Merely measuring an adequate peak inspiratory flow, although a big step forward from solely measuring activation, is still not a guarantee of adequate use.

Measurement of medication levels is a potentially attractive marker of adherence, but in clinical practice is applicable only for children prescribed theophylline or maintenance prednisolone (both now hardly ever the case). Levels need to be measured within six hours of taking prednisolone, within two hours of standard theophylline, and within 12 hours of a slow-release preparation [36]. If the child is prescribed alternate-day glucocorticoids, measuring levels on the off day for dosing is not useful. Two surrogates for adherence to regular oral prednisolone are serum cortisol and the short synacthen test. Serum cortisol should be low, and the synacthen test abnormal, if the child has been consistently taking prednisolone. However, it must be said that, with the increased use of the asthma biologic, treatment of a child with long-term oral glucocorticoids is rarely deployed. Measurement of blood levels of ICS is still a research tool only [37, 38].

Finally, for research purposes only, the use of exhaled breath may be useful to quantify adherence [39]. Exhaled breath contains thousands of compounds, which in this study were analysed by gas chromatography coupled with time-of-flight mass spectrometry. The investigators showed some correlation between urinary levels of salbutamol and oral corticosteroids and profiles of exhaled breath analytes. The strengths of the study included the use of discovery and validation cohorts. For this technique to be practical in the future, the discrimination will need to be improved, and a rapid turnaround of results ensured. Although this is a long way from reality, in the future a breath test may be useful for delineating adherence, in addition to identifying specific asthma phenotypes and potentially endotypes [40].

14.6 UNDERSTANDING THE REASONS FOR POOR ADHERENCE

The perceptions and practicalities (PAPA) framework [41] is conceptually useful. Perceptions may lead to a deliberate, active decision not to take medication. These include a lack of understanding of the correct usage; the failure to understand that the lack of immediate and obvious benefit from inhaled corticosteroids does not mean that they are unhelpful in controlling asthma and concerns regarding side effects. There may also be a false perception that if there are no symptoms of asthma, then treatment is not needed. Practical considerations include forgetfulness, which may be compounded by a hectic and chaotic lifestyle, and difficulty in making time for supervision of medication inhalation. The complexity of the regime, including the devices for inhalation, may be another barrier. Finally, children do not like to be seen as being different or may be teased for being a "druggie" if they take medication in front of their friends.

14.7 HOW CAN POOR ADHERENCE BE IMPROVED: IMPLEMENTING CHANGE?

A general point about adherence interventions is that many studies are predicated on the assumption that improving adherence is an end in itself, not a means to the end of improving disease outcomes. Indeed, if a study demonstrates improved adherence but no change in clinical outcomes, it calls into question whether the study patients needed to improve adherence or whether the findings of poor outcomes are truly related to poor adherence. Therefore, it is important to review adherence studies through this critical lens.

Most important is for all concerned to understand that the issue of adherence should not be discussed in a blame culture or finger-pointing way but as an effort by everyone to work together to improve adherence and hence asthma outcomes. Perceptions and practicalities are not mutually exclusive, as both may be present and the contribution of each may vary over time, especially during the teenage years [42]. A qualitative study in teenagers who had undergone a period of electronic monitoring identified a number of key themes relating to perceptions and motivations. These included poor understanding of the nature of asthma and the reasons for treatment with ICS; worries about side effects and over-reliance on inhalers; the societal impact including social stigma among peers; the trivialization of asthma; and the poor understanding of those who do not have asthma. Practical barriers identified included the importance of routine; the effect of family (parental reminders, ordering repeat prescriptions); and forgetfulness [43]. The importance of routine is underscored by the fact that, counter-intuitively, adherence is often worse on weekends despite the fact there are generally fewer time pressures.

Clearly both perceptions and practicalities need an individual approach; if a child is convinced that ICS are unnecessary or harmful, simplifying the regime is unlikely to increase adherence. Adherence interventions should likely target both perceptions and practicalities to give the best chance of success. Perceptions need to be understood from an open discussion and addressed with asthma educational input. Ignoring the important issue of patient beliefs will surely reduce the chances of success. If practicalities are identified, these also need an individualized approach. Some young people find that setting up alerts on their phone is helpful in improving adherence. Simplification of the regime may involve using a combination inhaler that is needed only once a day, for example a combination of fluticasone furoate and vilanterol. Another strategy is to use a single inhaler for maintenance and relief (SMART regime), in which a combined budesonide and formoterol inhaler (usually the 100/6 strength, occasionally 200/6 for more severe disease) is used once or twice daily regularly and also as reliever therapy. This approach is supported by multiple studies in young people aged 12 years and over [44] and a single study in 6- to 11-year-olds [45]. This avoids the very dangerous situation of a child not using ICS while using short-acting β2-agonists to control symptoms and attacks.

Another area of complexity is the choice of the medication delivery device. It is relatively easy for a skilled nurse to teach good technique in the clinic. However, transferring this skill to real life outside is more challenging [34, 46]; it can take any weeks of directly observed therapy by video link before the correct technique is achieved. The optimal device is the one the child can use and is prepared to use. We advocate for spacers especially when using high-dose ICS, but some young people think these are "babyish" and just use the metered dose inhaler directly into the mouth. In such cases, whatever the theoretical advantages of spacers, a dry powder device should be prescribed.

A Cochrane review [47], which combined studies in adults and children (40 studies, 1527 participants), reported on digital interventions to improve adherence to maintenance asthma medications. In most, the primary end-point was improved adherence, but not improved outcomes, although these were frequently reported as secondary outcomes. Most effective were electronic monitoring devices and short text messages. Digital interventions may result in a large increase in adherence (electronic monitoring devices 23% over control, seven studies), and with short messages 12% over control, four studies) (low-certainty evidence). There was moderate-certainty evidence that digital adherence interventions may result in clinically significant improvements in asthma control and also improve quality of life, but there was no clinically significant improvement in lung function. There was little evidence of a reduction in asthma attacks. It was thought that there was some evidence that in-person components and feedback on adherence may improve asthma control and adherence, respectively.

A recent systematic review and meta-analysis [48] of adherence interventions identified 240 possibly relevant studies, of which only 25 were eligible for inclusion and only 13 were categorized as being highly reliable. Nine of 13 interventions increased adherence, of which six used a PAPA intervention. The techniques utilized targeting in successful interventions included rewards, reminders, feedback and monitoring of adherence, pharmacological support, education on how to take medication, and knowledge about symptom triggers. Behaviour-changing techniques were also used in effective interventions. Ideally, any intervention will have effects lasting long after the end of the intervention. Certainly, in clinical practice, checking and supporting adherence is an ongoing issue, not a one-off at the initial consultation. Effective interventions can be delivered by a range of professionals, including pharmacists, nurses, specialist physicians, community health workers [49], and researchers, any of whom are commonly underutilized in asthma care.

The review documented a number of potential behaviour-changing techniques:

- **Reward and Threat:** Financial rewards will be discussed in more detail, but threats, in my experience, do not work; young persons have to work out for themselves that taking the medication leads to, e.g. better sports results, but in my experience, they will not believe threats of what may or may not happen if treatment is not taken. (When you are a teenager, you know you are impregnable and immortal!)
- **Prompts and Cues:** For example, mobile phone alerts.
- **Feedback and Monitoring:** If adherence data are fed back to the young person, this may motivate improved adherence.
- **Pharmacological Support:** Free treatment may be provided, but that is not relevant in all healthcare systems.
- **Instruction and Teaching:** For example, on correct inhaler use.
- **Education About the Nature of Asthma:** For example, that the risk may be high even in the absence of current symptoms.

Another meta-analysis [50] reported on 33 studies with diverse interventions including asthma education, written asthma plans, electronic monitoring, text messages, lung function monitoring reports, and parental support groups. There was an initial small but significant initial benefit with a number of different interventions, but this was not sustained at follow-up. Again, the focus was improving adherence, not improving outcomes.

Financial incentives to change behaviour are increasingly being used in a number of healthcare contexts, including promoting better health behaviours such as vaccination uptake, physical activity, and smoking cessation including reducing passive exposure in children [51], with varying degrees of success [49]. Most studies are in adults, but there are increasing numbers of studies in children, for example the prevention of repeat adolescent pregnancies and improved healthy eating for schoolchildren. Importantly, a non-randomized study in children with diabetes showed that financial incentives led to sustained behaviour change post-intervention, supported by better clinical outcomes [52]. A UK pilot feasibility study in which financial incentives were provided to adolescents with both poor adherence and asthma control reported some improvements in adherence to ICS; any change in clinical outcomes could not be assessed due to lack of power [42]. However, the use of financial incentives in this context was found to be feasible and acceptable. More evidence is needed, and the use of financial inducements to improve outcomes in paediatric asthma cannot yet be recommended in clinical practice, but they do seem to have the potential to form a habit of adherence which persists long term. One study showed that submitting adherence metrics to a cluster analysis unsurprisingly showed poor adherence was associated with decline in symptom control, indicating that adherence habits can persist over time [34]. Whether adherence habits could be changed and the change sustained over time was not studied. Nonetheless, attempting behavioural change seems worth trying. Of course, there are those who feel it is unethical to reward bad behaviour (i.e. poor adherence) The author's personal viewpoint is that unethical behaviour of providing financial incentive for improved adherence outweighs the significant morbidity and potential mortality associated with poor adherence.

In summary, it is likely that a bespoke treatment approach is needed for each individual, depending on the mix of perceptions and practicalities that are important. The specific perceptions that hinder adherence need to be identified, understood by the asthma team, addressed by an education programme, and the practical barriers identified and removed as much as possible.

14.8 SUSTAINING CHANGE: CAN IMPROVED ADHERENCE BE MAINTAINED?

As with all aspects of asthma care, achieving a good position and maintaining it are two very different challenges. Adherence is notoriously difficult to sustain. The STAAR trial randomized children to electronic monitoring with feedback regarding ICS use or electronic monitoring only [53]. Adherence in the intervention group was 70% versus 49% in the control group, despite them knowing they were being monitored. The intervention group had fewer admissions and corticosteroid bursts but no change in quality of life.

14.9 ARE THERE ADHERENCE PHENOTYPES, AND DO THEY HELP US CLINICALLY?

A phenotype is defined as "the set of observable characteristics of an individual resulting from the interaction of its genotype with the environment," and it is arguable whether this is a useful term in adherence studies as the term "patterns" may be more appropriate. As before, one must be aware that patterns may change over time. One useful division of patterns combines use and techniques, namely regular use, good technique; regular use, frequent critical technique errors; irregular use, good technique; and irregular use, frequent critical errors [54]. Unsurprisingly, in a chronic obstructive pulmonary disease (COPD) study, the last group did worst.

14.10 REFRACTORY DIFFICULT ASTHMA: WHAT IF ADHERENCE CANNOT BE IMPROVED?

A proportion of paediatric patients continue to be nonadherent even despite intensive interventions, a category we have described elsewhere as refractory difficult asthma despite ruling out or treating comorbid illnesses in conjunction with asthma [2]. Whereas it is the right of any mentally competent adult to refuse treatment, it is unethical to permit an under-age young person to be exposed to the risk of death because they are not receiving treatment. The child safeguarding team may need to be involved, and indeed safeguarding is an important factor with many children when asthma is apparently not responding to treatment.

Directly observed therapy is one option, most usually at school; once-daily therapy is best if the child is eligible. This means only five days of treatment per week at best and assumes the child will actually attend school. It is essential to precede this with a thorough detailed discussion with the school nurse or teacher. One young person told us that she went as planned to the school nurse's room, but when she took the inhaler, the nurse actually had her back turned to her because she was filling in forms on her computer and did not actually observe anything at all! There is also the problem of what to do on school holidays. Observation of therapy by video link using mobile phones is another but more labour-intensive strategy [45].

Finally, we have argued that the use of a biological (e.g. the anti-IgE monoclonal omalizumab, the anti-IL5 mepolizumab, or the anti-IL4/13 dupilumab) that has to be given by injection is justified in those children with refractory nonadherence [55]. Licencing states that these high-cost agents should be reserved for those who have poor asthma outcomes despite good adherence, but these agents can prevent harm in those young people who are unable or unwilling to use conventional medications, and they should not be withheld. We believe it is the parent's responsibility to ensure under-age children receive treatment, and it is unethical to withhold potentially life-saving treatment because of abrogation of parental responsibility by adults. Receiving an injectable medication removes the issue of adherence as a cause of poor outcomes and provides the added benefit for the child to be regularly assessed by the asthma team. Prior to the advent of biologicals, depot intramuscular triamcinolone could be given monthly to ensure adherence was not an issue, but the side effect profile of this therapy is much less favourable than biologicals and is now seldom used as a long-term treatment strategy.

14.11 SUMMARY AND CONCLUSIONS: ADHERENCE AND OUTCOMES

Unquestionably, adherence to asthma medications is difficult for many young people and a very common cause of poor asthma outcomes. A systematic approach is recommended. Firstly, it is important to be sure that the reported symptoms are due to asthma and not another glucocorticoid-resistant condition, because in this latter case, nonadherence is rational. In the young person with genuinely poor asthma outcomes, the wrong approach is to continue to escalate therapy without asking why response is poor. One of the commonest reasons is that appropriate medications are not being taken. Part of this is to remember that children with asthma may apparently have asthma-related symptoms that are in fact due to another underlying cause, for example breathlessness due to deconditioning. There is a suite of techniques for assessing adherence, most of which are imperfect. The least useful is asking the young person and family about whether medications are being used. Barriers to adherence include perceptions (e.g. "I do not need this treatment") and practicalities (e.g. "the regime is so complex I cannot master it"). If the barriers can be identified, a bespoke programme to support adherence may improve the situation. If this fails, then directly observed therapy or the use of an injectable biological if the young person is eligible is recommended to reduce the risk of a severe asthma attack and death. There are still many unmet needs and gaps in knowledge that require investigation to better understand and ameliorate poor adherence in young people with asthma.

REFERENCES

1. Lødrup Carlsen KC, Hedlin G, Bush A, et al; on behalf of the PSACI (Problematic Severe Asthma in Childhood Initiative) group. Assessment of problematic severe asthma in children. *Eur Respir J*. 2011; 37: 432–440.
2. Cook J, Beresford F, Fainardi V, Hall P, Housley G, Jamalzadeh A, Nightingale M, Winch D, Bush A, Fleming L, Saglani S. Managing the paediatric patient with refractory asthma: a multidisciplinary approach. *J Asthma Allergy*. 2017; 10: 123–130.
3. Bush A, Fleming L, Saglani S. Severe asthma in children. *Respirology*. 2017; 22: 886–897
4. Chan AHY, Horne R, Hankins M, Chisari C. The Medication Adherence Report Scale: A measurement tool for eliciting patients' reports of nonadherence. *Br J Clin Pharmacol*. 2020: 86: 1281–1288.
5. http://apps.who.int/iris/bitstream/handle/10665/42682/9241545992.pdf;jsessionid=7D6AFC0CCEE5F8DCA7BF46B959D9D3A4?sequence=1
6. Fischer MA, Stedman MR, Lii J, Vogeli C, Shrank WH, Brookhart MA, Weissman JS. Primary medication non-adherence: analysis of 195,930 electronic prescriptions. *J Gen Intern Med*. 2010; 25: 284–290.
7. Bracken MB, Fleming L, Hall P, Van Stiphout N, Bossley CJ, Biggart E, Wilson NM, Bush A. The importance of nurse led home visits in the assessment of children with problematic asthma. *Arch Dis Child*. 2009; 94: 780–784.
8. Sharples J, Gupta A, Fleming L, Bossley CJ, Bracken-King M, Hall P, Hayward A, Puckey M, Balfour-Lynn IM, Rosenthal M, Bush A, Saglani S. Long-term effectiveness of a staged assessment for paediatric problematic severe asthma [Research Letter]. Eur Respir J. 2012; 40: 264–267.
9. Strunk RC, Bacharier LB, Phillips BR, Szefler SJ, Zeiger RS, Chinchilli VM, Martinez FD, Lemanske RF Jr, Taussig LM, Mauger DT, Morgan WJ, Sorkness CA, Paul IM, Guilbert T, Krawiec M, Covar R, Larsen G; CARE Network. Azithromycin or montelukast as inhaled corticosteroid-sparing agents in moderate-to-severe childhood asthma study. *J Allergy Clin Immunol*. 2008; 122: 1138–1144.
10. Williams LK, Peterson EL, Wells K, Ahmedani BK, Kumar R, Burchard EG, Chowdhry VK, Favro D, Lanfear DE, Pladevall M. Quantifying the proportion of severe asthma exacerbations attributable to inhaled corticosteroid nonadherence. *J Allergy Clin Immunol*. 2011; 128: 1185–1191.
11. Engelkes M, Janssens HM, de Jongste JC, Sturkenboom MCJM, Verhamme KMC. Medication adherence and the risk of severe asthma exacerbations: A systematic review. *Eur Respir J*. 2015; 45: 396–407.
12. Szefler SJ, Chmiel JF, Fitzpatrick AM, Giacoia G, Green TP, Jackson DJ, Nielsen HC, Phipatanakul W, Raissy HH. Asthma across the ages: Knowledge gaps in childhood asthma. *J Allergy Clin Immunol*. 2014; 133: 3–13.
13. Szefler SJ, Chipps B. Challenges in the treatment of asthma in children and adolescents. *Ann Allergy Asthma Immunol*. 2018; 120: 382–388.
14. Melani AS, Bonavia M, Cilenti V, Cinti C, Lodi M, Martucci P, Serra M, Scichilone N, Sestini P, Aliani M, Neri M; Gruppo Educazionale Associazione Italiana Pneumologi Ospedalieri. Inhaler mishandling remains common in real life and is associated with reduced disease control. *Respir Med*. 2011; 105: 930–938.
15. Dekhuijzen PNR, Levy ML, Corrigan CJ, Hadfield RM, Roche N, Usmani OS, Barnes PJ, Scullion JE, Lavorini F, Corbetta L, Kocks JWH, Cosio BG, Buhl R, Pedersen SE; ADMIT Working Group. Is inhaler technique adequately assessed and reported in clinical trials of asthma and chronic obstructive pulmonary disease therapy? A systematic review and suggested best practice checklist. *J Allergy Clin Immunol Pract*. 2022; 10: 1813–1824.
16. Heaney LG, Busby J, Hanratty CE, et al; investigators for the MRC Refractory Asthma Stratification Programme. Composite type-2 biomarker strategy versus a symptom-risk-based algorithm to adjust corticosteroid dose in patients with severe asthma: A multicentre, single-blind, parallel group, randomised controlled trial. *Lancet Respir Med*. 2021; 9: 57–68.
17. Saglani S, Bingham Y, Balfour-Lynn I, Goldring S, Gupta A, Banya W, Moreiras J, Fleming L, Bush A, Rosenthal M. Blood eosinophils in managing preschool wheeze: Lessons learnt from a proof-of-concept trial. *Pediatr Allergy Immunol*. 2022; 33: e13697.
18. Looijmans-van den Akker I, van Luijn K, Verheij T. Overdiagnosis of asthma in children in primary care: a retrospective analysis. *Br J Gen Pract*. 2016; 66: e152–e157. https://doi.org/10.3399/bjgp16X683965.
19. Yang, CL, Simons E, Foty RG, Subbarao P, To T, Dell SD. Misdiagnosis of asthma in schoolchildren. *Pediatr Pulmonol*. 2017; 52: 293–302.
20. Halvorsen T, Halvorsen T, Walsted ES, Bucca C, Bush A, Cantarella G, Friedrich G, Herth FJF, Hull JH, Jung H, Maat R, Nordang L, Remacle M, Rasmussen N, Wilson JA, Heimdal JH. Inducible laryngeal obstruction: an official joint European Respiratory Society and European Laryngological Society statement. *Eur Respir J*. 2017; 50: 1602221.
21. Johansson H, Norlander K, Berglund L, et al. Prevalence of exercise-induced bronchoconstriction and exercise-induced laryngeal obstruction in a general adolescent population. *Thorax*. 2015; 70: 57–63.

22. Williams LK, Peterson EL, Wells K, Ahmedani BK, Kumar R, Burchard EG, Chowdhry VK, Favro D, Lanfear DE, Pladevall M. Quantifying the proportion of severe asthma exacerbations attributable to inhaled corticosteroid nonadherence. *J Allergy Clin Immunol.* 2011; 128: 1185–1191.
23. Hatter L, Bruce P, Braithwaite I, Holliday M, Fingleton J, Weatherall M, Beasley R. ICS-formoterol reliever *versus* ICS and short-acting β_2-agonist reliever in asthma: A systematic review and meta-analysis. *ERJ Open Res.* 2021; 7: 00701–2020.
24. Couillard S, Laugerud A, Jabeen M, Ramakrishnan S, Melhorn J, Hinks T, Pavord I. Derivation of a prototype asthma attack risk scale centred on blood eosinophils and exhaled nitric oxide. *Thorax.* 2022; 77: 199–202.
25. Nagakumar P, Gambir N, Sanghani N, Hall P, Jamalzadeh A, Beresford F, Saglani S, Bush A, Fleming L. Role of a prolonged inpatient admission when evaluating children with problematic severe asthma. *Eur Respir J.* 2018; 51:1701061.
26. www.ginasthma.org
27. Escamilla-Gil JM, Fernandez-Nieto M, Acevedo N. Understanding the cellular sources of the fractional exhaled nitric oxide (FeNO) and its role as a biomarker of type 2 inflammation in asthma. *Biomed Res Int.* 2022; 2022: 5753524.
28. Loewenthal L, Menzies-Gow A. FeNO in Asthma. *Semin Respir Crit Care Med.* 2022; 43: 635–645.
29. Hoffmeyer F, Beine A, Lehnert M, Berresheim H, Taeger D, van Kampen V, Sander I, Zahradnik E, Brüning T, Raulf M. The Pattern of Sensitization Influences Exhaled and Nasal Nitric Oxide Levels in Young Adults. *Adv Exp Med Biol.* 2020; 1279: 15–26.
30. Payne DNR, Wilson NM, James A, Hablas H, Agrafioti C, Bush A. Evidence for different subgroups of difficult asthma in children. *Thorax* 2001; 56: 345–350.
31. Alahmadi F, Peel A, Keevil B, Niven R, Fowler SJ. Assessment of adherence to corticosteroids in asthma by drug monitoring or fractional exhaled nitric oxide: A literature review. *Clin Exp Allergy.* 2021; 51: 49–62.
32. Chrystyn H, Audibert R, Keller M, Quaglia B, Vecellio L, Roche N. Real-life inhaler adherence and technique: Time to get smarter! *Respir Med.* 2019; 158: 24–32.
33. Jochmann A, Artusio L, Jamalzadeh A, Nagakumar P, Delgado-Eckert E, Saglani S, Bush A, Frey U, Fleming L. Electronic monitoring of adherence to inhaled corticosteroids: An essential tool in identifying severe asthma in children. *Eur Respir J.* 2017; 50: 1700910.
34. Jochmann A, Artusio L, Jamalzadeh A, et al. Electronic monitoring of adherence to inhaled corticosteroids: An essential tool in identifying severe asthma in children. *Eur Respir J.* 2017; 50: 1700910.
35. Sulaiman I, Seheult, MacHale E, et al. A method to calculate adherence to inhaled therapy that reflects the changes in clinical features of asthma. *Ann Am Thorac Soc.* 2016; 13: 1894–1903.
36. Robinson DS, Campbell DA, Durham SR, Pfeffer J, Barnes PJ, Chung KF; Asthma and Allergy Research Group of the National Heart and Lung Institute. Systematic assessment of difficult-to-treat asthma. *Eur Respir J.* 2003; 22: 478–483.
37. George KE, Ryan DM, Keevil B, Niven R, Fowler SJ. A pilot study to investigate the use of serum inhaled corticosteroid concentration as a potential marker of treatment adherence in severe asthma. *J Allergy Clin Immunol.* 2017; 139: 1037–1039.
38. Alahmadi FH, Simpson AJ, Gomez C, Ericsson M, Thörngren JO, Wheelock CE, Shaw DE, Fleming LJ, Roberts G, Riley J, Bates S, Sousa AR, Knowles R, Bansal AT, Corfield J, Pandis I, Sun K, Bakke PS, Caruso M, Chanez P, Dahlén B, Horvath I, Krug N, Montuschi P, Singer F, Wagers S, Adcock IM, Djukanovic R, Chung KF, Sterk PJ, Dahlen SE, Fowler SJ; U-BIOPRED Study Group. Medication Adherence in Patients With Severe Asthma Prescribed Oral Corticosteroids in the U-BIOPRED Cohort. *Chest.* 2021; 160: 53–64.
39. Brinkman P, Ahmed WM, Gómez C, Knobel HH, Weda H, Vink TJ, Nijsen TM, Wheelock CE, Dahlen SE, Montuschi P, Knowles RG, Vijverberg SJ, Maitland-van der Zee AH, Sterk PJ, Fowler SJ; U-BIOPRED Study Group. Exhaled volatile organic compounds as markers for medication use in asthma. *Eur Respir J.* 2020; 55: 1900544.
40. Ibrahim B, Basanta M, Cadden P, Singh D, Douce D, Woodcock A, Fowler SJ. Non-invasive phenotyping using exhaled volatile organic compounds in asthma. *Thorax.* 2011; 66: 804–809.
41. Horne R, Cooper V, Wileman V, Chan A. Supporting adherence to medicines for long-term conditions: A perceptions and practicalities approach based on an extended commonsense model. *European Psychologist* 2019; 24: 82–96.
42. De Simoni A, Fleming L, Holliday L, Horne R, Priebe S, Bush A, Sheikh A, Griffiths C. Electronic reminders and rewards to improve adherence to inhaled asthma treatment in adolescents: A non-randomised feasibility study in tertiary care. *BMJ Open.* 2021; 11: e053268.
43. Pearce CJ, Chan AHY, Jackson T, Fleming L, Foot H, Bush A, Horne R. Features of successful interventions to improve adherence to inhaled corticosteroids in children with asthma. *Pediatr Pulmonol.* 2022; 57: 822–847.
44. Hatter L, Bruce P, Braithwaite I, Holliday M, Fingleton J, Weatherall M, Beasley R. ICS-formoterol reliever *versus* ICS and short-acting β_2-agonist reliever in asthma: A systematic review and meta-analysis. *ERJ Open Res.* 2021; 7: 00701–2020.
45. Bisgaard H, Le Roux P, Bjåmer D, Dymek A, Vermeulen JH, Hultquist C. Budesonide/formoterol maintenance plus reliever therapy: A new strategy in pediatric asthma. *Chest.* 2006; 130: 1733–1743.
46. Shields MD, F AL, Rivey MP, McElnay JC. Mobile direct observation of therapy (MDOT)—A rapid systematic review and pilot study in children with asthma. *PLOS ONE.* 2018; 13: e0190031.
47. Chan A, De Simoni A, Wileman V, Holliday L, Newby CJ, Chisari C, Ali S, Zhu N, Padakanti P, Pinprachanan V, Ting V, Griffiths CJ. Digital interventions to improve adherence to maintenance medication in asthma. *Cochrane Database Syst Rev.* 2022; 6(6): CD013030.
48. Pearce CJ, Chan AHY, Jackson T, Fleming L, Foot H, Bush A, Horne R. Features of successful interventions to improve adherence to Inhaled Corticosteroids in children with asthma. *Pediatr Pulmonol.* 2022; 57: 822–847.
49. Fidler A, Sweenie R, Ortega A, Cushing CC, Ramsey R, Fedele D. Meta-analysis of adherence promotion interventions in pediatric asthma. *J Pediatr Psychol.* 2021; 46: 1195–1212.
50. Jassal MS, Lewis-Land C, Thompson RE, Butz A. Randomised pilot trial of cash incentives for reducing paediatric asthmatic tobacco smoke exposures from maternal caregivers and members of their social network. *Arch Dis Child.* 2021; 106: 345–354.

51. Hoskins K, Ulrich CM, Shinnick J, Buttenheim AM. Acceptability of financial incentives for health-related behavior change: An updated systematic review. *Prev Med.* 2019; 126: 105762.
52. Kenyon CC, Flaherty C, Floyd GC, Jenssen BP, Miller VA. Promoting healthy childhood behaviors with financial incentives: A narrative review of key considerations and design features for future research. *Acad Pediatr.* 2022 Mar; 22(2): 203–209.
53. Morton RW, Elphick HE, Rigby AS, Daw WJ, King DA, Smith LJ, Everard ML. STAAR: A randomised controlled trial of electronic adherence monitoring with reminder alarms and feedback to improve clinical outcomes for children with asthma. *Thorax.* 2017; 72: 347–354.
54. Cushen B, Sulaiman I, Greene G, et al. The clinical impact of different adherence behaviors in patients with severe chronic obstructive pulmonary disease. *Am J Respir Crit Care Med.* 2018; 197: 1630–1633.
55. Bush A, Saglani S, Fleming L. Severe asthma: Looking beyond the amount of medication. *Lancet Respir Med.* 2017; 5: 844–846.

15 Inhaler Devices

Federico Lavorini, Alessandra Sorano, and Mark L. Levy

CASE PRESENTATIONS

1. *Jane, a 45-year-old woman with a 10-year history of asthma, visited the clinic due to worsening symptoms, including shortness of breath, wheezing, and frequent night-time awakenings. Despite regularly using her salbutamol MDI for quick relief and Fluticasone MDI for maintenance, she saw little improvement.*

   During her visit, Jane demonstrated how she used her inhalers. It became evident that she was making several common mistakes. She wasn't shaking the inhaler before use, held it incorrectly, and failed to coordinate pressing the canister with inhaling. Additionally, she inhaled too quickly and didn't hold her breath long enough after inhaling, reducing the medication's effectiveness.

   We provided Jane with detailed instructions on the correct technique: shaking the inhaler before use, holding it correctly, starting to breathe in slowly before pressing the canister, taking a slow and deep breath, and holding her breath for 10 seconds after inhalation. Jane practiced this under supervision until she was comfortable with the new method. We also gave her written instructions and scheduled a follow-up visit.

   Two weeks later, Jane reported significant improvements. She experienced fewer night-time awakenings and used her rescue inhaler less frequently. Her technique had markedly improved, leading to better asthma control.

2. *Robert, a 65-year-old man with a 10-year history of asthma-COPD overlap syndrome, came into the clinic complaining of worsening shortness of breath, frequent exacerbations, and persistent coughing. Despite using his prescribed salbutamol MDI for quick relief and Fluticasone DPI + Tiotropium DPI for daily maintenance, his symptoms had progressively worsened over the past few months.*

   During our discussion, it became apparent that Robert was confused about the proper use of his inhalers. He admitted that he often mixed up the techniques for the MDI and DPI, using the technique of one inhaler type for the other, which likely contributed to his deteriorating condition. When he demonstrated how he used his inhalers, several mistakes stood out. For the salbutamol MDI, Robert wasn't shaking the inhaler before use, leading to inconsistent dosing. He also had poor coordination, pressing the canister too late after starting to inhale, and inhalations were too rapid rather than the recommended slow, deep breaths, causing most of the medication to deposit in his throat instead of his lungs. For both the Fluticasone and Tiotropium DPIs, Robert frequently failed to load the dose correctly and took shallow breaths instead of the forceful inhalation required to disperse the powder properly. He also tried to use the DPI like an MDI, pressing and inhaling simultaneously, which is unnecessary for DPIs.

   Recognizing these issues, we spent time demonstrating the correct techniques for both types of inhalers, also clarifying the differences between MDI and DPI usage. Robert practiced these techniques under our supervision until he felt comfortable and confident with both. We provided written instructions and scheduled a follow-up visit to reassess his technique and monitor his disease control. When Robert returned two weeks later, he reported significant improvements. He experienced fewer exacerbations and better control of his breathlessness. His inhaler technique had markedly improved, leading to better management of his symptoms.

Comment

These clinical cases highlight the critical role of proper inhaler technique in managing chronic respiratory obstructive diseases such as asthma and COPD. Both Jane and Robert experienced worsening symptoms despite using their prescribed medications, primarily due to incorrect inhaler use. Proper inhaler technique is essential for effective respiratory disease management. By focusing on patient education and simplifying inhaler regimens, healthcare providers can significantly improve treatment outcomes and patient quality of life.

DOI: 10.1201/9781003287209-19

15.1 INTRODUCTION

The incidence of asthma has significantly increased globally, doubling over the past decade.[1,2] This surge has placed a substantial economic strain on healthcare systems. To address this, asthma management guidelines have been established in almost every country.[3] These guidelines aim to control the disease with the minimum necessary medication. Asthma guidelines recommend a stepwise approach to pharmacological treatment that involves increasing medication dosage and frequency as asthma symptoms worsen ("step up") and reducing them when asthma is under control ("step down"). More recently, the Global Initiative for Asthma (GINA)[3] recommended a fundamental change to the way mild asthma is managed by using a single inhaler "as needed" for symptoms; these devices contain an inhaled corticosteroid and formoterol, a fast-acting, long-acting beta-agonist bronchodilator. This system has been adopted by over 52 countries within their national guidelines worldwide. Once asthma is controlled and stable, a gradual reduction in maintenance therapy is advised to determine the minimum effective dose needed to maintain control. Despite these guidelines, the current level of asthma control is far from ideal.[4] Many patients experience daytime and night-time symptoms at least once a week, leading to frequent unscheduled visits and hospitalizations. A significant factor contributing to poor asthma control is the incorrect use of inhalers by patients,[5] which prevents them from getting the full benefit of their medication.

Common issues with inhaler use include poor coordination between actuation and inhalation with pressurized metered-dose inhalers (pMDIs) and exhaling into dry powder inhalers (DPIs), which results in loss of drug that is blown out of the device.[5] Additionally, patients occasionally misuse their inhalers in other less common ways.

Several inhaler types are currently available on the market; based on the method of producing the aerosol, inhalers can be classified as propellant-based pressurized metered dose inhaler devices (i.e. pMDIs and breath-actuated pMDIs), as non-propellant-based dry powder inhaler devices (i.e. DPIs), and as liquid-based devices (nebulizers and soft mist inhalers).[6] Each class of inhaler device has pros as well as cons (Table 15.1). Inhalers differ in their efficiency of drug delivery to the lower respiratory tract, depending on device design, its internal resistance, the formulation of the medication, its particle size, the velocity of the produced aerosol plume, and the ease with which patients can use the device.[6] The efficiency of drug delivery may also be influenced significantly by patients' preference, which, in turn, affects patients' adherence to treatment and, indeed, the subsequent long-term control of the disease.[7] There seems little point in prescribing an effective medication in an inhaler device that patients cannot use correctly. Thus the choice of the right inhaler for the patient is just as important as choosing the most effective medication.[7]

15.2 AEROSOL DELIVERY DEVICES

15.2.1 Pressurized Metered-Dose Inhalers

Introduced in the mid-20th century, pMDIs remain the most commonly prescribed device for delivering inhaled therapy.[8] The pressurized metered-dose inhaler (pMDI) consists of an aluminium canister housed in a plastic holder, containing a pressurized suspension or solution of micronized drug particles dispersed in propellants.[9] The crucial component of the pMDI is the metering valve, which accurately delivers a known volume of propellant containing the micronized drug with each actuation. The fundamental operation of contemporary pMDIs remains similar to the original 1950s design: pressing the canister into the actuator seat releases the formulation from the metering valve, creating a heterogeneous aerosol of droplets. These droplets consist of drug particles within a shell of propellant that evaporates over time and distance, reducing particle size (Figure 15.1). This process uses a pressurized propellant to generate a metered dose of aerosol through an atomization nozzle.[9]

Initially, pMDIs used chlorofluorocarbon (CFC) propellants, which were replaced by hydrofluoroalkane (HFA) propellants due to environmental concerns over CFCs' damage to the ozone layer. HFA-based pMDI formulations are generally categorized as either suspension or solution technologies. Since drugs commonly used in pMDIs are not readily soluble in HFAs, a co-solvent is required.[10] Ethanol is often used, as it is miscible with HFAs and a good solvent for many hydrophobic drugs. Solution-based pMDIs utilizing volatile co-solvents result in higher fine-particle respirable fractions due to the small particle size of the dried aerosol. The particle size of solution-based pMDIs can be adjusted by adding non-volatile agents that dissolve in the HFA co-solvent system but do not evaporate during aerosolization, thus increasing the final particle size.[11]

Some HFA-driven pMDIs have been extensively modified to produce aerosols with small (mass median aerodynamic diameter ~1.3 μ) particle sizes.[12] These pMDIs deliver small aerosol particles and achieve higher rates of pulmonary drug deposition compared to conventional pMDIs that do not emit small aerosol particles.[12] Generally, the velocity of the HFA spray is slower than that of the CFC, allowing better distribution of drugs along the respiratory airways and potentially making these devices more functional, especially for elderly patients.[13]

Correct use of the pMDI involves holding the inhaler correctly and performing a series of coordinated steps, which can be challenging for some patients.[5,6] Suspension pMDIs also need to be shaken before use, a step often overlooked by both patients and healthcare professionals. Efficient aerosol delivery to the lungs requires slow, deep inhalation (an inspiratory flow rate of about 30 L/min, corresponding to a total inhalation time of 4–5 seconds) starting just before device activation, followed by a brief breath-hold of up to 10 seconds.[5,6] Unfortunately, many patients struggle

TABLE 15.1
Strengths and Weaknesses of Each Inhaler Device Type

	Strengths	Weaknesses
pMDI	Compact and portable; Dose consistency; Multidose; Cannot contaminate contents; Wide range of therapies; Relatively cheap	Contains propellant; Requires good coordination of actuation and inhalation
BA-pMDI	Compact and portable; Multidose; Cannot contaminate contents; Breath actuated (no coordination needed)	Few drugs available; "Cold Freon" effect; Requires a minimum (>20 L/min) flow to be triggered
DPI Single dose	Compact and portable; Wide range of therapies; No propellants; Breath actuated (no coordination needed); Cheap	Some are moisture-sensitive; Requires a minimum (>30 L/min) inspiratory flow; Requires many (>5) steps for preparation; Requires a minimum inspiratory flow; May not be appropriated during exacerbation
Multiple dose	Compact and portable; Multidose; Wide range of therapies; No propellants; Breath actuated (no coordination needed); Dose counter	Some are moisture-sensitive; Requires some (<5) steps for preparation; Requires a minimum inspiratory flow; May not be appropriated during exacerbation; Expensive
SMI*	Portable and compact; Multidose; High lung deposition; Does not contain propellants	Few drugs available; Not breath actuated; Requires some coordination of actuation and inhalation; Requires priming before first use; Expensive
Nebulizers	No specific inhalation technique required; May be used at any age; Vibrating mesh is portable and does not require an outside energy source; High lung deposition (mesh nebulizers)	Jet and ultrasonic nebulizers require an outside energy source; Treatment times can be long; performance varies between nebulizers; Risk of bacterial contamination; Expensive (vibrating mesh)

pMDI, pressurized metered dose inhaler; BA-pMDI, breath-actuated pMDI; DPI, dry powder inhaler; SMI, soft mist inhaler.
*Respimat.

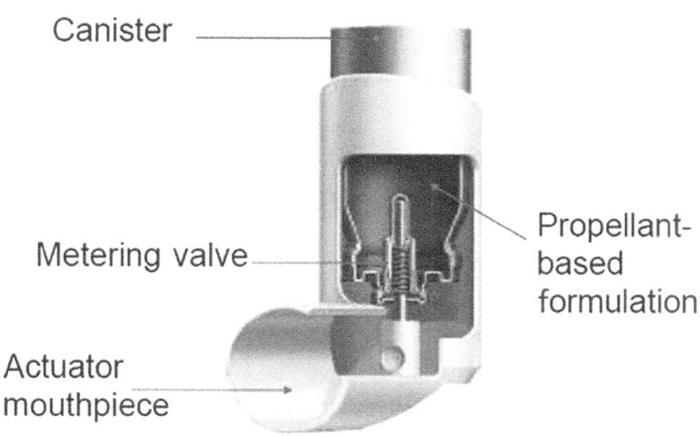

FIGURE 15.1 Representation of a pressurized metered-dose inhaler with its main components.

to coordinate inhaler activation with inhalation and/or cannot generate a sufficiently deep inhalation, inhale too quickly, or fail to hold their breath long enough, even after repeated training.[5, 6] Misuse of pMDIs is associated with poorer asthma control and increased exacerbations.[14] To address the issues associated with poor pMDI use, spacers[15] and breath-actuated pMDIs are available.[16, 17]

Spacer devices attach to the mouthpiece of a pMDI and have volumes ranging from 50 to 800 ml. Many spacers feature a one-way valve that prevents the patient from blowing away the dose after actuation.[15] These devices help patients inhale medication without needing to synchronize with the device's activation. Spacers act as aerosol reservoirs, reducing aerosol velocity and increasing the distance between the pMDI actuator and the patient's mouth.[15] This allows particle size to decrease, leading to better lung deposition of the aerosol. Additionally, spacers trap large particles (up to 80% of the dose), reducing oropharyngeal deposition and associated side effects like throat irritation, dysphonia, and oral candidiasis.[15] There are three primary spacer designs: open tube, holding chamber, and reverse flow (where the pMDI is fired away from the patient). Valved holding chambers with face masks are used for neonates, young children, and elderly patients. Key factors for optimal aerosol delivery include a tight, comfortable mask fit and minimized mask dead space. Some spacers incorporate a whistle to provide feedback if inspiration is too fast, helping patients optimize their inhalation technique.[15] Spacers can enhance the clinical effectiveness of inhaled medications, particularly for patients unable to use a pMDI correctly.[15] They may improve the response to short-acting beta-adrenergic bronchodilators even in patients with proper inhalation techniques.[18–21] However, spacers make the inhalation system less portable and compact, which can reduce patient compliance, especially in children. Electrostatic charge can cause medication to deposit on the spacer walls, leading to inconsistent drug delivery.[15] Spacers made from non-electrostatic materials or those washed with a low concentration of dishwashing liquid and allowed to drip dry can minimize this issue. Cleaning recommendations vary, generally ranging from once a week to once a month, and patients should follow the manufacturer's instructions. The proportion of the drug dose inhaled can vary significantly with different spacers, and data from studies with one drug and pMDI may not apply to others.[22]

Breath-actuated (BA) pMDIs, such as the Autohaler® (3M Healthcare Ltd, United States of America), the K-haler® (Mundipharma International Ltd, Cambridge, United Kingdom), the Easibreathe® (Teva Pharmaceutical Industries Ltd, Petach Tikva, Israel), and the Syncrobreathe® (Cipla Ltd, India) are alternatives to standard pMDIs that have been developed to overcome the problem of poor coordination of pMDI actuation and inhalation.[16, 17] BA pMDIs have different flow-triggered systems that release the dose during inhalation, so that firing and inhaling are automatically coordinated.[16, 17] These inhalation devices can achieve good lung deposition and clinical efficacy in patients unable to use a pMDI correctly because of coordination difficulties.[16, 17] Errors when using a BA pMDI are less frequent than when using a standard pMDI.[17] An increased use of BA pMDIs might improve asthma control and reduce the overall cost of asthma therapy compared with conventional pMDIs.[17] On the negative side, BA pMDIs still contain fluorinated propellants that are very strong greenhouse gases; in addition, most BA-pMDI are available only with one drug or combination.[16, 17]

15.2.2 Dry Powder Inhalers

Dry powder inhalers (DPIs), similar to pMDIs, are small, portable, and available as single-dose or multiple-dose devices.[23, 24] DPI doses can be premetered in the form of single capsules or foil blisters or as multi-single unit dose disks; alternatively, device metering of bulk powder can be achieved through the use of reservoir devices (Figure 15.2).[23, 24] Unlike pMDIs, all DPIs require a pre-inhalation dose-loading step for proper functionality. DPIs are activated by the patient's inspiratory flow, eliminating the need for synchronization between inhaler actuation and inhalation, thus simplifying their use for most patients.[23, 24]

DPIs typically contain drug particles attached to excipient carrier molecules like lactose or in the form of agglomerated pellets.[23] These devices are designed with internal resistance that must be overcome by a forceful inhalation to generate turbulent flow, de-aggregate the drug particles, and produce fine particles for inhalation.[23, 24] The physical design of a DPI establishes its specific resistance to airflow (measured as the square root of the pressure drop across the device divided by the flow rate through the device), with current designs having specific resistance values ranging from about 0.02 to 0.05 $kPa^{0.5}L/min^{-1}$ (Figure 15.3).[6, 25] The internal resistance of DPIs varies and is classified based on the inhalation flow required to produce a 4 kPa pressure drop. The force needed to overcome this resistance and create an aerosol depends on the patient's inhalation flow and the device's internal resistance.[23–25]

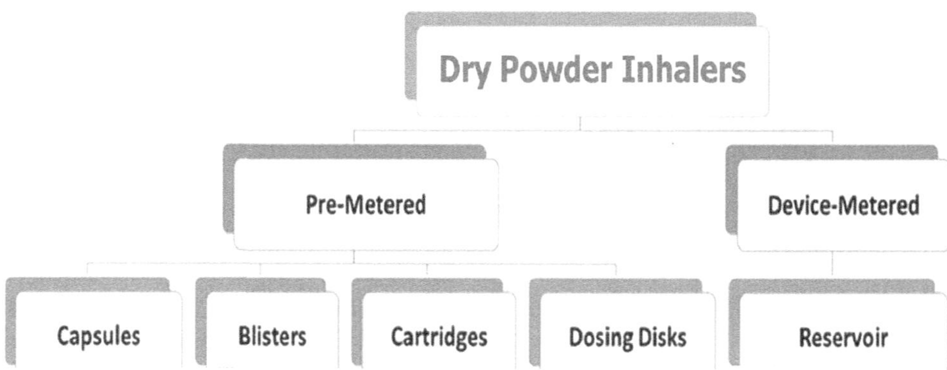

FIGURE 15.2 Classification of different types of dry powder inhalers.

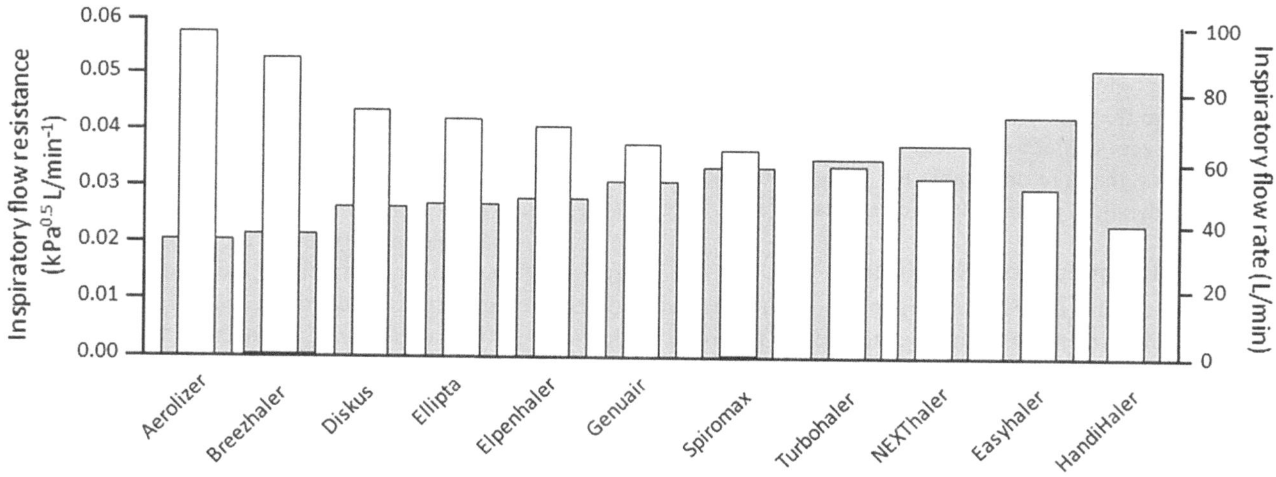

FIGURE 15.3 Inspiratory resistance of dry powder inhalers (filled bars) and the corresponding flow (empty bars) required to achieve a 4 kPa pressure drop. (Adapted from Lavorini F., Mannini C., Chellini E., Fontana G.A. Optimising inhaled pharmacotherapy for elderly patients with chronic obstructive pulmonary disease: the importance of delivery devices. *Drugs Aging* 2016; 33:461–473.)

Lung deposition with DPIs is a balance between generating sufficient power for particle de-aggregation and avoiding increased oropharyngeal deposition at higher aerosol velocities.[23–25] A limitation of DPIs is their dependence on the patient's ability to generate the necessary inspiratory force to efficiently de-aggregate the powder formulation and ensure effective drug delivery to the lungs.[23, 24] While most patients can generate enough flow to operate a DPI effectively, children under six years of age and patients with severe airway obstruction may struggle to achieve the required inspiratory force.[6] A systematic literature review revealed that up to 90% of patients did not use their DPI correctly.[26] Common errors made by patients included lack of exhalation before inhalation, incorrect positioning and loading of the inhaler, failure to inhale forcefully and deeply through the device, and patients' failure to breath-hold after inhalation.[26] All these errors may lead to insufficient drug delivery, which adversely influences drug efficacy and may contribute to inadequate disease control.[27]

15.2.3 Nebulizer Systems and Soft Mist Inhaler

Nebulizers are devices that convert liquid medications into small droplets that can be easily inhaled. These liquids can be either solutions, where the drug is dissolved in a carrier liquid, or suspensions, where solid drug particles are suspended in the liquid.[27] It is crucial to consider the entire "nebulizer system" because various components, beyond just the nebulizer itself, significantly influence aerosol delivery and its characteristics.[28] Key components include the compressor or line feed, fill volume, residual volume, driving gas flow, and the use of a face mask or mouthpiece. Each component affects the total drug delivered, the rate of aerosol output, and the particle size distribution. Altering any part of the nebulizer system can significantly change its aerosol output characteristics.[28] Unlike pMDIs and DPIs, no special inhalation techniques are needed for optimum delivery with nebulizers; tidal breathing with only occasional deep breaths is sufficient.[28, 29] Thus, for patients who are unable to master the proper pMDI technique despite repeated instruction, the proper use of a nebulizer probably improves drug delivery. However, nebulizers have some distinct disadvantages. Patients must load the device with the medication solution for each treatment, and bacterial contamination of the reservoir can cause respiratory infections, making regular cleaning important.[28, 29] Also, nebulizer treatments take longer than pMDIs and DPIs to administer (10–15 minutes for a jet nebulizer, five minutes for an ultrasonic or mesh nebulizer). Although they are relatively portable, a typical jet nebulizer must be plugged into a wall outlet or a power adaptor and thus cannot be used easily in transit. Newer nebulizer designs have enhanced patients' convenience.

There are three main types of nebulizers: jet nebulizers, ultrasonic wave nebulizers, and vibrating mesh nebulizers.

15.2.3.1 Jet Nebulizers

Jet nebulizers are the most commonly used nebulizers worldwide. They operate using compressed gas (usually air or oxygen) that draws medication through a capillary tube in the nebulizer chamber, creating an aerosol by shearing the liquid formulation and directing it toward a baffle. Coarse droplets impact the baffle, while smaller droplets can be inhaled or return to the reservoir for re-nebulization.[27, 28] The newer jet nebulizers (the so-called breath-enhanced or breath-actuated jet nebulizers) are designed to increase efficiency by delivering more aerosol to the patient and reducing wastage during exhalation.[27–29]

15.2.3.2 Ultrasonic Wave Nebulizers

Ultrasonic wave nebulizers use a rapidly vibrating (>1 MHz) piezoelectric crystal to generate aerosol particles.[27–29] The vibrations are transmitted to the surface of the drug solution, forming standing waves from which droplets break free and become aerosolized. The droplet size is determined by the frequency of the oscillation. Although ultrasonic nebulizers can nebulize solutions more quickly than jet nebulizers, they are unsuitable for suspensions and can heat the medication, potentially affecting its stability.[27–29]

15.2.3.3 Vibrating Mesh Nebulizers

Introduced around 2005, vibrating mesh nebulizers use ultrasonic vibrating mesh technology to address the limitations of conventional jet nebulizers, such as long treatment times and inefficient drug use.[30] These nebulizers feature a vibrating mesh plate with precision-formed holes that control the size and flow of aerosolized particles. An attached power supply provides electricity to a vibrating piezoelectric element. As the plate vibrates, the drug passes through the holes, creating a dense aerosol at low flow rates.[30] Examples include the AeroNeb® Pro (Aerogen, Ireland) and the eFlow® (Pari, Germany). These devices offer greater efficiency, precision, and consistency in drug delivery and are quieter and generally portable. However, they are more expensive and require significant maintenance and cleaning to prevent build-up, blockage, and pathogen colonization.[30]

The development of soft mist inhalers (SMIs) has opened up new opportunities for inhaled drug delivery. These inhalation devices use liquid formulations similar to those in nebulizers, but they are generally multidose devices that have the potential to compete with pMDIs and DPIs in the portable inhaler market. Currently, the only SMI marketed in some European countries is the Respimat inhaler.[31]

The Respimat soft mist inhaler operates without propellants, utilizing the energy from a compressed spring inside the device. It delivers individual doses through a precisely engineered nozzle system, producing a slow-moving aerosol cloud, which is referred to as a soft mist.[31] Scintigraphic studies have demonstrated that lung deposition with the Respimat is higher, reaching up to 50%, compared to CFC-based pMDIs. Clinical trials indicate that medications delivered by the Respimat are effective at lower doses for patients with obstructive airway diseases.[31] The Respimat functions as a "press and breathe" device, with an inhalation technique similar to that of a pMDI. While coordination between actuation and inhalation is necessary, the device's low spray velocity and the prolonged duration of the aerosol cloud (typically 1–1.5 seconds) make it easier for patients to synchronize their breathing with the actuation compared to a traditional pMDI.[31] Recently, a new reusable version of the Respimat has been launched in the market.[32] The reusable Respimat Soft Mist inhaler includes enhanced features that simplify its assembly and improve handling and ease of use.[32] The usability of the reusable Respimat inhaler compared with the original disposable inhaler has been improved in terms of handling and ease of use. Moreover, cartridge exchange was rated as intuitive and simple to manage. It has a reduced environmental impact versus the disposable inhaler.[32]

15.3 CHOICE OF AN INHALER DEVICE FOR ASTHMA THERAPY

More than 230 inhaled device-drug combinations are currently available in Europe for the treatment of asthma patients.[8] The number is likely to increase with the development of generic inhaled drugs delivered by relatively low-cost pMDIs and DPIs. Consequently, the level of confusion experienced by clinicians, nurses, and pharmacists when trying to choose the most appropriate device for each patient is increased. Thus physicians' experience is among the most important factors that influence decision-making in the choice of inhaler in asthma therapy. In fact, inhalers are often prescribed on an empirical basis rather than an evidence-based approach. Following their own experience, doctors are much more likely to prescribe the same old inhaler that they have always prescribed rather than new, improved inhaler devices. However, selecting and properly using inhalation devices is crucial in managing asthma.[33] Numerous challenges exist with inhaler usage, and no single device is suitable for every patient. These challenges can stem from the severity of lung disease and pulmonary function, as well as physical factors like manual dexterity and comorbidities such as arthritis. Additionally, patient engagement and satisfaction play vital roles in device selection and adherence. Issues with inhaler use are particularly prevalent among children and the elderly.[33] The criteria to be considered when choosing an inhaler device differ depending on the audience being addressed.[34] From the viewpoint of the respiratory therapist, consistent and safe dosing, sufficient drug deposition, and clinical effect should be the driving factors for the inhaler choice. The patient's ability to inhale through the device, the intrinsic airflow resistance of the device, and the degree of dependence of the drug release on inspiratory airflow variability are all important determinants when considering the constancy of dosing.[34] From the point of view of the clinician, clinical efficacy and safety should take precedence when choosing an inhaler.[34] However, in the real world, clinical efficacy must be balanced against cost-effectiveness, and inhalers with an insufficient performance may be prescribed simply because they are cheap. Patients' preferences and acceptance of the inhaler should also be considered when deciding on a specific inhaler, since these will have major implications for adherence.[33] The Aerosol Drug Management Improvement Team (ADMIT), a consortium of European respiratory physicians with a common interest in promoting the excellent delivery of inhaled drugs, has made a number of recommendations related to the delivery instructions for a correct inhalation technique for each inhaler device.[35–37] These evidence-based recommendations are summarized in Table 15.2. The ADMIT group has also proposed a practical algorithm in order to improve the

TABLE 15.2
Recommendations from ADMIT for Inhaler Choice and Correct Inhalation Technique

- Inhalers should be matched to the patient as much as possible.
- In young children, if pMDIs are prescribed, they should be used with a spacer device.
- An alternative to a pMDI should be considered in elderly patients with a mini-mental test score <23/30 or an ideomotor dyspraxia score <14/20, as they are unlikely to have a correct inhalation technique through a pMDI.
- The patient's peak inspiratory flow value should be considered before prescribing a DPI. Those patients with severe airflow obstruction, children, and the elderly would benefit from an inhaler device with a low airflow resistance.
- Before prescribing a DPI, check that the patient can inhale deeply and forcibly at the start of the inhalation maneuver because the airflow profile affects the particle size produced and hence drug deposition and efficacy.
- Where possible, one patient should have one type of inhaler.
- Establish an official board to compile instructions for the correct inhalation technique for each inhaler device currently on the market.
- Instructions for correct inhaler use should be made readily accessible on a dedicated website.
- Training in the correct inhalation technique is essential for patients and healthcare professionals.
- Inhalation techniques should be checked and reinforced at regular intervals.
- Teaching correct inhalation techniques should be tailored to the patient's needs and preferences: group instruction in correct inhalation techniques appears to be more effective than personal one-to-one instruction and equally as effective as video instruction; younger patients may benefit more from multimedia teaching methods; elderly patients respond well to one-to-one tuition.

Source: Modified from Crompton, G.K., Barnes, P.J., Broeders, M., et al., *Respir. Med.*, 2006; 100, 1479–1494.
Note: DPI, dry powder inhaler; PIF, peak inspiratory flow; pMDI, pressurized metered-dose inhaler.

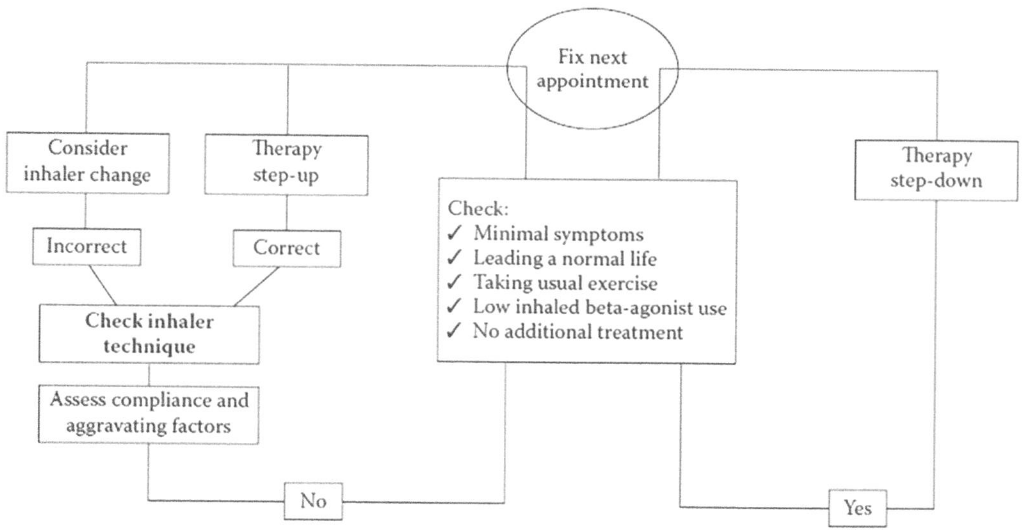

FIGURE 15.4 Asthma therapy adjustment flow chart. (Reprinted from Crompton, G.K., Barnes, P.J., Broeders, M., et al. *Respir. Med.*, 2006; 100: 1479–1494.)

instruction given to patients regarding the optimal use of their inhalers (Figure 15.4). At each consultation, the physician should establish the patient's current level of symptoms and control, and if the patient's asthma is well-controlled for at least three months, therapy should be stepped down gradually according to the treatment guidelines. Conversely, if the patient answers "no" to any of these checklist questions, then compliance and aggravating (trigger) factors should be assessed. Most importantly, the patient's inhalation technique should be assessed. If the patient is unable to use a particular inhaler correctly despite repeated attempts, a change in inhaler device should be considered. In the cases where ongoing, uncontrolled asthma persists despite correct inhaler technique, then asthma therapy should be stepped up according to the treatment guidelines and another appointment scheduled in order to recheck the symptoms.

15.4 FUTURE OF INHALATION THERAPY

In the last decade, the efficiency of inhalers, as gauged by total lung deposition, has surged from less than 10% to nearly 50% of the total dose. Nonetheless, less than half of the dose reaches the site of absorption in the alveoli. There is significant potential for new technologies to further improve these figures, and pharmaceutical companies are continually working to innovate and refine current inhalation technologies. The integration of modern technology into inhaler devices aims to enhance drug delivery, minimize device errors, boost patient adherence, and monitor and manage patients' conditions.[38]

A novel co-suspension technology employs low-density phospholipid particles to suspend micronized drug crystals in an HFA propellant, enabling the uniform administration of multiple drugs via a single pMDI.[39] These low-density phospholipid particles enhance the physicochemical stability of the drugs and can also reduce the impact of shake-fire delay. *In vitro* and *in vivo* studies have demonstrated highly reproducible and consistent drug delivery with effective lung deposition. This consistency is maintained across different flow rates, and drug delivery remains stable even with simulated patient handling errors, such as varied shake techniques and delays between shaking and actuation.[39]

One proposed solution to increase patient adherence to their treatments is the use of digital health solutions, including monitoring systems based on mobile applications (apps) and electronic sensors. The first built-in inhaler monitoring technology, developed in the 1980s, primarily aimed to assess medication adherence and has evolved over the years to include various other sensing functions.[40] The creation of the Smartinhaler® Tracker (Adherium) to log the dates and times of inhaler actuations led to the development of more advanced devices incorporating GPS or functions capable of monitoring parameters such as inhalation flow and volume.[40] Features like dose-memory and dose-reminder functions in inhalers can positively influence adherence and bolster confidence in self-management behaviors. Developments in digital health have also proved highly useful in managing device errors, offering detailed feedback on patients' device proficiency.[40] The SmartMist™ (Aradigm) and MDILog™ (Westmed Technologies) have incorporated sensing capabilities to facilitate the assessment of inhalation techniques. The MDILog™, widely used in clinical research, is designed to attach to the casing of standard inhalers. It includes an inhaler actuation sensor, an accelerometer to detect inhaler shaking, and a sensitive temperature sensor for assessing inhalation. The ProAir® Digihaler®[41] is a Food and Drug Administration (USA)-approved albuterol multidose dry powder inhaler (DPI) with an integrated electronic module that provides data on inhalation technique (peak inspiratory flow [PIF], inhalation volume, inhalation duration, and time to PIF), as well as a time-stamped recording every time the inhaler is used. Inhalation detection technologies such as these can coach patients on correct device techniques. This kind of technology, along with other innovative e-health developments such as mobile communication technology (mHealth), electronic reminders, telemedicine, and inhaler tracker interventions, has the potential to reduce the resource burden on healthcare systems and provide optimal and personalized asthma management to patients.[42]

The current crisis related to global warming has prompted some governments to consider banning the future use of HFA gas propellants in industry.[43] This could pose major problems for those people worldwide who depend upon pMDIs for delivery of their inhaled medication, mainly because a proportion of HFA has been allocated for medical use. As a result, manufacturers have a major challenge to urgently develop and produce sufficient new environment-friendly propellants with lower contribution to greenhouse gas emissions. At the time of writing, new HFAs are being developed and produced, and hopefully these will be available in the near future.

15.5 CONCLUSIONS

The pulmonary route of administration has demonstrated effectiveness in delivering a variety of drugs to treat asthma. Achieving successful pulmonary administration requires a harmonious interaction between the drug formulation, the inhaler device, and the patient. Inhalation products are inherently more complex compared to conventional dosage forms: the interconnected features of the device and formulation must work together to aerosolize the drug and deliver it to the target site.

In 2011, more than 230 different drug-device combinations were available in Europe,[8] and many new other device technologies are in development. These numbers reflect the ingenuity of technologists but do not necessarily translate into clinical improvements. Indeed, the biggest issue leading to a lack of desired effects or adverse outcomes is the incorrect use of the device. Moreover, the plethora of devices and the complex physics involved in drug delivery make it challenging for clinicians to choose the appropriate device for their patients. An ideal inhaler should deliver precise and consistent doses to targeted lung regions and maintain the stability of the delivered drugs. It is also desirable for devices to be compact and simple enough for patients to use easily. Dry powder inhalers (DPIs) are gaining popularity due to their ease of use; however, pMDIs still face challenges related to formulation and design. Nebulizers are being redesigned to expand their applicability. Currently, no single device meets all the requirements for delivering drugs with varying physicochemical properties. Medical personnel must thoroughly understand the capabilities of each inhaler and match them to the needs of the patient, according to their health condition, to achieve the best therapeutic outcomes. Ongoing and repeated education for both healthcare professionals and patients on the correct inhalation technique is crucial, with regular reassessments. Significant improvements in educational efforts are needed, specifically targeting general practitioners and asthma nurses, who are typically responsible for teaching patients how to use their inhalers properly. It is important to recognize that frequently changing inhaler devices that deliver the same medication is not a solution, as this can erode patients' confidence in both the device and the medication, leading to decreased adherence to therapy. An inhaler should only be prescribed when there is absolute certainty that the patient can use it correctly.

REFERENCES

1. Cao Y, Chen S, Chen X et al. Global trends in the incidence and mortality of asthma from 1990 to 2019: An age-period-cohort analysis using the global burden of disease study 2019. *Front Public Health*. 2022:10:1036674.
2. Xie, M., Liu, X., Cao, X. et al. Trends in prevalence and incidence of chronic respiratory diseases from 1990 to 2017. *Respir Res*. 2020;21:49.
3. Global Initiative for Asthma. GINA Report, Global Strategy for Asthma Management and Prevention, 2024. Accessed July 14, 2024. https://ginasthma.org/.
4. Murphy KR, Schatz M. Asthma management and control in children, adolescents, and adults. *Lancet Respir Med*. 2020;8:1012–1025.
5. Usmani OS, Lavorini F, Marshall J et al Critical inhaler errors in asthma and COPD: A systematic review of impact on health outcomes. *Respir Res*. 2018;19(1):10.
6. Laube BL, Janssens HM, de Jongh FHC, et al. What the pulmonary specialist should know about the new inhalation therapies. *Eur Respir J*. 2011;37:1308–1331.
7. Lavorini F, Janson C, Braido F. What to consider before prescribing inhaled medications: a pragmatic approach. *Ther Adv Respir Dis*. 2019;13:1753466619884532
8. Lavorini F, Corrigan CJ, Barnes PJ, et al. Retail sales of inhalation devices in European countries: So much for a global policy. *Respir Med*. 2011;98:1099–1013.
9. Roche N, Dekhuijzen PNR. The evolution of pressurized metered-dose inhalers from early to modern devices. *J Aerosol Med Pulm Drug Deliv*. 2016;29:1–17.
10. Ganderton D, Lewis D, Davies R, Meakin B, Brambilla G, Church T. Modulite: a means of designing the aerosols generated by pressurized metered dose inhalers. *Respir Med*. 2002;96(Suppl D):S3–S8.
11. Buttini F, Miozzi M, Balducci AG, et al. Differences in physical chemistry and dissolution rate of solid particle aerosols from solution pressurised inhalers. *Int J Pharm*. 2014;465(1–2):42–51.
12. Lavorini F, Pedersen S, Usmani OS. Dilemmas, confusion, and misconceptions related to small airways directed therapy. *Chest*. 2017;151:1345–1355.
13. Lavorini F, Mannini C, Chellini E, Fontana GA. Optimising inhaled pharmacotherapy for elderly patients with chronic obstructive pulmonary disease: the importance of delivery devices. *Drugs Aging*. 2016;33:461–473.
14. Price DB, Román-Rodríguez M, McQueen RB, et al. Inhaler Errors in the CRITIKAL Study: Type, Frequency, and Association with Asthma Outcomes. *J Allergy Clin Immunol Pract*. 2017;5:1071–1081.
15. Lavorini F, Fontana GA. Targeting drugs to the airways: The role of spacer devices. *Expert Opin Drug Deliv*. 2009;6:91–102.
16. Lavorini F, Fontana GA, Usmani OS. New inhaler devices—the good, the bad and the ugly. *Respiration*. 2014; 88:3–15.
17. Lavorini F, Usmani OS, Salvi S, et al. A narrative review on the Synchrobreathe™: A novel breath-actuated pressurised metered-dose inhaler for the treatment of obstructive airway diseases. *Respir Med*. 2023:219:107435.
18. Fontana GA, Lavorini F, Chiostri M, et al. Large and small airway responses to procaterol hydrochloride administered through different extension devices in asthmatic patients. *J Aerosol Med*. 1999;12:177–185.
19. Lavorini F, Geri P, Luperini M, et al. Clinical and functional responses to salbutamol inhaled via different devices in asthmatic patients with induced bronchoconstriction. *Brit J Clin Pharmacol*. 2004;58:512–520.
20. Lavorini F, Geri P, Mariani L et al. Speed of onset of bronchodilator response to salbutamol inhaled via different devices in asthmatics. A bioassay based on functional antagonism *Brit J Clin Pharmacol*. 2006;62:403–411.
21. Lavorini F, Geri P, Camiciottoli G, Pistolesi M, Fontana GA. Agreement between two methods for assessing bioequivalence *Pulm Pharmacol Ther*. 2008;21:380–384.
22. Lavorini F, Barreto C, van Boven Job FM et al. Spacers and valved holding chambers-the risk of switching to different chambers. *J Allergy Clin Immunol Pract*. 2020;8:1569–1573.
23. De Boer AH, Hagedoorn P, Hoppentocht M, et al. Dry powder inhalation: past, present and future. *Expert Opin Drug Deliv*. 2017; 14(4):499–512.
24. Levy ML, Carroll W, Izquierdo Alonso JL, et al. Understanding dry powder inhalers: key technical and patient preference attributes. *Adv Ther*. 2019; 36: 2547–2557.
25. Azouz W, Chrystyn H. Clarifying the dilemmas about inhalation techniques for dry powder inhalers: Integrating science with clinical practice. *Prim Care Respir J* 2012;21:208–213.
26. Lavorini F, Magnan A, Dubus JC, et al. Effect of incorrect use of dry powder inhalers on management of patients with asthma and COPD. *Respir Med*. 2008;102:593–604.
27. Carvalho TC, McConville JT. The function and performance of aqueous aerosol devices for inhalation therapy. *J Pharmacy Pharmacol*, 2016;68:556–578.
28. Dolovich MB Assessing nebulizer performance. *Respir Care*. 2002;47:1290–1301.
29. Hess DR. Nebulizers: principles and performance. *Respir Care*. 2000;45:609–622.
30. Dhand R. Nebulisers that use a vibrating mesh or plate with multiple apertures to generate aerosol. *Respir Care*. 2002;47:1406–1416.
31. Dalby R, Spallek M, Voshaar T. A review of the development of respimat soft mist inhaler. *Int J Pharm*. 2004;283:1–9.
32. Dhand R, Eicher J, Hänsel M et al. Improving usability and maintaining performance: human-factor and aerosol-performance studies evaluating the new reusable Respimat inhaler. *Int J COPD*. 2019;14:509–523.
33. Usmani OS. Choosing the right inhaler for your asthma or COPD patient *Ther Clin Risk Manag*. 2019;15:461–472.
34. Virchow JC. What plays a role in the choice of inhaler device for asthma therapy? *Curr Med Res Opin*. 2005;21(Suppl.):s19–s25.
35. Broeders ME, Sanchis J, Levy ML, Crompton GK, Dekhuijzen PN; ADMIT Working Group. The ADMIT series—issues in inhalation therapy. 2. Improving technique and clinical effectiveness. *Prim Care Respir J*. 2009;18(2):76–82.
36. Vincken W, Dekhuijzen PR, Barnes P; ADMIT Group. The ADMIT series—Issues in inhalation therapy. 4) how to choose inhaler devices for the treatment of COPD. *Prim Care Respir J*. 2010;19(1):10–20.
37. Levy ML, Dekhuijzen PN, Barnes PJ, et al. Inhaler technique: facts and fantasies. A view from the Aerosol Drug Management Improvement Team (ADMIT). *Prim Care Respir Med*. 2016;26:16017.

38. Rogueda P, Traini D The future of inhalers: how can we improve drug delivery in asthma and COPD? *Expert Rev Respir Med.* 2016;10:1041–1044.
39. Ferguson GT, Hickey AJ, Dwivedi S. Co-suspension delivery technology in pressurized metered-dose inhalers for multi-drug dosing in the treatment of respiratory diseases. *Respir Med.* 2018;134:16–23.
40. Kikidis D, Konstantinos V, Tzovaras D et al. The digital asthma patient: the history and future of inhaler based health monitoring devices. *J Aerosol Med Pulm Drug Deliv.* 2016;29:219–232.
41. Levy ML, Kocks JWH, Bosnic-Anticevich et al. Uncovering patterns of inhaler technique and reliever use: the value of objective, personalized data from a digital inhaler. *NPJ Prim Care Respir Med.* 2024;34(1):23.
42. Bonini M, Usmani OS. Novel methods for device and adherence monitoring in asthma. *Curr Opin Pulm Med.* 2018; 24:63–69
43. Levy ML, Bateman ED, Allan K, et al. Global access and patient safety in the transition to environmentally friendly respiratory inhalers: the global initiative for Asthma perspective. *The Lancet.* 2023;402(10406):1012–1016.

Section V

Asthma Management and Treatments

16 Management of Pediatric Asthma

Jeffrey R. Stokes and Leonard B. Bacharier

16.1 BRIEF CASE REPORT

A four-year-old boy presents for evaluation of recurrent episodes of cough and wheezing since one year of age. His initial episode, at age three months, was in the setting of a viral illness characterized by coryza, low-grade fever, and wheezing. For two years, he has experienced cough and wheeze with nearly all upper respiratory tract infections. Over the past year, his mother has noticed coughing and wheezing while he played soccer in addition to similar symptoms during upper respiratory tract infections. He awakens due to cough or wheeze approximately twice monthly. Albuterol consistently provides prompt, albeit transient, symptom relief. Oral corticosteroids have been prescribed twice yearly for the most significant episodes. No emergency department visits or hospitalizations have been required.

His past medical history is notable for an itchy rash over the ante-cubital and popliteal fossae since one year of age, which improved with topical corticosteroids. He has never had pneumonia or croup. His only current medication is albuterol by nebulization as needed. His environment contains a cat and wall-to-wall carpeting throughout the home. The family history is notable for asthma in the father and allergic rhinitis in the mother.

On physical examination, he is alert, interactive, and not distressed. His weight is at the 45th percentile, and his height is at the 40th percentile. Heart rate is 100/min, and respiratory rate 16/minute. He has infra-orbital shiners, edematous and pale nasal turbinates, no tonsillar enlargement, and his chest exam is clear without adventitious lung sounds or evidence of increased work of breathing. His skin exam discloses erythematous papules and excoriation in the ante-cubital fossae bilaterally.

A chest radiograph is normal without infiltrates or hyperinflation.

His parents wonder what can be done to prevent him from experiencing further episodes of cough and wheeze.

16.2 GOALS OF ASTHMA MANAGEMENT IN PRESCHOOL AND SCHOOL-AGE CHILDREN

The principles of asthma management in preschool and school-age children have evolved substantially over the past two decades to the current approach, which is guided by the goals of attainment and maintenance of asthma control (see Chapter 5 of this volume). In contrast to asthma severity, which defines the intrinsic intensity of asthma as assessed without use of controller therapy, asthma control reflects the degree to which the signs and symptoms of asthma are minimized. Thus successful asthma management achieves multiple goals, including (1) minimization of day-to-day asthma-related symptomatology (i.e. reduction in the current impairment domain of asthma), (2) reduction or elimination of asthma exacerbations, (3) minimization of treatment-related side effects, and, ideally, (4) the prevention of impaired lung growth and progressive decline in lung function (i.e. reduction in the future risk domain of asthma).

Preschool-aged children often exhibit asthma that is more exacerbation-prone than impairment-dominant, while school-age children begin to demonstrate elements of both impairment and risk. Recognition of these different phenotypes and of patterns of asthma expression has directed research examining different treatment strategies in these two age groups, with exacerbation prevention and disease modification being major focuses in preschool children, while exacerbation prevention has been coupled with impairment reduction and interventions to prevent declines in lung function among school-age children.

16.3 HETEROGENEITY OF EARLY CHILDHOOD WHEEZING AND ASTHMA

Recurrent wheezing in the preschool-age group is a highly heterogeneous disorder, with multiple phenotypes of disease based upon age of onset, age, and likelihood of remission, concomitant risk factors (especially atopy), and triggering factors (such as viral infections). These multiple different phenotypic expressions of early childhood asthma are likely due to different underlying immunopathophysiologic mechanisms, which may confer differential responses to therapeutic strategies. The heterogeneity of early childhood wheezing and asthma complicates the interpretation of much of the early research done in this population, as most early studies enrolled highly heterogeneous populations of subjects rather than specific wheezing phenoytpes. Fortunately, several recent studies have begun to focus on more well-defined and homogeneous

DOI: 10.1201/9781003287209-21

populations, providing evidence to guide decision-making in this challenging age group.

16.4 STEPWISE APPROACH TO ASTHMA CARE

Over the past decade, several asthma guidelines have been developed that provide carefully developed treatment recommendations for children with asthma, including the National Asthma Education and Prevention Program (NAEPP) [1, 2], the Global Initiative for Asthma (GINA) [3], and the European Respiratory Society (ERS) Task Force [4]. All of these guidelines have proposed algorithms for the pharmacologic management of asthma using stepwise approaches, with the steps of care being aligned with the levels of both asthma severity and control. While the guidelines differ in terms of number of steps of care and the order of preferences of treatments within each step, there is consensus that achievement of asthma control is the major goal of therapy and that an individualized approach for each child is necessary based upon the level of control achieved (Tables 16.1, 16.2, and 16.3).

16.5 MANAGEMENT OF INTERMITTENT DISEASE (STEP 1 CARE)

According to the NAEPP Guidelines [2], children with intermittent asthma under the age of 12 years should receive Step 1 care, which includes as-needed use of a short-acting beta-agonist. The phenotype of intermittent asthma is most apparent in the preschool population, where it has been referred to using various terminology, including severe intermittent asthma and episodic viral wheeze. This phenotype exemplifies exacerbation-dominant disease with minimal to no intercurrent symptomatology. However, given the substantial morbidity experienced during these episodes, therapeutic strategies aiming to prevent or attenuate episode severity, ranging from daily preventative therapy to episodic therapy, have been studied. In recognition of this symptom pattern, and since publication of the NAEPP Guidelines in 2007 [1], several studies have clarified and broadened the treatment possibilities for young children with intermittent/episodic disease, including episodic use of controller medications at episode onset to attenuate symptom progression as well as examination of daily controller therapy intended to prevent exacerbations.

16.5.1 Episodic Controller Therapy

The intermittent and episodic nature of this condition has led parents, physicians, and investigators to consider the potential efficacy of intermittent use of controller therapies just during periods of increased asthma symptomatology, such as viral respiratory tract infections. The use of high-dose ICS therapy (fluticasone propionate 750 mcg twice daily) in one- to six-year-old children, started at the early signs of a developing respiratory tract illness, reduced the risk of oral corticosteroid use by approximately 50% but was associated with statistically significant reductions in both height and weight gain [5]. In contrast, two studies examining budesonide used intermittently (either 1 mg twice daily for seven days at the earliest signs of respiratory tract illness or 400 mcg daily beginning three days after onset of respiratory tract symptoms) did not demonstrate reduction in exacerbations requiring oral corticosteroids [6, 7] but did result in modest reductions in symptomatology during illnesses.[6] Based on these studies, the 2020 NAEPP guideline update recommends the use of a short course of high-dose ICS at the start of a respiratory tract infection in preschool children with viral-induced wheezing but are otherwise asymptomatic [2]. The 2023 GINA report considers this therapeutic approach when the provider is confident that the treatment would be used appropriately given the concerns about potential growth side effects with high-dose ICS [3].

Episodic use of montelukast at the early signs of respiratory tract illnesses also produced modest reductions in symptomatology without reducing the need for systemic corticosteroids [6].

The updated 2023 GINA report expresses concern about underlying inflammation in school-age children with asthma, thus recommending the use of low-dose ICS whenever SABAs are used as an alternative to daily low-dose ICS [8, 9], based in part due to inconsistent adherence with daily ICS by children with infrequent symptoms [3].

16.5.2 Daily Controller Therapy

Given the severity of episodes experienced by many children with intermittent disease, studies of daily controller therapy aimed at episode prevention have also been conducted. Daily treatment with low-dose inhaled corticosteroids (fluticasone propionate 88 mcg twice daily) for two years in children 2–3 years of age with recurrent wheeze, absent evidence of ongoing asthma impairment, and risk factors for persistence of asthma (positive modified Asthma Predictive Index) resulted in significantly fewer oral corticosteroid courses and more episode-free days than did placebo over a Two-year period [10]. A meta-analysis of 29 studies of infants and preschool children with recurrent wheeze or asthma demonstrated approximately a 40% reduction in the risk of exacerbations associated with daily ICS therapy as well as improved symptom burden and lung function [11]. Daily therapy with the montelukast produced a significant reduction in asthma exacerbations relative to placebo among two- to five-year-old children with intermittent asthma but did not impact the frequency of oral corticosteroid use [12]. A study in preschool children compared the efficacy of daily low-dose ICS (budesonide 0.5 mg daily) to episodic use of high-dose ICS (budesonide 1 mg twice daily started at the early signs of a respiratory illness) among 12- to 53-month-old children with recurrent wheeze, positive modified Asthma Predictive Indices, and an exacerbation in the previous year and demonstrated no difference between the two treatment strategies in terms of oral corticosteroid use, episode severity, indicators of daily asthma impairment, or linear growth [13]. At present, there are no studies directly comparing daily ICS and daily LTRA therapy in intermittent asthma

TABLE 16.1
Management of asthma in preschool children (0–4 years EPR-4, 0–5 years GINA)

		Step 1	Step 2	Step 3	Step 4	Step 5	Step 6
		Intermittent	**Persistent**				
EPR-4 2020	Preferred Controller	At the start of URI: add short course daily ICS	Daily Low Dose ICS	Daily Med Dose ICS	Daily Med Dose ICS-LABA	Daily High Dose ICS-LABA	Daily High Dose ICS-LABA + OCS
	Alternative Controller		Daily montelukast or Cromolyn		Daily Med dose ICS+montelukast	Daily High Dose ICS+montelukast	Daily High Dose ICS+montelukast + OCS
	Rescue	SABA					
GINA 2023	Preferred Controller		Daily Low Dose ICS	Double "Low Dose"	Continue controller & refer for specialist assessment	No Step 5 or 6	
	Other Controller Options	Consider intermittent short course ICS at onset of viral illness	Daily LTRA, or intermittent short course ICS at onset of viral illness	Low Dose ICS + LTRA Consider specialist referral	Add LTRA, or increase ICS frequency, or add intermittent ICS		
	Reliever	SABA					

ICS: Inhaled Corticosteroids, LABA: Long-Acting Beta-Agonist, Form: Formoterol, OCS: Oral Corticosteroids, LAMA: Long-Acting Muscarinic Antagonist, MART: Maintenance and reliever therapy

TABLE 16.2

Management of asthma in school age children (5–11 years EPR-4, 6–11 years GINA)

		Step 1	Step 2	Step 3	Step 4	Step 5	Step 6
		Intermittent	**Persistent**				
EPR-4 2020	Controller		Daily Low Dose ICS	Daily and PRN Low Dose ICS-Form	Daily and PRN Med Dose ICS-Form	Daily High Dose ICS-LABA	Daily High Dose ICS-LABA + OCS
	Alternative Controller		Daily LTRA, or Cromolyn, or Nedocromil, or Theophylline	Daily Med Dose ICS, or Daily Low Dose ICS-LABA, or Daily Low Dose ICS+LTRA, or Daily Low Dose ICS+theophylline	Daily Med Dose ICS-LABA, or Daily Med dose ICS+LTRA, or Daily Med Dose ICS+Theophylline	Daily High Dose ICS+LTRA, or Daily High Dose ICS+ Theophylline	Daily High Dose ICS+LTRA+OCS, or Daily High Dose ICS+Theophylline+OCS
	Rescue	SABA		ICS-Form (max 8 puffs/day)		SABA	
GINA 2023	Controller	Low Dose ICS take whenever SABA taken	Daily Low Dose ICS	Low Dose ICS-LABA OR Medium Dose ICS ***OR*** Very low dose ICS-Form (MART)	Med Dose ICS-LABA OR Low Dose ICS-Form MART Refer for expert advice	Refer for phenotypic assessment +/- higher dose ICS-LABA or add-on therapy (e.g anti-IgE, anti-I L4R, anti-IL5)	No Step 6
	Other controller options	Consider daily low dose ICS	Daily LTRA or low dose ICS taken whenever SABA is taken	Low dose ICS + LTRA	Add tiotropium or add LTRA	At last resort, consider add-on OCS, but consider side effects	
	Reliever	As Needed SABA		As Needed SABA or ICS-Form in MART		As Needed SABA	

TABLE 16.3
Management of asthma in adolescents and adults (12+ Years)

		Step 1	Step 2	Step 3	Step 4	Step 5	Step 6
		Intermittent	**Persistent**				
EPR-4 2020	Preferred Controller		Low Dose ICS or PRN concomitant ICS and SABA	Daily and PRN Low Dose ICS-Form (MART)	Daily and PRN Med Dose ICS-Form (MART)	Daily Med-High Dose ICS-LABA + LAMA	Daily High Dose ICS-LABA + OCS
	Alternative Controller		Daily LTRA, or Cromolyn, or Nedocromil, or Zileuton, or Theophylline	Daily Med Dose ICS, or Daily Low dose ICS-LABA, or Daily Low Dose ICS+LAMA or Daily Low Dose ICS + Theophylline or Zileuton	Daily Med Dose ICS-LABA, or Dialy Med Dose ICS+LAMA, or Dialy Med Dose ICS+Theophylline or Daily Med Dose ICS+Zileuton	Daily Med-High Dose ICS-LABA, or Daily High Dose ICS+LTRA	
	Rescue	SABA	SABA or PRN ICS with SABA	ICS-Form (Max 12 puffs/day)		SABA	
GINA 2023	Preferred Controller and Reliever	As-needed-only Low Dose ICS-Form		Low Dose Maintenance ICS-Form	Med Dose Maintenance ICS-Form	Add on LAMA Refer for phenotypic assessment +/- biologic therapy. Consider High Dose ICS-Form	No Step 6
		Reliever: As needed Low Dose ICS-formoterol					
	Alternative Controller	Take ICS whenever SABA is taken	Low Dose Maintenance ICS	Low Dose Maintenance ICS-LABA	Med-High Dose Maintenance ICS-LABA	Add on LAMA Refer for phenotypic assessment +/- biologic therapy. Consider High Dose ICS-LABA	
		Reliever: As needed SABA or as-needed ICS-SABA					

in preschool children to determine the relative efficacies of these approaches. In school-age children with asthma, the use of a daily low-dose ICS can also be considered as an option in those children requiring Step 1 care [3].

16.6 MANAGEMENT OF PERSISTENT ASTHMA (STEP 2 CARE)

16.6.1 Daily Inhaled Corticosteroid Therapy

There is consensus among guidelines that children with persistent asthma should receive daily controller therapy to reduce the elements of asthma impairment and risk. Nearly all guidelines endorse low-dose ICS therapy as the preferred controller for the management of mild persistent asthma (Step 2), based upon a multitude of trials in preschool and school-age populations that demonstrate improvements in nearly all facets of asthma impairment and risk. Daily ICS therapy has consistently been shown to reduce days and nights with asthma symptoms, exacerbations requiring oral corticosteroids, healthcare utilization, urgent care visit, hospitalizations, as well as physiologic measures such as bronchial hyperresponsiveness and exhaled nitric oxide levels. While many studies have shown improvement in lung function (FEV_1) over relatively short time intervals (12 weeks), the Childhood Asthma Management Program (CAMP) demonstrated that among children 5–12 years of age with mild-moderate asthma, and despite significant improvements in multiple clinical measures of asthma control, there was no significant difference in lung function after 4.3 years of low-dose ICS therapy (budesonide 200 mcg twice daily) relative to placebo [14], nor was there a difference in lung function 4.8 years after stopping daily ICS therapy [15].

ICS therapy is generally well-tolerated by most pediatric patients. However, potential side effects of ICS therapy, which are generally dose-dependent, include alterations in skeletal growth, bone density, hypothalamic-pituitary-adrenal axis function, and local side effects including oral candidiasis and hoarseness. The clearly established clinical benefits provided by daily ICS therapy must be weighed against the potential risks associated with this approach in preschool children. The effect of ICS therapy on linear growth may be dependent on multiple factors, including age, weight, ICS dosing, specific ICS product, and delivery system. Multiple studies in school-age children have consistently demonstrated a clinically modest but statistically significant effect in linear growth (typically ~1.1 cm over the first year of therapy) with budesonide and beclomethasone, while studies in preschool-age children have been less consistent, demonstrating either similar growth effects [10, 16] or no statistically significant effects of ICS therapy [17–19] on growth velocity. Long-term follow-up reveals that the growth-suppressive effects of ICS therapy in children are generally small on average and appear to improve over time in most children, but there remain subgroups of children who experience greater than expected reductions in linear growth. Regular monitoring of growth in children receiving ICS therapy remains appropriate, with titration of the ICS dosing to the minimally effective dose.

16.6.2 Daily Leukotriene Receptor Antagonist Therapy

Among preschool children with persistent asthma, montelukast given daily over 12 weeks significantly reduces asthma symptom frequency, rescue albuterol use, oral corticosteroid use, peripheral blood eosinophil levels, bronchial hyperreactivity, and fractional exhaled nitric oxide levels [20–22]. Similarly, among school-age children montelukast therapy reduced asthma symptoms and rescue albuterol use while improving pulmonary function, quality of life, and peripheral blood eosinophil counts over an eight-week period in children 6–14 years of age with moderate asthma compared with placebo [23] as well as inhibiting exercise-induced bronchoconstriction in school-age children with mild to moderate asthma [24].

Montelukast therapy in children has achieved an excellent overall safety experience in pediatric patients, with upper respiratory tract infection, worsening asthma, pharyngitis, and fever reported as the most commonly reported side effects [25]. Neuropsychiatric events have been reported infrequently in patients of all ages taking montelukast, with preschool and school-age children not appearing to be more susceptible to such effects than older individuals [26]. Recently, the US Food and Drug Administration inserted a black box warning on montelukast to reflect this concern.

The NAEPP/EPR4 Guidelines [2] recommend low-dose ICS as the preferred controller at Step 2, with montelukast identified as an alternative based upon several comparative trials and supported by a meta-analysis demonstrating greater efficacy for ICS therapy in general, compared to LTRA in terms of markers of asthma control, including symptom reduction, exacerbation prevention, and lung function improvements [27–32]. However, not all patients achieve superior asthma control with ICS relative to LTRA, with recent research confirming that patient characteristics may identify patients who may experience a differential response to ICS and LTRA. A cross-over trial found that children with lower levels of lung function or high levels of markers of allergic inflammation (exhaled nitric oxide levels or greater airway hyperresponsiveness) were more likely to experience greater improvements in lung function (FEV_1) and other indicators of asthma control with ICS therapy than with LTRA [27, 28], suggesting that ICS may be preferred over LTRA in children with these features. However, children aged less than 10 years and those with urinary leukotriene C4 levels >100 pg/mg were more likely to experience at least a 7.5% improvement in FEV_1 while receiving montelukast over an eight-week period, but they did not experience comparable improvements while receiving ICS, further emphasizing the significant heterogeneity in response to asthma therapies. Based upon their overall efficacy relative to ICS, LTRAs may be considered an alternative to ICS as monotherapy at Step 2, if therapy is not desirable.

16.7 APPROACHES FOR CHILDREN NOT WELL CONTROLLED WITH STEP 2 (AND ABOVE) THERAPY

Among children with persistent asthma, most will achieve asthma control with Step 2 therapy. When children fail to achieve asthma control with either daily low-dose ICS or LTRA therapy, considerations should include (1) heterogeneity of drug response (and thus a trial of an alternate agent in Step 2), (2) suboptimal adherence to the medical regimen, (3) improper drug administration techniques (e.g. ineffective or incorrect inhalation technique), (4) comorbid conditions (e.g. rhinosinusitis, gastroesophageal reflux, and obesity), (5) ongoing trigger exposure (e.g. aeroallergens, environmental tobacco smoke, viral infections), and (6) psychosocial factors (e.g. maternal and/or child stress and/or depression). If consideration and modification of these factors does not produce asthma control, a step-up to Step 3 is indicated.

16.7.1 Step 3 Care and Above

For children 0–4 years of age, the NAEPP/EPR4 Guidelines recommend escalating therapy to medium-dose ICS therapy in patients not controlled with low-dose ICS therapy (Step 3), rather than the institution of combination therapy recommended in school-age children, in an effort to maximize the likelihood that an effective dose of ICS delivered to the lower airways before consideration of adjunctive (i.e. combination) therapy [2]. If use of medium-dose ICS therapy does not achieve well-controlled asthma in children 0–4 years of age, the NAEPP/EPR4 Guidelines suggest the following options for Step 4 care: the initiation of combination controller therapy with a medium-dose ICS along with either a long-acting beta-agonist (LABA) or alternatively with montelukast [2]. There are limited data in this age group to firmly support these recommendations in preschool children, and thus these recommendations are largely based on extrapolation from studies in older children and adults. One randomized trial demonstrated improved lung function but not reduction in asthma symptoms or rescue medication use among four- to seven-year-old children with multiple-trigger wheeze treated with ICS plus a LABA relative to ICS treatment alone, although participants who received ICS within the previous six months were excluded from this trial, and thus it is not clear if these participants would have demonstrated inadequate control while receiving ICS alone to warrant consideration of the addition of the LABA salmeterol [33]. Due to the sparsity of evidence in preschool children, the 2023 GINA guidelines prefer increasing the ICS dose if not well-controlled on low-dose ICS or adding montelukast rather than adding a LABA [3]. Clearly, additional adequately designed and powered prospective controlled trials of ICS+LABA therapy must be conducted in this age group to determine the appropriate role for LABA therapy.

For school-age children not well-controlled on low-dose ICS, both the NAEPP/EPR4 and GINA 2023 recommend the use of an ICS combined with formoterol for maintenance and reliever therapy (MART) [2, 3]. This is the NAEPP/EPR4 preferred option with other choices including (1) low-dose ICS + LABA, (2) low-dose ICS + LTRA, (3) low-dose ICS + theophylline, or (4) medium-dose ICS, although relatively limited data for these approaches are available in this age group [2]. For the children still having significant symptoms despite Step 3 therapy of very low-dose ICS + formoterol, low-dose ICS-LABA, or low-dose ICS + LTRA, GINA recommends advancing therapy to low-dose ICS + formoterol MART or medium-dose ICS-LABA, other alternatives including the addition of tiotropium or montelukast [3].

The role of the addition to LABA to ICS therapy in school-age children has been clarified over the past decade. An early trial demonstrated no difference in clinical or physiologic outcomes among children who received medium-dose ICS compared to those treated with low-dose ICS+LABA [34], and a more recent non-inferiority study demonstrated no differences in lung function, exacerbations, or adverse events between children treated with low-dose ICS+LABA and those treated with medium-dose ICS [35]. Two recent Cochrane Reviews concluded that the effect of addition of LABA therapy to ICS, when compared to either the same dose of ICS alone or with a higher dose of ICS alone, is not certain and may be associated with an increased risk of oral corticosteroid-treated exacerbations and hospitalizations [36, 37]. In children with persistent asthma, the addition of LABA to ICS was superior for improving lung function compared with the same or higher doses of ICS, while there was no difference in exacerbation rates [38]. Greater growth was seen with the use of ICS and LABA compared with a higher ICS dose [38]. In contrast, a meta-analysis concluded that there is insufficient evidence to determine whether the addition of LTRA to ICS improves asthma outcomes [32]. A prospective trial examined three step-up options among children 6–18 years of age with asthma inadequately controlled with low-dose ICS [39]. The addition of LABA to low-dose ICS was the approach most likely to produce the best response in terms of a composite outcome that included asthma exacerbations, episode-free days, and lung function. However, either of the other two therapies studied, the addition of an LTRA to low-dose ICS or an increase to medium-dose ICS, was the therapy most likely to produce the best response among substantial proportions of participants. These findings suggest that all three treatment strategies are indeed effective as step-up strategies among children with asthma inadequately controlled with low-dose ICS, since nearly all children respond best to one of these strategies. African American children were the least likely to show the best response to the addition of LTRA, and children without eczema were most likely to have the best response to LABA. Unfortunately, other predictors for which therapy is best for a given individual could not be clearly delineated. Thus, if a patient is inadequately controlled with a given Step 3 regimen, these data suggest changing to a different Step 3 approach before moving to Step 4.

The benefits associated with LABA therapy must be balanced against the potential risks of this class of therapeutics. Largely based upon trials in adolescents and adults, there appeared to be an increased risk of asthma-related death among patients who receive a LABA relative to those not treated with a LABA, although the largest studies demonstrating these effects did not mandate concomitant ICS use and provided LABA in a separate inhaler device, making it unclear whether concurrent ICS use mitigates the increased risk associated with LABA. As noted, while the evidence for efficacy of LABA therapy in school-age children appears generally supportive of this approach, several studies failed to demonstrate significant improvement with ICS+LABA therapy. An early study concluded that the use of a LABA-containing therapy was associated with increased likelihood of asthma-related death, intubation, and hospitalization among children, and that additional data are required to determine the risks of LABA in conjunction with ICS therapy [40]. In 2010, the FDA mandated that the four companies marketing LABAs for asthma perform prospective, randomized, controlled trials comparing the safety of combination therapy with a LABA plus an inhaled glucocorticoid with that of an inhaled glucocorticoid alone in adolescents (12–17 years of age) and adults. A joint oversight committee performed a combined analysis of the four trials comparing an inhaled glucocorticoid plus a LABA (combination therapy) with an inhaled glucocorticoid alone in 36,010 patients (3,608 children 12–17 years of age) [41]. The conclusion was that a combination therapy with a LABA plus an inhaled glucocorticoid did not result in a significantly higher risk of serious asthma-related events than treatment with an inhaled glucocorticoid alone but resulted in significantly fewer asthma exacerbations. In an international trial, 6208 children aged 4–11 years with asthma and an exacerbation in the previous year were randomized to LABA or placebo plus twice-daily ICS for 26 weeks. There was no significant difference between the ICS/LABA and ICS monotherapy groups in the primary safety end-point of a serious asthma-related event death, intubation, or hospitalization [42].

16.7.2 Temporary Step-Up in Anticipation of Exposure to Predictable Triggers

Asthma exacerbations consistently increase in prevalence in the month of September, presumably due to a combination of return to school and emergence of fall allergens and viral infections. Given the predictability of this increase, augmentation of therapy with montelukast in anticipation of this increase in risk has been evaluated. While one trial studying the addition of montelukast or placebo to usual asthma therapy from September 1 to October 15 among 2- to 14-year-olds demonstrated significant reductions in days with worse asthma symptoms (53% fewer) and unscheduled physician visits (78% fewer) [43], a second trial was unable to identify a clinically relevant effect of the addition of montelukast to standard therapy just prior to return to school in school-age children [44]. A trial among inner-city children with asthma examined an increase in ICS dosing prior to return to school in the fall and failed to demonstrate a protective effect in terms of exacerbation reduction during the fall season [45]. Thus it is unclear if such temporary step-up approaches provide consistent protection from the fall-time increase in asthma exacerbations.

16.7.3 Immunotherapy

The NAEPP/ERP4 Guidelines suggest that allergen immunotherapy be considered for patients five years and older with persistent asthma for whom there is a clear relationship between symptoms and exposure to an allergen to which the patient is sensitive [2]. A meta-analysis and an evidence-based review both concluded that specific immunotherapy is effective in the management of selected patients with allergic asthma [46, 47], particularly those with sensitization to a single allergen. In contrast, a large placebo-controlled trial evaluating the efficacy of multi-allergen immunotherapy for two years in asthmatic children did not demonstrate a benefit among children receiving appropriate medical treatment for asthma [48]. An early trial demonstrated that immunotherapy in monosensitized children with seasonal allergic rhinitis without asthma may prevent the subsequent development of asthma [49], suggesting that immunotherapy may allow for asthma prevention in children with sensitization to inhalant allergens.

16.8 MANAGEMENT OF SEVERE ASTHMA IN CHILDREN

The evaluation and management of the child who appears to have asthma that does not respond as expected to the Stepwise Approach to Asthma Care involves several considerations, as described in "Approaches for Children Not Well Controlled with Step 2 (and Above) Therapy," prior to further escalating Stepwise Care. However, should these additional strategies fail to bring asthma under control, further escalation of care becomes challenging due to a relative paucity of data to guide decision-making.

For children aged 0–4 years with severe asthma (i.e. those requiring Step 5 or 6 care), the NAEPP/EPR4 Guidelines recommend, based upon extrapolation from limited data in older children, the use of high-dose ICS therapy in combination with either a LABA or LTRA, and the addition of oral corticosteroids in the most extreme cases [2]. GINA recommends, for preschool children, to double the "low-dose" ICS and add LTRA if needed [3]. At this point, consider referral to a specialist. If despite these changes, the preschool child still is symptomatic, increase the ICS frequency or add intermittent ICS. GINA does not recommend adding LABAs in this age range due to lack of data and suggests increasing the frequency of ICS administration or adding intermittent ICS during the period of symptomatic worsening.

Similarly, for children 5–11 years of age with severe asthma, the NAEPP/EPR4 Guidelines recommend, based largely upon extrapolation from data in older children, the use of high-dose ICS therapy in combination with a LABA as preferred therapy at Step 5, with ICS+LTRA or ICS + theophylline as alternatives, and the addition of oral corticosteroids to ICS+LABA in those patients requiring Step 6 care [2]. At Step 5, GINA recommends referral for phenotypic assessment along with a trial of high-dose ICS therapy, consideration of add-on biologic therapy, or, as a last resort, consideration of OCS while carefully considering the side effect profile [3].

16.8.1 Omalizumab

The anti-IgE monoclonal antibody omalizumab is currently FDA approved for children with moderate to severe persistent asthma six years of age and older with perennial aeroallergen sensitivity and symptoms that are inadequately controlled with inhaled corticosteroids. Omalizumab effectively, rapidly, and significantly reduces circulating levels of IgE. Repeated subcutaneous administration of omalizumab has been demonstrated to be safe [50] and effective in permitting reduction of ICS dosing while preventing asthma exacerbations [51, 52] and improving asthma-related quality of life [53] in placebo-controlled trials involving children aged 6–12 years with moderate–severe persistent allergic asthma receiving ICS. A large trial conducted in 419 inner-city children and adolescents with asthma demonstrated that omalizumab therapy for 60 weeks produced a significant reduction in days with asthma symptoms and risk of exacerbation despite reductions in ICS and LABA use [54]. A small trial also demonstrated the ability of omalizumab to permit reduction in oral corticosteroid dosing in children 5–16 years of age receiving maintenance oral corticosteroids therapy [55]. Omalizumab is recommended by both the GINA and NAEPP/EPR4 guidelines as an optional adjunctive therapy for children six years of age and older with moderate–severe persistent allergic asthma whose symptoms are inadequately controlled with ICS therapy [2, 3].

16.8.2 Mepolizumab

Mepolizumab is an interleukin-5 (IL-5) antagonist monoclonal antibody that inhibits IL-5 signaling, thus reducing the production and survival of eosinophils. Mepolizumab has been demonstrated to reduce asthma exacerbation risk in adults and adolescents with severe eosinophilic asthma (DREAM [56], MENSA [57]) and was initially approved for use in children 6–11 years of age based upon a small open-label study focused on pharmacokinetics and pharmacodynamics [58]. Subsequently, the year-long MUPPITS2 trial in 290 inner-city children aged 6–17 years with severe eosinophilic, exacerbation-prone asthma demonstrated that the addition of mepolizumab to guideline-based care reduced the risk of severe exacerbations by 27% relative to placebo but did not impact other measures of asthma control or lung function [59]. GINA 2023 identifies mepolizumab as an alternative option at Step 5, whereas NAEPP/EPR4 does not comment on the role of mepolizumab in this age group [2, 3].

16.8.3 Dupilumab

Dupilumab is recombinant human IgG4 monoclonal anti-IL-4Rα antibody that inhibits both IL-4 and IL-13 pathways. A recent phase 3, randomized, double-blind, placebo-controlled trial involved 408 children between the ages of 6 and 11 years who had uncontrolled moderate to severe asthma to receive either dupilumab or placebo for 52 weeks [60]. Among patients with type 2 inflammation (blood eosinophils >=150 cells/uL or FeNO >=20pppb) or with blood eosinophils >=300 cells/uL, dupilumab significantly reduced this risk of severe asthma exacerbations by >50% and improved lung function and asthma control in these children with moderate to severe asthma. In 2021, the FDA expanded the approval of dupilumab to include children aged 6–11 years with moderate to severe asthma, and this is reflected in the 2023 GINA guidelines as a preferred option at Step 5 [3].

16.9 MANAGEMENT OF ASTHMA EXACERBATIONS

Exacerbations are often the dominant manifestation of asthma in young (i.e. preschool) children, and, while exacerbations tend to become less frequent as children age through adolescence, they remain a major source of morbidity. Viral infections, most notably human rhinoviruses, are the dominant trigger for acute exacerbations in childhood, with allergen-triggered exacerbations occurring less frequently.

An exacerbation may be defined as either moderate or severe [61], with moderate exacerbations consisting of events that are troublesome to the patient, do not represent the patient's usual day-to-day symptom variation, are not severe, but require prompt modification of treatment. A severe exacerbation is one that requires urgent action in order to prevent a serious outcome, such as asthma-related hospitalization or death.

The development of an exacerbation generally evolves over a period of days, highlighting the importance of the recognition of early changes in asthma status as antecedents to exacerbations. In addition to increases in typical asthma symptoms such as cough, wheeze, shortness of breath, other signs and symptoms often precede asthma exacerbations, including emergence of upper respiratory tract infectious symptoms, behavioral changes, and other non-specific symptoms [62, 63], and thus attention should be focused on the occurrence of such factors as a warning sign for impending asthma worsening.

16.10 QUICK RELIEVER MEDICATIONS

16.10.1 Beta-2 Adrenergic Agonists

Rapid-acting inhaled β_2-adrenergic receptor agonists produce bronchodilation and serve as the preferred treatment for acute symptoms and exacerbations of asthma. Several different β_2-agonists are currently available and have comparable efficacy and safety properties. As noted earlier, formoterol, a long-acting β_2-adrenergic receptor agonist, also has rapid onset properties that allows for use as a quick reliever.

16.10.2 Anticholinergic Agents

The parasympathetic nervous system contributes to the control of airway tone. In general, the degree of bronchodilation achieved with anticholinergic agents (such as atropine and ipratropium bromide) is less than that produced by inhaled β_2-agonists. The addition of ipratropium bromide to inhaled β_2-agonists in the emergency department during moderate–severe acute exacerbations of asthma in children decreases the rates of hospitalization [64] and duration of time in the emergency department [65], but no evidence supports the use of ipratropium in hospitalized patients.

16.10.3 Systemic Corticosteroids

Systemic corticosteroids may be considered quick-reliever medications due to their efficacy in moderate to severe acute exacerbations of asthma among school-age children. Systemic corticosteroids accelerate the resolution of acute exacerbations of asthma in school-age children, and emergency department administration of corticosteroids decreases asthma admission rates [66] and shortens the duration of hospitalization. In contrast, recent studies in preschool children with recurrent wheezing do not consistently demonstrate clinical improvement with systemic corticosteroids [67], and thus their use in wheezing exacerbations in this age group is currently uncertain [68]. Dosing recommendations for acute asthma range from 1 to 2 mg/kg of body weight per day of prednisone, with no significant difference in the efficacy of oral or parenteral corticosteroids in acute asthma [69], unless the child is unable to tolerate oral medications due to vomiting. Clinically relevant suppression of the HPA axis does not typically occur following short "bursts" of systemic corticosteroids for acute exacerbations of asthma, and tapering of the dose is not required with courses less than 10–14 days in duration.

16.11 MONITORING AND REASSESSMENT

The effective management of the child with asthma is an ongoing process, requiring frequent reassessments to determine the degree of asthma control achieved with a treatment regimen. In addition to general inquiry into the parent's and patient's perceptions of asthma status, several validated tools permit the longitudinal quantification of asthma control, including the Test for Respiratory and Asthma Control in Kids (TRACK) [70], the Childhood Asthma Control Test (C-ACT) [71, 72], and the Asthma Control Questionnaire (ACQ) [73].

Serial examination of pulmonary function via spirometry is an integral component of asthma monitoring and can generally be performed well by children over five years of age, and occasionally by four-year-old children. Spirometry measures the forced vital capacity (FVC), forced expiratory volume in one second (FEV_1), the ratio of FEV_1/FVC, as well as other measures of airflow including the forced expiratory flow between 25% and 75% of FVC (FEF_{25-75}). The FEV_1 is the most used and reproducible measure of pulmonary function, whereas the FEF_{25-75} demonstrates much more intrapatient variability. Standards are widely available for most spirometric measures and allow for correction based upon patient age, gender, race, and height. The FEV_1/FVC ratio is an indicator of airflow obstruction and may be more sensitive in identifying airflow abnormalities in asthma than the FEV_1, as most children with asthma have FEV_1 within the normal range, even in the presence of severe disease (see section on classification of asthma severity). Effective asthma therapy should lead to an improvement in, and ideally normalization of, the FEV_1 and the FEV_1/FVC ratio.

An assessment of the level of asthma symptom control, asthma-related morbidity as reflected by activity limitation, and school absences should be an integral component of every asthma visit. The frequency of rescue albuterol use and how frequently a canister of albuterol needs to be refilled due to use of the contents of a canister (200 actuations = 100 doses) are effective surrogate indicators of asthma control. The effect on the clinical course caused when the patient misses a dose (or several doses) of medications often provides valuable insight into disease activity.

16.11.1 Step-Down Therapy

If asthma is well-controlled for a period of at least three months, consideration should be given to a step-down in therapy [1]. Circumstances that may preclude a step-down even in the setting of well-controlled asthma include the impending exposure to a known trigger, such as return to school or an upcoming allergen or viral season, which has historically been associated with declines in asthma control. The general approach for step-down is to reduce therapy by one step at a time, although very little clinical trial evidence provides guidance as to the best strategy for this approach or how to best identify patients most likely to tolerate a step-down without deterioration in asthma control.

16.11.2 Step-Down to As-Needed Administration of ICS in Children with Mild Asthma

Recent attention has been directed to the use of ICS therapy on an as-needed basis, with ICS being administered whenever the child has asthma symptoms that require short-acting beta-agonist rescue therapy. Two trials have examined the use of ICS+ SABA use to daily ICS therapy. In a trial involving 288 children 5–18 years of age with mild persistent asthma that was demonstrated to be well-controlled on low-dose ICS therapy alone (beclomethasone 40 mcg twice daily), continuation of daily low-dose ICS therapy was superior to discontinuation of ICS in terms of exacerbations requiring oral corticosteroids but was associated with a 1.1 cm reduction in linear growth over the 44-week trial [8]. However, stepping down from daily ICS therapy to an ICS+SABA (beclomethasone 80 mcg whenever albuterol was used) resulted in fewer exacerbations than did discontinuation of ICS and was not associated with an adverse effect on linear growth. This study suggests that, among school-age children with mild asthma that is well-controlled on low-dose ICS, the use of ICS as rescue medication with albuterol might be an effective step-down strategy, as it is more effective than albuterol alone and avoids the ICS-related growth effects seen with daily ICS therapy. Similarly, in a trial involving 276 children 1–4 years of age with frequent wheeze, daily treatment with ICS (beclomethasone 400 mcg twice daily) was superior to as-needed SABA alone in terms of symptom-free days, SABA use, nocturnal awakenings, and time to first oral corticosteroid use [74]. However, there was not a statistically significant difference in these outcomes between the as-needed ICS+SABA group (beclomethasone 800 mcg each time albuterol was used) and the daily ICS group.

16.12 CONCLUSIONS

The evidence supporting treatment decision-making in the child with asthma has expanded substantially over the past decade. Optimal management entails continual reassessment focusing on the appropriate recognition and classification of disease severity and level of control and will result in minimization of asthma-related impairment and risk. Using an approach to stepwise care, attention should be paid to the need for step-up in care in the setting of suboptimal control as well as the potential step-down in care when disease control is achieved and maintained.

REFERENCES

1. National Asthma Education and Prevention Program, *Expert panel report III: Guidelines for the diagnosis and management of asthma*. Publication No. 08–4051. 2007. Bethesda, MD: US Department of Health and Human Services.
2. National Asthma Education and Prevention Program Committee, et al., *2020 Focused updates to the asthma management guidelines: A report from the national asthma education and prevention program coordinating committee expert panel working group*. J Allergy Clin Immunol, 2020. **146**(6): p. 1217–1270.
3. Global Initiative for Asthma. *Global strategy for asthma management and prevention, 2023*, 20 December 2023. Available from: www.ginasthma.org.
4. Brand, P.L., et al., *Definition, assessment and treatment of wheezing disorders in preschool children: an evidence-based approach*. Eur Respir J, 2008. **32**(4): p. 1096–1110.
5. Ducharme, F.M., et al., *Preemptive use of high-dose fluticasone for virus-induced wheezing in young children*. N Engl J Med2009. **360**(4): p. 339–353.
6. Bacharier, L.B., et al., *Episodic use of an inhaled corticosteroid or leukotriene receptor antagonist in preschool children with moderate-to-severe intermittent wheezing*. J Allergy Clin Immunol, 2008. **122**(6): p. 1127–1135 e8.
7. Bisgaard, H., et al., *Intermittent inhaled corticosteroids in infants with episodic wheezing*. N Engl J Med, 2006. **354**(19): p. 1998–2005.
8. Martinez, F.D., et al., *Use of beclomethasone dipropionate as rescue treatment for children with mild persistent asthma (TREXA): a randomised, double-blind, placebo-controlled trial*. Lancet, 2011. **377**(9766): p. 650–657.
9. Fitzpatrick, A.M., et al., *Individualized therapy for persistent asthma in young children*. J Allergy Clin Immunol, 2016. **138**(6): p. 1608–1618 e12.
10. Guilbert, T.W., et al., *Long-term inhaled corticosteroids in preschool children at high risk for asthma*. N Engl J Med, 2006. **354**(19): p. 1985–1997.
11. Castro-Rodriguez, J.A. and G.J. Rodrigo, *Efficacy of inhaled corticosteroids in infants and preschoolers with recurrent wheezing and asthma: a systematic review with meta-analysis*. Pediatrics, 2009. **123**(3): p. e519–e525.
12. Bisgaard, H., et al., *Montelukast reduces asthma exacerbations in 2- to 5-year-old children with intermittent asthma*. Am J Respir Crit Care Med, 2005. **171**(4): p. 315–322.
13. Zeiger, R.S., et al., *Daily or intermittent budesonide in preschool children with recurrent wheezing*. N Engl J Med, 2011. **365**(21): p. 1990–2001.
14. Childhood Asthma Management Program Group, *Long-term effects of budesonide or nedocromil in children with asthma*. N Engl J Med, 2000. **343**(15): p. 1054–1063.
15. Strunk, R.C., et al., *Mild to moderate asthma affects lung growth in children and adolescents*. J Allergy Clin Immunol, 2006. **118**(5): p. 1040–1047.
16. Skoner, D.P., et al., *Longitudinal growth in infants and young children treated with budesonide inhalation suspension for persistent asthma*. J Allergy Clin Immunol, 2000. **105**(2 Pt 1): p. 259–268.
17. Bisgaard, H., et al., *Twelve-month safety and efficacy of inhaled fluticasone propionate in children aged 1 to 3 years with recurrent wheezing*. Pediatrics, 2004. **113**(2): p. e87–94.
18. Baker, J., et al., *A multiple-dosing, placebo-controlled study of budesonide inhalation suspension given once or twice daily for treatment of persistent asthma in young children and infants*. Pediatrics, 1999. **103**: p. 414–421.
19. Shapiro, G., et al., *Efficacy and safety of budesonide inhalation suspension (Pulmicort Respules) in young children with inhaled steroid-dependent asthma*. J Allergy Clin Immunol, 1998. **102**: p. 789–796.
20. Knorr, B., et al., *Montelukast, a leukotriene receptor antagonist, for the treatment of persistent asthma in children aged 2 to 5 years*. Pediatrics, 2001. **108**(3): p. E48.
21. Hakim, F., et al., *The effect of montelukast on bronchial hyperreactivity in preschool children*. Chest2007. **131**(1): p. 180–186.
22. Moeller, A., et al., *Effects of montelukast on subjective and objective outcome measures in preschool asthmatic children*. Pediatr Pulmonol, 2008. **43**(2): p. 179–186.
23. Knorr, B., et al., *Montelukast for chronic asthma in 6- to 14-year-old children: a randomized, double-blind trial. Pediatric Montelukast Study Group*. Jama, 1998. **279**(15): p. 1181–1186.

24. Kemp, J.P., et al., *Montelukast once daily inhibits exercise-induced bronchoconstriction in 6- to 14-year-old children with asthma*. J Pediatr, 1998. **133**(3): p. 424–428.
25. Bisgaard, H., et al., *Safety and tolerability of montelukast in placebo-controlled pediatric studies and their open-label extensions*. Pediatr Pulmonol, 2009. **44**(6): p. 568–579.
26. Philip, G., et al., *Analysis of behavior-related adverse experiences in clinical trials of montelukast*. J Allergy Clin Immunol, 2009. **124**(4): p. 699–706 e8.
27. Szefler, S.J., et al., *Characterization of within-subject responses to fluticasone and montelukast in childhood asthma*. J Allergy Clin Immunol, 2005. **115**(2): p. 233–242.
28. Zeiger, R.S., et al., *Response profiles to fluticasone and montelukast in mild-to-moderate persistent childhood asthma*. J Allergy Clin Immunol, 2006. **117**(1): p. 45–52.
29. Garcia Garcia, M.L., et al., *Montelukast, compared with fluticasone, for control of asthma among 6- to 14-year-old patients with mild asthma: the MOSAIC study*. Pediatrics, 2005. **116**(2): p. 360–369.
30. Ostrom, N.K., et al.. *Comparative efficacy and safety of low-dose fluticasone propionate and montelukast in children with persistent asthma*. J Pediatr, 2005. **147**(2): p. 213–220.
31. Sorkness, C.A., et al., *Long-term comparison of 3 controller regimens for mild-moderate persistent childhood asthma: The pediatric asthma controller trial*. J Allergy Clin Immunol, 2007. **119**(1): p. 64–72.
32. Castro-Rodriguez, J.A. and G.J. Rodrigo, *The role of inhaled corticosteroids and montelukast in children with mild-moderate asthma: results of a systematic review with meta-analysis*. Arch Dis Child, 2010. **95**(5): p. 365–370.
33. Makela, M.J., et al., *Salmeterol and fluticasone in young children with multiple-trigger wheeze*. Ann Allergy Asthma Immunol, 2012. **109**(1): p. 65–70.
34. Verberne, A.A., et al., *Addition of salmeterol versus doubling the dose of beclomethasone in children with asthma. The Dutch asthma study group*. Am J Respir Crit Care Med, 1998. **158**(1): p. 213–219.
35. Vaessen-Verberne, A.A., et al., *Combination therapy salmeterol/fluticasone versus doubling dose of fluticasone in children with asthma*. Am J Respir Crit Care Med, 2010. **182**(10): p. 1221–1227.
36. Ducharme, F.M., et al., *Addition of long-acting beta2-agonists to inhaled corticosteroids versus same dose inhaled corticosteroids for chronic asthma in adults and children*. Cochrane Database Syst Rev, 2010(5): p. CD005535.
37. Ducharme, F.M., et al., *Addition of long-acting beta2-agonists to inhaled steroids versus higher dose inhaled steroids in adults and children with persistent asthma*. Cochrane Database Syst Rev, 2010(4): p. CD005533.
38. Chauhan, B.F., et al., *Addition of long-acting beta2-agonists to inhaled corticosteroids for chronic asthma in children*. Cochrane Database Syst Rev, 2015. **2015**(11): p. CD007949.
39. Lemanske, R.F., Jr., et al., *Step-up therapy for children with uncontrolled asthma receiving inhaled corticosteroids*. N Engl J Med, 2010. **362**(11): p. 975–985.
40. McMahon, A.W., et al., *Age and risks of FDA-approved long-acting beta(2)-adrenergic receptor agonists*. Pediatrics, 2011. **128**(5): p. e1147–1154.
41. Busse, W.W., et al., *Combined analysis of asthma safety trials of long-acting beta(2)-agonists*. N Engl J Med, 2018. **378**(26): p. 2497–2505.
42. Stempel, D.A., S.J. Szefler, and S.J. Pascoe, *Salmeterol and fluticasone propionate in children with asthma*. N Engl J Med, 2016. **375**(22): p. e46.
43. Johnston, N.W., et al., *Attenuation of the September epidemic of asthma exacerbations in children: a randomized, controlled trial of montelukast added to usual therapy*. Pediatrics, 2007. **120**(3): p. e702–e712.
44. Weiss, K.B., et al., *The back to school asthma study: the effect of montelukast on asthma burden when initiated prophylactically at the start of the school year*. Ann Allergy Asthma Immunol, 2010. **105**(2): p. 174–181.
45. Teach, S.J., et al., *Preseasonal treatment with either omalizumab or an inhaled corticosteroid boost to prevent fall asthma exacerbations*. J Allergy Clin Immunol, 2015. **136**(6): p. 1476–1485.
46. Abramson, M.J., R.M. Puy, and J.M. Weiner, *Injection allergen immunotherapy for asthma*. Cochrane Database Syst Rev, 2010(8): p. CD001186.
47. Larenas-Linnemann, D.E., D.R. Pietropaolo-Cienfuegos, and M.A. Calderon, *Evidence of effect of subcutaneous immunotherapy in children: complete and updated review from 2006 onward*. Ann Allergy Asthma Immunol, 2011. **107**(5): p. 407–416 e11.
48. Adkinson, N.F., Jr., et al., *A controlled trial of immunotherapy for asthma in allergic children*. N Engl J Med, 1997. **336**(5): p. 324–331.
49. Jacobsen, L., et al., *Specific immunotherapy has long-term preventive effect of seasonal and perennial asthma: 10-year follow-up on the PAT study*. Allergy, 2007. **62**(8): p. 943–948.
50. Berger, W., et al., *Evaluation of long-term safety of the anti-IgE antibody, omalizumab, in children with allergic asthma*. Ann Allergy Asthma Immunol, 2003. **91**(2): p. 182–188.
51. Milgrom, H., et al., *Treatment of childhood asthma with anti-immunoglobulin E antibody (omalizumab)*. Pediatrics, 2001. **108**(2): p. E36.
52. Lanier, B., et al., *Omalizumab for the treatment of exacerbations in children with inadequately controlled allergic (IgE-mediated) asthma*. J Allergy Clin Immunol, 2009. **124**(6): p. 1210–1216.
53. Lemanske, R.F., Jr., et al., *Omalizumab improves asthma-related quality of life in children with allergic asthma*. Pediatrics, 2002. **110**(5): p. e55.
54. Busse, W.W., et al., *Randomized trial of omalizumab (anti-IgE) for asthma in inner-city children*. N Engl J Med, 2011. **364**(11): p. 1005–1015.
55. Brodlie, M., et al., *The oral corticosteroid-sparing effect of omalizumab in children with severe asthma*. Arch Dis Child, 2012. **97**(7): p. 604–609.
56. Pavord, I.D., et al., *Mepolizumab for severe eosinophilic asthma (DREAM): a multicentre, double-blind, placebo-controlled trial*. Lancet, 2012. **380**(9842): p. 651–659.
57. Ortega, H.G., et al., *Mepolizumab treatment in patients with severe eosinophilic asthma*. N Engl J Med, 2014. **371**(13): p. 1198–1207.
58. Gupta, A., et al., *Subcutaneous mepolizumab in children aged 6 to 11 years with severe eosinophilic asthma*. Pediatr Pulmonol, 2019. **54**(12): p. 1957–1967.
59. Jackson, D.J., et al., *Mepolizumab for urban children with exacerbation-prone eosinophilic asthma in the USA (MUPPITS-2): a randomised, double-blind, placebo-controlled, parallel-group trial*. Lancet, 2022. **400**(10351): p. 502–511.
60. Bacharier, L.B., et al., *Dupilumab in children with uncontrolled moderate-to-severe asthma*. N Engl J Med, 2021. **385**(24): p. 2230–2240.
61. Reddel, H.K., et al., *An official American thoracic society/European respiratory society statement: asthma control and*

exacerbations: standardizing endpoints for clinical asthma trials and clinical practice. Am J Respir Crit Care Med, 2009. **180**(1): p. 59–99.
62. Rivera-Spoljaric, K., et al., *Caregivers report a wide variety of early signs and symptoms of impending asthma exacerbations that are not different between preschool and school-aged children*. J Allergy Clin Immunol, 2011. **128**(5): p. 1109–1111 e1–5.
63. Garbutt, J., et al., *Detection and home management of worsening asthma symptoms*. Ann Allergy Asthma Immunol, 2009. **103**(6): p. 469–473.
64. Qureshi, F., et al., *Effect of nebulized ipratropium on the hospitalization rates of children with asthma*. N Engl J Med, 1998. **339**(15): p. 1030–1035.
65. Zorc, J.J., et al., *Ipratropium bromide added to asthma treatment in the pediatric emergency department*. Pediatrics, 1999. **103**(4 Pt 1): p. 748–752.
66. Scarfone, R.J., et al., *Controlled trial of oral prednisone in the emergency department treatment of children with acute asthma*. Pediatrics, 1993. **92**(4): p. 513–518.
67. Panickar, J., et al., *Oral prednisolone for preschool children with acute virus-induced wheezing*. N Engl J Med, 2009. **360**(4): p. 329–338.
68. Guilbert, T.W. and L.B. Bacharier, *Controversies in the treatment of the acutely wheezing infant*. Am J Respir Crit Care Med, 2011. **183**(10): p. 1284–1285.
69. Becker, J.M., et al., *Oral versus intravenous corticosteroids in children hospitalized with asthma*. J Allergy Clin Immunol, 1999. **103**(4): p. 586–590.
70. Murphy, K.R., et al., *Test for respiratory and asthma control in kids (TRACK): a caregiver-completed questionnaire for preschool-aged children*. J Allergy Clin Immunol, 2009. **123**(4): p. 833–839 e9.
71. Liu, A.H., et al., *Development and cross-sectional validation of the childhood asthma control test*. J Allergy Clin Immunol, 2007. **119**(4): p. 817–825.
72. Liu, A.H., et al., *The childhood asthma control test: retrospective determination and clinical validation of a cut point to identify children with very poorly controlled asthma*. J Allergy Clin Immunol, 2010. **126**(2): p. 267–273, 273 e1.
73. Juniper, E.F., et al., *Development and validation of a questionnaire to measure asthma control*. Eur Respir J, 1999. **14**(4): p. 902–907.
74. Papi, A., et al., *Regular vs prn nebulized treatment in wheeze preschool children*. Allergy, 2009. **64**(10): p. 1463–1471.

17 Management of Adolescent Asthma

Laura Chen, Beverley J. Sheares, and Jean-Marie Bruzzese

CASE PRESENTATION

Jessica is a 15-year-old female who was diagnosed with asthma at five years of age. She has never had a severe asthma exacerbation or been hospitalized. Her mother, Anna, was vigilant about monitoring Jessica's symptoms and had consistently administered her daughter's daily inhaled corticosteroid until a year ago when Jessica started high school. Jessica has now started her sophomore year and has just made the basketball team. She leaves for school very early in the morning and often misses dinner due to basketball practice. On the weekends, she spends time with her friends. Because Jessica has been a straight-A student, her mother believes that she is responsibly balancing school with extracurricular activities. She assumes that Jessica is also taking her asthma medications and is symptom-free, as she is able to participate in sports and has not complained of symptoms. One day, Anna receives a call from Jessica's basketball coach telling her that Jessica is in an ambulance en route to the local emergency department. He reports that while at practice Jessica started coughing, became short of breath, and could barely speak. He also notes that Jessica had a cold two weeks previously and since then has been coughing during practice and has had wheezing and shortness of breath on occasion. However, she rests, and the symptoms abate. At the emergency department, Jessica is evaluated and treated for status asthmaticus. She is admitted to the pediatric intensive care unit for further management.

When her condition improves, after repeated questioning by the medical team, she casually acknowledges that with her long days and rigorous schedule, she often forgets to take her controller medication. Since she was feeling well and was able to succeed at basketball, she did not think much about missing the doses. In retrospect, Jessica recalls that she had noticed some increased night-time cough, as well as cough, chest tightness, and shortness of breath during the day that were worse during basketball practice, but she did not link this to her asthma. When asked, she reports that she tried vaping nicotine on a couple of occasions with her friends. Her understanding was that cigarettes trigger asthma but did not think e-cigarettes would be as harmful. She also did not want to feel left out or different from her friends who vaped.

Since the beginning of sophomore year, schoolwork has been getting increasingly harder, and Jessica endorses feeling anxious about maintaining her grades while trying out for the basketball team. Playing on the basketball team has been a priority for Jessica. Out of fear of isolation from the rest of her team members, she has been too embarrassed to take albuterol prior to or during practice in the presence of her peers.

Jessica's condition improves, and she is ready for discharge. Her mother threatens to resume responsibility for administering Jessica's asthma medications; however, Jessica protests that she is too old to have her mother give her medicine like she is a child. Both Jessica and her mother are left with many questions on how to manage Jessica's asthma at this stage in her development.

17.1 INTRODUCTION

The successful, ongoing treatment of asthma in adolescents presents numerous challenges because adolescence is a time of profound and rapid change. It is marked by the development of new cognitive skills, independent decision-making, and increased peer pressure. Delivering effective care to reduce asthma morbidity and mortality and improve the quality of life and health of adolescents with asthma requires clinicians to have knowledge and effectively implement state-of-the-art asthma care while understanding the role that cognitive and psychosocial development play in asthma management by this age group. To that end, this chapter reviews the epidemiology and natural history of asthma related to adolescents, discusses updates in clinical management, and examines how the developmental features of adolescence affect self-management and treatment of asthma. We also review the literature focused on asthma in adolescents belonging to different identity groups and the role of social and structural drivers of health on asthma morbidity in adolescents.

17.2 EPIDEMIOLOGY

Adolescence is defined as individuals aged 11–21 years[1] and is divided into three age groups: (1) early adolescents (11–14 years), (2) middle adolescents (15–17 years), and (3) late adolescents (18–21 years).[2] While asthma prevalence has leveled off in younger children, this is not true of adolescence where there is a rise in prevalence.[3] Compared to

DOI: 10.1201/9781003287209-22

children 0–10 years old, early and middle adolescents have a higher asthma prevalence.[4, 5] Adolescents are at increased risk of asthma-related morbidities.[4, 6, 7] Routine asthma care use among adolescents is less than optimal,[8–10] which may contribute to these morbidities.

Several groups of adolescents are also at greater risk for asthma and asthma-related morbidities. Non-Hispanic Black and Hispanic adolescents,[4, 5, 11–13] as well adolescents living below the Federal Poverty Level,[4, 5] are at increased risk of having asthma and the deleterious effects of the disease. Most recently, data has supported asthma disparities among sexual and gender minority adolescents (SGM: e.g. lesbian, gay, bisexual, queer, transgender, non-binary), with SGM youth being at greater risk for ever being diagnosed with asthma[14] and having non-remitting asthma.[15]

17.3 FACTORS CONTRIBUTING TO MORBIDITY

While there are noted differences in asthma prevalence and outcomes among racial and ethnic marginalized groups and low-resourced families, data now suggests that the factors most cited—older housing stock, greater population density, environmental exposures,[16] and decreased access to specialty care[17]—are closely linked with historical and contemporary structural and systemic racism that worsens asthma outcomes in patients from marginalized groups.[18] Racist and discriminatory practices in the healthcare system are linked to mistrust of clinicians.[19, 20] In a recent study among rural adolescents with asthma, Black adolescents reported significantly more medical mistrust, particularly suspicion of and lack of support from clinicians.[21]

The connection between poverty and asthma has been well described. Adolescents living in neighborhoods that have been subjected to divestment with few resources, with a shortage of high-quality, healthy housing, increased indoor triggering environmental exposures, high population density, communities overburdened by outdoor pollution near highways, and those lacking access to high-quality asthma care, are more likely to have poorly controlled asthma.[22] A recent study showed that moving children and adolescents from high-poverty to low-poverty neighborhoods resulted in significant improvements in days with asthma symptoms and exacerbations.[23] Moreover, measures of stress including social cohesion, neighborhood safety, and urban stress all improved significantly after moving.[23] These findings suggest that anti-poverty structural changes, although expensive and intensive, may address one of the root causes for ongoing asthma disparities among adolescents living in poverty.

Asthma disparities among SGM adolescents may be explained in part by the increased use of inhaled substances (e.g. cigarettes, electronic vaping products, synthetic marijuana).[14] Factors related to weight and stress due to bullying may also contribute to these disparities.[15] Asthma disparities experienced by SGM adolescents may be also attributed to discrimination associated with SGM identity. The Minority Stress Model postulates that minority stress, or the combined effect of stressors that occur due to SGM identity, impacts both physical and mental health.[24] Stressors are exacerbated when multiple systems of oppression (e.g. SGM identity, race, ethnicity, class) converge or intersect.[25] Adolescents with multiple marginalized identities may be at greatest risk for disparate asthma outcomes.[15]

Stress has been well described as influencing asthma outcomes in adolescents.[26, 27] One of the effects of repeated stressful life events, including adverse childhood experiences and interpersonal racism, is dysregulation of allostasis,[28] the process by which the body maintains physiological homeostasis as it responds to external stress. Stress activates inflammation in asthma. When patients with asthma encounter chronic stress, cortisol levels increase, which results in a state of increased inflammation. This in turn can worsen asthma symptoms and control. Allostatic load refers to the cumulative burden exacted on the body through repetitive adaptation to physical and emotional stress.[29] Everyday discrimination is increasingly recognized as a significant contributor to stress and adverse outcomes in asthma that lead to disparities.[30, 31]

17.4 NATURAL HISTORY OF ASTHMA IN ADOLESCENCE

A commonly held notion that asthma remits during adolescence is drawn mostly from clinical anecdotal experience. It is unclear if the improvement or lack of symptoms indicates remission of asthma as there are various phenotypes of asthma. Population longitudinal cohort studies have shown that children with transient wheeze during infancy rarely continue to have or develop asthma in later childhood or adolescence;[32] however, persistent wheezing and airway hyperresponsiveness at age six and beyond is associated with persistent wheezing in adolescence through adulthood.[33, 34] Moreover, even if fewer asthma symptoms are seen during adolescence, pulmonary function test (PFT) abnormalities such as airway hyperresponsiveness may still be present.[32] Adolescents with persistent airway hyperresponsiveness are at increased risk of airflow obstruction and potential chronic obstructive pulmonary disease in adulthood.[34] Thus airway hyperresponsiveness seen on PFTs are important predictors of persistent asthma and symptoms during adolescence.[34, 35] However, an absence of symptoms, no use of inhaled and systemic corticosteroids for long periods of time, lack of airway hyperresponsiveness, or unimpaired lung function may suggest complete remission.[32]

Risk factors associated with persistent asthma and wheezing during adolescence, which affects about 3–5% of individuals with asthma, are multifactorial.[32] Such risk factors include parental history of asthma, persistent atopy, eosinophilia in the airways, air pollution exposure, certain respiratory tract infections early in childhood, hormonal changes, and genetic influences.[32, 36] During puberty, changes in androgen levels may mediate smooth muscle airway activity. For example, a rise in testosterone is associated with increased smooth muscle relaxation with anti-inflammatory properties,[32] whereas higher estrogen levels may be associated with higher beta-2 adrenergic receptor density, thereby increasing smooth muscle activity.[35] The presence of genetic polymorphisms and epigenetics may also play a role in persistent asthma.[37–39] A longitudinal study of parents and children with asthma has shown that upregulation of the gasdermin B or orosomucoid like 3 genes located on chromosome 17q21 (*GSDMB* and *ORMDL3*) may have a significant effect on persistent wheezing through adulthood.[40] Three independent population birth cohort studies have also demonstrated that lower levels of circulating Club Cell Secretory Protein (CC16), which is found abundantly in airway secretions but may be measured in serum, is associated with persistent asthma symptoms from childhood into adulthood and may be an important emerging biomarker of persistent asthma.[41]

17.5 GUIDELINES FOR THE TREATMENT OF ADOLESCENT ASTHMA

The most recent guidelines from the updated Expert Panel Report 3 (EPR-3) in the United States[42–44] and the International Global Initiative for Asthma[45] guidelines emphasize the need to achieve control of asthma symptoms, thereby reducing impairment and risk for future morbidity—all goals that are most pertinent to the adolescent patient. These guidelines provide tools to help clinicians assess the patient's level of asthma severity prior to the start of treatment, as well as the patient's level of asthma control once on medications. Figures 17.1 and 17.2 provide the updated EPR-3 criteria to assess the severity and control among different age groups including adolescents.[43]

As detailed in Figure 17.2, the two main domains of asthma control are impairment and risk. The prevention of chronic, recurrent symptoms, the reduction in beta-agonist use, the maintenance of normal or near-normal lung function, the resumption or maintenance of activities of daily living (including exercise) as measured by validated questionnaire such as the Asthma Control Test, and meeting the patient's and family's expectations and satisfaction with care are the goals of reducing the patient's impairment from asthma. Reducing the risk for future adverse effects includes the prevention of recurrent exacerbations and a reduction in the need for emergency department visits and hospitalizations, the prevention of the loss of lung function, and the provision of an optimal medication regimen with minimal adverse effects that the patient can follow.[42, 43]

A stepwise approach to medications is recommended in order to get asthma symptoms under control as reflected in the 2020 updates to the EPR3 (see Figure 17.3 for a stepwise plan).[46] The type, amount, and frequency of medications are determined by the level of asthma severity. The level of severity provides a guide for the initiation of therapy in a patient who is not currently taking long-term controller medications. A key approach to reducing asthma symptoms is to select a medication regimen corresponding to the highest level of asthma severity for the patient and, once their asthma symptoms, lung function, and activity levels are optimized, step down the therapy to the least amount of medicine required to maintain adequate asthma control and to reduce medication side effects. Once the patient is taking long-term controller medications, the response to the therapy and the control of the symptoms should guide the clinician's decision-making regarding which step of care is appropriate.

Key changes were made in 2020 to the EPR3. Adolescents with mild persistent asthma who fall under Step 2 (Figure 17.3 and Figure 17.4) are recommended to be either on a daily low-dose ICS and an as-needed SABA or to be on an as-needed ICS and SABA when having an acute exacerbation.[46] Patients who may be under- or over-perceivers of their asthma symptoms are not advised to use as-needed ICS and SABA, as they may benefit more from daily controller use.[46] The preferred therapy for adolescents with asthma with moderate to severe persistent asthma who fall under Steps 3 and 4 is an inhaled ICS-formoterol, to be used as a "single maintenance and reliever therapy," or SMART therapy.[46] Patients whose asthma is well-controlled on a daily ICS and as-needed SABA are recommended to continue this regimen, but if their asthma is not well or is poorly controlled on this regimen, SMART therapy is preferred prior to stepping up therapy. Evidence in support of SMART therapy versus same-dose ICS or ICS-formoterol in adolescents has shown an overall reduction in asthma exacerbations and decrease in inhaled and systemic corticosteroid use when SMART therapy is used.[47–49]

Close monitoring is essential to ensure that asthma control is achieved. Lung function monitoring is an invaluable tool in the adolescent population when symptoms may be unrecognized and underreported. It is also useful for monitoring disease progression over time and for monitoring the response and adherence to medications.[45, 46] As studies show that adolescents with asthma demonstrate a tendency toward under-perception of their symptoms[50] and inaccurate perception of asthma control,[50] objective measures of lung function are helpful.

It is recommended that patients receive a written asthma action plan that details the day-to-day management of their asthma, how to recognize and respond to specific symptoms, and when to seek medical care.[45, 46] There should be consideration of the patient's health literacy level when providing specific instructions for the administration of medications and engaging in discussions regarding the management of exercise-induced symptoms, and the identification and avoidance of specific triggers.[51] A copy should be provided to the patient's school nurse.[45, 46]

The adolescent patient should be directly involved in the formulation of the asthma treatment plan in establishing goals for therapy, and the plan should be realistic and achievable. To accomplish these goals, it is recommended that the adolescent meet with the clinician without the

	Components of Severity	Intermittent			Persistent: Mild			Persistent: Moderate			Persistent: Severe		
		Ages 0–4 years	Ages 5–11 years	Ages ≥12 years	Ages 0–4 years	Ages 5–11 years	Ages ≥12 years	Ages 0–4 years	Ages 5–11 years	Ages ≥12 years	Ages 0–4 years	Ages 5–11 years	Ages ≥12 years
Impairment	Symptoms	≤2 days/week			>2 days/week but not daily			Daily			Throughout the day		
	Nighttime awakenings	0	≤2x/month		1–2x/month	3–4x/month		3–4x/month	>1x/week but not nightly		>1x/week	Often 7x/week	
	SABA* use for symptom control (not to prevent EIB*)	≤2 days/week			>2 days/week but not daily	>2 days/week but not daily and not more than once on any day		Daily			Several times per day		
	Interference with normal activity	None			Minor limitation			Some limitation			Extremely limited		
	Lung function		Normal FEV_1 between exacerbations	Normal FEV_1 between exacerbations									
	➔ FEV_1* (% predicted)	Not applicable	>80%	>80%	Not applicable	>80%	>80%	Not applicable	60–80%	60–80%	Not applicable	<60%	<60%
	➔ FEV_1/FVC*		>85%	Normal†		>80%	Normal†		75–80%	Reduced 5%†		<75%	Reduced >5%†
Risk	Asthma exacerbations requiring oral systemic corticosteroids‡	0–1/year			≥2 exacerb. in 6 months, or wheezing ≥4x per year lasting >1 day AND risk factors for persistent asthma	≥2/year		Generally, more frequent and intense events indicate greater severity. (0–4 years)			Generally, more frequent and intense events indicate greater severity. (5–11 and ≥12 years)		
		Consider severity and interval since last asthma exacerbation. Frequency and severity may fluctuate over time for patients in any severity category. Relative annual risk of exacerbations may be related to FEV_1.*											
Recommended Step for Initiating Therapy	(See "Stepwise Approach for Managing Asthma Long Term," page 7.) The stepwise approach is meant to help, not replace, the clinical decision making needed to meet individual patient needs.	Step 1			Step 2			Step 3	Step 3 Medium-dose ICS* option	Step 3	Step 3	Step 3 Medium-dose ICS* option or Step 4	Step 4 or 5
								Consider short course of oral systemic corticosteroids.					
		In 2–6 weeks, depending on severity, assess level of asthma control achieved and adjust therapy as needed. For children 0–4 years old, if no clear benefit is observed in 4–6 weeks, consider adjusting therapy or alternate diagnoses.											

FIGURE 17.1 Initial visit: Classifying asthma severity and initiating therapy: Level of severity (Columns 2–5) is determined by events listed in Column 1 for both impairment (frequency and intensity of symptoms and functional limitations) and risk (of exacerbations). Assess impairment by patient's or caregiver's recall of events during the previous 2–4 weeks; assess risk over the last year. Recommendations for initiating therapy based on level of severity are presented in the last row. *Abbreviations: EIB: exercise-induced bronchospasm; FEV_1: forced expiratory volume in 1 second; FVC, forced vital capacity; ICS, inhaled corticosteroid; SABA, short-acting beta$_2$-agonist. †Normal FEV_1/FVC by age: 8–19 years, 85%; 20–39 years, 80%; 40–59 years, 75%; 60–80 years, 70%. ‡Data are insufficient to link frequencies of exacerbations with different levels of asthma severity. Generally, more frequent and intense exacerbations (e.g. requiring urgent care, hospital or intensive care admission, and/or oral corticosteroids) indicate greater underlying disease severity. For treatment purposes, patients with ≥2 exacerbations may be considered to have persistent asthma, even in the absence of impairment levels consistent with persistent asthma. (From National Heart, Lung, and Blood Institute; National Institutes of Health; US Department of Health and Human Services.)

	Components of Control	Well Controlled			Not Well Controlled			Very Poorly Controlled		
		Ages 0–4 years	Ages 5–11 years	Ages ≥12 years	Ages 0–4 years	Ages 5–11 years	Ages ≥12 years	Ages 0–4 years	Ages 5–11 years	Ages ≥12 years
Impairment	Symptoms	≤2 days/week	≤2 days/week but not more than once on each day	≤2 days/week	>2 days/week	>2 days/week or multiple times on ≤2 days/week	>2 days/week	Throughout the day		
	Nighttime awakenings	≤1x/month		≤2x/month	>1x/month	≥2x/month	1–3x/week	>1x/week	≥2x/week	≥4x/week
	Interference with normal activity	None			Some limitation			Extremely limited		
	SABA* use for symptom control (not to prevent EIB*)	≤2 days/week			>2 days/week			Several times per day		
	Lung function									
	➔ FEV_1* (*% predicted*) or peak flow (*% personal best*)	Not applicable	>80%	>80%	Not applicable	60–80%	60–80%	Not applicable	<60%	<60%
	➔ FEV_1/FVC*		>80%	Not applicable		75–80%	Not applicable		<75%	Not applicable
	Validated questionnaires† ➔ ATAQ* ➔ ACQ* ➔ ACT*	Not applicable	Not applicable	0 ≤0.75‡ ≥20	Not applicable	Not applicable	1–2 ≥1.5 16–19	Not applicable	Not applicable	3–4 Not applicable ≤15
Risk	Asthma exacerbations requiring oral systemic corticosteroids§	0–1/year			2–3/year	≥2/year		>3/year	≥2/year	
		Consider severity and interval since last asthma exacerbation.								
	Reduction in lung growth/Progressive loss of lung function	Not applicable	Evaluation requires long-term follow-up care.		Not applicable	Evaluation requires long-term follow-up care.		Not applicable	Evaluation requires long-term follow-up care.	
	Treatment-related adverse effects	*Medication side effects can vary in intensity from none to very troublesome and worrisome. The level of intensity does not correlate to specific levels of control but should be considered in the overall assessment of risk.*								
Recommended Action for Treatment	*(See "Stepwise Approach for Managing Asthma Long Term," page 7)* *The stepwise approach is meant to help, not replace, the clinical decision-making needed to meet individual patient needs.*	*Maintain current step.* *Regular follow-up every 1–6 months.* *Consider step down if well controlled for at least 3 months.*			Step up 1 step	Step up at least 1 step	Step up 1 step	*Consider short course of oral systemic corticosteroids.* *Step up 1–2 steps.* *Reevaluate in 2 weeks to achieve control.*		
					Reevaluate in 2–6 weeks to achieve control. *For children 0–4 years, if no clear benefit observed in 4–6 weeks, consider adjusting therapy or alternative diagnoses.*					
					Before step up in treatment: Review adherence to medication, inhaler technique, and environmental control. If alternative treatment was used, discontinue and use preferred treatment for that step. For side effects, consider alternative treatment options.					

FIGURE 17.2 Follow-up visits: Assessing asthma control and adjusting therapy. Level of control (Columns 2–4) is based on the most severe component of impairment (symptoms and functional limitations) or risk (exacerbations). Assess impairment by patient's or caregiver's recall of events listed in Column 1 during the previous 2–4 weeks and by spirometry and/or peak flow measures. Symptom assessment for longer periods should reflect a global assessment, such as inquiring whether the patient's asthma is better or worse since the last visit. Assess risk by recall of exacerbations during the previous year and since the last visit. Recommendations for adjusting therapy based on level of control are presented in the last row.

Abbreviations: ACQ, Asthma Control Questionnaire©; ACT, Asthma Control Test™; ATAQ, Asthma Therapy Assessment Questionnaire©; EIB, exercise-induced bronchospasm; FVC, forced vital capacity; FEV_1, forced expiratory volume in 1 second; SABA, short-acting $beta_2$-agonist.

†Minimal important difference: 1.0 for the ATAQ; 0.5 for the ACQ; not determined for the ACT.

‡ACQ values of 0.76–1.4 are indeterminate regarding well-controlled asthma.

§Data are insufficient to link frequencies of exacerbations with different levels of asthma control. Generally, more frequent and intense exacerbations (e.g. requiring urgent care, hospital or intensive care admission, and/or oral corticosteroids) indicate poorer asthma control.

(From National Heart, Lung, and Blood Institute; National Institutes of Health; US Department of Health and Human Services.)

	Intermittent Asthma	Management of Persistent Asthma in Individuals Ages 12+ Years				
Treatment	STEP 1	STEP 2	STEP 3	STEP 4	STEP 5	STEP 6■
Preferred	PRN SABA	Daily low-dose ICS and PRN SABA or PRN concomitant ICS and SABA▲	Daily and PRN combination low-dose ICS-formoterol▲	Daily and PRN combination medium-dose ICS-formoterol▲	Daily medium-high dose ICS-LABA + LAMA and PRN SABA▲	Daily high-dose ICS-LABA + oral systemic corticosteroids + PRN SABA
Alternative		Daily LTRA* and PRN SABA or Cromolyn,* or Nedocromil,* or Zileuton,* or Theophylline,* and PRN SABA	Daily medium-dose ICS and PRN SABA or Daily low-dose ICS-LABA, or daily low-dose ICS + LAMA,▲ or daily low-dose ICS + LTRA,* and PRN SABA or Daily low-dose ICS + Theophylline* or Zileuton,* and PRN SABA	Daily medium-dose ICS-LABA or daily medium-dose ICS + LAMA, and PRN SABA▲ or Daily medium-dose ICS + LTRA,* or daily medium-dose ICS + Theophylline,* or daily medium-dose ICS + Zileuton,* and PRN SABA	Daily medium-high dose ICS-LABA or daily high-dose ICS + LTRA,* and PRN SABA	
		Steps 2–4: Conditionally recommend the use of subcutaneous immunotherapy as an adjunct treatment to standard pharmacotherapy in individuals ≥ 5 years of age whose asthma is controlled at the initiation, build up, and maintenance phases of immunotherapy▲			Consider adding Asthma Biologics (e.g. anti-IgE, anti-IL5, anti-IL5R, anti-IL4/IL13)**	

Assess Control

- First check adherence, inhaler technique, environmental factors,▲ and comorbid conditions.
- **Step up** if needed; reassess in 2–6 weeks.
- **Step down** if possible (if asthma is well controlled for at least 3 consecutive months)

Consult with asthma specialist if Step 4 or higher is required. Consider consultation at Step 3.

Control assessment is a key element of asthma care. This involves both impairment and risk. Use of objective measures, self-reported control, and healthcare utilization are complementary and should be employed on an ongoing basis, depending on the individual's clinical situation.

FIGURE 17.3 Stepwise approach for management of asthma in individuals ages 12 years and older. Abbreviations: ICS, inhaled corticosteroid; LABA, long-acting beta$_2$-agonist; LAMA, long-acting muscarinic antagonist; LTRA, leukotriene receptor antagonist; SABA, inhaled short-acting beta$_2$-agonist.▲Updated based on the 2020 guidelines.

***Cromolyn, nedocromil, LTRAs including zileuton and montelukast, and theophylline were not considered for this update and/or have limited availability for use in the United States and/or have an increased risk of adverse consequences and need for monitoring that make their use less desirable. The FDA issued a boxed warning for montelukast in March 2020.**

****The AHRQ systematic reviews that informed this report did not include studies that examined the role of asthma biologics (e.g. anti-IgE, anti-IL5, anti-IL5R, anti-IL4/IL13). Thus this report does not contain specific recommendations for the use of biologics in asthma in Steps 5 and 6. ▪ Data on the use of LAMA therapy in individuals with severe persistent asthma (Step 6) were not included in the AHRQ systematic review, and thus no recommendation is made.**

(From National Heart, Lung, and Blood Institute; National Institutes of Health; US Department of Health and Human Services).

parents or caregivers present at the beginning of the visit. This allows adolescent patients to assume more control and take more responsibility for their asthma management. Parents or caregivers should be brought in at the end of the visit to review the plan together so that they can support the patient's efforts. The plan should encompass goals that personally benefit the adolescent, such as looking and feeling better (self-image), fully participating in physical activities and organized sports, or reduction of symptoms when around friends (peer acceptance). These types of rewards are important to adolescent patients, and achieving asthma control provides positive feedback that reinforces their efforts.

Using PFTs may be helpful when assessing asthma control (Figure 17.2). Traditionally, PFT normative reference values have been dependent on equations based on a

Quick-relief medications	• Use SABA as needed for symptoms. The intensity of treatment depends on the severity of symptoms: up to three treatments at 20-minute intervals as needed. • In Steps 3 and 4, the preferred option includes the use of ICS-formoterol one to two puffs as needed up to a maximum total daily maintenance and rescue dose of 12 puffs (54 mcg).▲ • **Caution:** Increasing use of SABA or use >2 days a week for symptom relief (not prevention of EIB) generally indicates inadequate control and may require a step up in treatment.
Each step: Assess environmental factors, provide patient education, and manage comorbidities▲	• In individuals with sensitization (or symptoms) related to exposure to pests:‡ conditionally recommend integrated pest management as a single or multicomponent allergen-specific mitigation intervention.▲ • In individuals with sensitization (or symptoms) related to exposure to identified indoor allergens, conditionally recommend a multicomponent allergen-specific mitigation strategy.▲ • In individuals with sensitization (or symptoms) related to exposure to dust mites, conditionally recommend impermeable pillow/mattress covers only as part of a multicomponent allergen-specific mitigation intervention but not as a single component intervention.▲

FIGURE 17.4 Notes for individuals ages 12+ years diagram in Figure 17.3. Abbreviations: EIB, exercise-induced bronchoconstriction; FeNO, fractional exhaled nitric oxide; ICS, inhaled corticosteroid; LABA, long-acting beta$_2$-agonist; SABA, inhaled short-acting beta$_2$-agonist. ▲Updated based on the 2020 guidelines.

‡Refers to mice and cockroaches, which were specifically examined in the Agency for Healthcare Research and Quality systematic review. The terms ICS-LABA and ICS-formoterol indicate combination therapy with both an ICS and a LABA, usually and preferably in a single inhaler. Where formoterol is specified in the steps, it is because the evidence is based on studies specific to formoterol. In individuals ages 12 years and older with persistent allergic asthma in which there is uncertainty in choosing, monitoring, or adjusting anti-inflammatory therapies based on history, clinical findings, and spirometry, FeNO measurement is conditionally recommended as part of an ongoing asthma monitoring and management strategy that includes frequent assessment. Bronchial thermoplasty was evaluated in Step 6. The outcome was a conditional recommendation against the therapy. (From National Heart, Lung, and Blood Institute; National Institutes of Health; US Department of Health and Human Services.)

patient's age, height, race, and ethnicity. Using race- and ethnicity-based PFT average reference equations has been found to underestimate severity of, miss, or delay diagnoses in people of color.[52] In 2021, the American Thoracic Society evaluated the use of race and ethnicity in PFT interpretation and currently recommends using race-neutral average reference equations.[52] As race is a social construct, it does not infer biological characteristics and fails to consider the effects of structural determinants of health (e.g. stress, racism, and housing, economic, and educational policies) on lung health. Additionally, lung health is impacted by downstream social determinants of health, such as increased risk of preterm birth, early exposure to respiratory infections due to overcrowding, air pollution, or secondhand smoke.

In transgender youth, there is currently little data on how to interpret spirometry, especially in adolescents undergoing gender-affirming hormone therapy. As mentioned previously, hormones may affect airway smooth muscle activity. More research is needed to understand the impact of higher levels of testosterone or the use of testosterone blockers on lung function. Although there are currently no formal recommendations on spirometry interpretation in transgender non-binary individuals, it is proposed that those who undergo gender-affirming hormone therapy during early puberty will likely have lung function that closely aligns with their affirmed gender. The availability of spirometry with both gender reference ranges may also be helpful to clinicians.[53]

17.6 ADOLESCENTS WHO DO NOT RESPOND TO THERAPY

The diagnosis of asthma requires episodic symptoms consistent with airflow obstruction or hyperresponsiveness and airway obstruction that are at least partially reversible. Additionally, alternative diagnoses should be excluded. Although patients with asthma present in different ways, most share common clinical and historical features that support the diagnosis. The use of lung function measurements, bronchial challenges, exercise challenges, and allergy skin tests to support the diagnosis is helpful, and, in some cases, it is necessary. Adolescent patients often describe symptoms of chest tightness with colds, chest congestion, and bronchitis. The symptoms occur more often at night and in the early morning hours and improve throughout the day.[54] Patients may also only present with exercise-induced dyspnea.[55] However, because many adolescents either deny their symptoms, or they underestimate or are unaware of the severity of their symptoms, the respiratory problem may not be diagnosed, or, if it is diagnosed, it may be undertreated.[56]

For some adolescents, their history, clinical findings, response to therapy, and ancillary test results are inconsistent with a diagnosis of asthma. In these cases, alternative diagnoses should be considered, including cystic fibrosis, primary ciliary dyskinesia, immunodeficiency, lung restriction, congenital malformations, and congenital heart disease.[55, 56]

Other more common differentials to consider that may also coexist with asthma include gastroesophageal reflux and allergic rhinitis.[54] Reflux of acid or non-acid contents in the distal esophagus may lead to cough and bronchospasm mediated via stimulation of the vagal nerve or possibly via micro-aspiration of gastric material.[54] Allergic rhinitis may result in postnasal drip and cough. Emerging evidence has shown that there may be a common inflammatory and immune process between allergic rhinitis and asthma triggered by allergies.[54]

Special attention should be given to paradoxical vocal fold motion (PVFM), otherwise known as vocal cord dysfunction, or by its physiologic term, inducible laryngeal obstruction. PVFM is a condition where the vocal cords will paradoxically and intermittently adduct during inspiration, resulting in upper airflow obstruction, and signs and symptoms such as stridor, shortness of breath, and wheezing.[57] PVFM may frequently be mistaken for or coexist with asthma, with about a 20% overlap of asthma in patients with PVFM.[58] It is more common among female adolescents and has been described in elite athletes.[58, 59] Triggers of PVFM include social stressors, anxiety, and participating in high-performance or competitive sports.[60] Patients with PVFM exhibit loud wheezing over the trachea, often have supraglottic retractions, and complain of chest tightness. Despite the wheezing, patients with PVFM have a poor response to bronchodilators, are generally asymptomatic when asleep, and their oxygen saturations are usually normal.[54] Adolescents in particular tend to complain more of shortness of breath and chest/throat tightness compared to younger children.[60] Diagnostic studies during an acute episode include (1) spirometry, which may demonstrate a flat inspiratory loop of the flow volume curve; and (2) flexible laryngoscopy with or without videostroboscopy, which may demonstrate adduction of the vocal cords during phonation. PVFM may be undetectable at rest when asymptomatic.[54] Treatment of PVFM is aimed at relaxation of the vocal cords, including glottic airway and inspiratory muscle training with the help of a speech therapist and/or psychologist.[57] For more difficult-to-treat cases, biofeedback, vocal fold botulinum toxin injections, and low-dose amitriptyline have been associated with improvement in symptoms.[57, 59] The accurate diagnosis and treatment of VCD can reduce morbidity and result in an overall decrease in asthma medication use.[61]

Another disorder that is commonly mistaken for asthma is habit or tic cough syndrome.[62] A habit cough typically begins during a viral upper respiratory illness and persists after the acute illness has resolved. Male and female adolescents are equally affected, with the majority of cases affecting children 8–14 years of age.[62] Symptoms include a loud, barky, abrasive, and repetitive cough that attracts considerable attention and is usually absent when asleep.[54, 62] The cornerstone of therapy includes suggestion therapy and self-hypnosis.[62] These treatments distract the patient from the cough and help patients gain confidence that they can suppress and break the cycle of the repetitive cough.[62]

17.7 ADOLESCENT ASTHMA MANAGEMENT: DEVELOPMENTAL CONSIDERATIONS

The developmental changes that define adolescence present unique opportunities as well as challenges to asthma management. Clinicians should consider these developmental changes when guiding adolescents through asthma self-management. In this section, we focus on how cognitive development, peer relations, risk-taking behaviors, and mental health may impact asthma and offer suggestions on improving adherence among adolescent patients.

17.7.1 Cognitive Development

Adolescence marks the onset of significant changes to the way youth think and process information.[2] Some of these changes render them ready to care for their asthma. Adolescents can think systematically about logical operations. As abstract thinking develops, adolescents can weigh and consider multiple perspectives and can think about the future. The hallmarks of asthma are chronic airway inflammation and bronchoconstriction. With more sophisticated thinking, adolescents can understand inflammation, something they cannot necessarily see or feel. They can also begin to link the sensation of chest tightness to the concept of airway constriction. Moreover, they can understand the different roles of rescue medications and anti-inflammatory medications. Clinicians should begin to teach adolescents about the pathophysiology of asthma and how bronchodilators and anti-inflammatory medications work. Being able to think about the future allows adolescents to better understand the chronic nature of asthma and that symptoms may persist in the future unless they take steps to control them. Their improved cognitive skills allow them to understand and use treatment plans that require stepping up or stepping down medications in response to changes in symptoms or exposure to specific triggers.

Adolescents also develop more refined decision-making skills.[2] They also spend more time away from parents or caregivers who may no longer be fully aware of their adolescent's symptoms. Thus members of the healthcare team should engage the adolescent in shared decision-making where they seek adolescent participation in discussions, along with their caregiver, in making treatment decisions. Symptom history, medication use, and trigger avoidance techniques should be elicited from the adolescent before engaging in a joint discussion with parents or caregivers. The adolescent's improved decision-making skills are also essential as they navigate social situations that could impair their asthma. For example, they are better equipped to weigh the risks and benefits of smoking or vaping or being near peers who are engaging in these behaviors. Thus it is important for clinicians to teach adolescents about the deleterious effects of smoking and vaping.

17.7.2 Peer Relations

Adolescents spend increased time with peers, and friendships become more intense.[2] They report being embarrassed about having asthma and taking medication in front of friends,[63] often denying they have asthma.[64] Their embarrassment leads to nonadherence with medications, particularly in front of friends.[65, 66] Clinicians may want to address these issues with adolescents during the visit.

17.7.3 Risk-Taking in Adolescents

Risk-taking behaviors, such as tobacco, alcohol, and drug use increase during adolescence.[2] Despite the increased harms of cigarettes and e-cigarettes to respiratory health, nationally, adolescents with asthma are more likely to smoke cigarettes than those without asthma.[14, 67–72] Similarly, vaping is more prevalent among those with asthma,[14, 67, 68, 73–75] and this association is independent of cigarette use.[70, 76] Additionally, Black, Hispanic, and Indigenous adolescents and SGM adolescents, who bear a disproportionate burden of asthma,[4, 5, 11–15] have relatively high rates of cigarette and e-cigarette use.[13, 14, 77–80]

Smoking and exposure to secondhand smoke complicate asthma management. Teenagers with asthma who actively smoke or who have passive smoke exposure have more asthma symptoms,[81, 82] have more exacerbations requiring steroids,[81] and are more likely to have acute medical visits or overnight hospital stays.[83] They also have reduced lung function.[84] Recent reviews have documented that adolescents who vape also have worse respiratory health, including more symptoms, increased risk of having an asthma exacerbation, and worse lung function, even after adjusting for cigarette smoking.[85, 86]

It is suggested that clinicians ask the adolescent about their smoking and vaping behaviors and provide appropriate counseling regarding the specific asthma-related dangers associated with smoking cigarettes and vaping. Moreover, they should recommend interventions or refer the patient to appropriate cessation programs. It is important to inquire about exposure to smoke not only at home but also in vehicles and in other places the adolescent may frequent. Reviewing strategies to avoid exposure is also recommended, including possible smoking cessation programs for parents and other family members who may smoke.

The American Academy of Pediatrics recommends screening in a confidential manner for smoking and e-cigarette use in children starting at age 11.[87] Inquiry about specific products rather than asking about "e-cigarettes" along with pictures may be more helpful in gathering information, as adolescents may not view vaping as related to nicotine or other harmful substance use.[87] Screening questionnaires such as the CRAFFT 2.1+N (https://crafft.org), distributed before or at the clinical visit, may be helpful to determine substance use.[87]

Employment of motivational interviewing may be helpful to determine whether the adolescent is ready to quit. Those who are not ready to stop smoking or vaping and who state they can quit at any time may be tasked with a "two-week challenge," where they are asked to stop smoking or vaping for two weeks to determine if cessation is feasible. Cessation support should include behavioral support potentially alongside nicotine replacement and nonnicotine medication use.[88] Behavioral cessation support should be tailored to the level of dependence including the use of multiple hotlines, text message support, web-based interventions, smartphone apps, and in-person counseling.[88] As nicotine replacement therapy is currently not FDA approved for adolescents under 18 years of age, a prescription may be required.[87] When supporting patients in smoking or vaping cessation, follow-up is most important.

17.7.4 Mental Health and Asthma

The developmental changes adolescents experience can make them vulnerable to mental health problems. Anxiety and depression are common psychiatric conditions in adolescents,[89, 90] and both are comorbid with asthma. Increased anxiety and depressive symptoms are associated with worse asthma severity, poor asthma control, and asthma-related morbidity.[91–95] Anxiety and depression may result in worse outcomes by impeding asthma self-management. A recent review examining associations of mental health and asthma self-management found that youth with anxiety symptoms were more likely to smoke cigarettes, overuse quick-reliever medication, and have worse adherence.[96] Results regarding depression are mixed, with several studies finding adolescents with depressive symptoms implementing worse trigger control.[96] Given the associations between asthma and mental health, screening of adolescent mental health should be incorporated in routine asthma care. Clinicians should also make referrals to appropriate psychosocial services when warranted.

17.8 SUMMARY

The management of asthma in adolescents is a complex undertaking that requires clinicians' awareness of medical therapies and diagnostic tests, as well as a deeper understanding of the structural and social determinants of health, as well as the psychosocial changes that adolescents undergo. As knowledge of these intricate issues increases, clinicians can work with adolescent patients and their families using shared decision principles to help the adolescent live a healthy, active, and symptom-free life.

REFERENCES

1. Alderman EM, Breuner CC, AAP Committee on Adolescence. Unique needs of the adolescent. *Pediatrics*. 2019;144(6):e20193150. https://doi.org/10.1542/peds.2019-3150.
2. Kuther TL. *Adolescence in Context: Lives in Context*. Thousand Oaks, CA: Sage Publications; 2020.
3. Akinbami LJ, Simon AE, Rossen LM. Changing trends in asthma prevalence among children. *Pediatrics*. 2016;137(1):1–7. https://doi.org/10.1542/peds.2015-2354.
4. Centers for Disease Control and Prevention. Most Recent National Asthma Data (2021). https://www.cdc.gov/asthma/most_recent_national_asthma_data.htm.
5. Zahran H, Bailey C, Damon S, Garbe P, Breysse P. Vital signs: asthma in children—United States, 2001–2016.

MMWR Morb Mortal Wkly Rep. 2018;67(5):149–155. https://doi.org/10.15585/mmwr.mm6705e1.
6. Bitsko MJ, Everhart RS, Rubin BK. The adolescent with asthma. *Paediatr Respir Rev.* 2014;15(2):146–153. https://doi.org/10.1016/j.prrv.2013.07.003.
7. Schneider T. Asthma and academic performance among children and youth in North America: a systematic review. *J Sch Health.* 2020;90(4):319–342.
8. Leonard S, Turi E, Céspedes A, Liu J, Powell J, Bruzzese JM. Asthma knowledge, self-efficacy, and self-management among rural adolescents with poorly controlled asthma. *J Sch Nurs.* 2022 Jul 25:10598405221116017.
9. Bruzzese J-M, Stepney C, Fiorino EK, et al. Asthma self-management is sub-optimal in urban Hispanic and African American/Black early adolescents with uncontrolled persistent asthma. *J Asthma.* 2012;49(1):90–7. https://doi.org/10.3109/02770903.2011.637595.
10. Netz M, Fedele DA, Sweenie R, Baker D, Light M, McQuaid EL. Asthma management responsibility, control, and quality of life among emerging adolescents. *J Pediatr Psychol.* 2020;45(1):40–49. https://doi.org/10.1093/jpepsy/jsz069.
11. Forno E, Ortega VE, Celedón JC. Asthma and chronic obstructive pulmonary disease. *Clin Chest Med.* 2023;44(3):519–530. https://doi.org/10.1016/j.ccm.2023.03.008.
12. Bruzzese J-M, Kingston S, Bruzelius E, Falletta KA, Poghosyan L. Individual and neighborhood factors associated with undiagnosed asthma among urban adolescents. *J Urban Health.* 2019;96(2):252–261. https://doi.org/10.1007/s11524-018-00340-2.
13. Curry CW, Felt D, Beach LB, Ruprecht MM, Wang X, Phillips GL, 2nd. Lifetime asthma prevalence and correlates among US youths by sexual identity and race/ethnicity, 2009–2017. *Am J Public Health.* 2020;110(7):e1–e8. https://doi.org/10.2105/ajph.2020.305664.
14. Veldhuis CB, George M, Everett BG, Liu J, Hughes TL, Bruzzese JM. The association of asthma, sexual identity, and inhaled substance use among U.S. adolescents. *Ann Am Thorac Soc.* 2021;18(2):273–280. https://doi.org/10.1513/AnnalsATS.202001-062OC.
15. Curry CW, Felt D, Kan K, et al. Asthma remission disparities among US youth by sexual identity and race/ethnicity, 2009–2017. *J Allergy Clin Immunol Pract.* 2021;9(9):3396–3406. https://doi.org/10.1016/j.jaip.2021.04.046.
16. Khan S, Bajwa S, Brahmbhatt D, et al. Multi-level socioenvironmental contributors to childhood asthma in New York City: a cluster analysis. *J Urban Health.* 2021;98(6):700–710. https://doi.org/10.1007/s11524-021-00582-7.
17. Mitchell SJ, Bilderback AL, Okelo SO. Racial disparities in asthma morbidity among pediatric patients seeking asthma specialist care. *Acad Pediatr.* 2016;16(1):64–7. https://doi.org/10.1016/j.acap.2015.06.010.
18. Zanobetti A, Ryan PH, Coull B, et al. Childhood asthma incidence, early and persistent wheeze, and neighborhood socioeconomic factors in the ECHO/CREW Consortium. *JAMA Pediatr.* 2022;176(8):759–767. https://doi.org/10.1001/jamapediatrics.2022.1446.
19. Jaiswal J. Whose responsibility is it to dismantle medical mistrust? Future directions for researchers and health care providers. *Behav Med.* 2019;45(2):188–196. https://doi.org/10.1080/08964289.2019.1630357.
20. Wheldon CW, Kolar SK, Hernandez ND, Daley EM. Factorial invariance and convergent validity of the group-based medical mistrust scale across gender and ethnoracial identity. *J Health Care Poor Underserved.* 2017;28(1):88–99. https://doi.org/10.1353/hpu.2017.0011.
21. Leonard SI, Pizii CT, Zhao Y, Céspedes A, Kingston S, Bruzzese JM. Group-based medical mistrust in adolescents with poorly controlled asthma living in rural areas. *Health Promot Pract.* 2023:15248399221150913. https://doi.org/10.1177/15248399221150913.
22. Federico MJ, McFarlane AE, 2nd, Szefler SJ, Abrams EM. The impact of social determinants of health on children with asthma. *J Allergy Clin Immunol Pract.* 2020;8(6):1808–1814. https://doi.org/10.1016/j.jaip.2020.03.028.
23. Pollack CE, Roberts LC, Peng RD, et al. Association of a housing mobility program with childhood asthma symptoms and exacerbations. *JAMA.* 2023;329(19):1671–1681. https://doi.org/10.1001/jama.2023.6488.
24. Meyer IH. Prejudice, social stress, and mental health in lesbian, gay, and bisexual populations: conceptual issues and research evidence. *Psychol Bull.* 2003;129(5):674–697. https://doi.org/10.1037/0033-2909.129.5.674.
25. Crenshaw K. Mapping the margins—Intersectionality, identity politics, and violence against women of color. *Stanford Law Rev.* 1993;42:1241–1299.
26. Luria CJ, Sitarik AR, Havstad S, et al. Association between asthma symptom scores and perceived stress and trait anxiety in adolescents with asthma. *Allergy Asthma Proc.* 2020;41(3):210–217. https://doi.org/10.2500/aap.2020.41.200017.
27. Landeo-Gutierrez J, Celedón JC. Chronic stress and asthma in adolescents. *Ann Allergy Asthma Immunol.* 2020;125(4):393–398. https://doi.org/10.1016/j.anai.2020.07.001.
28. Helminen EC, Scheer JR, Edwards KM, Felver JC. Adverse childhood experiences exacerbate the association between day-to-day discrimination and mental health symptomatology in undergraduate students. *J Affect Disord.* 2022;297:338–347. https://doi.org/10.1016/j.jad.2021.10.058.
29. Duru OK, Harawa NT, Kermah D, Norris KC. Allostatic load burden and racial disparities in mortality. *J Natl Med Assoc.* 2012;104(1–2):89–95. https://doi.org/10.1016/s0027-9684(15)30120-6.
30. Malleske DT, Bryant-Stephens TC, Montoya-Williams D. Childhood asthma disparities—Race, place, or not keeping pace? *JAMA Pediatr.* 2022;176(8):739–740. https://doi.org/10.1001/jamapediatrics.2022.1457.
31. Asthma and Allergy Foundation of America. Asthma disparities in America: A roadmap to reducing burden on racial and ethnic minorities. https://www.aafa.org/asthmadisparities.
32. Fuchs O, Bahmer T, Rabe KF, von Mutius E. Asthma transition from childhood into adulthood. *Lancet Respir Med.* 2017;5(3):224–234. https://doi.org/10.1016/S2213-2600(16)30187-4.
33. Stern DA, Morgan WJ, Halonen M, Wright AL, Martinez FD. Wheezing and bronchial hyper-responsiveness in early childhood as predictors of newly diagnosed asthma in early adulthood: a longitudinal birth-cohort study. *Lancet.* 2008;372(9643):1058–1064.
34. McGeachie MJ, Yates KP, Zhou X, et al. Patterns of growth and decline in lung function in persistent childhood asthma. *N Engl J Med.* 2016;374(19):1842–1852. https://doi.org/10.1056/NEJMoa1513737.
35. Strachan DP, Griffiths JM, Johnston ID, Anderson HR. Ventilatory function in British adults after asthma or wheezing illness at ages 0–35. *Am J Respir Crit Care Med.* 1996;154(6 Pt 1):1629–1635. https://doi.org/10.1164/ajrccm.154.6.8970346.
36. Ross KR, Teague WG, Gaston BM. Life cycle of childhood asthma: prenatal, infancy and preschool, childhood, and

adolescence. *Clin Chest Med*. 2019;40(1):125–147. https://doi.org/10.1016/j.ccm.2018.10.008.
37. Moffatt MF, Gut IG, Demenais F, et al. A large-scale, consortium-based genomewide association study of asthma. *N Engl J Med*. 2010;363(13):1211–1221. https://doi.org/10.1056/NEJMoa0906312.
38. Moffatt MF, Kabesch M, Liang L, et al. Genetic variants regulating ORMDL3 expression contribute to the risk of childhood asthma. *Nature*. 2007;448(7152):470–473. https://doi.org/10.1038/nature06014.
39. Kabesch M. Epigenetics in asthma and allergy. *Curr Opin Allergy Clin Immunol*. 2014;14(1):62–68. https://doi.org/10.1097/ACI.0000000000000025.
40. Granell R, Henderson AJ, Timpson N, et al. Examination of the relationship between variation at 17q21 and childhood wheeze phenotypes. *J Allergy Clin Immunol*. 2013;131(3):685–694. https://doi.org/10.1016/j.jaci.2012.09.021.
41. Voraphani N, Stern DA, Ledford JG, et al. Circulating CC16 and asthma: a population based, multi-cohort study from early childhood through adult life. *Am J Respir Crit Care Med*. 2023. https://doi.org/10.1164/rccm.202301-0041OC.
42. Expert Panel Report 3 (EPR-3): Guidelines for the Diagnosis and Management of Asthma. NIH Publication No. 07-4051. Bethesda, MD, U.S. Department of Health and Human Services; National Institutes of Health; National Heart, Lung and Blood Institute, National Asthma Education and Prevention Program; 2007. http://www.ncbi.nlm.nih.gov/pubmed/17983880.
43. National Asthma Education Prevention Program. *Asthma Care Quick Reference Diagnosing and Managing Asthma*. National Heart, Lung, and Blood Institute; National Institutes of Health; U.S. Department of Health and Human Services; 2012.
44. Cloutier MM, Baptist AP, Blake KV, et al. 2020 focused updates to the asthma management guidelines: a report from the national asthma education and prevention program coordinating committee expert panel working group. *J Allergy Clin Immunol*. 2020;146(6):1217–1270. https://doi.org/10.1016/j.jaci.2020.10.003.
45. Reddel HK, Bacharier LB, Bateman ED, et al. Global initiative for Asthma strategy 2021: executive summary and rationale for key changes. *Eur Respir J*. 2022;59(1). https://doi.org/10.1183/13993003.02730-2021.
46. Expert Panel Working Group of the National Heart Lung Blood Institute. 2020 focused updates to the asthma management guidelines: a report from the national asthma education and prevention program coordinating committee expert panel working group. *J Allergy Clin Immunol*. 2020;146(6):1217–1270. https://doi.org/10.1016/j.jaci.2020.10.003.
47. Papi A, Corradi M, Pigeon-Francisco C, et al. Beclometasone-formoterol as maintenance and reliever treatment in patients with asthma: a double-blind, randomised controlled trial. *Lancet Respir Med*. 2013;1(1):23–31. https://doi.org/10.1016/S2213-2600(13)70012-2.
48. Rabe KF, Pizzichini E, Stallberg B, et al. Budesonide/formoterol in a single inhaler for maintenance and relief in mild-to-moderate asthma: a randomized, double-blind trial. *Chest*. 2006;129(2):246–256. https://doi.org/10.1378/chest.129.2.246.
49. Jenkins CR, Eriksson G, Bateman ED, et al. Efficacy of budesonide/formoterol maintenance and reliever therapy compared with higher-dose budesonide as step-up from low-dose inhaled corticosteroid treatment. *BMC Pulm Med*. 2017;17(1):65. https://doi.org/10.1186/s12890-017-0401-y.
50. Rhee H, Belyea MJ, Elward KS. Patterns of asthma control perception in adolescents: associations with psychosocial functioning. *J Asthma*. 2008;45(7):600–606. https://doi.org/10.1080/02770900802126974.
51. Sadof M, Kaslovsky R. Adolescent asthma: a developmental approach. *Curr Opin Pediatr*. 2011;23(4):373–378. https://doi.org/10.1097/MOP.0b013e32834837cb.
52. Bhakta NR, Bime C, Kaminsky DA, et al. Race and ethnicity in pulmonary function test interpretation: an official American Thoracic Society statement. *Am J Respir Crit Care Med*. 2023;207(8):978–995. https://doi.org/10.1164/rccm.202302-0310ST.
53. Roth KA. Spirometry for transgender and nonbinary patients. *Ann Am Thorac Soc*. 2023;20(7):944–946. https://doi.org/10.1513/AnnalsATS.202301-033IP.
54. Wilmott RW, Deterding R, Li A, et al. *Kendig and Chernick's Disorders of the Respiratory Tract in Children*, 9th ed. Philadelphia, PA: Elsevier; 2019.
55. de Benedictis D, Bush A. Asthma in adolescence: Is there any news? *Pediatr Pulmonol*. 2017;52(1):129–138. https://doi.org/10.1002/ppul.23498.
56. de Benedictis D, Bush A. The challenge of asthma in adolescence. *Pediatr Pulmonol*. 2007;42(8):683–692. https://doi.org/10.1002/ppul.20650.
57. Mahoney J, Hew M, Vertigan A, Oates J. Treatment effectiveness for vocal cord dysfunction in adults and adolescents: a systematic review. *Clin Exp Allergy*. 2022;52(3):387–404. https://doi.org/10.1111/cea.14036.
58. Zhang C, Hicks M, Ospina MB, et al. The impact of identifying laryngeal obstruction syndromes on reducing treatment of pediatric asthma: a systematic review. *Pediatr Pulmonol*. 2022;57(6):1401–1415. https://doi.org/10.1002/ppul.25910.
59. Marcinow AM, Thompson J, Chiang T, Forrest LA, deSilva BW. Paradoxical vocal fold motion disorder in the elite athlete: experience at a large division I university. *Laryngoscope*. 2014;124(6):1425–1430. https://doi.org/10.1002/lary.24486.
60. Yi JS, Davis AC, Pietsch K, et al. Demographic differences in clinical presentation of pediatric paradoxical vocal fold motion (PVFM). *J Voice*. 2021. https://doi.org/10.1016/j.jvoice.2021.08.017.
61. Ivancic R, Matrka L, Wiet G, Puckett A, Haney J, deSilva B. Reduced asthma medication use after treatment of pediatric paradoxical vocal fold motion disorder. *Laryngoscope*. 2021;131(7):1639–1646. https://doi.org/10.1002/lary.29283.
62. Weinberger M, Lockshin B. When is cough functional, and how should it be treated? *Breathe (Sheff)*. 2017;13(1):22–30. https://doi.org/10.1183/20734735.015216.
63. De Simoni A, Horne R, Fleming L, Bush A, Griffiths C. What do adolescents with asthma really think about adherence to inhalers? Insights from a qualitative analysis of a UK online forum. *BMJ Open*. 2017;7(6):e015245. https://doi.org/10.1136/bmjopen-2016-015245.
64. Kaplan A, Price D. Treatment adherence in adolescents with asthma. *J Asthma Allergy*. 2020;13:39–49. https://doi.org/10.2147/jaa.S233268.
65. Mulvaney SA, Ho YX, Cala CM, et al. Assessing adolescent asthma symptoms and adherence using mobile phones. *J Med Internet Res*. 2013;15(7):e141. https://doi.org/10.2196/jmir.2413.
66. Braido F, Chrystyn H, Baiardini I, et al. "Trying, but failing"—the role of inhaler technique and mode of delivery in respiratory medication adherence. *J Allergy Clin Immunol Pract*. 2016;4(5):823–832. https://doi.org/10.1016/j.jaip.2016.03.002.
67. Fedele DA, Barnett TE, Dekevich D, Gibson-Young LM, Martinasek M, Jagger MA. Prevalence of and beliefs about

electronic cigarettes and hookah among high school students with asthma. *Ann Epidemiol.* 2016;26(12):865–869. https://doi.org/10.1016/j.annepidem.2016.10.004.
68. Han YY, Rosser F, Forno E, Celedón JC. Electronic vapor products, marijuana use, smoking, and asthma in US adolescents. *J Allergy Clin Immunol.* 2020;145(3):1025–1028.e6. https://doi.org/10.1016/j.jaci.2019.12.001.
69. Vázquez-Nava F, Vázquez-Rodríguez EM, Vázquez-Rodríguez CF, Castillo Ruiz O, Peinado Herreros J. Epidemiological profile of smoking and nicotine addiction among asthmatic adolescents. *Public Health.* 2017;149:49–56. https://doi.org/10.1016/j.puhe.2017.04.012.
70. Wills TA, Choi K, Pagano I. E-cigarette use associated with asthma independent of cigarette smoking and marijuana in a 2017 national sample of adolescents. *J Adolesc Health.* 2020;67(4):524–530. https://doi.org/10.1016/j.jadohealth.2020.03.001.
71. Jordão E, Kuschnir FC, Figueiredo VC, et al. ERICA: smoking is associated with more severe asthma in Brazilian adolescents. *J Pediatr (Rio J).* 2019;95(5):538–544. https://doi.org/10.1016/j.jped.2018.05.010.
72. Turner E, Fedele DA, Thompson L, Salloum RG. Patterns of electronic cigarette use in youth with asthma: results from a nationally representative sample. *Ann Allergy Asthma Immunol.* 2018;120(2):220–222. https://doi.org/10.1016/j.anai.2017.11.020.
73. Xian S, Chen Y. E-cigarette users are associated with asthma disease: a meta-analysis. *Clin Respir J.* 2021;15(5):457–466. https://doi.org/10.1111/crj.13346.
74. Clapp PW, Jaspers I. Electronic cigarettes: their constituents and potential links to asthma. *Curr Allergy Asthma Rep.* 2017;17(11):79. https://doi.org/10.1007/s11882-017-0747-5.
75. Li X, Zhang Y, Zhang R, Chen F, Shao L, Zhang L. Association between e-cigarettes and asthma in adolescents: a systematic review and meta-analysis. *Am J Prev Med.* 2022;62(6):953–960. https://doi.org/10.1016/j.amepre.2022.01.015.
76. Schweitzer RJ, Wills TA, Tam E, Pagano I, Choi K. E-cigarette use and asthma in a multiethnic sample of adolescents. *Prev Med.* 2017;105:226–231. https://doi.org/10.1016/j.ypmed.2017.09.023.
77. Kamke K, Sabado-Liwag M, Rodriquez EJ, Pérez-Stable EJ, El-Toukhy S. Adolescent smoking susceptibility: gender-stratified racial and ethnic differences, 1999–2018. *Am J Prev Med.* 2020;58(5):666–674. https://doi.org/10.1016/j.amepre.2019.11.023.
78. Lanza ST, Russell MA, Braymiller JL. Emergence of electronic cigarette use in US adolescents and the link to traditional cigarette use. *Addict Behav.* 2017;67:38–43. https://doi.org/10.1016/j.addbeh.2016.12.003.
79. Dai H, Ramos AK, Faseru B, Hill JL, Sussman SY. Racial disparities of e-cigarette use among US youths: 2014–2019. *Am J Public Health.* 2021;111(11):2050–2058. https://doi.org/10.2105/ajph.2021.306448.
80. Barrington-Trimis JL, Bello MS, Liu F, et al. Ethnic differences in patterns of cigarette and e-cigarette use over time among adolescents. *J Adolesc Health.* 2019;65(3):359–365. https://doi.org/10.1016/j.jadohealth.2019.04.002.
81. Merianos AL, Jandarov RA, Mahabee-Gittens EM. Association of secondhand smoke exposure with asthma symptoms, medication use, and healthcare utilization among asthmatic adolescents. *J Asthma.* 2019;56(4):369–379. https://doi.org/10.1080/02770903.2018.1463379.
82. Cheng ZR, Tan YH, Teoh OH, Lee JH. Keeping pace with adolescent asthma: a practical approach to optimizing care. *Pulm Ther.* 2022;8(1):123–137. https://doi.org/10.1007/s41030-021-00177-2.
83. Merianos AL, Jandarov RA, Mahabee-Gittens EM. Secondhand smoke exposure and pediatric healthcare visits and hospitalizations. *Am J Prev Med.* 2017;53(4):441–448. https://doi.org/10.1016/j.amepre.2017.03.020.
84. Kamga A, Rochefort-Morel C, Guen YL, Ouksel H, Pipet A, Leroyer C. Asthma and smoking: a review. *Respir Med Res.* 2022;82:100916. https://doi.org/10.1016/j.resmer.2022.100916.
85. Afolabi F, Rao DR. E-cigarettes and asthma in adolescents. *Curr Opin Allergy Clin Immunol.* 2023;23(2):137–143. https://doi.org/10.1097/aci.0000000000000891.
86. Di Cicco M, Sepich M, Ragazzo V, Peroni DG, Comberiati P. Potential effects of e-cigarettes and vaping on pediatric asthma. *Minerva Pediatr.* 2020;72(5):372–382. https://doi.org/10.23736/s0026-4946.20.05973-3.
87. Tobacco Use: Considerations for Clinicians. *American Academy of Pediatrics.* March 8, 2022. https://www.aap.org/en/patient-care/tobacco-control-and-prevention/youth-tobacco-cessation/tobacco-use-considerations-for-clinicians/.
88. Behavioral Cessation Supports for Youth and Young Adults. *American Academy of Pediatrics*, April 25, 2023. https://www.aap.org/en/patient-care/tobacco-control-and-prevention/youth-tobacco-cessation/behavioral-cessation-supports-for-youth/.
89. Kowalchuk A, Gonzalez SJ, Zoorob RJ. Anxiety disorders in children and adolescents. *Am Fam Physician.* 2022;106(6):657–664.
90. Rikard-Bell C, Hunt C, McAulay C, et al. Adolescent depression from a developmental perspective: the importance of recognizing developmental distress in depressed adolescents. *Int J Environ Res Public Health.* 2022;19(23). https://doi.org/10.3390/ijerph192316029.
91. Cobham VE, Hickling A, Kimball H, Thomas HJ, Scott JG, Middeldorp CM. Systematic review: anxiety in children and adolescents with chronic medical conditions. *J Am Acad Child Adolesc Psychiatry.* 2020;59(5):595–618. https://doi.org/10.1016/j.jaac.2019.10.010.
92. Fidler A, Lawless C, LaFave E, et al. Anxiety among adolescents with asthma: relationships with asthma control and sleep quality. *Clin Pract Pediatr Psychol.* 2019;7(2):151–156. https://doi.org/10.1037/cpp0000267.
93. Licari A, Ciprandi R, Marseglia G, Ciprandi G. Anxiety and depression in adolescents with severe asthma and in their parents: preliminary results after 1 year of treatment. *Behav Sci.* 2019;9(7). https://doi.org/10.3390/bs9070078.
94. Bardach NS, Neel C, Kleinman LC, et al. Depression, anxiety, and Emergency Department use for asthma. *Pediatrics.* 2019;144(4):e20190856. https://doi.org/10.1542/peds.2019-0856.
95. Kulikova A, Lopez J, Antony A, et al. Multivariate association of child depression and anxiety with asthma outcomes. *J Allergy Clin Immunol Pract.* 2021;9(6):2399–2405. https://doi.org/10.1016/j.jaip.2021.02.043.
96. Leonard SI, Turi ER, Powell JS, Usseglio J, MacDonell KK, Bruzzese JM. Associations of asthma self-management and mental health in adolescents: a scoping review. *Respir Med.* 2022;200:106897. https://doi.org/10.1016/j.rmed.2022.106897.

18 Management of Adult Asthma

S. Shahzad Mustafa, Sara Patrawala, and Thomas B. Casale

CASE PRESENTATION

A 47-year-old female presented to the allergy office complaining of difficulty breathing. Although she had not previously been diagnosed with asthma, her primary care provider prescribed her an albuterol inhaler five months earlier for similar complaints without lung function testing performed. She had used albuterol sporadically until recently, when her symptoms worsened.

Her current symptoms consisted of coughing, wheezing, shortness of breath, chest tightness, and occasional production of clear mucus. She experienced symptoms at rest, but her symptoms were particularly notable with exertion. Her activity was limited due to her respiratory complaints, and she had stopped hobbies such as walking and gardening. She also had disturbed sleep due to night-time symptoms and was also waking up at night and using albuterol, with very little relief. She reported she had used albuterol 6–8 times daily over the past week, with each use providing only temporary and modest relief from symptoms.

Additionally, she also complained of postnasal drip, nasal congestion, and itchy/watery eyes. She had a good sense of smell. Her nasal symptoms were present throughout the year but more troublesome in the spring and fall. She wondered if her nasal symptoms worsened her respiratory status. She had no history of recurrent infections and tolerated all food groups. She had no known drug allergies and tolerated NSAIDs without difficulty.

Her past medical history was significant for hyperlipidemia treated with atorvastatin 20 mg daily and allergic rhinitis treated with cetirizine 10 mg daily. Her family history was positive for allergic rhinitis in her mother, but there was no history of asthma in the family. She was a lifelong non-smoker but was briefly exposed to secondhand cigarette smoke as a child. Her review of systems was unremarkable other than her upper and lower respiratory tract symptoms.

Examination of the patient's vital signs revealed the following: pulse = 88 beats/minute, respiratory rate = 18 breaths/minute, blood pressure (BP) = 130/80 mmHg, height 65 inches, and weight 155 pounds. She was breathing comfortably and in no distress. Her head, eyes, ears, nose, and throat examination was remarkable for pale, boggy nasal turbinates, and posterior pharyngeal cobblestoning consistent with postnasal drainage. There were no visible nasal polyps. Her cardiac examination was within the normal limits. Her lung examination revealed a prolonged expiratory phase and bilateral wheezing diffusely throughout all lung fields.

Her screening Asthma Control Test (ACT) revealed a score of 6 (i.e., severely impaired asthma control). Spirometry revealed a forced vital capacity (FVC) of 2.08 L (62% predicted), a forced expiratory volume in 1 second (FEV_1) of 1.23 L (45% predicted), and an FEV_1/FVC ratio of 0.59. She received bronchodilator treatment with four puffs of albuterol and her FEV_1 improved to 1.52 (55% predicted), indicating significant reversibility. Her exhaled nitric oxide (FeNO) was 64 ppb. The patient was determined to have poorly controlled asthma along with allergic rhino-conjunctivitis.

She was treated with prednisone 40 mg orally every morning for seven days; and also started on fluticasone/salmeterol 250/50 mcg one puff twice daily; along with fluticasone nasal spray two sprays in each nostril once per day, and continuation of cetirizine. One week later, she returned to the office and had a marked decrease in her asthma symptoms. She denied any coughing, shortness of breath, wheezing, or chest tightness. She was able to sleep through the night. Her physical examination had essentially normalized, with normal breath sounds with good aeration and resolution of wheezing. A spirometry revealed a FVC of 2.75 L (69% predicted), an FEV_1 of 2.26 L (76% predicted), and an FEV_1/FVC ratio of 0.88. Her FeNO was 29 ppb. The patient's prednisone was discontinued, and her fluticasone/salmeterol 250/50 mcg was continued, along with nasal fluticasone and cetirizine.

The patient was seen six weeks later, and at that time she indicated that her breathing was better than it had been in the last four years. She also reported resolution of her nasal symptoms. Her ACT was 25. She had only used her rescue inhaler once in the previous six weeks, and she denied any daytime or nocturnal symptoms. She was able to exercise and be active as she wished. Her physical examination was unremarkable with clear lung fields. Her spirometry revealed an FEV_1 of 2.48 L (84% of predicted).

This case illustrates several important points.

DOI: 10.1201/9781003287209-23

1. **The importance of objective lung function testing with spirometry in diagnosing and assessing the severity of asthma:** *This patient never had a spirometry prior to her initial visit to the allergy office. If a spirometry had been obtained when she was first prescribed albuterol, the diagnosis and the assessment of her asthma severity could have been made sooner, thereby preventing the marked impairment and risk factors that led to her presentation.*
2. **The utility of the Expert Panel Report 3 (EPR-3) asthma classification for judging asthma severity and guiding therapy decisions, including the assessment of impairment using standardized patient questionnaires such as the ACT.**
3. **The utility of FeNO in assessing lung inflammation and responsiveness to corticosteroids:** *This patient presented with a significantly elevated FeNO that was much improved after one week of treatment with oral and inhaled corticosteroids (OCS, ICS). Typically, higher FeNO levels occur with an eosinophilic asthma phenotype, which tends to respond better to corticosteroids.*
4. **The overuse of albuterol associated with uncontrolled asthma:** *Patients using as much albuterol as this patient are at a higher risk for catastrophic asthma events, including an increased risk of death.*
5. **The utility of OCS and ICS to quickly reduce the symptoms of asthma and improve spirometry and lower lung inflammation as assessed by FeNO.**
6. **The utility of spirometry and ACT to monitor control in patients.**
7. **The importance of addressing upper airway inflammation when managing asthma and optimizing respiratory status.**
8. **Appropriate treatment can considerably improve the quality of life for patients with asthma and reverse many of the impairments and risk factors for future exacerbations and poor outcomes.**

18.1 OVERVIEW

Asthma is an inflammatory obstructive airway disease, with a complicated pathophysiology, and is multifactorial in etiology. The onset of asthma can occur at any time during a person's lifetime but commonly occurs in childhood or early adolescence. According to data from the United States Centers for Disease Control, the disease burden has been on the rise for the past 20 years, with a reported prevalence of 7.8% in 2020 [1]. Approximately 3800 deaths per year are from asthma, and asthma has been a contributing factor in another 7000 deaths per year. In adults, asthma is the fourth leading cause of work absenteeism and results in almost $3 billion per year in lost productivity. Lower socioeconomic classes and African American populations have higher rates of mortality and morbidity [2]. Close monitoring of disease progression, timely intervention in acute settings, and making sure that patients are on adequate therapy for their stage/control of disease to prevent exacerbations all contribute to the prevention of morbidity and mortality.

18.2 CLINICAL PRESENTATION AND EVALUATION

Common symptoms of asthma include wheezing, chest tightness, dyspnea, and cough, often at night or early in the morning. These symptoms tend to be episodic in nature with near complete remission between episodes in most cases. Exertional symptoms are also common, most commonly occurring late in exertion or even during the cool-down phase. It is important to keep in mind the following differential diagnoses, since these disorders can present with similar signs and symptoms: chronic obstructive pulmonary disease (COPD; emphysema and chronic bronchitis); cardiac etiologies such as congestive heart failure or coronary artery disease, mechanical obstruction of the upper or lower airways (malignant and benign tumors); obstructive sleep apnea (OSA); vocal cord dysfunction; tracheomalacia; hyperventilation with panic attacks; gastro-esophageal reflux disease (GERD), cough due to angiotensin converting enzyme (ACE) inhibitors; and other pulmonary conditions such as interstitial lung disease. In patients with difficult to control asthma, comorbid conditions such as GERD, rhinosinusitis, OSA, obesity, and allergic bronchopulmonary aspergillosis (ABPA) should be recognized early and adequately treated. The triggers for worsening asthma should be documented and include allergens, irritants (e.g. environmental and tobacco smoke), respiratory viruses, and occupational exposures.

Each office visit should include an evaluation of asthma control, adherence with medications along with proper inhaler technique, and the success of pharmacotherapy. A questionnaire encompassing various symptoms, duration, frequency, and severity can be used, and objective testing with spirometry and/or FeNO should be considered.

A physical examination during routine visits is often normal but may be useful in recognizing an exacerbation and in identifying comorbid conditions, particularly upper airway inflammation. On nasopharyngeal examination, there could be increased induration and erythema in the nasal turbinates and cobblestoning in the retropharynx from a postnasal drip in patients with chronic rhinosinusitis. Evaluating for nasal polyps is also important. On lung examination, patients can have wheezing, prolonged end-expiration, and decreased air movement. Patients could also present with a normal lung examination. A silent chest may actually indicate a severe exacerbation.

In the initial evaluation of new onset of asthma symptoms in adults, a chest X-ray should be completed to rule out other etiologies of dyspnea [3]. In asthma, the chest X-ray is usually within normal limits or occasionally shows hyperinflation and air trapping from mucus plugs. Spirometry is an integral part of assessing asthma severity and control. If feasible, spirometry should be performed prior to initiating treatment to establish the presence and severity of baseline airway obstruction. The initial spirometry should also include measurements before and after inhalation of a short-acting bronchodilator (SABA) to assess reversibility, especially in patients with significant airway obstruction. Spirometry is generally recommended over measurements by a peak flow meter. Peak expiratory flow (PEF) meters are more appropriate for monitoring than they are as diagnostic tools, but a home PEF diary may be helpful in diagnosing patients with a suggestive history of asthma when the lung function is normal in the office. PEF completed at home can also help differentiate between different causes of dyspnea, such as anxiety.

When completing spirometry, the ratio of FEV_1/FVC is typically less than 70% in asthma. The FEV_1 is also characteristically low in asthma, below 80%. Reversibility is defined as a 12% improvement and an increase of 200 cc in FEV_1 in comparison to the baseline. Spirometry should be done to determine airflow obstruction and should be correlated with the symptom profile. Many patients do not perceive airway obstruction; therefore, spirometry is especially useful in individuals that under-report symptoms. There are guidelines for the technique and the equipment to be used while performing office spirometry [4, 5]. Patient age, gender, height, race, and ethnic background should be taken into account when interpreting the results. In patients with a normal spirometry, airway hyperresponsiveness (AHR) can be assessed using methacholine or mannitol bronchoprovocation challenge testing. A positive bronchoprovocation test does not confirm the diagnosis of asthma; however, a negative test makes asthma highly unlikely.

Laboratory testing can help in understanding an individual's asthma phenotype. Total immunoglobulin E (IgE) can be elevated or normal, but population studies indicate a higher probability of AHR and asthma with elevated IgE levels [6]. Elevated blood eosinophil levels are not diagnostic for asthma but are predictive of better responses to ICS and many of the currently approved biologics, and higher levels are also predictive of a higher risk of future exacerbation [7].

An evaluation for sensitization to common aeroallergens should be considered for all patients with persistent asthma. This is ideally completed through skin or *in vitro* testing, since this has the better sensitivity and specificity as compared to total serum IgE testing. Environmental allergies are significant triggers for asthma in ≥80% of children and 50–60% of adults.

TABLE 18.1
Strategies to Understand an Individual's Asthma Phenotype

Characteristic or Biomarker	Consideration
Age of onset	Younger age tends to be T2 high. Older age of onset is more often T2 low.
Race	Blacks and Hispanics have worse outcomes as compared to Caucasian counterparts.
BMI	Higher BMI associated with decreased steroid responsiveness.
Lung function	Reversible obstruction tends to be T2 high, whereas fixed obstruction is more often T2 low.
FeNO	Elevated FeNO associated with T2 high and increased steroid and dupilumab responsiveness.
Allergic sensitizations	Associated with T2 high.
Total IgE	Higher levels associated with T2 high.
Peripheral eosinophil count	Higher levels associated with T2 high, and increased risk of future exacerbation.

FeNO can be helpful in certain instances. Guidelines [8] indicate that it can be used to assist in assessing the etiology of respiratory symptoms; to help in identifying the eosinophilic asthma phenotype; to assess the potential response or failure to respond to anti-inflammatory agents, notably corticosteroids and certain biologics (e.g. dupilumab); to establish a baseline during clinical stability for subsequent monitoring of persistent asthma; to guide changes in doses of anti-inflammatory medications: step-down dosing, step-up dosing, or discontinuation of anti-inflammatory medications; to assist in the evaluation of adherence to anti-inflammatory medications; and to assess whether airway inflammation is contributing to poor asthma control. Table 18.1 summarizes considerations on how to best identify an individual's asthma phenotype.

18.3 INTERMITTENT ASTHMA

The treatment of mild intermittent asthma is essentially SABAs, which are used for bronchodilation, as a rescue inhaler [9]. As-needed SABA is the current NHBLI guideline, but it is important to note that the most recent Global Initiative for Asthma (GINA) guidelines do not recommend SABA alone but instead prefer as-needed LABA (formoterol) in combination with a low-dose ICS. If this cannot be achieved, GINA guidelines then recommend concurrent low-dose ICS administration whenever SABA is taken [10].

18.4 MILD AND MODERATE PERSISTENT ASTHMA

ICS are key controller agents for patients with chronic persistent asthma [3] and should be used in all patients with moderate to severe asthma. For mild asthma, ICS plus as-needed SABA or as-needed concurrent ICS and LABA (formoterol) are the preferred treatment. Agents aimed at the leukotriene pathway, such as leukotriene receptor antagonists (LTRA) (montelukast and zafirlukast) or 5-lipooxygenase inhibitors (zileuton) can also be used but are not preferred controllers. Theophylline is no longer routinely utilized as a controller medication. If symptoms are still uncontrolled, the preferred next step up is to use daily and as-needed combination low-dose ICS-formoterol. Previously, low-dose ICS plus any LABA (not specifically formoterol), long-acting anticholinergics (LAMA), LTRA or theophylline, or medium-dose ICS were recommended. Step-up therapy from there includes increasing to medium-dose ICS in combination with formoterol (preferred) or other LABA, LAMA, LTRA, zileuton, or theophylline [9].

18.5 SEVERE PERSISTENT ASTHMA

In patients with uncontrolled symptoms despite high doses of ICS plus LABA and/or LAMA or high-dose ICS plus LTRA, biologics have now essentially replaced OCS as the next step in management [9].

18.5.1 Pharmacotherapy: Summary of the Individual Asthma Therapies

18.5.1.1 Short-Acting Beta-2 Adrenergic Agonists (SABAs)

Beta-2 agonists stimulate beta-2 adrenergic receptors and increase cyclic adenosine monophosphate (cAMP), causing a relaxation of the airway smooth muscles and thus reversing bronchoconstriction. Albuterol, salbutamol, levalbuterol, and pirbuterol are all drugs of choice for the immediate relief of symptoms. SABAs should only be used as rescue medications or prophylaxis for exercise-induced symptoms and not continuously for disease control. Higher frequency usage is a warning sign for loss of disease control and an increased risk for an exacerbation and puts patients at increased risk of poor outcomes, including death [11].

18.5.1.2 Long-Acting Beta-2 Adrenergic Agonists (LABAs)

LABAs have an increased lipophilic nature and thus have prolonged retention in the lung tissue with a duration of action of up to 24 hours. Salmeterol has a slower onset of action than formoterol, which some studies support using as a rescue inhaler when combined with ICS. Side effects include tachycardia, a prolonged QTC interval, and hypokalemia [12, 13]. LABAs should not be used as monotherapy, and, when used with ICS, there is an improvement in both the impairment and risk domains. Although the US Food and Drug Administration (FDA) has issued a black box warning about LABAs, noting that their use may increase the risk of severe asthma exacerbation or death, this is only in the setting of monotherapy with LABA and is not clinically meaningful when using a LABA in combination with an ICS.

18.5.1.2.1 Single Maintenance and Reliever Therapy (SMART) Therapy

Initially approved in Europe and Canada and now used in over 120 countries worldwide, formoterol plus ICS for both reliever and maintenance therapy has demonstrated a greater reduction in asthma exacerbations at a lower overall corticosteroid load compared with fixed-dose ICS/LABA in patients over 12 years of age (with limited evidence in 4- to 11-year-olds) [9]. Coined SMART (single maintenance and reliever therapy) therapy, studies have focused on ICS and specifically formoterol as the LABA as it has a rapid onset of action, producing bronchodilation in less than 15 minutes. While current GINA guidelines recommend SMART therapy, its use in the United States has been limited due to lack of FDA approval for this regimen [10]. Despite the demonstrated safety and efficacy of SMART therapy, additional work is needed to evaluate other ICS-LABA combinations. Furthermore, its use will continue to be limited to patients with a clear understanding of asthma self-management as well be limited by national or local payer coverage of these medications [14].

18.5.1.2.2 Corticosteroids

Corticosteroids have multiple mechanisms of action: suppressing cytokine release, decreasing the recruitment of airway eosinophils, and inhibiting the release of inflammatory mediators. They help diminish AHR and decrease lung inflammation [15]. Corticosteroids can be administered via different routes: inhaled, oral, intramuscular, or intravenous. There is an increased bioavailability of ICS, requiring lower doses and thus lowering the incidence of adverse reactions with their usage. Local adverse effects include oral candidiasis, dysphonia (seen in higher doses and in vocal stress), reflex cough, and bronchospasm (from the faster rate of inhalation). Oral candidiasis and dysphonia can be controlled by washing the mouth after each use and by using a spacer. Severe and difficult to control asthma warrants the possibility of using OCS for long-term symptom control; however, this is less and less the case due to the availability of multiple biologics. Prolonged use of systemic side effects is limited by a myriad of side effects, such as adrenal suppression, hypertension, hyperglycemia, cataracts, fatty liver, proximal muscle weakness, and increased infection risk [3]. Corticosteroid insensitivity is a result of various molecular mechanisms and varies in different patient phenotypes. If asthma is poorly controlled despite high-dose ICS and OCS, corticosteroid insensitivity should be considered [16]. Decreased responsiveness has been shown with smoking (active and passive) or asthma with predominantly neutrophilic inflammation.

18.5.1.2.3 Leukotriene Modifiers

Montelukast and zafirlukast block the effects of the CysLT1 receptor (approved for use in childhood asthma) and zileuton ($\geq$ 12 years) inhibits the 5-lipoxygenase pathway. The use of zileuton requires close monitoring of liver function tests, as 3% of individuals may experience drug-induced hepatitis. Leukotriene modifiers can be used in mild, persistent asthma as a monotherapy and in addition to ICS for more severe disease, but they are not the preferred adjunctive therapy [9]. In 2020, the FDA issued a black box warning for montelukast, stating that serious neuropsychiatric events that may include suicidal thoughts or actions have been reported. Certain phenotypes show a better response, including patients with a smoking history and thus ICS insensitivity, exercise-induced asthma, obesity, and aspirin-exacerbated disease.

18.5.1.2.4 Anticholinergic Agents

Ipratropium bromide inhibits muscarinic cholinergic receptors and reduces the intrinsic vagal tone of airways. This is a quick-relief medication used either as an additive to SABA or as an alternative to SABA in patients who cannot tolerate SABAs. Long-acting antimuscarinics (LAMAs) are also available as controller treatment of asthma in individuals 12 years and older. Studies have shown similar efficacy with the addition of a LABA to ICS when compared to LAMA plus ICS in exacerbation rates, asthma control, quality of life, use of rescue medications, and quality of life. However, in one specific trial looking at Blacks (the BELT study), they found a 2.6-fold higher risk of asthma-related hospitalizations in the ICS plus LAMA arm and, although the death rate was small, both deaths occurred in the ICS plus LAMA group [17]. Therefore, current guidelines recommend against ICS plus LAMA for patients 12 years and older with uncontrolled asthma. In patients where ICS plus LABA cannot be used (due to side effects, cost, etc.), LAMA plus ICS is recommended in place of the same dose of ICS alone. Additionally, in patients with uncontrolled persistent asthma on ICS plus LABA, the addition of a LAMA is recommended as it offers a benefit in asthma control and quality of life [9].

18.5.1.2.5 Omalizumab

Omalizumab is a recombinant IgG humanized monoclonal antibody (mAb) to the Fc3 portion of the IgE antibody and was the first biologic available to treat moderate to severe asthma. Approved initially in 2003 for patients 12 years of age and older, it is now available to those six years and older with moderate to severe persistent asthma with perennial allergic sensitization whose symptoms are not controlled with ICS therapy. Omalizumab reduces free IgE by 95%, thus downregulating the FcεRI expression on basophils, mast cells, dendritic cells, monocytes, and airway submucosal cells [18, 19]. Its dosing is determined by baseline IgE levels and body weight, and it is administered subcutaneously (SQ) every 2–4 weeks either at home or in the office [20]. Omalizumab decreases asthma exacerbation rates as well as hospitalizations, improves quality of life (QoL), and has an ICS sparing effect [21–23]. Studies also indicate that omalizumab in adolescents and adults leads to improved lung function, especially in patients with airway reversibility [22, 24]. Now with long-term safety data, omalizumab has proven itself safe and well tolerated with no increased risk of malignancy [25–28]. Additionally, it is the only biologic with significant pregnancy data demonstrating no risk of congenital abnormalities when used during pregnancy [29]. In addition to asthma, omalizumab is also FDA-approved for chronic, spontaneous urticaria, and chronic rhinosinusitis with nasal polyposis (CRSwNP).

18.5.1.2.6 Anti-Interleukin 5 (IL-5) Biologics: Mepolizumab, Reslizumab, Benralizumab

IL-5 is considered the central cytokine in the recruitment, survival, and effector function of eosinophils and therefore plays a pivotal role in the pathophysiology of eosinophilic asthma. Drugs that target the IL-5 pathway have been successful in the treatment of eosinophilic asthma. The first drug in this class approved for patients with severe eosinophilic asthma, for ages six years and older, was mepolizumab, a humanized mAb against IL–5. It is dosed based on age given SQ every four weeks either in the office or at home [30]. Benefits of mepolizumab include a reduction in exacerbation rates in patients and in daily OCS use as well as improvement in lung function, QoL, and asthma control [31–34]. Minimal serious AE to mepolizumab have been reported [31]. In addition to asthma, mepolizumab is also FDA-approved for CRSwNP, hypereosinophilic syndrome (HES), and eosinophilic granulomatosis with polyangiitis (EGPA).

The next mAb against IL-5 that was approved is reslizumab, which is indicated for add-on maintenance therapy for patients 18 years and older with severe eosinophilic asthma [35]. Its use in clinical practice is limited by the need to dose it intravenously every four weeks. Similar to other biologics, however, it decreases exacerbations while improving lung function and QoL [36, 37].

Different from the prior IL-5 agents, benralizumab acts as a competitive inhibitor of the IL-5 receptor by binding to the receptor's alpha subunit. Approved for patients 12 years and older with eosinophilic asthma, it is given SQ at home or in office every four weeks for three doses, then every eight weeks after that [38]. It too decreases asthma exacerbations and improves asthma control and lung function with low serious AE rates [39, 40]. Additionally, it leads to a reduction in OCS dose [41].

18.5.1.2.7 Dupilumab

Dupilumab, a mAb targeting the alpha subunit of the interleukin-4 (IL-4) receptor, thus blocking signaling of Il-4 and interleukin-13 (IL-13), is approved for the treatment of moderate to severe asthma in patients six years and older with an eosinophilic phenotype or with OCS-dependent asthma. It is administered SQ every 2–4 weeks at home or in the office with dosing depending on age and weight. IL-4 and IL-13 are cytokines thus implicated in T2 inflammation by blocking them; dupilumab is thought to decrease exacerbation rates, improve asthma control, reduce total OCS dose, and increase lung function [42–45]. Minimal AE have been reported with dupilumab, but elevated blood eosinophils occurs early in the course. Dupilumab is not associated with an increased risk of conjunctivitis as noted in patients treated for atopic dermatitis. In addition to asthma, dupilumab is also FDA-approved for atopic dermatitis, CRSwNP, and eosinophilic esophagitis.

18.5.1.2.8 Tezepelumab

Tezepelumab is the most recently FDA-approved biologic for the treatment of severe uncontrolled asthma. Tezepelumab is administered SQ every four weeks in office (not yet approved for home administration). A human mAb, tezepelumab targets thymic stromal lymphopoietin (TSLP), which is one of several "alarmin" cytokines released from damaged epithelium leading to T2 inflammation [46]. In a recent phase 3 trial, tezepelumab decreased asthma exacerbations, improved lung function, and resulted in better quality of life in patients with severe asthma [47, 48]. Tezepelumab, unlike other biologics, appears beneficial even at lower eosinophil counts (<150 cells/microliter), although maximum benefit was seen in patients with higher eosinophil levels. Tezepelumab is well tolerated with a low AE rate [47].

18.5.1.2.9 Methylxanthines

Theophylline is a competitive nonselective phosphodiesterase inhibitor and nonselective adenosine receptor antagonist that acts as a bronchodilator in the treatment of asthma. It has a narrow therapeutic window requiring close lab monitoring as side effects include arrhythmias and seizures. Due these factors, its use is less desirable and is not preferred in add-on therapy for asthma [3].

18.5.1.2.10 Cromolyn Sodium and Nedocromil

Cromolyn and nedocromil exert their mechanism of action by blocking chloride channels and modulating the release of mast cell mediators and eosinophil recruitment. Both agents inhibit bronchospasm caused by exercise or cold air and prophylactically prevent allergen-induced asthma worsening. Their safety profile is very good, and they can be used as a maintenance therapy especially in childhood asthma [3]. However, they are no longer available in the United States because nonchlorofluorocarbon (CFC) formulations have not been approved.

18.5.1.2.11 Allergen Immunotherapy

Current NHLBI guidelines recommend the use of subcutaneous immunotherapy (SCIT) for the adjunctive treatment of asthma in patients who demonstrate allergic sensitization and worsening of asthma symptoms in relation to exposure to these antigens. SCIT improves exacerbation rates, asthma control, and QoL in patients. Studies show a reduction in rescue and controller medication use. Asthma control must be optimized before initiating SCIT as uncontrolled asthma is the most significant risk factor for fatal anaphylaxis from SCIT. Sublingual immunotherapy (SLIT) is not recommended specifically for the treatment of allergic asthma. That said, in patients with concurrent allergic rhinitis, SLIT for this indication may also reduce symptoms of allergic asthma. Anaphylaxis is of less concern for SLIT; however, the same recommendation regarding asthma control prior to initiation holds true [9]. Studies in children have shown a decrease in the incidence of asthma exacerbations with SCIT, the ability to prevent new sensitizations, and the progression to newly diagnosed asthma in patients with allergic rhinitis [49].

18.5.1.2.12 Bronchial Thermoplasty (BT)

BT has been studied as another add-on therapy to patients with uncontrolled moderate to severe asthma. It involves a bronchoscopy and administering thermal energy to the airways and is believed to work by reducing the airway smooth muscle mass. The majority of data on the risks and benefits of BT come from three randomized control trials enrolling a total of only 432 patients with follow-up extending to five years [50–52]. Adverse events of BT included bronchial irritation, chest discomfort, cough, nocturnal awakenings, wheezing during the treatment as well as ongoing symptoms up to five years following treatment [53–55]. Pulmonary-related hospitalizations (worsening asthma, respiratory infections, pulmonary artery complications, etc.) were also higher in the treatment arm than the placebo during and after BT therapy. NHLBI guidelines do not recommend BT, as improvements are small and harm is moderate. Long-term follow-up to assess clinical response is also lacking. At this time, BT is reserved for patients who, after careful, shared decision-making, feel the risk benefit ratio is favorable [9].

18.5.1.3 How to Select the Optimal Treatment for the Patient

Asthma is a heterogeneous condition, and therapy must be tailored to individuals based on their specific asthma phenotype, access to care, and financial state. Initial therapy will focus with ICS/LABA as needed or SMART therapy. ICS will be used in all patients with moderate to severe asthma. Whereas some patients may benefit from higher doses of ICS, such as when FeNO is elevated, others may benefit from the addition of a LABA or LAMA at a lower dose of ICS, especially in the absence of detectable eosinophilic airway inflammation. LTRAs are often used as adjunctive therapy. When patients remain poorly controlled despite typical therapies, biologics have been shown to improve outcomes with favorable safety profiles. Choosing the optimal biologic depends on a myriad of factors, including age, asthma phenotype, comorbidities, goals of therapy (e.g. decrease in chronic OCS use versus improved lung function), potential asthma triggers (e.g. viral infections versus allergic rhinitis), and adverse effect profile (Figure 18.1). To date, there are no head-to-head trials demonstrating superiority of one biologic over another, and these decisions require shared decision-making between the clinician and patient. To maximize asthma control, comorbidities must

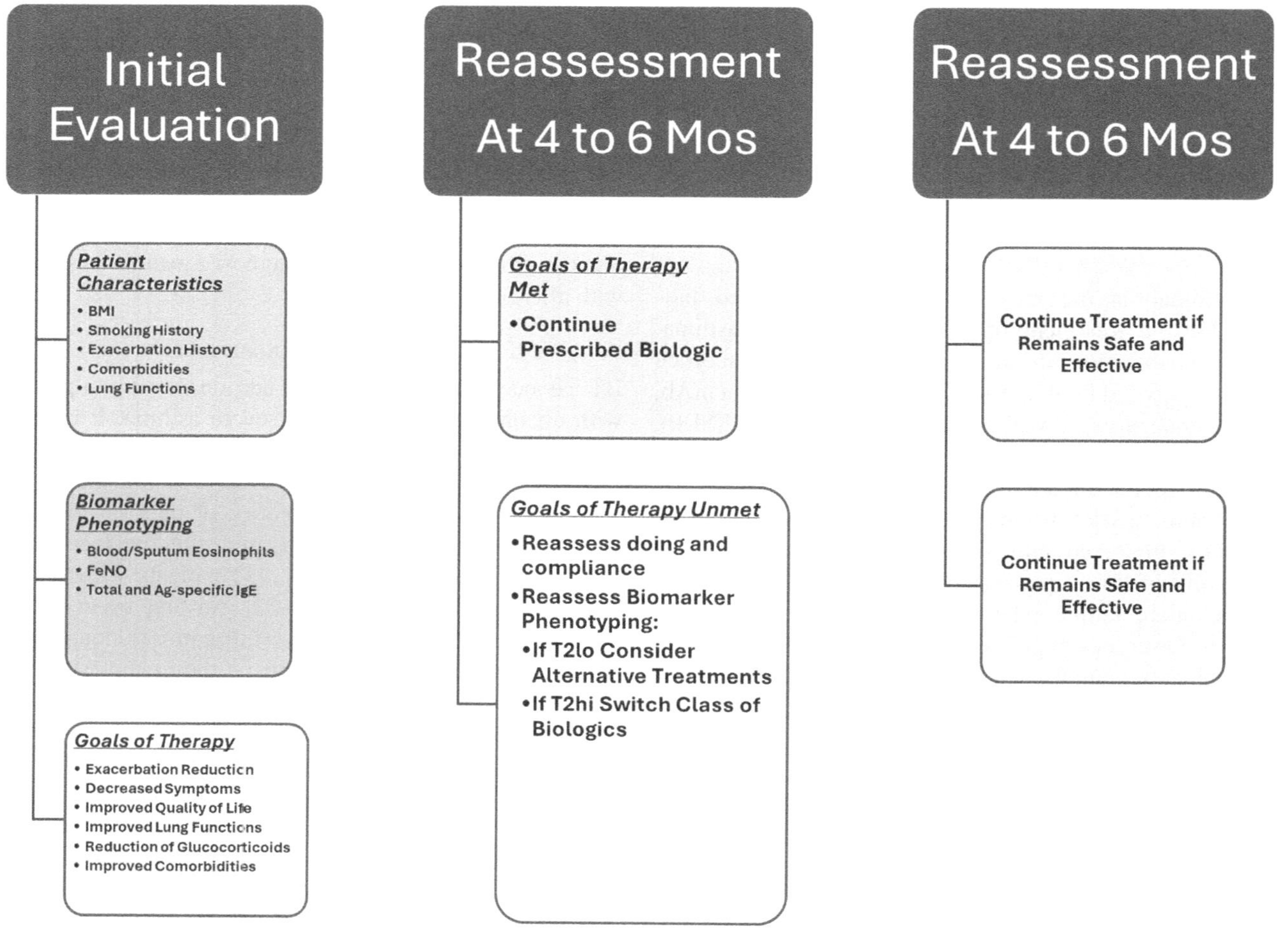

FIGURE 18.1 Choosing the optimal biologic drug.

also be addressed, such as allergic rhino conjunctivitis and CRSwNP. In a patient who has asthma and a comorbid condition also treated by a biologic, the use of this biologic makes sense.

18.5.1.4 Emergency Management

The evaluation of an acute exacerbation of asthma starts with a history. Recent multiple emergency room visits and current oral corticosteroids may indicate an exacerbation that has become refractory to outpatient management, mandating a hospital admission. A previous exacerbation leading to respiratory failure requiring intubation or an attack that has previously caused seizures may indicate that the disease has progressed to severe uncontrolled asthma (see Chapters 21 and 22). The severity of an attack cannot be clearly assessed by the intensity of wheezing, and sometimes a fatal attack can present without any wheezing and with only silent lung sounds on auscultation. Pulsus paradoxus is another indicator of the severity of the disease. An altered mental status in a patient with an acute exacerbation may require intubation.

If possible, spirometry should be done to assess the severity of the airway obstruction and to help determine if admission is needed. A markedly low FEV_1 without response to bronchodilator can indicate the need for admission into hospital. Arterial blood gases and/or O_2 saturation should be done if there is a severe attack, as values can help decisions on admission or discharge. Management consists of intensive bronchodilator therapy, oxygen, and systemic corticosteroids. Approximately one-third of patients in the emergency department (ED) might show no bronchodilator response to albuterol.

18.5.2 How Do You Wean Asthma Medications in Patients with Well-Controlled Symptoms?

While considerable effort has been made to outline asthma step-up therapy, the process of step-down therapy is less clear. Current guidelines recommend that the current step in asthma therapy be maintained until control is achieved for a minimum of three months, at which time step-down therapy should be considered. In patients who are on medium to high doses of ICS with a LABA, the question arises whether one should step off the LABA or step down the ICS. In 2010, the US FDA recommended that the LABA should be stepped off. However, there are no data to support this approach.

A systematic review published in the *Archives of Internal Medicine* in 2012 showed that a meta-analysis of studies to date favored the continued use of LABA [56]. Thus although there is controversy over the safety of LABAs, there is a considerable amount of evidence supporting their use for patients with asthma. A separate randomized clinical trial published in 2018 did not show a difference in time to treatment failure between reduced ICS/LABA and LABA step-off; however, lung function and hospitalization rates were higher in the LABA step-off group [57].

18.5.3 Miscellaneous Considerations

18.5.3.1 Aspirin-Exacerbated Respiratory Disease/NSAID-Exacerbated Respiratory Disease (NERD)

Aspirin (acetylsalicylic acid [ASA])-induced asthma is associated with rhinosinusitis, nasal polyps, and asthma [ASA triad or Sampter's triad]), which is precipitated by aspirin and other nonsteroidal anti-inflammatory drugs (NSAIDs). This is more commonly seen in females and often presents in patients around 30–40 years of age. Aspirin-sensitive patients have increased eosinophilic inflammation and increased levels of urinary LTE4. Atopy is not a risk factor for NERD. Aspirin and cross-reacting COX1 nonsteroidal anti-inflammatory agents should be avoided in such patients and, if this cannot be done, desensitization, preferably post-polypectomy is an option [58]. Several biologics indicated for the treatment of moderate to severe asthma have also been shown efficacious in improving upper respiratory tract symptoms of AERD [59]. Currently, omalizumab, mepolizumab, and dupilumab are all FDA-approved for the treatment of chronic rhinosinusitis with nasal polyps. Dupilumab, however, is the only biologic with prospective data showing efficacy in a small case series of a patient with NERD [60] and may also decrease NSAID sensitivity in patients with NERD [61]. There has also been indication that certain dietary modifications can also lead to reduced symptoms of AERD including one high in omega-3 fatty acids. LTD4 blockers as well as zileuton, the 5-lipoxygenase inhibitor discussed previously, are useful therapeutic interventions [59].

18.6 ASTHMA IN PREGNANCY AND LACTATION (SEE CHAPTER 25)

Asthma has been shown to affect up to 8% of pregnant women and is probably one of the most common medical causes of morbidity in pregnancy. Better control of asthma lowers the risk of pregnancy complications and mortality associated with asthma. Limited information is available on pharmacotherapy in pregnancy. Most studies have shown that it is safer to use medications to keep asthma under control, rather than have an acute exacerbation during pregnancy and while lactating. Although no studies of asthma biologics have intentionally included pregnant patients, a safety registry for omalizumab has shown no increase for major congenital malformations, prematurity, or low birth weight [62]. It is essential to identify and avoid any exacerbating factors, including exposure to tobacco smoke and GERD [63].

18.7 OCCUPATIONAL ASTHMA (SEE CHAPTER 24)

Exposure to high molecular weight proteins and low molecular weight chemicals, followed by a latency period before symptom onset, has been demonstrated to cause occupational asthma in a previously healthy, susceptible worker or to exacerbate pre-existing asthma. Furthermore, acute or chronic exposure to irritants in the workplace can cause AHR and bronchial constriction, referred to as irritant-induced asthma or reactive airways dysfunction syndrome (RADS). The early identification of occupational asthma is required to prevent further exposure and to obtain good long-term outcomes [64].

18.8 EXERCISE-INDUCED BRONCHOCONSTRICTION (EIB) (SEE CHAPTER 12)

EIB is defined as a lower airway obstruction with symptoms of cough, wheezing, or dyspnea induced by exercise in patients without underlying asthma. Exercise-induced asthma is the same as EIB except that it occurs in patients with chronic asthma. Exercising causes hyperventilation of air that is dryer and cooler [65], and this loss of heat and moisture causes bronchoconstriction. The onset of EIB is usually minutes after beginning exercise, peaks around 10 minutes after stopping exercise, and lasts around 30–40 minutes. The diagnosis is based on a history of chest tightness, cough, and wheezing after exercising; also, exercise-challenge testing can be done. A 15% decrease in FEV_1 post-exercise is consistent with EIB [66]. Treatment usually involves the use of a SABA 15–30 minutes prior to exercise. Montelukast is also FDA-approved as a controller for EIB, but it may not prevent all symptoms, so rescue SABA should also be available [67].

REFERENCES

1. Prevention, C.F.D.C.A. *Most Recent National Asthma Data*. 2022 May 25, 2022 [cited 2022 July 25]. https://www.cdc.gov/asthma/most_recent_national_asthma_data.htm.
2. Akinbami, L.J., et al., *Trends in asthma prevalence, health care use, and mortality in the United States, 2001–2010*. NCHS Data Brief, 2012(94): p. 1–8.
3. National Heart, L., and Blood Institute, National Institutes of Health. National Asthma Education and Prevention Program, *Expert panel report 3: Guidelines for the diagnosis and management of asthma*. NIH Publication No. 07–4051, 2007.
4. Miller, M.R., et al., *Standardisation of spirometry*. Eur Respir J, 2005. **26**(2): p. 319–38.

5. Levy, M.L., et al., *Diagnostic spirometry in primary care: Proposed standards for general practice compliant with American Thoracic Society and European Respiratory Society recommendations: a General Practice Airways Group (GPIAG)1 document, in association with the Association for Respiratory Technology & Physiology (ARTP)2 and Education for Health3 1* www.gpiag.org 2 www.artp.org 3 www.educationforhealth.org.uk. Prim Care Respir J, 2009. **18**(3): p. 130–47.
6. Burrows, B., et al., *Association of asthma with serum IgE levels and skin-test reactivity to allergens.* N Engl J Med, 1989. **320**(5): p. 271–7.
7. Price, D.B., et al., *Blood eosinophil count and prospective annual asthma disease burden: a UK cohort study.* Lancet Respir Med, 2015. **3**(11): p. 849–58.
8. Dweik, R.A., et al., *An official ATS clinical practice guideline: interpretation of exhaled nitric oxide levels (FENO) for clinical applications.* Am J Respir Crit Care Med, 2011. **184**(5): p. 602–15.
9. Cloutier, M.M., et al., *2020 Focused updates to the asthma management guidelines: a report from the national asthma education and prevention program coordinating committee expert panel working group.* J Allergy Clin Immunol, 2020. **146**(6): p. 1217–70.
10. Reddel, H.K., et al., *Global Initiative for Asthma Strategy 2021: executive summary and rationale for key changes.* Eur Respir J, 2022. **59**(1).
11. Nelson, H.S., et al., *The salmeterol multicenter asthma research trial: a comparison of usual pharmacotherapy for asthma or usual pharmacotherapy plus salmeterol.* Chest, 2006. **129**(1): p. 15–26.
12. Nelson, H.S., et al., *Update on the safety of long-acting beta-agonists in combination with inhaled corticosteroids for the treatment of asthma.* Ann Allergy Asthma Immunol, 2009. **102**(1): p. 11–15.
13. Ostrom, N.K., *Tolerability of short-term, high-dose formoterol in healthy volunteers and patients with asthma.* Clin Ther, 2003. **25**(11): p. 2635–46.
14. Reddel, H.K., et al., *A practical guide to implementing SMART in asthma management.* J Allergy Clin Immunol Pract, 2022. **10**(1s): p. S31–s38.
15. Masoli, M. and R. Beasley, *Asthma exacerbations and inhaled corticosteroids.* Lancet, 2004. **363**(9416): p. 1236.
16. Tantisira, K.G., et al., *Genomewide association between GLCCI1 and response to glucocorticoid therapy in asthma.* N Engl J Med, 2011. **365**(13): p. 1173–83.
17. Wechsler, M.E., et al., *Anticholinergic vs long-acting β-Agonist in combination with inhaled corticosteroids in black adults with asthma: the BELT randomized clinical trial.* JAMA, 2015. **314**(16): p. 1720–30.
18. MacGlashan, D.W., Jr., et al., *Down-regulation of Fc(epsilon)RI expression on human basophils during in vivo treatment of atopic patients with anti-IgE antibody.* J Immunol, 1997. **158**(3): p. 1438–45.
19. Beck, L.A., et al., *Omalizumab-induced reductions in mast cell FcεRI expression and function.* J Allergy Clin Immunol, 2004. **114**(3): p. 527–30.
20. US Food and Drug Administration, *XOLAIR® (omalizumab) injection, for subcutaneous use Initial U.S. Approval: 2003.* US Food and Drug Administration, Accessed August 24, 2021.
21. Normansell, R., et al., *Omalizumab for asthma in adults and children.* Cochrane Database Syst Rev, 2014(1): p. Cd003559.
22. Busse, W., et al., *Omalizumab, anti-IgE recombinant humanized monoclonal antibody, for the treatment of severe allergic asthma.* J Allergy Clin Immunol, 2001. **108**(2): p. 184–90.
23. Buhl, R., et al., *The anti-IgE antibody omalizumab improves asthma-related quality of life in patients with allergic asthma.* Eur Respir J, 2002. **20**(5): p. 1088–94.
24. Busse, W.W., et al., *Effect of omalizumab on lung function and eosinophil levels in adolescents with moderate-to-severe allergic asthma.* Ann Allergy Asthma Immunol, 2020. **124**(2): p. 190–6.
25. Agache, I., et al., *Efficacy and safety of treatment with biologicals (benralizumab, dupilumab, mepolizumab, omalizumab and reslizumab) for severe eosinophilic asthma. A systematic review for the EAACI Guidelines—recommendations on the use of biologicals in severe asthma.* Allergy, 2020. **75**(5): p. 1023–42.
26. Mansur, A.H., et al., *Longterm clinical outcomes of omalizumab therapy in severe allergic asthma: Study of efficacy and safety.* Respir Med, 2017. **124**: p. 36–43.
27. Busse, W., et al., *Omalizumab and the risk of malignancy: results from a pooled analysis.* J Allergy Clin Immunol, 2012. **129**(4): p. 983–9.e6.
28. Long, A., et al., *Incidence of malignancy in patients with moderate-to-severe asthma treated with or without omalizumab.* J Allergy Clin Immunol, 2014. **134**(3): p. 560–67. e4.
29. Namazy, J.A., et al., *Pregnancy outcomes in the omalizumab pregnancy registry and a disease-matched comparator cohort.* J Allergy Clin Immunol, 2020. **145**(2): p. 528–36.e1.
30. US Food and Drug Administration, *NUCALA® (mepolizumab) injection, for subcutaneous use initial U.S. Approval: 2015.* US Food and Drug Administration, Accessed July 9, 2021.
31. Ortega, H.G., et al., *Mepolizumab treatment in patients with severe eosinophilic asthma.* N Engl J Med, 2014. **371**(13): p. 1198–207.
32. Ortega, H.G., et al., *Severe eosinophilic asthma treated with mepolizumab stratified by baseline eosinophil thresholds: a secondary analysis of the DREAM and MENSA studies.* Lancet Respir Med, 2016. **4**(7): p. 549–56.
33. Harrison, T., et al., *Real-world mepolizumab in the prospective severe asthma REALITI-A study: initial analysis.* Eur Respir J, 2020. **56**(4).
34. Bel, E.H., et al., *Oral glucocorticoid-sparing effect of mepolizumab in eosinophilic asthma.* N Engl J Med, 2014. **371**(13): p. 1189–97.
35. US Food and Drug Administration, *CINQAIR® (reslizumab) injection, for intravenous use Initial U.S. Approval: 2016.* US Food and Drug Administration, Accessed October 9, 2021.
36. Castro, M., et al., *Reslizumab for inadequately controlled asthma with elevated blood eosinophil counts: results from two multicentre, parallel, double-blind, randomised, placebo-controlled, phase 3 trials.* Lancet Respir Med, 2015. **3**(5): p. 355–66.
37. Castro, M., et al., *Reslizumab for poorly controlled, eosinophilic asthma: a randomized, placebo-controlled study.* Am J Respir Crit Care Med, 2011. **184**(10): p. 1125–32.
38. US Food and Drug Administration, *FASENRA® (benralizumab) injection, for subcutaneous use Initial U.S. Approval: 2017.* US Food and Drug Administration, Accessed July 9, 2021.
39. Bleecker, E.R., et al., *Efficacy and safety of benralizumab for patients with severe asthma uncontrolled with high-dosage inhaled corticosteroids and long-acting β(2)-agonists*

(SIROCCO): a randomised, multicentre, placebo-controlled phase 3 trial. Lancet, 2016. **388**(10056): p. 2115–27.
40. Busse, W.W., et al., *Long-term safety and efficacy of benralizumab in patients with severe, uncontrolled asthma: 1-year results from the BORA phase 3 extension trial*. Lancet Respir Med, 2019. **7**(1): p. 46–59.
41. Nair, P., et al., *Oral glucocorticoid–sparing effect of benralizumab in severe asthma*. N Engl J Med, 2017. **376**(25): p. 2448–58.
42. Castro, M., et al., *Dupilumab efficacy and safety in moderate-to-severe uncontrolled asthma*. N Engl J Med, 2018. **378**(26): p. 2486–96.
43. Corren, J., et al., *D201 Dupilumab efficacy in patients with uncontrolled, moderate-to-severe asthma and serologic evidence of allergic bronchopulmonary aspergillosis*. Ann Allergy Clin Immunol, 2019. **123**(5): p. S15.
44. Agache, I., et al., *Efficacy and safety of treatment with dupilumab for severe asthma: A systematic review of the EAACI guidelines-Recommendations on the use of biologicals in severe asthma*. Allergy, 2020. **75**(5): p. 1058–68.
45. Zayed, Y., et al., *Dupilumab safety and efficacy in uncontrolled asthma: a systematic review and meta-analysis of randomized clinical trials*. J Asthma, 2019. **56**(10): p. 1110–19.
46. Porsbjerg, C.M., et al., *Anti-alarmins in asthma: targeting the airway epithelium with next-generation biologics*. Eur Respir J, 2020. **56**(5).
47. Menzies-Gow, A., et al., *Tezepelumab in adults and adolescents with severe, uncontrolled asthma*. N Engl J Med, 2021. **384**(19): p. 1800–9.
48. Menzies-Gow, A., et al., *NAVIGATOR: a phase 3 multicentre, randomized, double-blind, placebo-controlled, parallel-group trial to evaluate the efficacy and safety of tezepelumab in adults and adolescents with severe, uncontrolled asthma*. Respir Res, 2020. **21**(1): p. 266.
49. Cox, L., et al., *Allergen immunotherapy: a practice parameter third update*. J Allergy Clin Immunol, 2011. **127**(1 Suppl): p. S1–55.
50. Pavord, I.D., et al., *Safety and efficacy of bronchial thermoplasty in symptomatic, severe asthma*. Am J Respir Crit Care Med, 2007. **176**(12): p. 1185–91.
51. Castro, M., et al., *Effectiveness and safety of bronchial thermoplasty in the treatment of severe asthma: a multicenter, randomized, double-blind, sham-controlled clinical trial*. Am J Respir Crit Care Med, 2010. **181**(2): p. 116–24.
52. Cox, G., et al., *Asthma control during the year after bronchial thermoplasty*. N Engl J Med, 2007. **356**(13): p. 1327–1337.
53. Thomson, N.C., et al., *Long-term (5 year) safety of bronchial thermoplasty: Asthma Intervention Research (AIR) trial*. BMC Pulm Med, 2011. **11**: p. 8.
54. Wechsler, M.E., et al., *Bronchial thermoplasty: Long-term safety and effectiveness in patients with severe persistent asthma*. J Allergy Clin Immunol, 2013. **132**(6): p. 1295–302.
55. Pavord, I.D., et al., *Safety of bronchial thermoplasty in patients with severe refractory asthma*. Ann Allergy Asthma Immunol, 2013. **111**(5): p. 402–7.
56. Brozek, J.L., et al., *Long-acting β2-agonist step-off in patients with controlled asthma*. Arch Intern Med, 2012. **172**(18): p. 1365–75.
57. Rogers, L., et al., *Step-down therapy for asthma well controlled on inhaled corticosteroid and long-acting beta-agonist: a randomized clinical trial*. J Allergy Clin Immunol Pract, 2018. **6**(2): p. 633–43.el.
58. Chang, J.E., et al., *Aspirin-exacerbated respiratory disease: burden of disease*. Allergy Asthma Proc, 2012. **33**(2): p. 117–21.
59. Laidlaw, T.M., *Clinical updates in aspirin-exacerbated respiratory disease*. Allergy Asthma Proc, 2019. **40**(1): p. 4–6.
60. Mustafa, S.S., et al., *Dupilumab as add-on therapy for chronic rhinosinusitis with nasal polyposis in aspirin exacerbated respiratory disease*. Am J Rhinol Allergy, 2021. **35**(3): p. 399–407.
61. Mustafa, S.S. and K. Vadamalai, *Dupilumab increases aspirin tolerance in aspirin-exacerbated respiratory disease*. Ann Allergy Asthma Immunol, 2021. **126**(6): p. 738–39.
62. Bonham, C.A., K.C. Patterson, and M.E. Strek, *Asthma outcomes and management during pregnancy*. Chest, 2018. **153**(2): p. 515–27.
63. Louik, C., et al., *Asthma in pregnancy and its pharmacologic treatment*. Ann Allergy Asthma Immunol, 2010. **105**(2): p. 110–7.
64. Nicholson, P.J., et al., *Evidence based guidelines for the prevention, identification, and management of occupational asthma*. Occup Environ Med, 2005. **62**(5): p. 290–9.
65. Anderson, S.D., *Exercise-induced bronchoconstriction in the 21st century*. J Am Osteopath Assoc, 2011. **111**(11 Suppl 7): p. S3–10.
66. Anderson, S.D., et al., *Responses to bronchial challenge submitted for approval to use inhaled beta2-agonists before an event at the 2002 Winter Olympics*. J Allergy Clin Immunol, 2003. **111**(1): p. 45–50.
67. Carver, T.W., *Exercise-induced asthma: critical analysis of the protective role of montelukast*. J Asthma Allergy, 2009. **2**: p. 93–103.

19 Management of Asthma in Older Adults

Tolly E.G. Epstein, Alan P. Baptist, Anil Nanda, Andrew M. Smith, Deborah Lee, and Jenny J. Lee

CASE STUDY

A 72-year-old female presents with coughing, wheezing, and shortness of breath. Symptoms began 10 years ago and are worse with exertion and viral illnesses. She's had recurrent sinus infections 3–4 times per year since her 50s. She has comorbid hypertension, diabetes, depression, gastroesophageal reflux disease (GERD), and high cholesterol and has been prescribed nine medications for these conditions; she admits to nonadherence due to cost. She smoked one pack of cigarettes per day for 10 years and quit 40 years ago. Her body mass index is 40.

19.1 EPIDEMIOLOGY

Asthma is frequently considered a disease of children and young adults, yet it affects a significant portion of adults age 65 years and older. More than 4 million older adults (7.8%) have asthma in the US, making the prevalence of asthma in this population similar to other age groups.[1] As the population ages, up to 20% of asthmatics may be age 65 or older by 2050.[2] Morbidity and mortality from asthma are much higher for older adults. Based on data from the Centers for Disease Control from 2020, the fatality rate from asthma among those age 65 years and older was 30.7 (standard error [SE] = 0.74) per million individuals, versus the next highest rate of 13.8 (SE = 0.33) among those ages 35–64 years old.[1] Hospitalizations, emergency room visits, and utilization of other healthcare resources are also higher among older asthmatics than for other age groups, and asthma-related quality of life is lower.[3–5] Older adults are more likely to have very poorly controlled asthma, persistent asthma, and require one or more controller medications for asthma.[6]

The burden of asthma in older adults is higher among certain demographic populations. Older women have higher morbidity and mortality than men from asthma.[7] A survey of more than 14,076 older adults with asthma found that older female asthmatics were more likely than men to be African American and to have household incomes <$25,000.[6] Female gender was also associated with not having a primary care physician or being able to afford asthma medications. In addition, female older asthmatics were more likely to have comorbid chronic obstructive pulmonary disease (COPD), depression, and obesity. A surveillance survey of 4700 asthmatics age 55 years or older found that, even after controlling for educational level, income, impaired access to care due to cost, and gaps in health insurance coverage, older African American and Hispanic asthmatics were twice as likely to have an emergency room visit for asthma.[2]

Different asthma phenotypes may be more prominent in older adults, which impacts severity and response to treatment. Several studies have performed cluster analyses aimed at identifying high-risk phenotypes in this population.[8–10] Various characteristics have been evaluated, including age of asthma onset, duration of symptoms, asthma and COPD overlap syndrome (ACOS), atopy, and baseline and post-bronchodilator forced expiratory volume in 1 second (FEV_1). Obesity and hormonal changes associated with aging may also impact phenotypic presentations of asthma. Biomarkers such as sputum neutrophilia may be associated with more severe disease, but findings have not been consistent.[11, 12] Although distinct phenotypes exist in older adults, the clinical and therapeutic implications of these phenotypes remains poorly understood. The ACO syndrome also has unique pathophysiologic and phenotypic features that impact responses to treatment but is beyond the scope of this chapter.

19.2 IMMUNOLOGIC CHANGES WITH AGING

With age, the total amount of hematopoietic tissue in the bone marrow, and the ability of hematopoietic stem cells to proliferate decreases.[13] Subsequently, fewer pro-B cells are generated and progress to differentiation steps, and lower numbers of mature B cells leave the bone marrow.[14] Macrophages and macrophage precursors are also significantly reduced in the bone marrow.[15] In contrast to some other immune cells, natural killer cell numbers increase in older adults; however, there are significant reductions in NK cell function.[16] Several functional defects in dendritic cells

DOI: 10.1201/9781003287209-24

have been observed with age, including reduced capacity for phagocytosis, and defects in migration and micropinocytosis.[17] Most studies report that the number of neutrophils in the blood of healthy adults remain unchanged with age, but phagocytic capacity is significantly decreased, particularly in response to opsonized *S. aureus* and *S. pneumoniae*.[18] While the number of blood monocytes does not decrease with age, there are significant decreases in the number of macrophages in the bone marrow of older adults and in their phagocytic ability.[19] In addition, the respiratory burst in older adults is reduced, resulting in impairment of intracellular killing.[20]

The major change in immunosenescence of T cells is the involution of the thymus by 40–50 years of age.[21] After age 70, there is a significant contraction in the T cell repertoire due to a dramatic decline in diversity.[22] Unlike naïve T cells, peripheral B cell numbers do not decline with age. With the accumulation of memory B cells, there is a clonal expansion of particular B cell specificities, and a limited repertoire may develop.[23] In addition, intrinsic defects in class-switch recombination develop, and antibody production shifts in isotype from IgG to IgM with age, which leads to lower affinity.[24]

Elevation of multiple cytokines, chemokines, and other pro-inflammatory signals has been reported in older adults.[25] Increased plasma cytokine expression is thought to contribute to continuous immune system stimulation, which leads to a subclinical inflammatory state known as inflammaging.[26] A number of different environmental and metabolic factors may influence inflammaging. [27] Persistent latent viral infection can impact T cells in older adults. These environmental factors may interact with genetic and epigenetic changes in concert with immunosenescence to modulate or mediate the outcomes of the underlying inflammatory state.[28]

19.3 CLINICAL PRESENTATION AND DIAGNOSIS OF ASTHMA IN THE OLDER ADULT

The symptoms of asthma in older adults are the same as those in younger individuals. Despite this, asthma remains under-diagnosed in the older adult. Older adults are frequently poor perceivers of asthmatic symptoms and may minimize the significance of chronic respiratory symptoms, attributing them to deconditioning or natural aging.[29] Psychosocial factors such as depression and poor health literacy also impact whether older adults seek care for asthmatic symptoms.[30] Physicians often don't consider asthma as a principal consideration in older adults presenting with chest symptoms. This is in part due to the perception by some that asthma only begins in childhood or young adulthood and because of initial consideration for other illnesses that are also common in older adults.[3] In addition, older patients are more likely than younger individuals to have more than one comorbid illness causing respiratory symptoms, further confounding diagnosis.

Ultimately, the diagnosis of asthma in older adults is still based on clinical evaluation, but testing should still be attempted.[31] A detailed medical history is paramount, and classic symptoms can include wheezing, cough, and shortness of breath.[32] Physical examination may reveal wheezing or prolonged expiration time but can be completely normal, as with younger asthmatics.[31] There is an extensive differential diagnosis in older adults, including heart disease, COPD, pulmonary embolism, pulmonary hypertension, gastroesophageal reflux disease (GERD), and vocal cord dysfunction.[31] Evaluation for age-related comorbid illnesses may need to be conducted simultaneously with evaluation for asthma. Testing includes pulmonary function testing and spirometry, methacholine challenge, fractional exhaled nitric oxide (FeNO), and chest radiograph X-ray. Achieving quality end-points can be more challenging due to physical and cognitive impairments, and additional time and coaching may be needed.[33] Pulmonary function testing in asthma patients can reveal variable expiratory flow obstruction with a reduced forced expiratory volume in 1 second (FEV_1) and reduced FEV_1/FVC (forced vital capacity) ratio.[34] Interpretation of test results must include consideration for the normal reduction in FEV_1 due to aging and the increased possibility of fixed obstruction in asthmatics with long-standing disease.[35] Bronchodilator reversibility (>12% or absolute 200 mL increase in baseline FEV_1) is often one of the diagnostic criteria in asthma; however, this can underestimate asthma in older adults.[34] Methacholine challenge utilizes inhaled increasing amounts of methacholine, with a subsequent decrease of >20% in FEV_1 considered a positive test.[34] FeNO measures nitric oxide produced by inflammatory and epithelial cells of the lung and an elevation (usually greater than 50) usually indicate asthma.[31] Chest X-ray imaging is often normal but can show bronchial thickening.[31] Allergy testing utilizing skin prick method or specific IgE can determine if there is an allergic asthma component.[10] In situations where it may be difficult to distinguish asthma from COPD based on lung function alone, factors such as the age of onset, smoking history, atopic status, diffusing capacity for carbon monoxide, and exhaled nitric oxide may prove useful in establishing the diagnosis.[36]

19.4 UNIQUE FACTORS OF ASTHMA MANAGEMENT IN OLDER ADULTS (TABLE 19.1)

The goals of asthma management in older adults are not different from those in younger patients: to control asthma in both impairment and risk domains to improve overall well-being and quality of life and to prevent exacerbations.[35] However, asthma management may look different in older adults due to differing physical, functional, cognitive, psychosocial, and economic factors affecting their health. Multidimensional assessment of these specific needs for individual older adults is essential to achieving optimal asthma control.[37]

TABLE 19.1
Unique Factors to Consider When Treating Older Adults with Asthma

Barriers to Care	Helpful Strategies
Cognitive impairment and memory loss	• Utilize written asthma action plans.
	• Review patient's social support system and clarify caregiver role in asthma management.
	• Educate patient and their caregiver on identifying asthma symptoms and self-management strategies.
	• Utilize teach-back methods and reinforce/repeat education.
	• Use shared decision-making to come up with a medication schedule that patient can adhere to.
Physical function impairment	• Use larger fonts for medication instructions and asthma action plans.
Impaired vision	• Review inhaler techniques in clinic to verify proper use of inhalers.
Poor inhaler use technique due to musculoskeletal diseases or poor breathing coordination	• Use spacers for MDIs.
	• Consider using breath-actuated inhalers, DPIs, or nebulizers.
Comorbidities Polypharmacy	• Review all medications and identify any medications that may worsen bronchospasm or cough (NSAIDs, nonselective beta-blockers, and ACE-Is).
Comorbidities that can cause symptoms similar to asthma	• Simplify medication schedule by limiting dose frequency and number of medications, if possible.
	• Discuss patient's concerns regarding medication side effects.
	• Consider nonpharmacologic therapies such as breathing exercises and pulmonary rehabilitation, if appropriate.
	• Identify any psychiatric comorbidities that may hinder optimal asthma control, such as depression and anxiety, and treat them appropriately.
	• Review medications used for acute symptoms of different comorbidities (especially diuretics and bronchodilators).
Use of complementary/alternative medications	• Review all complementary medications and alternative home remedies used.
Transportation issues	• Assess patient's need for transportation and provide virtual follow-up, if appropriate.
	• Involve social worker and/or case manager, who can arrange transportation for patient.
	• Schedule medical visits on the same day as other medical appointments.
Limited or fixed income	• Consider cost of prescription medications.
	• Involve social worker and/or case manager, who can provide financial resources to patient.

19.4.1 Menopause/HRT

The female predominance in asthma prevalence after elementary school age is thought to be associated with hormonal changes during puberty, and this continues into the later years of life. There is conflicting data on new-onset asthma incidence during menopause.[38] The prevalence of atopic asthma decreases with age.[39] A case series published by Barbaro et al.[40] concluded that asthma with menopausal onset is more likely non-atopic. In this study, 40 women with perimenopausal-onset asthma had a higher percentage of neutrophils and a lower percentage of eosinophils in their sputum when compared with the sputum from 35 women with premenopausal-onset asthma.

More recently, a 17-year longitudinal cohort study from the United Kingdom of over 30,000 women with asthma aged 46–70 found that previous but not current use of HRT was associated with an increased risk of severe asthma exacerbations.[41] The longer that the women had used HRT, the greater the risk of a severe reaction. The authors suggest that the drop in estrogen after discontinuing HRT may predispose to asthma exacerbations.

19.4.2 Memory Loss and Cognitive Impairment

The prevalence of memory and cognitive impairment increase with age. One neuro-epidemiologic study notes that the prevalence of cognitive impairment after 70 years of age is approximately 22.2% and as high as 39% in adults above age 90.[42]

Memory loss and cognitive impairment in older adults can lead to many adverse outcomes including unintentional medication non-compliance, increased healthcare utilization, and greater costs. Aging is one of the strong predictors for medication nonadherence.[43] A three-year prospective cohort study of 758 non-nursing home adults found that the older adults who reported subjective memory complaints had increased cost of healthcare utilization by 60%.[44] Polypharmacy is extremely common in older adults, and this poses a significant challenge to those with cognitive impairment. Polypharmacy with complex medication instructions, such as inhalers that require multiple puffs, multiple times a day, in older adults with cognitive impairment can contribute to unintentional medication nonadherence.

19.4.3 Functional Status

Functional status decline is a natural part of aging. A longitudinal household survey reported 70% of adults who live beyond age 65 developed severe long-term service and support needs including paid home care, residential care, and/or nursing home care.[45] Many develop disabilities such as difficulty with mobility (reported by 40% of adults age 65 and older), hearing (31%), cognition (27%), and vision (22%), requiring help from their family members or other caregivers.[46] However, one study of 46 older adults with asthma found that the majority of participants did not have anyone who regularly helped with their asthma self-management. Even when caregivers' help is available, many older adults still prefer to have autonomy over their own medical care. In one study, a majority of older adults with asthma reported they preferred not to ask for help or inform their family members of their asthma symptoms.[47]

19.4.4 Caregiver Roles

Despite declining functional status, older adults often take on caregiving roles of others, including their aging spouse with significant medical or cognitive needs, their children who may be living at home, or their grandchildren while their parents are at work.[48] Increased caregiving stress is associated with worse self-reported health and greater use of healthcare services.[49] It is also associated with increased caregiver anxiety and depression.[50] One survey-based study of 169 caregivers to geriatric patients with dementia reported a high prevalence of caregivers' unmet needs; 87% of these caregivers reported at least one unmet need, some in emotional well-being and others in their own health. Caregiver burden and stress can have increased negative impact on older adults' well-being. This has been demonstrated among older adults with asthma, especially women, who reported that they put the needs of their family members above their own health and may forget to take asthma medications.

19.4.5 Transportation

Access to transportation can be problematic for older adults. The National Institute on Aging lists stiff joints and muscles, trouble seeing, trouble hearing, dementia, slow reaction time and reflexes, and medications that can affect driving as factors that may impact the safety of an older adult's driving.[51] It is common for older adults to lose their ability to drive with aging, and this can lead to limited autonomy and independence, adding another barrier to their asthma care.

19.4.6 Fixed Income

Older adults' asthma management can be affected by limited financial resources as a great proportion of the US older adults live in poverty and/or with fixed income. In 2019, nearly 1 in 10 older adults aged 65 and older lived below the poverty level. A greater proportion of ethnic minority groups were experiencing poverty: 18% of African American, 17.1% of Hispanic, and 9.3% of Asian American older adults compared to 6.8% of the non-Hispanic White older adults.[46] One survey-based study conducted on cost-associated medication restriction among older adults above age 70 showed that medication restriction due to financial burden was very common.[52]

19.5 PHARMACOLOGIC STRATEGIES

The cornerstone controller therapy for asthma, an inflammatory condition, is inhaled corticosteroids (ICS). The side effect profile is much more favorable compared to systemic corticosteroids in terms of diabetes, bone density, and immune suppression with chronic doses.[31] ICS can cause oral thrush. In addition to ICS, long-acting beta-agonist (LABA) therapy can be added, as well as long-acting muscarinic antagonists (LAMA), or anticholinergics, with ICS-LABA-LAMA combination therapy.[53] LABA therapy can cause nervous system side effects, such as agitation or tremors.[31] LAMA therapy has been associated with worsening of acute angle glaucoma and urinary issues.[31] Short-acting beta-agonists (SABA) can be useful for fast-acting therapy and can cause similar side effects to LABA therapy.[31]

The 2020 National Asthma Education and Prevention Program Coordinating Committee Expert Panel Working Group (NAEPP) and 2021 Global Initiative for Asthma (GINA) recently published updated guidelines for the treatment of asthma.[54] There is an increased emphasis on single-inhaler maintenance and reliever therapy (SMART) using the ICS-LABA combination, budesonide-formoterol; however, this use is not currently approved by the United States (US) Food and Drug Administration (FDA).[54]

Biologic therapies are the most recent advances in asthma therapy, currently approved for moderate to severe asthma, and include omalizumab (anti-IgE), mepolizumab (anti-IL-5), reslizumab (anti-IL-5), benralizumab (anti-IL5ra), dupilumab (anti-IL4ra), and tezepelumab (anti-TSLP [thymic stromal lymphopoietin] therapy).[55–62] These therapies are systemic corticosteroid sparing, are usually added to ICS-based asthma therapy, and generally have a favorable side effect profile. Several studies have shown that omalizumab is safe and effective for older adults with severe asthma, although it may be more effective in younger individuals.[56, 57, 63] In a sub-analysis of 80 older adults with severe asthma on mepolizumab, there was a 76% reduction in exacerbations compared to placebo; there were also improvements in quality of life end-points, and a good safety profile among older adults.[64] Reslizumab has shown similar safety and effectiveness among older adults compared to younger asthmatics.[65, 66] Benralizumab also has proven safety and efficacy for adults age 65 years and older with severe asthma and elevated eosinophils, although only nine patients age 75 years and older were included in clinical trials.[67] Some studies regarding dupilumab and severe asthma have included a small number of adults age 65 years and older, but additional data are needed in this age group.[68, 69] Studies for the newest asthma biologic, Tezepelumab, have included adults age 65 years and older, although comparative data relative to younger individuals are lacking.[70]

19.6 NONPHARMACOLOGIC STRATEGIES

Given the unique challenges of older adults with asthma as just discussed, a number of nonpharmacologic strategies can improve outcomes, including pulmonary rehabilitation and breathing techniques.[71, 72] Providing multidimensional care is important in older adults because their health is closely connected to the cognitive, functional, biological, psychological, and socioeconomic domains of their lives.[73] Given the significant effects of depression on asthma outcomes in older adults, screening for depression should be considered. Comorbidities and polypharmacy, when combined with declining cognitive and physical functions, may pose great challenges to asthma control. Careful review of medications should be done to minimize drug–drug interactions and side effects of medications while obtaining optimal asthma control. The use of NSAIDS and nonselective beta-blockers in older adults is common for controlling aches and pains and coronary artery disease, respectively, and may worsen asthma. Review of complementary and alternative medications should be performed, as they may be ineffective and potentially harmful.[47]

Medication nonadherence is a common and complex problem in older adults related to multiple factors as just listed: limited financial resources, concerns about side effects, impaired inhaler technique, cognitive impairment, poor understanding of medications, polypharmacy, and depression/other comorbidities.[37] Identifying barriers to optimal medical care and devising a feasible plan is critical. Some barriers, especially those associated with finances and transportation, may require social workers and case managers. Because many older adults desire independence and autonomy despite declining functional and cognitive status, involving caregivers in their asthma care-planning must be done with respect and consideration. Studies show that patient education can be effective in older adults, but it may be necessary to repeat and reinforce medication instructions and management plans to ensure good asthma control over time.[48, 74]

19.7 ENVIRONMENTAL CONTROL STRATEGIES

Older adults with asthma may be more susceptible to the impact of various environmental triggers, including indoor allergens, respiratory infections, and both indoor and outdoor air pollutants. As with all asthmatics, obtaining an environmental history is an important aspect of asthma management. Interventions targeted toward environmental exposures can be especially useful in older adults, given the potential for poorer responses to medications.

Although atopic sensitization declines with age, a significant portion of older adult asthmatics remain atopic.[75] Indoor allergens have been shown to be especially problematic, given that older adults often spend a significant amount of time indoors and may live in older homes with greater exposure to dust mites, cockroaches, mold, and rodents.[6, 76] Pet allergen exposure has also specifically been linked to poorer asthma outcomes among sensitized older adults.[77] Mitigation of indoor allergen triggers has been shown to decrease asthma severity including improvements in lung function and reductions in emergency room visits and hospitalizations.[78] Strategies to reduce allergen exposure are similar to those in younger individuals, although additional consideration for cost and ease of implementation may be needed.[79–81]

Older adults are also more susceptible to both indoor and outdoor air pollutants due to increased time spent at home, increased likelihood of living in impoverished areas with greater exposure to outdoor pollutants, and age-related decline in anti-oxidant defenses.[82, 83] Indoor air pollutants include tobacco smoke, cooking-related pollutants, pesticide sprays, cleaning materials (volatile organic compounds), and furniture and building materials (aldehydes).[84, 85] Acute and/or chronic exposure to outdoor air pollutants such as nitrogen dioxide, ozone, and particulate matter increases the risk for asthma hospitalizations and death, with greater effects seen among older adults relative to younger individuals.[83, 86] Ideally, impacted individuals would remove themselves from settings with increased exposure to pollutants; however, when this is not feasible, other strategies such as HEPA (high-efficiency particulate air) filtration may be considered.[87]

19.8 INFECTIONS AND VACCINATION

Older asthmatics experience increased morbidity and mortality from respiratory infections due to multiple factors, including immune senescence, physiological changes associated with aging, and increased exposures to infectious agents among those living in group settings.[75] Although non-asthmatic older adults are also at greater risk for adverse outcomes with viral and bacterial pathogens, the impact is even greater among those with asthma.[88] In particular, influenza and pneumococcal disease are vaccine-preventable illnesses associated with significant morbidity and mortality among asthmatics. It is therefore strongly recommended that asthmatics age 65 years and older annually receive a high-dose, quadrivalent influenza vaccine.[89] Starting at age 65, those who have not previously received pneumococcal conjugate vaccination are recommended to receive Prevnar PCV13 or PCV20 followed in one year by Pneumovax PPSV23 vaccination.[90]

19.9 OLDER ADULTS WITH ASTHMA AND COVID-19

Older adults with asthma may have vulnerabilities regarding infection with SARS-CoV-2. While the effect that asthma has on outcomes related to COVID remains unclear, older age is an established risk factor for COVID-19-related morbidity and mortality.[91, 92] Underlying changes in immunocompetence have been described that partially explain differences in outcomes among older patients with COVID−19.[93] A retrospective observational study among older adults with asthma found that comorbidities, male sex, and oral corticosteroid dependence correlated with outcomes such as hospitalization, respiratory failure, and death from COVID−19.[91]

Special considerations for older adults with asthma regarding the COVID-19 pandemic should include a thorough assessment of asthma control, comorbidities, and optimization of pharmacologic and nonpharmacologic therapies.[31] Incorporation of mental health screening and addressing mental health needs may decrease the burden of asthma especially for socially isolated older adults with asthma during the COVID-19 pandemic.[2, 94] Structured behavioral interventions and asthma action plans to improve autonomy and self-management have been shown to improve outcomes.[95] Technology such as video chatting and texting has beneficial roles in the care of older adults with improved communication, decreasing feelings of loneliness, and improving healthcare access.[96] However, further studies are necessary to understand how racial and ethnic minority older adults with asthma may experience these challenges and interventions in the setting of the COVID-19 pandemic, as well as the effects of technology access and health equity.

The role of vaccination for older adults with asthma is critical in the prevention of COVID-19-related morbidity and mortality. A recent modeling study estimated that around 27 million SARS-CoV-2 infections, 1.6 million hospitalizations, and 235,000 deaths due to COVID-19 were prevented in the US in 2021 due to vaccinations, with the greatest effect found among adults ages 65 and older.[97] Furthermore, COVID-19 vaccination and boosters were effective in protecting against death, especially among adults aged 50 years and older as Delta and Omicron SARS-CoV-2 variants predominated in late 2021.[98] The risk of adverse reactions to COVID-19 vaccinations is very rare for older adults with asthma. Real-world analysis in the US showed extremely low rates of anaphylaxis at around 0.3% after the first dose of either mRNA-based COVID-19 vaccines (BNT162b2 by Pfizer-BioNTech and mRNA-1273 by Moderna) and 0.2% after one dose of JNJ-78436735, including those among older adults and adults with asthma.[99] A discussion of COVID-19 vaccination is an important consideration for the care of older adults with asthma given its safety and the significant reduction in morbidity and mortality.

REFERENCES

1. Center for Disease Control and Prevention. most recent national asthma data 2022 [updated May 25, 2022; cited 2022 Jul 30]. Available from: https://www.cdc.gov/asthma/most_recent_national_asthma_data.htm.
2. Cremer NM, Baptist AP. Race and asthma outcomes in older adults: results from the national asthma survey. *J Allergy Clin Immunol Pract*. 2020;8(4):1294–301 e7. Epub February 5, 2020. https://doi.org/10.1016/j.jaip.2019.12.014. PubMed PMID: 32035849.
3. Hanania NA, King MJ, Braman SS, Saltoun C, Wise RA, Enright P, Falsey AR, Mathur SK, Ramsdell JW, Rogers L, Stempel DA, Lima JJ, Fish JE, Wilson SR, Boyd C, Patel KV, Irvin CG, Yawn BP, Halm EA, Wasserman SI, Sands MF, Ershler WB, Ledford DK, Asthma in elderly workshop p. Asthma in the elderly: current understanding and future research needs—a report of a National Institute on Aging (NIA) workshop. *J Allergy Clin Immunol*. 2011;128(3 Suppl):S4–24. https://doi.org/10.1016/j.jaci.2011.06.048. PubMed PMID: 21872730; PMCID: PMC3164961.
4. Enright PL, McClelland RL, Newman AB, Gottlieb DJ, Lebowitz MD. Underdiagnosis and undertreatment of asthma in the elderly. *Chest*. 1999;116(3):603–13. https://doi.org/10.1378/chest.116.3.603. PubMed PMID: 10492260.
5. Kannan JA, Bernstein DI, Bernstein CK, Ryan PH, Bernstein JA, Villareal MS, Smith AM, Lenz PH, Epstein TG. Significant predictors of poor quality of life in older asthmatics. *Ann Allergy Asthma Immunol*. 2015;115(3):198–204. Epub July 21, 2015. https://doi.org/10.1016/j.anai.2015.06.021. PubMed PMID: 26208758; PMCID: PMC4567431.
6. Hsu J, Chen J, Mirabelli MC. Asthma morbidity, comorbidities, and modifiable factors among older adults. *J Allergy Clin Immunol Pract*. 2018;6(1):236–43 e7. Epub July 26, 2017. https://doi.org/10.1016/j.jaip.2017.06.007. PubMed PMID: 28756082; PMCID: PMC5760447.
7. Baptist AP, Hamad A, Patel MR. Special challenges in treatment and self-management of older women with asthma. *Ann Allergy Asthma Immunol*. 2014;113(2):125–30. https://doi.org/10.1016/j.anai.2014.05.013. PubMed PMID: 25065349; PMCID: PMC4153393.
8. Moore WC, Meyers DA, Wenzel SE, Teague WG, Li H, Li X, D'Agostino R, Jr., Castro M, Curran-Everett D, Fitzpatrick AM, Gaston B, Jarjour NN, Sorkness R, Calhoun WJ, Chung KF, Comhair SA, Dweik RA, Israel E, Peters SP, Busse WW, Erzurum SC, Bleecker ER, National Heart L, Blood Institute's Severe Asthma Research P. Identification of asthma phenotypes using cluster analysis in the Severe Asthma Research Program. *Am J Respir Crit Care Med*. 2010;181(4):315–23. Epub November 5, 2009. https://doi.org/10.1164/rccm.200906-0896OC. PubMed PMID: 19892860; PMCID: PMC2822971.
9. Park HW, Song WJ, Kim SH, Park HK, Kim SH, Kwon YE, Kwon HS, Kim TB, Chang YS, Cho YS, Lee BJ, Jee YK, Jang AS, Nahm DH, Park JW, Yoon HJ, Cho YJ, Choi BW, Moon HB, Cho SH. Classification and implementation of asthma phenotypes in elderly patients. *Ann Allergy Asthma Immunol*. 2015;114(1):18–22. Epub October 24, 2014. https://doi.org/10.1016/j.anai.2014.09.020. PubMed PMID: 25455518.
10. Baptist AP, Hao W, Karamched KR, Kaur B, Carpenter L, Song PXK. Distinct asthma phenotypes among older adults with asthma. *J Allergy Clin Immunol Pract*. 2018;6(1):244–9 e2. Epub July 27, 2017. https://doi.org/10.1016/j.jaip.2017.06.010. PubMed PMID: 28757370; PMCID: PMC5897052.
11. Jatakanon A, Uasuf C, Maziak W, Lim S, Chung KF, Barnes PJ. Neutrophilic inflammation in severe persistent asthma. *Am J Respir Crit Care Med*. 1999;160(5 Pt 1):1532–9.

https://doi.org/10.1164/ajrccm.160.5.9806170. PubMed PMID: 10556116.
12. Nyenhuis SM, Schwantes EA, Evans MD, Mathur SK. Airway neutrophil inflammatory phenotype in older subjects with asthma. *J Allergy Clin Immunol.* 2010;125(5):1163–5. Epub April 9, 2010 https://doi.org/10.1016/j.jaci.2010.02.015. PubMed PMID: 20381851; PMCID: PMC3298970.
13. Hartsock RJ, Smith EB, Petty CS. Normal variations with aging of the amount of hematopoietic tissue in bone marrow from the anterior iliac crest: a study made from 177 cases of sudden death examined by necropsy. *Am J Clin Pathol.* 1965;43:326–31. https://doi.org/10.1093/ajcp/43.4.326. PubMed PMID: 14275849.
14. Cancro MP. B cells and aging: gauging the interplay of generative, selective, and homeostatic events. *Immunol Rev.* 2005;205:48–59. https://doi.org/10.1111/j.0105-2896.2005.00272.x. PubMed PMID: 15882344.
15. Plowden J, Renshaw-Hoelscher M, Engleman C, Katz J, Sambhara S. Innate immunity in aging: impact on macrophage function. *Aging Cell.* 2004;3(4):161–7. https://doi.org/10.1111/j.1474-9728.2004.00102.x. PubMed PMID: 15268749.
16. Iwasa H, Kikuchi S, Mine S, Sugita K, Miyagishima H, Hasegawa S. Functional significance of stimulatory GTP-binding protein in hippocampus is associated with kindling-elicited epileptogenesis. *Psychiatry Clin Neurosci.* 2000;54(2):191–7. https://doi.org/10.1046/j.1440-1819.2000.00657.x. PubMed PMID: 10803814.
17. Agrawal A, Agrawal S, Gupta S. Dendritic cells in human aging. *Exp Gerontol.* 2007;42(5):421–6. Epub December 19, 2006. https://doi.org/10.1016/j.exger.2006.11.007. PubMed PMID: 17182207; PMCID: PMC1909691.
18. Wenisch C, Patruta S, Daxbock F, Krause R, Horl W. Effect of age on human neutrophil function. *J Leukoc Biol.* 2000;67(1):40–5. https://doi.org/10.1002/jlb.67.1.40. PubMed PMID: 10647996.
19. Cuervo AM, Macian F. Autophagy and the immune function in aging. *Curr Opin Immunol.* 2014;29:97–104. Epub June 12, 2014. https://doi.org/10.1016/j.coi.2014.05.006. PubMed PMID: 24929664; PMCID: PMC4119564.
20. Plackett TP, Boehmer ED, Faunce DE, Kovacs EJ. Aging and innate immune cells. *J Leukoc Biol.* 2004;76(2):291–9. Epub March 23, 2004. https://doi.org/10.1189/jlb.1103592. PubMed PMID: 15039467.
21. George AJ, Ritter MA. Thymic involution with ageing: obsolescence or good housekeeping? *Immunol Today.* 1996;17(6):267–72. https://doi.org/10.1016/0167-5699(96)80543-3. PubMed PMID: 8962629.
22. Goronzy JJ, Weyand CM. T cell development and receptor diversity during aging. *Curr Opin Immunol.* 2005;17(5):468–75. https://doi.org/10.1016/j.coi.2005.07.020. PubMed PMID: 16098723.
23. Weksler ME, Szabo P. The effect of age on the B-cell repertoire. *J Clin Immunol.* 2000;20(4):240–9. https://doi.org/10.1023/a:1006659401385. PubMed PMID: 10939711.
24. Frasca D, Landin AM, Riley RL, Blomberg BB. Mechanisms for decreased function of B cells in aged mice and humans. *J Immunol.* 2008;180(5):2741–6. https://doi.org/10.4049/jimmunol.180.5.2741. PubMed PMID: 18292491.
25. Bruunsgaard H, Andersen-Ranberg K, Hjelmborg J, Pedersen BK, Jeune B. Elevated levels of tumor necrosis factor alpha and mortality in centenarians. *Am J Med.* 2003;115(4):278–83. https://doi.org/10.1016/s0002-9343(03)00329-2. PubMed PMID: 12967692.
26. Franceschi C, Bonafe M, Valensin S, Olivieri F, De Luca M, Ottaviani E, De Benedictis G. Inflamm-aging. An evolutionary perspective on immunosenescence. *Ann N Y Acad Sci.* 2000;908:244–54. https://doi.org/10.1111/j.1749-6632.2000.tb06651.x. PubMed PMID: 10911963.
27. Calder PC, Bosco N, Bourdet-Sicard R, Capuron L, Delzenne N, Dore J, Franceschi C, Lehtinen MJ, Recker T, Salvioli S, Visioli F. Health relevance of the modification of low grade inflammation in ageing (inflammageing) and the role of nutrition. *Ageing Res Rev.* 2017;40:95–119. Epub September 9, 2017. https://doi.org/10.1016/j.arr.2017.09.001. PubMed PMID: 28899766.
28. Fulop T, Larbi A, Pawelec G, Khalil A, Cohen AA, Hirokawa K, Witkowski JM, Franceschi C. Immunology of aging: the birth of inflammaging. *Clin Rev Allergy Immunol.* 2021. Epub September 18, 2021. https://doi.org/10.1007/s12016-021-08899-6. PubMed PMID: 34536213; PMCID: PMC8449217.
29. Ekici M, Apan A, Ekici A, Erdemoglu AK. Perception of bronchoconstriction in elderly asthmatics. *J Asthma.* 2001;38(8):691–6. https://doi.org/10.1081/jas-100107547. PubMed PMID: 11758898.
30. Ross JA, Yang Y, Song PX, Clark NM, Baptist AP. Quality of life, health care utilization, and control in older adults with asthma. *J Allergy Clin Immunol Pract.* 2013;1(2):157–62. Epub February 4, 2013. https://doi.org/10.1016/j.jaip.2012.12.003. PubMed PMID: 24565454.
31. Nanda A, Baptist AP, Divekar R, Parikh N, Seggev JS, Yusin JS, Nyenhuis SM. Asthma in the older adult. *J Asthma.* 2020;57(3):241–52. Epub January 18, 2019. https://doi.org/10.1080/02770903.2019.1565828. PubMed PMID: 30656998.
32. Lowhagen O. Diagnosis of asthma—new theories. *J Asthma.* 2015;52(6):538–44. Epub July 7, 2015. https://doi.org/10.3109/02770903.2014.991971. PubMed PMID: 25478896.
33. Yawn BP, Han MK. Practical considerations for the diagnosis and management of asthma in older adults. *Mayo Clin Proc.* 2017;92(11):1697–705. Epub January 1, 2017. https://doi.org/10.1016/j.mayocp.2017.08.005. PubMed PMID: 29101938.
34. Chotirmall SH, Watts M, Branagan P, Donegan CF, Moore A, McElvaney NG. Diagnosis and management of asthma in older adults. *J Am Geriatr Soc.* 2009;57(5):901–9. https://doi.org/10.1111/j.1532-5415.2009.02216.x. PubMed PMID: 19484848.
35. Cavallazzi R, Jorayeva A, Beatty BL, Antimisiaris D, Gopalraj R, Myers J, Folz RJ, Polivka BJ. Predicting asthma in older adults on the basis of clinical history. *Respir Med.* 2018;142:36–40. Epub July 20, 2018. https://doi.org/10.1016/j.rmed.2018.07.010. PubMed PMID: 30170799; PMCID: PMC6121730.
36. Fabbri LM, Romagnoli M, Corbetta L, Casoni G, Busljetic K, Turato G, Ligabue G, Ciaccia A, Saetta M, Papi A. Differences in airway inflammation in patients with fixed airflow obstruction due to asthma or chronic obstructive pulmonary disease. *Am J Respir Crit Care Med.* 2003;167(3):418–24. Epub November 8, 2002. https://doi.org/10.1164/rccm.200203-183OC. PubMed PMID: 12426229.
37. Gibson PG, McDonald VM, Marks GB. Asthma in older adults. *Lancet.* 2010;376(9743):803–13. Epub September 8, 2010. https://doi.org/10.1016/S0140-6736(10)61087-2. PubMed PMID: 20816547.
38. Zemp E, Schikowski T, Dratva J, Schindler C, Probst-Hensch N. Asthma and the menopause: a systematic review and meta-analysis. *Maturitas.* 2012;73(3):212–7.

Epub September 12, 2012. https://doi.org/10.1016/j.maturitas.2012.08.010. PubMed PMID: 22964072.
39. Busse PJ, Lurslurchachai L, Sampson HA, Halm EA, Wisnivesky J. Perennial allergen-specific immunoglobulin E levels among inner-city elderly asthmatics. *J Asthma*. 2010;47(7):781–5. Epub July 29, 2010. https://doi.org/10.3109/02770903.2010.489140. PubMed PMID: 20662744.
40. Foschino Barbaro MP, Costa VR, Resta O, Prato R, Spanevello A, Palladino GP, Martinelli D, Carpagnano GE. Menopausal asthma: a new biological phenotype? *Allergy*. 2010;65(10):1306–12. Epub June 19, 2010. https://doi.org/10.1111/j.1398-9995.2009.02314.x. PubMed PMID: 20557302.
41. Nwaru BI, Shah SA, Tibble H, Pillinger R, McLean S, Ryan D, Critchley H, Hawrylowicz CM, Simpson CR, Soyiri IN, Appiagyei F, Price D, Sheikh A. Hormone Replacement Therapy and Risk of Severe Asthma Exacerbation in Perimenopausal and Postmenopausal Women: 17-Year National Cohort Study. *J Allergy Clin Immunol Pract*. 2021;9(7):2751–60 e1. Epub March 12, 2021. https://doi.org/10.1016/j.jaip.2021.02.052. PubMed PMID: 33705997.
42. Plassman BL, Langa KM, Fisher GG, Heeringa SG, Weir DR, Ofstedal MB, Burke JR, Hurd MD, Potter GG, Rodgers WL, Steffens DC, Willis RJ, Wallace RB. Prevalence of dementia in the United States: the aging, demographics, and memory study. *Neuroepidemiology*. 2007;29(1–2):125–32. Epub November 3, 2007. https://doi.org/10.1159/000109998. PubMed PMID: 17975326; PMCID: PMC2705925.
43. Barr RG, Somers SC, Speizer FE, Camargo CA, Jr., National Asthma E, Prevention P. Patient factors and medication guideline adherence among older women with asthma. *Arch Intern Med*. 2002;162(15):1761–8. Epub August 3, 2002. https://doi.org/10.1001/archinte.162.15.1761. PubMed PMID: 12153380.
44. Waldorff FB, Siersma V, Waldemar G. Association between subjective memory complaints and health care utilisation: a three-year follow up. *BMC Geriatr*. 2009;9:43. Epub September 25, 2009. https://doi.org/10.1186/1471-2318-9-43. PubMed PMID: 19775441; PMCID: PMC2759924.
45. Johnson RW. What Is the Lifetime Risk of Needing and Receiving Long-Term Services and Supports? ASPE Reports 2019 April 3, 2019. Report No.: Contract No.: August 9.
46. Living TAfC. 2020 Profile of Older Americans. Online: 2021.
47. Baptist AP, Deol BB, Reddy RC, Nelson B, Clark NM. Age-specific factors influencing asthma management by older adults. *Qual Health Res*. 2010;20(1):117–24. Epub November 27, 2009. https://doi.org/10.1177/1049732309355288. PubMed PMID: 19940092.
48. Baptist AP, Busse PJ. Asthma Over the Age of 65: All's Well That Ends Well. *J Allergy Clin Immunol Pract*. 2018;6(3):764–73. Epub May 12, 2018. https://doi.org/10.1016/j.jaip.2018.02.007. PubMed PMID: 29747982; PMCID: PMC5951417.
49. Son J, Erno A, Shea DG, Femia EE, Zarit SH, Stephens MA. The caregiver stress process and health outcomes. *J Aging Health*. 2007;19(6):871–87. Epub January 1, 2008. https://doi.org/10.1177/0898264307308568. PubMed PMID: 18165286.
50. Del-Pino-Casado R, Priego-Cubero E, Lopez-Martinez C, Orgeta V. Subjective caregiver burden and anxiety in informal caregivers: A systematic review and meta-analysis. *PLOS ONE*. 2021;16(3):e0247143. Epub March 2, 2021. https://doi.org/10.1371/journal.pone.0247143. PubMed PMID: 33647035; PMCID: PMC7920375.
51. Aging NIo. Older Drivers [updated December 12, 2018August 9, 2022]. Available from: https://www.nia.nih.gov/health/infographics/concerned-about-driving-safety.
52. Steinman MA, Sands LP, Covinsky KE. Self-restriction of medications due to cost in seniors without prescription coverage. *J Gen Intern Med*. 2001;16(12):793–9. Epub March 21, 2002. PubMed PMID: 11903757; PMCID: PMC1495305.
53. Durrani S. Management of asthma in school-aged children and adolescents. *Pediatr Ann*. 2014;43(8):e184–91. https://doi.org/10.3928/00904481-20140723-08. PubMed PMID: 25102488.
54. Chipps BE, Murphy KR, Oppenheimer J. 2020 NAEPP Guidelines Update and GINA 2021-Asthma Care Differences, Overlap, and Challenges. *J Allergy Clin Immunol Pract*. 2022;10(1S):S19–S30. Epub October 27, 2021. https://doi.org/10.1016/j.jaip.2021.10.032. PubMed PMID: 34718214.
55. Humbert M, Busse W, Hanania NA, Lowe PJ, Canvin J, Erpenbeck VJ, Holgate S. Omalizumab in asthma: an update on recent developments. *J Allergy Clin Immunol Pract*. 2014;2(5):525–36 e1. Epub June 11, 2014. https://doi.org/10.1016/j.jaip.2014.03.010. PubMed PMID: 25213045.
56. Maykut RJ, Kianifard F, Geba GP. Response of older patients with IgE-mediated asthma to omalizumab: a pooled analysis. *J Asthma*. 2008;45(3):173–81. https://doi.org/10.1080/02770900701247277. PubMed PMID: 18415822.
57. Tat TS, Cilli A. Evaluation of long-term safety and efficacy of omalizumab in elderly patients with uncontrolled allergic asthma. *Ann Allergy Asthma Immunol*. 2016;117(5):546–9. Epub October 24, 2016. https://doi.org/10.1016/j.anai.2016.09.006. PubMed PMID: 27788886.
58. Pavord ID, Korn S, Howarth P, Bleecker ER, Buhl R, Keene ON, Ortega H, Chanez P. Mepolizumab for severe eosinophilic asthma (DREAM): a multicentre, double-blind, placebo-controlled trial. Lancet. 2012;380(9842):651–9. doi: 10.1016/S0140-6736(12)60988-X. PubMed PMID: 22901886.
59. Brusselle G, Germinaro M, Weiss S, Zangrilli J. Reslizumab in patients with inadequately controlled late-onset asthma and elevated blood eosinophils. Pulm Pharmacol Ther. 2017;43:39–45. Epub January 31, 2017. doi: 10.1016/j.pupt.2017.01.011. PubMed PMID: 28159511.
60. Laviolette M, Gossage DL, Gauvreau G, Leigh R, Olivenstein R, Katial R, Busse WW, Wenzel S, Wu Y, Datta V, Kolbeck R, Molfino NA. Effects of benralizumab on airway eosinophils in asthmatic patients with sputum eosinophilia. J Allergy Clin Immunol. 2013;132(5):1086–96.e5. Epub July 16, 2013. doi: 10.1016/j.jaci.2013.05.020. PubMed PMID: 23866823; PMCID: PMC4172321.
61. Wenzel S, Ford L, Pearlman D, Spector S, Sher L, Skobieranda F, Wang L, Kirkesseli S, Rocklin R, Bock B, Hamilton J, Ming JE, Radin A, Stahl N, Yancopoulos GD, Graham N, Pirozzi G. Dupilumab in persistent asthma with elevated eosinophil levels. N Engl J Med. 2013;368(26):2455–66. Epub May 21, 2013. doi: 10.1056/NEJMoa1304048. PubMed PMID: 23688323.
62. Menzies-Gow A, Wechsler ME, Brightling CE. Unmet need in severe, uncontrolled asthma: can anti-TSLP therapy with tezepelumab provide a valuable new treatment option? Respir Res. 2020;21(1):268. Epub October 15, 2020. doi: 10.1186/s12931-020-01505-x. PubMed PMID: 33059715; PMCID: PMC7560289.
63. Hammond C, Kurten M, Kennedy JL. Rhinovirus and asthma: a storied history of incompatibility. Curr Allergy Asthma Rep. 2015;15(2):502. doi: 10.1007/s11882-014-0502-0. PubMed PMID: 25612798; PMCID: PMC4327812.

64. Ortega HY, Katial R. Response to treatment with mepolizumab in elderly patients. Am J Respir Crit Care Med. 2015;191:A4177.
65. Bernstein JA, Virchow JC, Murphy K, Maspero JF, Jacobs J, Adir Y, Humbert M, Castro M, Marsteller DA, McElhattan J, Hickey L, Garin M, Vanlandingham R, Brusselle G. Effect of fixed-dose subcutaneous reslizumab on asthma exacerbations in patients with severe uncontrolled asthma and corticosteroid sparing in patients with oral corticosteroid-dependent asthma: results from two phase 3, randomised, double-blind, placebo-controlled trials. Lancet Respir Med. 2020;8(5):461–74. Epub February 14, 2020. doi: 10.1016/S2213-2600(19)30372-8. PubMed PMID: 32066536.
66. Bjermer L, Lemiere C, Maspero J, Weiss S, Zangrilli J, Germinaro M. Reslizumab for inadequately controlled asthma with elevated blood eosinophil levels: a randomized phase 3 study. Chest. 2016;150(4):789–98. Epub April 4, 2016. doi: 10.1016/j.chest.2016.03.032. PubMed PMID: 27056586.
67. Bleecker ER, FitzGerald JM, Chanez P, Papi A, Weinstein SF, Barker P, Sproule S, Gilmartin G, Aurivillius M, Werkstrom V, Goldman M, Investigators Ss. Efficacy and safety of benralizumab for patients with severe asthma uncontrolled with high-dosage inhaled corticosteroids and long-acting beta2-agonists (SIROCCO): a randomised, multicentre, placebo-controlled phase 3 trial. Lancet. 2016;388(10056):2115–27. Epub September 5, 2016. doi: 10.1016/S0140-6736(16)31324-1. PubMed PMID: 27609408.
68. Rabe KF, Nair P, Brusselle G, Maspero JF, Castro M, Sher L, Zhu H, Hamilton JD, Swanson BN, Khan A, Chao J, Staudinger H, Pirozzi G, Antoni C, Amin N, Ruddy M, Akinlade B, Graham NMH, Stahl N, Yancopoulos GD, Teper A. Efficacy and safety of dupilumab in glucocorticoid-dependent severe asthma. N Engl J Med. 2018;378(26):2475–85. Epub May 21, 2018. doi: 10.1056/NEJMoa1804093. PubMed PMID: 29782224.
69. Wechsler ME, Ford LB, Maspero JF, Pavord ID, Papi A, Bourdin A, Watz H, Castro M, Nenasheva NM, Tohda Y, Langton D, Cardona G, Domingo C, Park HS, Chapman KR, Mao X, Zhang Y, Khan AH, Deniz Y, Rowe PJ, Kapoor U, Khokhar FA, Mannent LP, Ruddy M, Laws E, Amin N, Hardin M. Long-term safety and efficacy of dupilumab in patients with moderate-to-severe asthma (TRAVERSE): an open-label extension study. Lancet Respir Med. 2022;10(1):11–25. Epub September 28, 2021. doi: 10.1016/S2213-2600(21)00322-2. PubMed PMID: 34597534.
70. Menzies-Gow A, Corren J, Bourdin A, Chupp G, Israel E, Wechsler ME, Brightling CE, Griffiths JM, Hellqvist A, Bowen K, Kaur P, Almqvist G, Ponnarambil S, Colice G. Tezepelumab in adults and adolescents with severe, uncontrolled asthma. N Engl J Med. 2021;384(19):1800–9. doi: 10.1056/NEJMoa2034975. PubMed PMID: 33979488.
71. Hall C, Nici L, Sood S, ZuWallack R, Castro M. Nonpharmacologic therapy for severe persistent asthma. J Allergy Clin Immunol Pract. 2017;5(4):928–35. Epub July 12, 2017. doi: 10.1016/j.jaip.2017.04.030. PubMed PMID: 28689843.
72. Zampogna E, Centis R, Negri S, Fiore E, Cherubino F, Pignatti P, Heffler E, Canonica GW, Sotgiu G, Saderi L, Migliori GB, Spanevello A, Visca D. Effectiveness of pulmonary rehabilitation in severe asthma: a retrospective data analysis. J Asthma. 2020;57(12):1365–71. Epub July 19, 2019. doi: 10.1080/02770903.2019.1646271. PubMed PMID: 31317799.
73. Pilotto A, Custodero C, Maggi S, Polidori MC, Veronese N, Ferrucci L. A multidimensional approach to frailty in older people. Ageing Res Rev. 2020;60:101047. Epub March 17, 2020. doi: 10.1016/j.arr.2020.101047. PubMed PMID: 32171786; PMCID: PMC7461697.
74. Buist AS, Vollmer WM, Wilson SR, Frazier EA, Hayward AD. A randomized clinical trial of peak flow versus symptom monitoring in older adults with asthma. Am J Respir Crit Care Med. 2006;174(10):1077–87. Epub August 26, 2006. doi: 10.1164/rccm.200510-1606OC. PubMed PMID: 16931634; PMCID: PMC2648108.
75. Yanez A, Cho SH, Soriano JB, Rosenwasser LJ, Rodrigo GJ, Rabe KF, Peters S, Niimi A, Ledford DK, Katial R, Fabbri LM, Celedon JC, Canonica GW, Busse P, Boulet LP, Baena-Cagnani CE, Hamid Q, Bachert C, Pawankar R, Holgate ST. Asthma in the elderly: what we know and what we have yet to know. World Allergy Organ J. 2014;7(1):8. Epub May 30, 2014. doi: 10.1186/1939-4551-7-8. PubMed PMID: 25152804; PMCID: PMC4137434.
76. Calhoun KH. Allergy in the geriatric population. Curr Opin Otolaryngol Head Neck Surg. 2015;23(3):235–9. doi: 10.1097/MOO.0000000000000157. PubMed PMID: 25943961.
77. Portnoy J, Kennedy K, Sublett J, Phipatanakul W, Matsui E, Barnes C, Grimes C, Miller JD, Seltzer JM, Williams PB, Bernstein JA, Bernstein DI, Blessing-Moore J, Cox L, Khan DA, Lang DM, Nicklas RA, Oppenheimer J. Environmental assessment and exposure control: a practice parameter—furry animals. Ann Allergy Asthma Immunol. 2012;108(4):223.e1–15. doi: 10.1016/j.anai.2012.02.015. PubMed PMID: 22469456; PMCID: PMC3519933.
78. O'Sullivan MM, Brandfield J, Hoskote SS, Segal SN, Chug L, Modrykamien A, Eden E. Environmental improvements brought by the legal interventions in the homes of poorly controlled inner-city adult asthmatic patients: a proof-of-concept study. J Asthma. 2012;49(9):911–7. Epub October 1, 2012. doi: 10.3109/02770903.2012.724131. PubMed PMID: 23020301.
79. Portnoy J, Chew GL, Phipatanakul W, Williams PB, Grimes C, Kennedy K, Matsui EC, Miller JD, Bernstein D, Blessing-Moore J, Cox L, Khan D, Lang D, Nicklas R, Oppenheimer J, Randolph C, Schuller D, Spector S, Tilles SA, Wallace D, Seltzer J, Sublett J, Joint Task Force on Practice P. Environmental assessment and exposure reduction of cockroaches: a practice parameter. J Allergy Clin Immunol. 2013;132(4):802–8.e1–25. Epub August 9, 2013. doi: 10.1016/j.jaci.2013.04.061. PubMed PMID: 23938214; PMCID: PMC3864888.
80. Phipatanakul W, Matsui E, Portnoy J, Williams PB, Barnes C, Kennedy K, Bernstein D, Blessing-Moore J, Cox L, Khan D, Lang D, Nicklas R, Oppenheimer J, Randolph C, Schuller D, Spector S, Tilles SA, Wallace D, Sublett J, Bernstein J, Grimes C, Miller JD, Seltzer J, Joint Task Force on Practice P. Environmental assessment and exposure reduction of rodents: a practice parameter. Ann Allergy Asthma Immunol. 2012;109(6):375–87. doi: 10.1016/j.anai.2012.09.019. PubMed PMID: 23176873; PMCID: PMC3519934.
81. Gautier C, Charpin D. Environmental triggers and avoidance in the management of asthma. J Asthma Allergy. 2017;10:47–56. Epub March 7, 2017. doi: 10.2147/JAA.S121276. PubMed PMID: 28331347; PMCID: PMC5349698.
82. Ciencewicki J, Trivedi S, Kleeberger SR. Oxidants and the pathogenesis of lung diseases. J Allergy Clin Immunol. 2008;122(3):456–68; quiz 69–70. doi: 10.1016/j.jaci.2008.08.004. PubMed PMID: 18774381; PMCID: PMC2693323.

83. Epstein TG, Ryan PH, LeMasters GK, Bernstein CK, Levin LS, Bernstein JA, Villareal MS, Bernstein DI. Poor asthma control and exposure to traffic pollutants and obesity in older adults. Ann Allergy Asthma Immunol. 2012;108(6):423–8.e2. Epub May 1, 2012. doi: 10.1016/j.anai.2012.04.009. PubMed PMID: 22626595; PMCID: PMC4715904.
84. Rayens MK, Burkhart PV, Zhang M, Lee S, Moser DK, Mannino D, Hahn EJ. Reduction in asthma-related emergency department visits after implementation of a smoke-free law. J Allergy Clin Immunol. 2008;122(3):537–41.e3. Epub August 9, 2008. doi: 10.1016/j.jaci.2008.06.029. PubMed PMID: 18692884.
85. Milner J, Chalabi Z, Vardoulakis S, Wilkinson P. Housing interventions and health: Quantifying the impact of indoor particles on mortality and morbidity with disease recovery. Environ Int. 2015;81:73–9. Epub May 25, 2015. doi: 10.1016/j.envint.2015.04.011. PubMed PMID: 25958127.
86. Ko FW, Tam W, Wong TW, Lai CK, Wong GW, Leung TF, Ng SS, Hui DS. Effects of air pollution on asthma hospitalization rates in different age groups in Hong Kong. Clin Exp Allergy. 2007;37(9):1312–9. doi: 10.1111/j.1365-2222.2007.02791.x. PubMed PMID: 17845411.
87. James C, Bernstein DI, Cox J, Ryan P, Wolfe C, Jandarov R, Newman N, Indugula R, Reponen T. HEPA filtration improves asthma control in children exposed to traffic-related airborne particles. Indoor Air. 2020;30(2):235–43. Epub December 8, 2019. doi: 10.1111/ina.12625. PubMed PMID: 31743467; PMCID: PMC7895332.
88. Iikura M, Hojo M, Koketsu R, Watanabe S, Sato A, Chino H, Ro S, Masaki H, Hirashima J, Ishii S, Naka G, Takasaki J, Izumi S, Kobayashi N, Yamaguchi S, Nakae S, Sugiyama H. The importance of bacterial and viral infections associated with adult asthma exacerbations in clinical practice. *PLOS ONE*. 2015;10(4):e0123584. Epub April 22, 2015. doi: 10.1371/journal.pone.0123584. PubMed PMID: 25901797; PMCID: PMC4406689.
89. Centers for Disease Control and Prevention. CDC Director Adopts Preference for Specific Flu Vaccines for Seniors. 2022 [cited 2022 Aug 14]. Available from: https://www.cdc.gov/media/releases/2022/s0630-seniors-flu.html.
90. Centers for Disease Control and Prevention. Pneumococcal Vaccination: What Everyone Should Know. 2022 [cited 2022 Aug 14]. Available from: https://www.cdc.gov/vaccines/vpd/pneumo/public/index.html#who-gets-vaccine.
91. Avdeev SN, Pozdnakova AA, Gaynitdinova VV, Chikina SY, Vlasenko AE. Asthma in older adults with severe coronavirus disease 2019: Clinical outcomes and predictors of mortality. Ann Allergy Asthma Immunol. 2022;128(2):213–5. Epub October 21, 2021. doi: 10.1016/j.anai.2021.10.016. PubMed PMID: 34670163; PMCID: PMC8520591.
92. Cummings MJ, Baldwin MR, Abrams D, Jacobson SD, Meyer BJ, Balough EM, Aaron JG, Claassen J, Rabbani LE, Hastie J, Hochman BR, Salazar-Schicchi J, Yip NH, Brodie D, O'Donnell MR. Epidemiology, clinical course, and outcomes of critically ill adults with COVID-19 in New York City: a prospective cohort study. Lancet. 2020;395(10239):1763–70. Epub May 23, 2020. doi: 10.1016/S0140-6736(20)31189-2. PubMed PMID: 32442528; PMCID: PMC7237188.
93. Lee GC, Restrepo MI, Harper N, Manoharan MS, Smith AM, Meunier JA, Sanchez-Reilly S, Ehsan A, Branum AP, Winter C, Winter L, Jimenez F, Pandranki L, Carrillo A, Perez GL, Anzueto A, Trinh H, Lee M, Hecht JM, Martinez-Vargas C, Sehgal RT, Cadena J, Walter EA, Oakman K, Benavides R, Pugh JA, South Texas Veterans Health Care System C-T, Letendre S, Steri M, Orru V, Fiorillo E, Cucca F, Moreira AG, Zhang N, Leadbetter E, Agan BK, Richman DD, He W, Clark RA, Okulicz JF, Ahuja SK. Immunologic resilience and COVID-19 survival advantage. J Allergy Clin Immunol. 2021;148(5):1176–91. Epub September 12, 2021. doi: 10.1016/j.jaci.2021.08.021. PubMed PMID: 34508765; PMCID: PMC8425719.
94. Patel PO, Patel MR, Baptist AP. Depression and Asthma Outcomes in Older Adults: Results from the National Health and Nutrition Examination Survey. J Allergy Clin Immunol Pract. 2017;5(6):1691–7.e1. Epub June 22, 2017. doi: 10.1016/j.jaip.2017.03.034. PubMed PMID: 28634102.
95. Baptist AP, Hao W, Song PX, Carpenter L, Steinberg J, Cardozo LJ. A behavioral intervention can decrease asthma exacerbations in older adults. Ann Allergy Asthma Immunol. 2020;124(3):248–53.e3. Epub December 27, 2019. doi: 10.1016/j.anai.2019.12.015. PubMed PMID: 31877361; PMCID: PMC7042081.
96. Rodrigues NG, Han CQY, Su Y, Klainin-Yobas P, Wu XV. Psychological impacts and online interventions of social isolation amongst older adults during COVID-19 pandemic: A scoping review. J Adv Nurs. 2022;78(3):609–44. Epub October 10, 2021. doi: 10.1111/jan.15063. PubMed PMID: 34625997; PMCID: PMC8661520.
97. Steele MK, Couture A, Reed C, Iuliano D, Whitaker M, Fast H, Hall AJ, MacNeil A, Cadwell B, Marks KJ, Silk BJ. Estimated Number of COVID-19 Infections, Hospitalizations, and Deaths Prevented Among Vaccinated Persons in the US, December 2020 to September 2021. *JAMA Netw Open*. 2022;5(7):e2220385. Epub July 7, 2022. doi: 10.1001/jamanetworkopen.2022.20385. PubMed PMID: 35793085; PMCID: PMC9260489.
98. Johnson AG, Ali AR, Hoots B, Cadwell BL, Arora S, Avoundjian T, Awofeso BO, Barnes J, Bayoumi NS, Busen K, Chang C, Cima M, Crockett M, Cronquist A. COVID-19 Incidence and Death Rates Among Unvaccinated and Fully Vaccinated Adults with and Without Booster Doses During Periods of Delta and Omicron Variant Emergence—25 U.S. Jurisdictions, April 4–December 25, 2021–2022. *MMWR Morb Mortal Wkly Rep*. 2022;71:132–8.
99. Beatty AL, Peyser ND, Butcher XE, Cocohoba JM, Lin F, Olgin JE, Pletcher MJ, Marcus GM. Analysis of COVID-19 Vaccine Type and Adverse Effects Following Vaccination. JAMA Netw Open. 2021;4(12):e2140364. Epub December 23, 2021. doi: 10.1001/jamanetworkopen.2021.40364. PubMed PMID: 34935921; PMCID: PMC8696570.

20 Severe Acute and Life-Threatening Asthma in Children

Adam Lawton, Andrew Nyman, and Louise Fleming

CASE STUDY

A 14-year-old boy presented to his local Emergency Department (ED) accompanied by his father. He has a past medical history significant for asthma and eczema. His regular medications consisted of Seretide and salbutamol inhalers. He was also prescribed emollients and mild topical steroids for his eczema.

He has had four courses of oral corticosteroids for worsening asthma symptoms in the past 12 months. Three of these episodes required hospital admissions for intravenous bronchodilators. He has never previously been admitted to the paediatric intensive care unit (PICU).

His parents no longer supervise his daily use of Seretide, and he admits that he had been missing all his evening doses and some of his morning doses for the past two weeks.

Three days ago, he began to experience some intermittent chest tightness, and yesterday he developed expiratory wheeze. He took his salbutamol inhaler as per the directions on his written personalised asthma management plan, but this provided only partial relief. Today he presented to ED after becoming acutely short of breath and using the maximum number of salbutamol puffs in his asthma plan.

His respiratory rate was 34 breaths per minute on arrival, and his oxygen saturation was 90% in air. He was too breathless to reliably provide a peak expiratory flow (PEF) measurement. His initial treatment consisted of inhaled salbutamol and oral prednisolone. His saturations did not improve, and he was cannulated and given IV aminophylline. Whilst intravenous access was obtained, a venous blood gas was taken, which revealed a pH of 7.29 and a pCO_2 of 6.2 kPa. He received a bolus of intravenous magnesium sulfate, and regular nebulised salbutamol and ipratropium. As he remained tachypnoeic with low oxygen saturations despite 40% supplemental oxygen via an air-entrainment mask, a second cannula was inserted, and a repeat venous blood gas was taken.

His pH had fallen to 7.19, and his pCO_2 had risen to 7.3 kPa. The decision was made to intubate and mechanically ventilate due to respiratory failure, and he required almost 24 hours of mechanical ventilation until his oxygen requirement fell, and he was extubated onto high-flow oxygen. He was subsequently weaned off intravenous aminophylline and continued on inhaled salbutamol and ipratropium for another four days until he had recovered and his peak flow had returned to 90% of his predicted value for age and height.

He completed a five-day course of oral prednisolone and was discharged with advice to take his preventer inhalers regularly as prescribed.

He had an urgent appointment scheduled with his respiratory paediatrician, at which they discussed adherence to monitoring devices and the initiation of single maintenance and reliever therapy (SMART). His mother also asked to hear more about the newer asthma treatments that she had recently read about—the biologic drugs that are taken by regular subcutaneous injection.

20.1 INTRODUCTION

This chapter will outline the definition, investigations, and management of an acute severe asthma attack. The global burden of asthma is significant. The prevalence in children and young people (CYP) is estimated at 113.7 million cases.[1] Although there have been improvements in overall incidence and mortality, there is huge regional variation with increasing hospital admissions in high-income countries such as the United Kingdom (UK).[2] Globally, over 50% of CYP have uncontrolled or partially controlled asthma,[3] increasing their risk of an attack. It is estimated that over 50% of children with a diagnosis of asthma in the US have an asthma attack per year.[4]

Although the overall incidence of asthma-related deaths in children is low and declining, each death of a child marks a tragic and preventable loss of life. In 2021, there were an estimated 11,093 asthma-related deaths in children globally.[1] Reviews of asthma deaths have highlighted deficiencies in asthma management and missed opportunities to improve care.[5] Particularly in children, the potential seriousness of asthma and risk of asthma death are vastly

DOI: 10.1201/9781003287209-25

underestimated. Whilst management of the acute attack is important and will be the focus of this chapter, the necessity to view asthma as a long-term condition and not as serious as acute episodes cannot be emphasised strongly enough.

20.2 RISK FACTORS FOR SEVERE ASTHMA ATTACKS

The strongest predictor of an asthma attack is a previous attack in the past year.[6] In the UK, almost 10% of children admitted for an asthma attack are readmitted within 30 days and almost 20% within 90 days.[7] This underscores the importance of recognising an asthma attack as a failure of long-term management. Once the acute attack has been appropriately treated, interventions must be put in place to optimise control and prevent further attacks.

Poor asthma control and inadequate access to care are associated with a greatly increased risk of an attack.[6] Suboptimal adherence to inhaled corticosteroids and short-acting beta-agonist (SABA) monotherapy overuse are also risk factors for attacks. Analysis of national primary care data has demonstrated that prescription of three or more SABA inhalers per year is associated with a twofold increased risk of an attack.[8] A third of children in that cohort were prescribed SABA only, and of those prescribed, ICS adherence was poor (median 33%). There are a number of plausible explanations for the association of increased SABA use and asthma attacks. High SABA use is a marker of poor control, an independent risk factor for attacks. When SABA is used alone, or if adherence to ICS is poor, inflammation is untreated, again leading to an increased risk. Furthermore, there is also evidence that regular or frequent SABA use—even for one to two weeks—is associated with adverse effects including beta-receptor downregulation, decreased broncho-protection, rebound hyperresponsiveness, and decreased bronchodilator response.[9] Since 2019, the Global Initiative for Asthma (GINA) has no longer recommended SABA therapy alone for the treatment of asthma[10] and now recommends so-called anti-inflammatory relievers (AIR), an ICS combined with a fast-acting beta-agonist such as formoterol, as the reliever of choice for all severities of asthma.[11]

20.3 ASTHMA-RELATED DEATHS IN CHILDREN

Asthma-related deaths in children are almost invariably preventable. There have been numerous reviews of asthma deaths over the past 30 years, including five in the United Kingdom alone, which depressingly highlight similar inadequacies in asthma care and missed opportunities for intervention.[5, 12–15] The National Review of Asthma Deaths[5] found potentially avoidable factors, relating to patients, their families, or the environment, in 90% of those under 10 years, and in 94% of those between 10 and 19 years—a much higher proportion than for adults who died. These enquiries are supported by individual patient stories, which put into sharp focus the devastating consequences of fragmented asthma care.[16] The risk factors identified are similar to those outlined for severe attacks, including overuse of reliever medicine, poor adherence to controller medication, as well as inadequate monitoring and the lack of a personal asthma action plan.

20.4 PATHOPHYSIOLOGY OF ASTHMA ATTACKS

The hallmarks of asthma attacks are airway hyperreactivity, increased inflammation, mucus hypersecretion, and impaired anti-viral responses triggered by stimuli such as viral infection, allergens, and environmental exposures (such as pollution or tobacco smoke) or, more often, a synergistic interaction between two or more of these (Figure 20.1).[17] A dichotomous timing in the duration of fatal and near fatal attacks has been described.[18] The most common is characterised by a gradual deterioration in patients with poorly controlled asthma and is associated with mucous plugging and eosinophilic inflammation. The second accounts for 15–20% of near fatal asthma, and there tends to be a more rapid progression, neutrophilic inflammation, and faster response to treatment. However, these data are largely based on adult cases. In a small paediatric case series of 12 fatal asthma cases, eosinophilic inflammation and mucous plugs were the predominant findings, in keeping with the slow-onset phenotype and highlighting the potentially preventable nature of these cases.[19]

20.5 PRESENTATION OF ACUTE ASTHMA

20.5.1 History of the Acute Episode

Adult data suggests that each asthma attack a person suffers permanently reduces lung function measurements such as peak expiratory flow rate.[20] As such, every attack should be taken extremely seriously, and preventing attacks is a key goal of asthma management.

An asthma attack can be defined as a worsening of respiratory symptoms or lung function from baseline.[21] It is worth considering the presenting features of an acute attack and exploring briefly the underlying pathophysiology.

Bronchoconstriction results in turbulent airflow, causing wheeze. Wheezing is an expiratory, high-pitched sound produced by the flow of air through a partially obstructed large airway. As such, it is a non-specific airway noise that is by no means unique to asthma and can be found in many other respiratory conditions that are occasionally misdiagnosed as asthma.

Acute cough is caused by stimulation of cough receptors found at the point where bronchi divide. Mucous hypersecretion is another hallmark of asthma. Cough receptors are stimulated by increased mucous production during an acute attack, with mucosal oedema due to airway inflammation also inhibiting normal mucociliary clearance mechanisms.

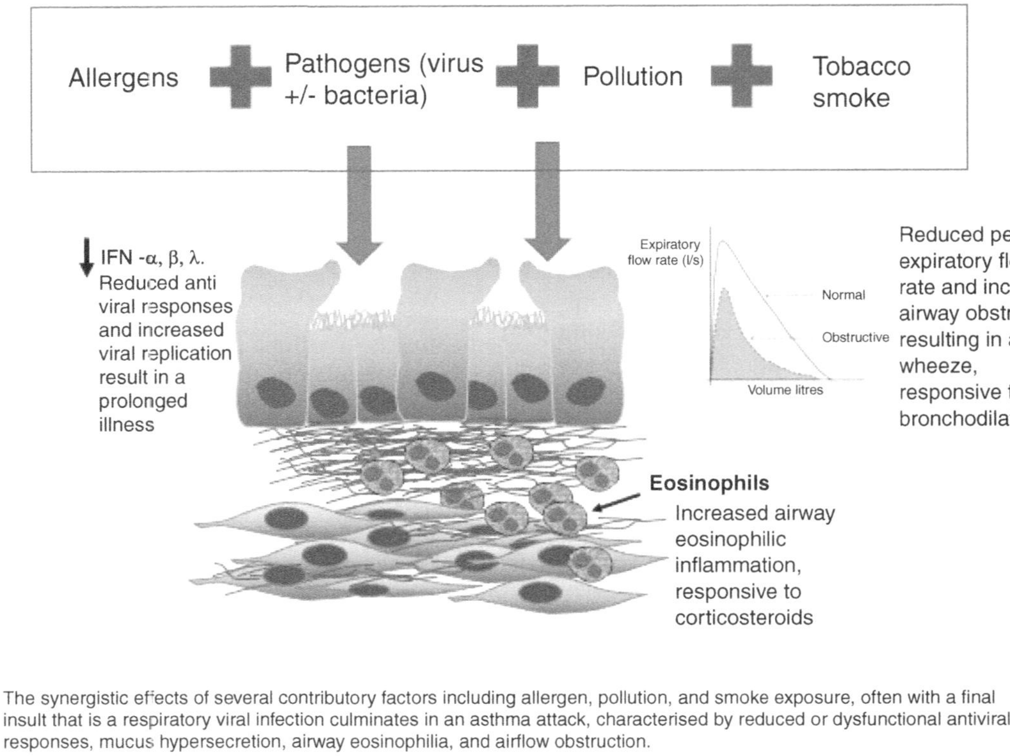

FIGURE 20.1 Pathogenesis of acute asthma attack: school-age children.

Finally, dyspnoea is due to airflow limitation and consequent failure of normal gas exchange. This is a multifactorial process caused in part by bronchoconstriction and in part by inflammation, mucosal oedema, and mucous plugging of airways. Hyperventilation will follow as homeostatic mechanisms attempt to compensate for inadequate gas exchange.

Poor asthma control and frequent symptoms are risk factors for an asthma attack; however, an attack can occur in the context of apparently good control.[22] Peak flow variability data suggests that poor control is characterised by wide diurnal peak expiratory flow variation, whereas in an acute attack there is a steep decline in peak flow, with no increased variability.[23] Whilst loss of baseline control is usually responsive to short-acting beta-agonists (SABA), severe attacks respond poorly to SABA and require corticosteroids. This suggests that an attack is not just a continuum of poor control and that there are distinct pathophysiological mechanisms characterised by loss of bronchodilator responsiveness and increased airway inflammation, which lead to a severe attack.

20.5.2 Physical Examination

The purpose of the physical examination is to rapidly assess the degree of respiratory distress and identify red flags for respiratory failure requiring urgent intervention. The child with acute asthma can be categorised as having an acute severe or life-threatening attack based on physical examination findings and clinical observations (see the section "Investigations in Acute Asthma"). Children unable to speak in full sentences are considered to have an acute severe asthma attack, and those with confusion are having a life-threatening attack.[24]

The first assessment that should be made of a child or young person having an asthma attack is of their level of consciousness and ability to talk in full sentences. This will give an idea of whether the patient has reached the point of respiratory failure and requires urgent intensive care management, as well as an understanding of the severity of the dyspnoea.

Secondly, an assessment should be made of both the degree of air movement in the chest and whether there are additional sounds. Infection is a trigger for acute asthma, and therefore focal bronchial breathing may be heard. Wheeze may be heard, especially in untreated acute asthma, but beware of patients in which air flow is so poor that wheeze is absent, and the chest is silent.

20.5.3 Investigations in Acute Asthma

20.5.3.1 Clinical Observations

Heart rate, respiratory rate, and oxygen saturation are all essential parameters to measure and can be used to risk-stratify patients into those having severe acute and those having life-threatening attacks.[24] Tachycardia is commonly seen in patients who have received salbutamol. However, this can be variable and so should not always be attributed to salbutamol use.

20.5.3.2 Blood Tests

The treatment of acute asthma should not be delayed whilst the results of blood tests are awaited. Patients can be identified and treated based on clinical presentation, observations, and examination findings alone. Many patients will respond well to first line inhaled and oral therapies and will not require blood tests during the admission.

In unwell patients where intravenous bronchodilators might be required, it is sensible to obtain secure intravenous access promptly, and this also provides an opportunity to take blood. Knowledge of the pH and pCO_2 will give a rapid understanding of the degree of concern that clinicians should have about a patient. Arterial blood gas sampling is often a painful procedure, and especially in children, it is reasonable to obtain a venous blood gas sample instead. The pH and pCO_2 from venous blood approximate well to that of arterial blood.[25]

Lactate will often be high in acute asthma, due to the synergistic effects of both corticosteroids and beta-agonists to raise plasma glucose levels.[26, 27] This excess blood glucose is converted by homeostatic mechanisms into pyruvate and then into lactate. Elevated lactate leads to increased respiratory effort to normalise the acidosis. This may be interpreted as worsening clinical condition and may result in increasing bronchodilator therapies, only worsening the clinical condition. Elevated lactate is one of the signs of beta-agonist toxicity, and, when it is identified, clinicians should consider decreasing this medication.

Inflammatory markers can be helpful to identify patients in whom concurrent infection is a concern and may help guide decisions regarding starting antibiotics alongside asthma therapies.

20.5.4 Imaging

20.5.4.1 Chest X-Ray

Routine chest X-ray is not recommended unless the physical examination raises concerns regarding the possibility of an alternate diagnosis such as inhaled foreign body or pneumothorax.

Most chest X-rays will be normal if performed in the setting of acute asthma, but hyperinflation may be seen due to air trapping. This occurs due to the reduced flow rate of air through narrowed airways. Areas of atelectasis or consolidation may also be present if there is coexisting infection. There is a wide spectrum of chest X-ray abnormalities depending on the severity of the attack, duration of asthma symptoms, and level of preceding asthma control.

20.5.4.2 Chest Ultrasound

Bedside lung ultrasound is an imaging modality that has become more popular in recent years, with increasing availability of more portable devices and increased training of emergency care and intensive care physicians in lung imaging protocols. The proposed benefits are the rapid bedside detection of some of the common differential diagnoses of acute asthma, such as pneumothorax, pleural effusion, and pneumonia. One study on children presenting with acute asthma demonstrated that positive findings on lung ultrasound correlated with increased rates of hospital admission and increased use of therapies such as antibiotics and supplemental oxygen.[28]

20.5.4.3 Lung Function Tests

There is value in determining the degree of airway narrowing during acute asthma in order to tailor initial treatment strategies and to plan ongoing emergency care. Forced expiratory volume in 1 second (FEV_1) and peak expiratory flow (PEF) are both valid bedside measurements of airway narrowing. PEF is generally more achievable during an asthma attack, as the emergency department staff are trained in their use and the devices are cheaper and more widely stocked than spirometry machines. The best of three peak flow measurements can be compared to the child's best value when well, or, if this is unknown, a percentage predicted value can be calculated from the child's age and height using widely available calculators, or it can be estimated using the equation PEFR in L/min = [(Height in cm − 100) × 5] + 100. The BTS guidelines on asthma use peak expiratory flow measurements to stratify acute events into life-threatening attacks (PEF < 33% best or predicted) or acute severe (33–50% best or predicted) attacks. Demonstration of reversible airflow obstruction at the time of an attack can also serve as a diagnostic test for asthma, and diagnostic yield is increased when spirometry and exhaled nitric oxide are measured close to an attack.[29]

20.6 GOALS OF ACUTE ASTHMA MANAGEMENT

The goals of management in acute asthma are, firstly, to confirm the diagnosis and to exclude common differential diagnoses, to reverse airway inflammation, to relieve bronchoconstriction, and to improve mucociliary clearance of airway mucous—all with the goal of preventing respiratory failure.

The immediate management steps therefore include applying supplemental oxygen so as to maintain normal oxygen saturations and delivering bronchodilator therapy (initially via a metered dose inhaler with a correctly sized spacer, or by nebulisation if supplemental oxygen is needed) alongside early use of corticosteroids to begin the process of reducing airway inflammation.

To arrange appropriate emergency therapy, assessment and categorisation of the severity of the attack are required. A multitude of national and international guidelines are available for the management of acute asthma, but there is no consistency regarding definitions or criteria required to differentiate an acute asthma attack from a life-threatening or near-fatal attack.[30] Greater consistency is required between guideline definitions to improve research into acute asthma.

There have been recent attempts to achieve consensus in defining the severity of attacks for research purposes. One recent international eDelphi study identified a near-fatal asthma attack as one that "occurs in a person who is exhausted, with severe dyspnoea, unable to speak with a silent chest. Respiratory arrest is considered imminent and invasive ventilation will likely be required. They will be responding poorly to emergency asthma therapies. This is associated with hypoxaemia, hypercarbia and a falling pH."[31]

20.7 INITIAL MANAGEMENT

The initial management of acute asthma is directed towards relieving bronchoconstriction and reducing airway inflammation whilst promoting normal oxygenation and ventilation.

The recognition that severe asthma attacks are life-threatening medical emergencies should prompt clinicians to rapidly assess patients using a standardised ABCDE approach.[32] Drowsiness, confusion, or a silent chest are findings that should prompt immediate escalation for ICU support (Figure 20.2).

Supplemental oxygen should be provided to children and young people as required to maintain oxygen saturations within the range of 94–98%. Short-acting beta-2 agonists (typically salbutamol) are administered early to reverse bronchoconstriction, and oral corticosteroids (prednisolone or dexamethasone, which may be better tolerated in younger children) to reverse airway inflammation.[33]

Other bronchodilators such as muscarinic antagonists (typically ipratropium bromide) can be considered alongside beta-2 agonists depending on the severity of the attack. Intravenous magnesium sulphate can also be considered for severe exacerbations. Ongoing deterioration despite these initial management steps should prompt clinicians to treat the attack as severe and to reconsider calling for ICU support. Measurements of lung function such as peak expiratory flow rate or FEV_1 after one hour of treatment will help guide clinicians as to where patients can be managed after the Emergency Department.

Continuous oxygen saturation monitoring should be utilised for all patients presenting with an asthma attack. Arterial blood gas measurements and chest X-rays are not routinely required, though they can be considered in deteriorating patients or those not responding to initial management strategies.

A list of the commonly used agents can be seen in Table 20.1. For more detailed guidance on the management of acute asthma attacks, we would direct the reader

TABLE 20.1
Pharmacological Management of Acute Asthma

Medication	Dose[35]	Route	Examples of Side Effects[35]
Beta-Receptor Agonists			
Salbutamol	100 µg over 0.5–1 minute for up to 10 doses, repeat every 10–20 minutes or when required	Inhaled (pMDI via spacer)	Arrhythmias, headache, muscle spasms, nasopharyngitis, oropharyngeal pain, palpitations, rash, tremor
	2.5–5 µg, repeat every 20–30 minutes or when required	Nebulised	
	1–2 µg/kg/minute, adjusted according to response and tolerance up to 5 µg/kg/minute	Continuous intravenous infusion	
Cholinergic agents			
Ipratropium bromide	20–40 µg 3–4 times per day	Inhaled	Arrhythmias, constipation, cough, dizziness, dry mouth, headache, nausea
	500 µg every 4–6 hours as required	Nebulised	
Corticosteroids			
Prednisolone	1–2 mg/kg, up to a maximum of 40 mg/day, for 3–5 days	Oral	Anxiety, abnormal behaviour, cataracts, impaired growth and healing, hypertension, increased risk of infection, peptic ulcer, psychotic disorder
Dexamethasone	0.3–0.6 mg/kg once daily, for 1–2 days	Oral	
Hydrocortisone	4 mg/kg every 6 hours, max. per dose 100 mg, until conversion to oral steroids is possible	Intravenous	
Other			
Magnesium sulphate	25–40 mg/kg over 20 min (maximum 2 g/dose)	Intravenous	Electrolyte imbalance
Aminophylline	1 month–11 years: 1mg/kg/hour 12–17 years: 500–700 µg/kg/hour	Intravenous infusion	Abdominal pain, anxiety, arrhythmia, diarrhoea, electrolyte imbalance, hyperventilation, hypotension, seizure, tachycardia, tremor, vomiting

to the latest edition of the Global Strategy for Asthma Management and Prevention report.[34]

Corticosteroids (inhaled versus IV), combination corticosteroid-bronchodilator treatment

20.8 PREVENTING RESPIRATORY FAILURE

It is important to recognise deterioration in severe asthma in order to adjust management with the goal of preventing respiratory failure. As progressive fatigue develops, patients may not have usual signs of agitation or tachypnoea. This may inadvertently result in the severity of the exacerbation being under-appreciated. Consensus guidelines on management are lacking for life-threatening exacerbations once corticosteroids and bronchodilators have been exhausted. In addition, there is wide variability in the monitoring and management of severe asthma where intensive care admission is required for respiratory failure.[36, 37] Many therapies have been tried to avoid intubation. It is worth being aware of salbutamol dosing and requirement to limit doses especially in older children. Current guidance recommends limiting total hourly dose of intravenous salbutamol to 20 μg/min.[35] Side effects include tachycardia, agitation, tremor, metabolic acidosis, myocardial injury, and nausea. These usually respond favourably to a reduction in salbutamol when observed.[26, 38, 39] Failure to respond to salbutamol may raise the question about use of aminophylline. Although there is limited evidence to support the use of aminophylline, blood levels are recommended to be taken on those patients who may be on regular oral theophylline therapies prior to commencing intravenous theophylline. Currently there is insufficient evidence to recommend aminophylline with the goal of reducing PICU admission and/or mechanical ventilation.[40] Adjunctive therapies such as inhaled helium-oxygen mixtures as well as non-invasive ventilatory support have been tried to avoid invasive ventilation. Non-invasive ventilation may improve respiratory distress; however, the effects are unpredictable and influenced by many factors such as mask fit and patient acceptance. There is insufficient evidence to support the use of helium-oxygen mixture or non-invasive ventilation in acute severe asthma in children.[41–43]

20.9 TREATING RESPIRATORY FAILURE

In treating respiratory failure, it is important to consider non-asthmatic causes of respiratory distress and wheeze. These would include but are not limited to foreign body aspiration, pneumothorax, pneumonia, congenital lung abnormalities, or cardiac pathologies. The decision to escalate therapy to invasive ventilation is a clinical one, and there are multiple indications for ventilation in acute asthma:

1. **Hypoxia:** Ventilation perfusion mismatch is common but is usually not severe due to effective hypoxic pulmonary vasoconstrictive responses. It usually responds very well to oxygen therapy.[44]
2. **Fatigue with Hypercarbia:** The work of breathing may be high when airflow limitation is severe and is inefficient with hyperinflated lungs due to diaphragmatic flattening. There is not a consensus threshold for pH or pCO_2 levels that should initiate invasive ventilation.
3. **Access to PICU and Need to Transfer the Patient:** Depending on co-location of PICU and/or the need to travel extended distances with a patient in respiratory failure, the decision to intubate and ventilate prior to transfer may be made on safety and risk versus benefit grounds.
4. **Confusion and Peri-Arrest Situations:** This may occur with both hypoxia and hypercarbia. In this group of patients, respiratory distress may not be severe, as respiratory drive is blunted.

During the induction of anaesthesia for patients with acute severe asthma, it is important to anticipate cardiovascular instability. Hypotension is a frequent complication and usually responds well to intravenous fluid administration and/or inotropic support. Anaesthetic agents that avoid hypotension are usually recommended such as ketamine and fentanyl, due to their haemodynamic profile. Use of end-tidal CO_2 monitoring is essential to confirm endotracheal placement, especially when identifying chest movement on clinical examination may be extremely challenging.[45]

An important strategy in the ventilation of patients with acute severe asthma is to avoid hypoxia and progressive air trapping, as these will both lead to a situation of escalating airway pressures, dynamic hyperinflation, cardiac instability, and complications such as air leaks and pneumothorax. Historic mortality of children ventilated for severe asthma was very high; however, this has improved since ventilation strategies have evolved to avoid normocarbia and rather tolerate controlled hypoventilation. Strategies that use lower respiratory rates allowing sufficient expiratory time, while also using high enough pressures to move to the chest ensuring sufficient minute ventilation, are recommended. These can be used while other therapies are utilised to improve airflow such as steroids, mucolytics, physiotherapy, and airway clearance.[46–48]

Numerous ventilatory modes and ventilators are currently available. Most would recommend pressure control modes in a paediatric population, as tidal volume estimates are variable and may be unreliable in paediatric and smaller patients. Pressure control has numerous advantages in asthma which have been well described.[49] High-frequency oscillation has been used in acute severe asthma; however, the use should be limited to those very familiar with its use in this group of patients. Refractory hypoxia and/or hypercarbia may be an indication for extra corporeal membrane oxygenation (ECMO), especially veno-venous. It is important to recognise, however, that refractory airflow limitation in severe cases is more likely to be due to excessive small and large airway mucous plugging than bronchospasm.[50, 51]

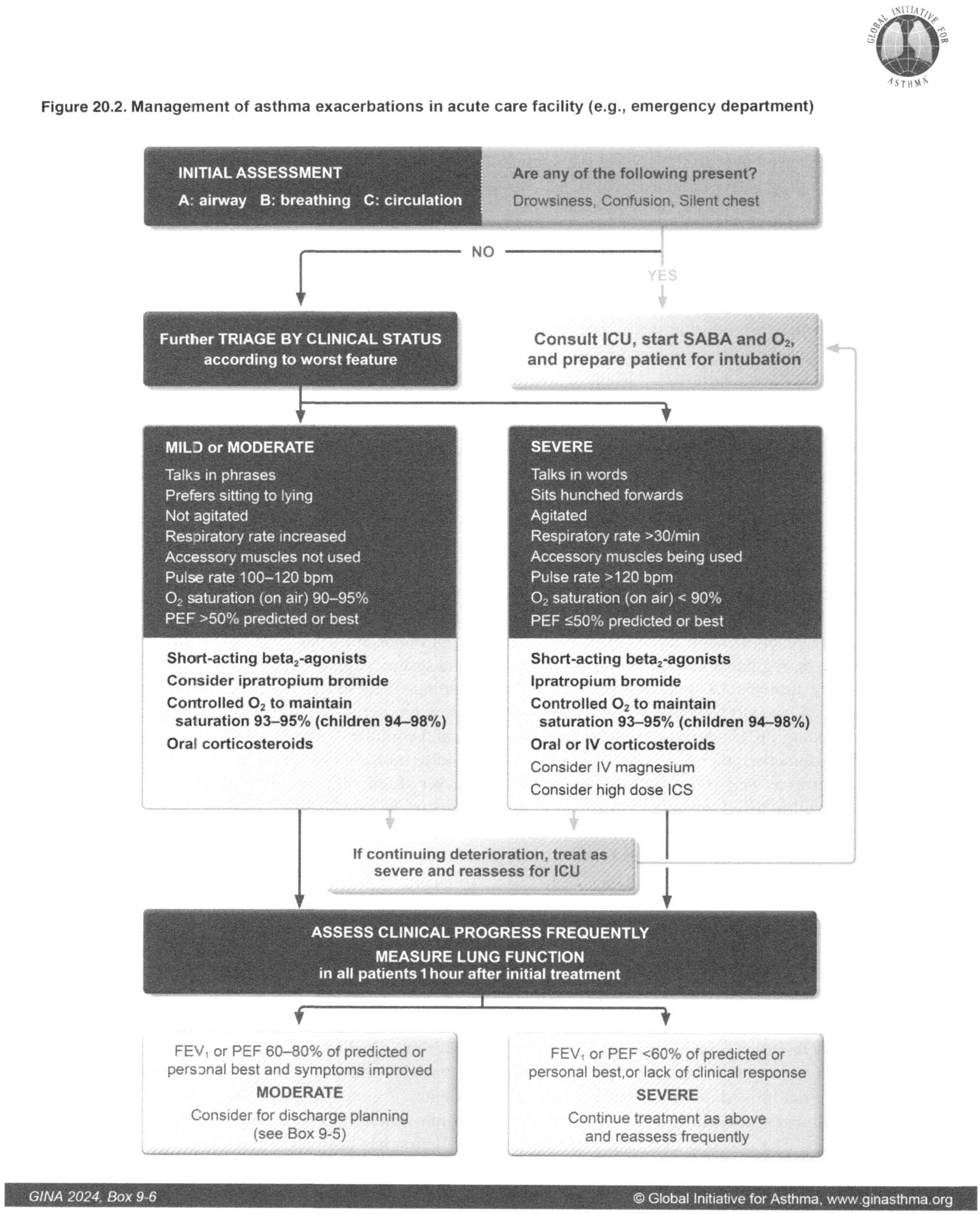

FIGURE 20.2 Global Initiative for Asthma: Emergency Department Management of Asthma Exacerbations. (Reproduced with permission from the Global Initiative for Asthma [GINA] [Ref 34].)

Children who have had an out-of-hospital arrest should have additional neurological monitoring and brain protective measures to prevent a hypoxic brain injury.

20.10 DISCHARGE PLANNING AND POST-ATTACK REVIEW

Discharge from hospital can be considered once IV therapy and supplemental oxygen are no longer needed and clinical parameters and examination are normalising. Prior to discharge it is important to ensure that the child is discharged on ICS-containing treatment, that inhaler technique has been checked, and that the child is issued with a Personal Asthma Action Plan. A post-attack review should be arranged within 2–7 days of discharge. The purpose of the post-attack review is twofold: firstly, to ensure the attack is resolving. If there is still a need for frequent reliever therapy or ongoing evidence of bronchoconstriction, a longer course of oral corticosteroids should be prescribed and further review arranged. Second is to explore the cause of the attack and to optimise management to prevent further attacks. This should include review of the asthma management plan, assessment of adherence to treatment (for example by review of prescription records), evaluation of allergic sensitisation and advice regarding minimising exposure where appropriate, taking steps to reduce other adverse environmental exposures (such as environmental tobacco smoke and mould), and ensuring the child has received the seasonal influenza vaccine.[17] All children should be reviewed by a paediatric asthma specialist following a severe attack. Additional monitoring will also be needed for those who have had an out-of-hospital arrest or required ECMO in order to assess for the sequalae of a hypoxic brain injury.

20.11 CONCLUSION

Severe asthma attacks in children have significant physiological and psychological sequalae. Prompt recognition of a severe attack and implementation of appropriate treatments is essential to prevent respiratory failure and asthma-related death. Optimising asthma management is essential to reduce the risk of asthma attacks and to ensure that asthma-related deaths in children are "never events."

REFERENCES

1. Shi H, Li Y, Yin Z, et al. Global, regional, and national burden of asthma in children and adolescents aged 0–20 years, 1990–2021: a systematic analysis for the global burden of disease study 2021. *Lancet Prepr.* Published online 2024. https://doi.org/10.2139/ssrn.5005772
2. NHS Digital—Statistical Hospital Admitted Patient Care Activity. Digital Health and Care Wales—A bespoke request for hospital admissions data.
3. The Global Asthma Report 2022. *Int J Tuberc Lung Dis.* 2022;26(Supp 1):1–104. https://doi.org/10.5588/ijtld.22.1010
4. Centers for Disease Control and Prevention. Vital Signs: Asthma in the US, May 2011. Available from: http://www.cdc.gov/vitalsigns/Asthma/
5. Royal College of Physicians London. National Review of Asthma Deaths (NRAD) London, 2014. Available from: https://www.rcplondon.ac.uk/projects/outputs/why-asthma-still-kills
6. Buelo A, McLean S, Julious S, et al. At-risk children with asthma (ARC): a systematic review. *Thorax.* 2018;73(9):813–824. https://doi.org/10.1136/thoraxjnl-2017-210939
7. Royal College of Physicians. *National Asthma and Chronic Obstructive Pulmonary Disease Audit Programme (NACAP). Outcomes of Patients Included in the Asthma and COPD Clinical Audit 2018/19 and/or 2019/20 Clinical Audit Reports.* Royal College of Physicians; 2023.
8. Morgan A, Maslova E, Kallis C, et al. Short-acting beta (2)-agonists and exacerbations in children with asthma in England: SABINA Junior. *ERJ Open Res.* 2023;9(2). https://doi.org/10.1183/23120541.00571-2022
9. Cockcroft DW. Clinical concerns with inhaled beta2-agonists: adult asthma. *Clin Rev Allergy Immunol.* 2006;31(2–3):197–208. https://doi.org/10.1385/CRIAI:31:2:197
10. Reddel HK, FitzGerald JM, Bateman ED, et al. GINA 2019: a fundamental change in asthma management: Treatment of asthma with short-acting bronchodilators alone is no longer recommended for adults and adolescents. *Eur Respir J.* 2019;53(6):1901046. https://doi.org/10.1183/13993003.01046-2019
11. Reddel HK, Bacharier LB, Bateman ED, et al. Global initiative for asthma strategy 2021: executive summary and rationale for key changes. *J Allergy Clin Immunol Pr.* 2022;10(1S):S1–S18. https://doi.org/10.1016/j.jaip.2021.10.001
12. Bucknall CE, Slack R, Godley CC, Mackay TW, Wright SC. Scottish confidential inquiry into asthma deaths (SCIAD), 1994–6. *Thorax.* 1999;54(11):978–984. https://doi.org/10.1136/thx.54.11.978
13. Burr ML, Davies BH, Hoare A, et al. A confidential inquiry into asthma deaths in Wales. *Thorax.* 1999;54(11):985–989. https://doi.org/10.1136/thx.54.11.985
14. Jones K, Berrill WT, Bromly CL, Hendrick DJ. A confidential enquiry into certified asthma deaths in the North of England, 1994–96: influence of co-morbidity and diagnostic inaccuracy. *Respir Med.* 1999;93(12):923–927. https://doi.org/10.1016/s0954-6111(99)90061-6
15. Anagnostou K, Harrison B, Iles R, Nasser S. Risk factors for childhood asthma deaths from the UK Eastern region confidential enquiry 2001–2006. *Prim Care Respir J.* 2012;21(1):71–77. https://doi.org/10.4104/pcrj.2011.00097
16. Levy ML, Fleming L, Warner JO, Bush A. Paediatric asthma care in the UK: fragmented and fatally fallible. *Br J Gen Pr.* 2019;69(685):405–406. https://doi.org/10.3399/bjgp19X704933
17. Saglani S, Fleming L, Sonnappa S, Bush A. Advances in the aetiology, management, and prevention of acute asthma attacks in children. *Lancet Child Adolesc Health.* 2019;3(5):354–364. https://doi.org/10.1016/S2352-4642(19)30025-2
18. Restrepo RD, Peters J. Near-fatal asthma: recognition and management. *Curr Opin Pulm Med.* 2008;14(1):13–23. https://doi.org/10.1097/MCP.0b013e3282f1982d
19. Malmstrom K, Lohi J, Sajantila A, et al. Immunohistology and remodeling in fatal pediatric and adolescent asthma. *Respir Res.* 2017;18(1):94. https://doi.org/10.1186/s12931-017-0575-0
20. Soremekun S, Heaney LG, Skinner D, et al. Asthma exacerbations are associated with a decline in lung function: a longitudinal population-based study. *Thorax.* 2023;78(7):643–652. https://doi.org/10.1136/thorax-2021-217032

21. Reddel HK, Taylor DR, Bateman ED, et al. An official American thoracic society/european respiratory society statement: asthma control and exacerbations: standardizing endpoints for clinical asthma trials and clinical practice. *Am J Respir Crit Care Med.* 2009;180(1):59–99. https://doi.org/10.1164/rccm.200801-060ST
22. Wu AC, Tantisira K, Li L, Schuemann B, Weiss ST, Fuhlbrigge AL. Predictors of symptoms are different from predictors of severe exacerbations from asthma in children. *Chest.* 2011;140(1):100–107. https://doi.org/10.1378/chest.10-2794
23. Reddel H, Ware S, Marks G, Salome C, Jenkins C, Woolcock A. Differences between asthma exacerbations and poor asthma control. *Lancet.* 1999;353(9150):364–369. https://doi.org/10.1016/S0140-6736(98)06128-5
24. SIGN. *British Guideline on the Management of Asthma.* SIGN; 2019. https://www.sign.ac.uk/media/2269/sign-158-2024-update-final.pdf
25. Chong WH, Saha BK, Medarov BI. Comparing central venous blood gas to arterial blood gas and determining its utility in critically Ill patients: narrative review. *Anesth Analg.* 2021;133(2):374–378. https://doi.org/10.1213/ane.0000000000005501
26. Meert KL, McCaulley L, Sarnaik AP. Mechanism of lactic acidosis in children with acute severe asthma: *Pediatr Crit Care Med.* 2012;13(1):28–31. https://doi.org/10.1097/PCC.0b013e3182196aa2
27. Meert KL, Clark J, Sarnaik AP. Metabolic acidosis as an underlying mechanism of respiratory distress in children with severe acute asthma*: *Pediatr Crit Care Med.* 2007;8(6):519–523. https://doi.org/10.1097/01.PCC.0000288673.82916.9D
28. Dankoff S, Li P, Shapiro AJ, Varshney T, Dubrovsky AS. Point of care lung ultrasound of children with acute asthma exacerbations in the pediatric ED. *Am J Emerg Med.* 2017;35(4):615–622. https://doi.org/10.1016/j.ajem.2016.12.057
29. Hakizimana A, Lo DKH, Roland D, et al. Effectiveness of paediatric asthma hubs: a clinical pilot study. *Arch Dis Child.* Published online 2024:archdischild-2023-326635. https://doi.org/10.1136/archdischild-2023-326635
30. Mcmurray A, Fleming L, Cunningham S. Defining acute asthma severity—how do worldwide asthma guidelines compare? *Eur Respir J.* 52(suppl 62):PA1288. https://doi.org/10.1183/13993003.congress-2018.PA1288
31. Mcmurray A, Cunningham S, Fleming L. Defining Near Fatal asthma—an international eDelphi study. *Eur Respir J.* 54(suppl 63):PA949. https://doi.org/10.1183/13993003.congress-2019.PA949
32. Soltan M, Kim M. The ABCDE approach explained. *BMJ.* 2016;355:i4512. https://doi.org/10.1136/sbmj.i4512
33. Cai KJ, Su SQ, Wang YG, Zeng YM. Dexamethasone versus prednisone or prednisolone for acute pediatric asthma exacerbations in the emergency department: a meta-analysis. *Pediatr Emerg Care.* 2021;37(12):e1139–e1144. https://doi.org/10.1097/PEC.0000000000001926
34. Global Initiative for Asthma (GINA). The global strategy for asthma management and prevention, 2024. Available from: http://www.ginasthma.org/reports
35. Joint Formulary Committee. *British National Formulary for Children.* BMJ and Pharmaceutical Press; 2024. Available from: https://bnfc.nice.org.uk
36. Bratton SL, Newth CJL, Zuppa AF, et al. Critical care for pediatric asthma: wide care variability and challenges for study. *Pediatr Crit Care Med.* 2012;13(4):407–414. https://doi.org/10.1097/PCC.0b013e318238b428
37. Roberts JS, Bratton SL, Brogan TV. Acute severe asthma: differences in therapies and outcomes among pediatric intensive care units*: *Crit Care Med.* 2002;30(3):581–585. https://doi.org/10.1097/00003246-200203000-00015
38. Sarnaik SM, Saladino RA, Manole M, et al. Diastolic hypotension is an unrecognized risk factor for β-Agonist-associated myocardial injury in children with asthma. *Pediatr Crit Care Med.* 2013;14(6):e273–e279. https://doi.org/10.1097/PCC.0b013e31828a7677
39. Tobin A. Intravenous salbutamol: too much of a good thing? *Crit Care Resusc J Australia's Acad Crit Care Med.* 2005;7(2):119–127.
40. Mitra AA, Bassler D, Watts K, Lasserson TJ, Ducharme FM. Intravenous aminophylline for acute severe asthma in children over two years receiving inhaled bronchodilators. Cochrane Airways Group, ed. *Cochrane Database Syst Rev.* Published online April 20, 2005. https://doi.org/10.1002/14651858.CD001276.pub2
41. Fernández MM, Villagrá A, Blanch L, Fernández R. Non-invasive mechanical ventilation in status asthmaticus. *Intensive Care Med.* 2001;27(3):486–492. https://doi.org/10.1007/s001340100853
42. Schaeffer EM, Pohlman A, Morgan S, Hall JB. Oxygenation in status asthmaticus improves during ventilation with helium-oxygen: *Crit Care Med.* 1999;27(12):2666–2670. https://doi.org/10.1097/00003246-199912000-00010
43. Korang SK, Baker M, Feinberg J, Newth CJ, Khemani RG, Jakobsen JC. Non-invasive positive pressure ventilation for acute asthma in children. Cochrane Central Editorial Service, ed. *Cochrane Database Syst Rev.* 2024;2024(10). https://doi.org/10.1002/14651858.CD012067.pub3
44. Rodriguez-Roisin R. Acute severe asthma: pathophysiology and pathobiology of gas exchange abnormalities. *Eur Respir J.* 1997;10(6):1359–1371. https://doi.org/10.1183/09031936.97.10061359
45. Deho A, Lutman D, Montgomery M, Petros A, Ramnarayan P. Emergency management of children with acute severe asthma requiring transfer to intensive care. *Emerg Med J.* 2010;27(11):834–837. https://doi.org/10.1136/emj.2009.082149
46. Leatherman JW, McArthur C, Shapiro RS. Effect of prolongation of expiratory time on dynamic hyperinflation in mechanically ventilated patients with severe asthma: *Crit Care Med.* 2004;32(7):1542–1545. https://doi.org/10.1097/01.CCM.0000130993.43076.20
47. Nyman A, Puppala K, Colthurst S, et al. Safety and efficacy of intratracheal DNase with physiotherapy in severe status asthmaticus. *Crit Care.* 2011;15(S1):P185, cc9605. https://doi.org/10.1186/cc9605
48. Durward A, Forte V, Shemie SD. Resolution of mucus plugging and atelectasis after intratracheal rhDNase therapy in a mechanically ventilated child with refractory status asthmaticus: *Crit Care Med.* 2000;28(2):560–562. https://doi.org/10.1097/00003246-200002000-00045
49. Sarnaik AP, Daphtary KM, Meert KL, Lieh-Lai MW, Heidemann SM. Pressure-controlled ventilation in children with severe status asthmaticus*: *Pediatr Crit Care Med.* 2004;5(2):133–138. https://doi.org/10.1097/01.PCC.0000112374.68746.E8
50. Kuyper LM, Paré PD, Hogg JC, et al. Characterization of airway plugging in fatal asthma. *Am J Med.* 2003;115(1):6–11. https://doi.org/10.1016/S0002–9343(03)00241–9
51. Carroll N, Carello S, Cooke C, James A. Airway structure and inflammatory cells in fatal attacks of asthma. *Eur Respir J.* 1996;9(4):709–715. https://doi.org/10.1183/09031936.96.09040709

21 Severe Acute and Chronic Life-Threatening Asthma in Adults

Engi Ahmed, Jérémy Charriot, Isabelle Vachier, Laureen Hurault, Clément Boissin, and Arnaud Bourdin

CASE STUDY

A 56-year-old man was intubated in the middle of a commercial center because of "asphyxia." Emergency services recorded bradycardia at 40/min, low blood pressure with a systolic at 70 mmHg, and a respiratory rate at 16/min with very limited thoracic expansion. Witnesses reported a phase of strong agitation before he lost consciousness. Two empty blue inhalers of salbutamol were found in his pockets together with a pack of cigarettes. Immediate intubation and massive fluid infusions couldn't prevent the need for continuous adrenaline support during transportation to ICU. At ICU admission, very high ventilation pressures were noted deserving a protective setting, curare, systemic corticosteroids, magnesium sulfate, and a maintained continuous infusion of adrenaline. Nasal swab PCR multiplex revealed high rhinovirus load. Spectacular improvement in less than 48 hours was unfortunately ruined by a ventilator-acquired pneumonia and a central venous catheter infection. A pneumothorax occurred at day 10, requiring drainage concomitantly with re-increasing ventilatory pressures. Blood eosinophil count increased to around 700/mm^3, and bronchoscopy found massive mucus plugging at the segmental level. Compassionate initiation of a biologic was decided after a multidisciplinary review. Successful extubation at day 17 revealed severe ICU-acquired neuromyopathy that took no less than three months to fully recover.

This patient explained he had always had asthma, neglected because of poorly perceived benefits of treatments and unacceptable side effects of oral corticosteroids (OCS). Because OCS were proposed at any outpatient clinic he attended, he decided to stop follow-up. He used to keep the door of his flat opened every night in the eventuality he couldn't speak or breathe to ease the way of emergency services, as he had a previous experience of dreadful asthma attack. The modifiable factors identified included cigarette smoking, polysensitization with massive exposure at home (in particular dust and mold), short-acting beta-agonist bronchodilator (SABA) overuse, absence of inhaled corticosteroid inhalers (ICS), high blood eosinophil count, ICU intubation in the past [1, 2]. After one year of multidisciplinary management in a tertiary center accompanying the initiation of the biologic, patient was deemed in "super response."

21.1 DISCUSSION

This case typically reflects the gaps between what is known, what is achievable, and what happens in real life in most dreadful circumstances. All warning signals were enlightened, but this unfortunately led nowhere else than in ICU. Major efforts in communication are needed, and the national review of asthma deaths in the UK (NRAD) identified that at least half of the asthma deaths could be preventable—indicating noteworthy that the other half couldn't [3]. All stakeholders from patients to pharmacists to physicians and any other people involved in the management of asthma (physiotherapist, nurses, relatives, psychologists, etc.) can combine their efforts in promoting modern and adapted messages. OCS and SABA still largely predominate the landscape of asthma medication sales in westernized countries, suggesting inappropriate overuse and over-reliance on rescue medications [4].

Although the clinical vignette depicted above led to positive outcomes, it also pinpoints the need for therapeutic improvements. Speed of onset of current medications is potentially insufficient and ICU-associated adverse events hard to totally prevent [5]. In chronic diseases, prevention of acute episodes—especially virally triggered exacerbations—is the main goal of the management, and GINA recommendations are fully dedicated for that.

21.2 ACUTE LIFE-THREATENING ASTHMA

Most of our understanding of these episodes is derived from autopsies of fatal asthma cases. Fortunately rare and becoming rarer still, these episodes were described to occur following two patterns according to the speed of onset, the assumption being the faster, the more related to bronchoconstriction, in contrast with the slower more related to inflammation [6]. Obviously, not all the clinical

DOI: 10.1201/9781003287209-26

characteristics of these cases could be fully reconstructed, leading to some lack of precision. Risk factors for severe exacerbation/life-threatening episodes are now well established (Table 21.1) [2].

Anyway, major findings that can distinguish between severe and life-threatening exacerbations are summarized in Figure 21.1.

TABLE 21.1
Risk Factors for Severe Exacerbation/Life-Threatening Episodes [2]

Risk factor for	Likely	Possible
Dying	β_2-agonist overuse No ICS treatment Age Virus infection Gender Drug and venom allergy Allergen exposure (including thunderstorm asthma)	Intubation outside ICU High number of ED visit Sports Alternaria and penicillium spores Nitrogen dioxide, ozone Severe asthma
ICU admission; near fatal asthma	No ICS treatment Severe asthma Virus infection Loss of elastic recoil Permanent airflow limitation Hyperinflation Menstruation Steroid dependence History of intubation Delayed systemic corticosteroid use	Heroin, cocaine
Severe exacerbation; ED admission	No ICS treatment Comorbidities Psychological issues Age Absence of ICS Virus infection	
Frequent severe exacerbations (≥2–3 OCS bursts per year)	No ICS treatment Virus infection High blood eosinophil count Smoking Genetic Atopy BMI BD responsiveness Chronic sinusitis	Low socioeconomic status GORD Aspirin sensitive Climate: thunderstorms during pollen season

Abbreviations: BD: bronchodilator, BMI: body mass gastro-oesophageal reflux disease, OCS, oral corticosteroids index, ED: emergency department, ICS: inhaled corticosteroids, ICU: intensive care unit

1. **Airway Hyperresponsiveness (AHR):** Life-threatening episodes are described by some as "bronchospasms." The distinction between ward-admitted and ICU-admitted episodes and episodes allowing for early discharge mostly depends on the extent of loss of airflow. High levels of airway hyperresponsiveness are known predictors for later asthma in children [7], poor lung function trajectories, and ICU admissions. Although present as early as one month of age (Figure 21.2) [8], AHR can vary with age and treatments, suggesting that it might be considered as a phenotypic and potentially treatable trait [9–11].

   The early phase of AHR recorded during a nonspecific challenge, for example with methacholine, reflects airway smooth muscle (ASM) behavior. Organized in bundles circling the airways until the bronchioles, the ASM plays a role during *in utero* growth through peristaltic waves helpful for determining airway caliber [12]. In one study of near-fatal asthma (NFA) and fatal asthma (FA) episodes, the ASM was found to be hyperplastic rather than hypertrophic [13]. After viewing recorded pictures of wonderful work during an airway challenge, the authors then modeled their findings, suggesting that severe/fatal loss of airflow during these episodes could be explained by spatial homogeneity as the difference of less severe episodes where bronchoconstriction occurred unevenly, as in natural disasters (Figure 21.3) [14, 15].

   Bronchial thermoplasty was found to potentially target the ASM but eventually at the price of bronchiectasis [16, 17]. Rac1 is supposed to be the key GTPases involved in ASM contractility and maintenance, and dedicated works are currently conducted for identifying pharmacological candidates [18]. Calcium metabolism is critical in ASM contractility, leading to successful proof of concept studies (Figure 21.4) [19].

   Interleukin 13 and thymic stromal lymphopoietin (TSLP) are also known to potentially promote ASM hyperplasia. The link between AHR and inflammation was largely suggested and tested so far even though the role of eosinophils and of eosinophilic depletion remains unclear [20]. A mast cell myositis [21] was recurrently reported supporting the role of histamine and other mast-released mediators as actors and the role of IgE and other mast-cell triggering signals as activators. Bronchoconstriction can lead to goblet cell hyperplasia and extra cellular matrix deposition in the airways even in absence of airway inflammation (Figure 21.5) [22].
2. **Inflammatory Pathways:** More or less all leucocytes have been found around or within the airways of patients who die from asthma. Neutrophils,

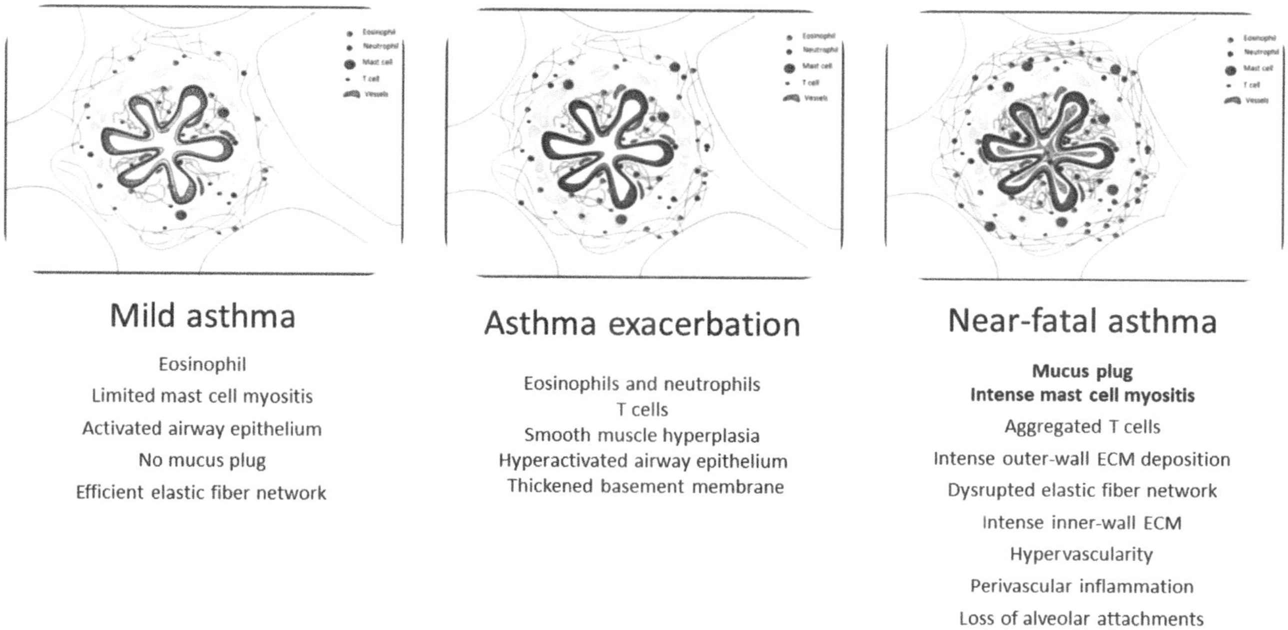

FIGURE 21.1 Summary of differences between mild asthma, asthma exacerbation, and near-fatal asthma findings at autopsy. In mild asthma, inflammation is mostly eosinophilic and the airway lumen free of mucus; during an asthma exacerbation, inflammation is more polymorphic with evidence of epithelial activation and features of remodeling. In near-fatal/fatal episodes, key findings are the presence of mucus plus occluding the airway lumen and an intense mast cell myositis. Other findings are also signs of remodeling including potential loss of alveolar attachments.

Airway hyperreactivity is present as soon as 1 month after birth

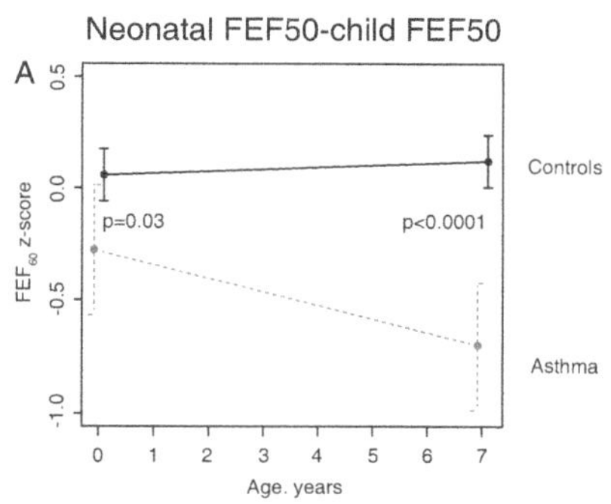

Forced expiratory flow (FEF) rate at 1 month and 7 years of age in children with (dashed line) and without (solid line) current asthma by age 7 years. Mean *z* score and 95% confidence interval.

COPSAC is a prospective clinical study of a birth cohort of 411 children. All mothers had a history of doctor's diagnosis of asthma after age 7. The newborns were enrolled in the first month of life.

Neonatal spirometry and bronchial responsiveness to methacholine were obtained by forced flow-volume measurements applying the raised volume rapid thoracic compression technique.

Neonatal Lung Function	Risk of Asthma* *(Odds Ratio per Interquartile Range)*	Neonatal Lung Function *Z* Score* *(Difference between Children with or without Asthma by Age 7)*
Neonatal-FEF_{50}	1.57 (1.04-2.37); *P* = 0.03	− 0.34; *P* = 0.03
Necnatal-$FEV_{0.5}$	1.41 (0.94-2.10); *P* = 0.09	− 0.29; *P* = 0.07
Neonatal-PD_{15} (TC_{02})	1.59 (1.11-2.28); *P* = 0.01	− 0.48; *P* = 0.005

Definition of abbreviation: FEF forced expiratory flow.
*Analyses are adjusted by sex and maternal smoking during third trimester of pregnancy.

FIGURE 21.2 Airway hyperreactivity is present as soon as one month after birth. A subset of 411 children with a strong mother asthma history was exposed to methacholine at age one month. PD15 at age one month was predictive of asthma at age seven.

eosinophils, mast cells, basophils, and T cells were found in excess at all airway levels, from proximal to distal [6, 23–25]. Actually, the improved understanding of viruses in promoting these episodes—rhinoviruses and RSV coming first [26]—led to a better description of the inflammatory cascade of events that occurred in asthmatic airways [27–30]. Impaired signaling at the CDHR3 rhinovirus receptor [31], impaired type III interferon response, and T2-preferred orientation of either the innate or adaptive immune systems through inappropriate epithelial response led to excessive ILC2 and Th2 activations and subsequent T2 inflammation. The role of anti-viral drugs needs confirmation [32].

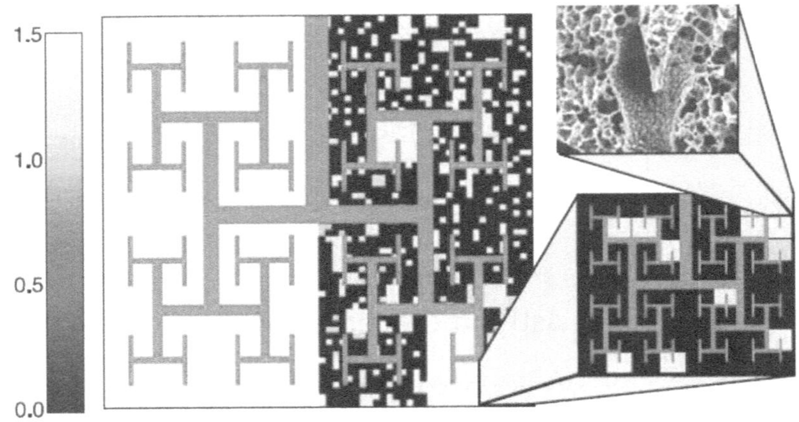

FIGURE 21.3 In the seminal paper from Venegas, fractal dimensions of airway closure during an episode of intense bronchoconstriction followed an heterogeneity law near the one seen in catastrophic shift, which includes preservation of some distal airspaces protecting against death.

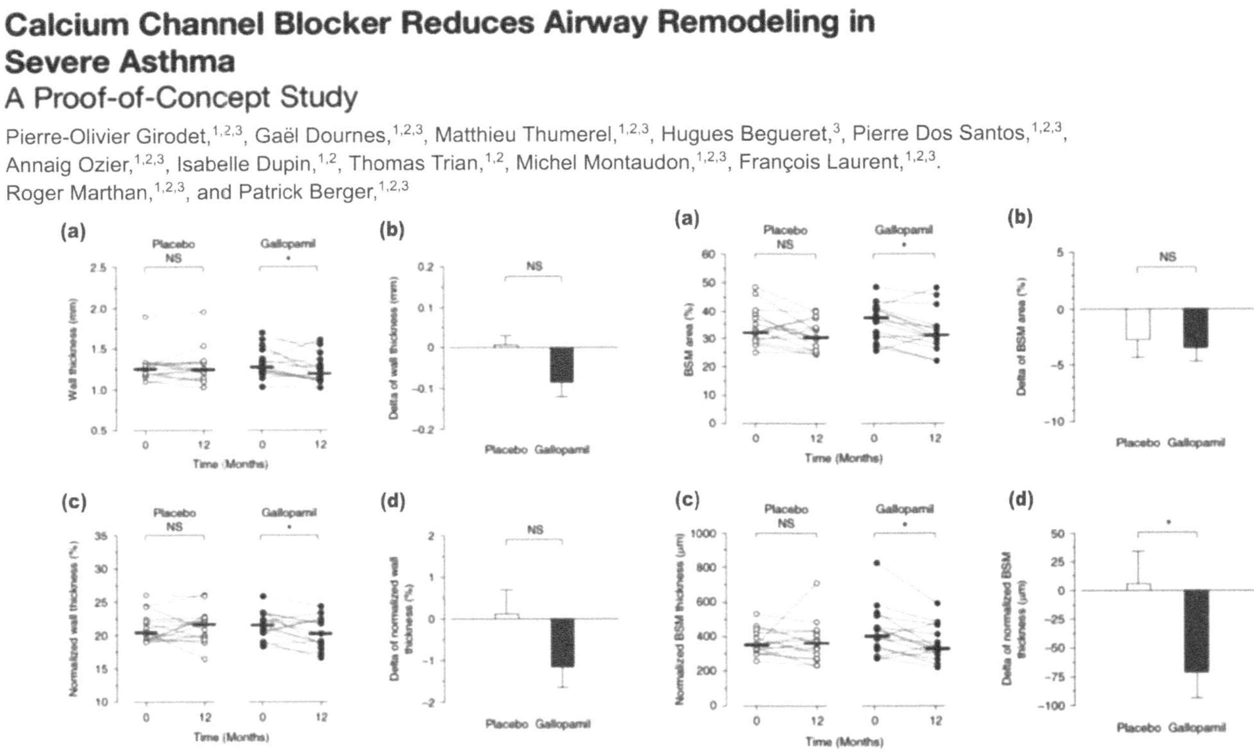

FIGURE 21.4 Gallopamil was able to prevent airway remodeling evidencing involvement of calcium in excessive contractility of the smooth muscle.

Neutrophils have been described as distinguishing NFA episodes from milder ones, but the role of corticosteroids and other potential confounders were hard to assess [33]. Finally, eosinophils and mast cells seem reasonable culprits and then reasonable targets to either prevent or treat these episodes. If corticosteroids are currently used as the gold standard, monoclonal antibodies targeting IL5-IL5R, IL4Ra, TSLP, and IgE are potentially worth assessing in ICU.

3. **Mucus Plugging:** There are many famous pictures of massive mucus casts matched with autopsy findings where pathologists consistently reported airway plugging at all levels (Figure 21.6) [5].

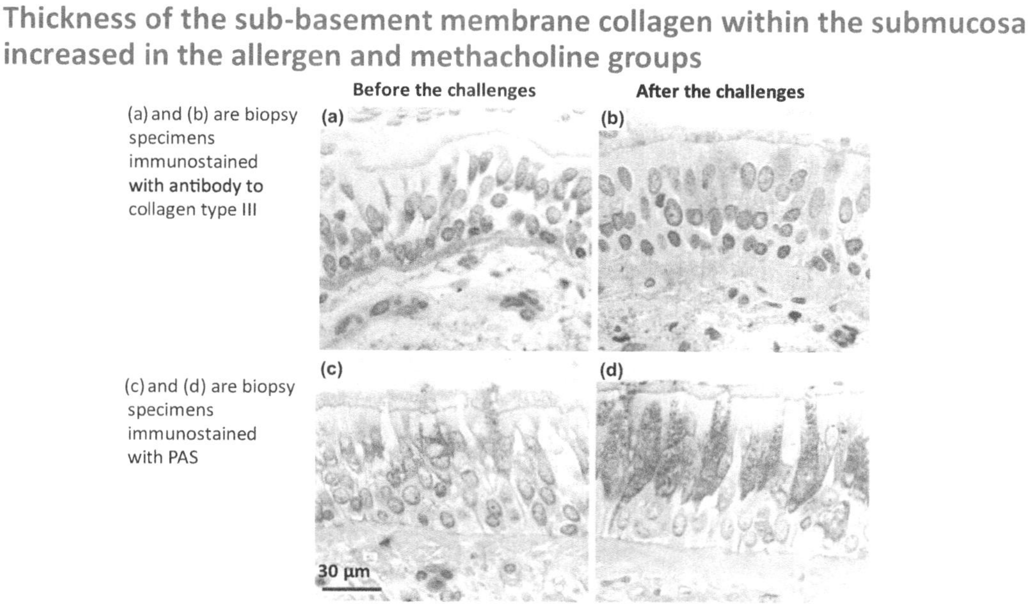

FIGURE 21.5 A methacholine challenge alone was able to induce thickening of the basement membrane and goblet cell hyperplasia in humans with asthma at a level similar to those challenged with allergens despite total absence of methacholine-induced eosinophilic inflammation.

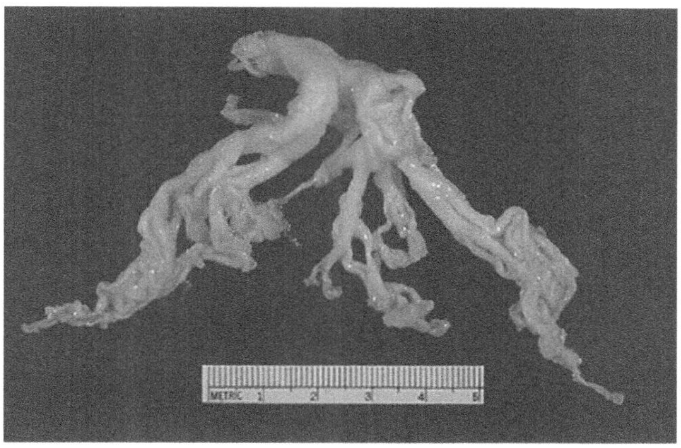

FIGURE 21.6 Mucus plug shaping a bronchial tree cast coughed by a patient. (With permission of Prof. Klatt.)

This might explain why intubation and non-invasive ventilation are not ideal breathing substitutes in these cases, leading some clinicians to propose ECMO [34] and other extracorporeal supports. Abnormal submucosal glands and goblet cell hyperplasia are supposed to contribute to excessive mucin release. More recently, these casts were described as T2-niches merging MUC5AC and eosinophil-dying Charcot–Leyden crystals (CLC), which plays a fascinating role of first aggregating mucins already organized in networks and second to worsen goblet hyperplasia and mucin release [35]. All these findings could be reversed *in vitro* and in an animal model by a specific monoclonal antibody able to accelerate dissolution of the CLC (Figure 21.7). The T2-cytokine environment, also involved as IL13, for example, is clearly involved in mucin release and in goblet cell hyperplasia [36].

21.3 CHRONIC LIFE-THREATENING ASTHMA

The apparent paradox is that asthmatics were reputed in the 18th and 19th centuries to live longer. From this period, it was shown that T2 inflammation may protect from potentially fatal cytokine thunderstorms as observed in septic shock or more recently during the COVID-19 outbreak. The TNF pathway may be involved in this regard given the observed difference in TNFAIP3 (or A20) between asthmatics and non-asthmatics who lived on the farm [37].

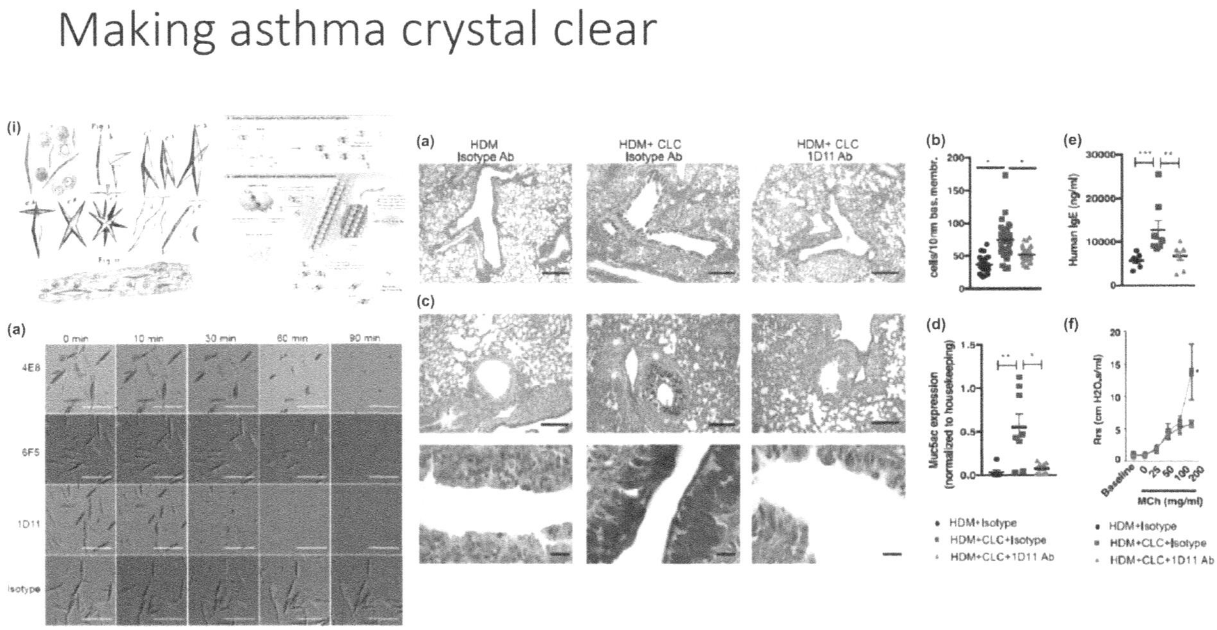

FIGURE 21.7 Charcot Leyden Crystals made of galectin-10, a protein released when eosinophils die, are able to increase mucus plugging by increasing mucus rheology by binding mucins. CLC targeting monoclonal antibodies could not only reverse mucus plugging but also reduce airway inflammation, mucus release, and airway hyperreactivity in mice.

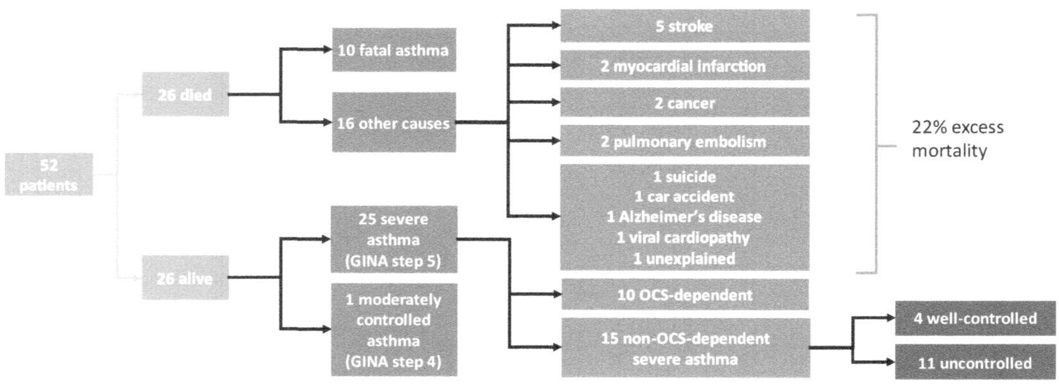

FIGURE 21.8 Chronic use of OCS rarely leads to success in severe asthma: 20-year follow-up; two of 52 patients successfully treated.

Epidemiological studies and some cohorts (Figure 21.8) nonetheless reported consistent loss of life expectancy in severe asthmatics [38].

Most of these early deaths could be associated with oral corticosteroids' adverse effects. Long-term consequences of OCS are still under-appreciated and under-reported, among which increased arterial and venous risks, renal impairment, increased risk of sepsis through diabetes or not, osteoporosis, and depression are all potential cause of premature deaths [39, 40]. Strokes, myocardial infarction, pulmonary embolism, suicides, etc. are more frequently recorded than expected in the course of OCS-maintained severe asthma patients, very often despite efforts of prevention. Limited reversibility of OCS adverse effects after withdrawal suggests the need for updating our current strategy [41]. Today, the word "severe" is given once patients are massively exposed to OCS through relapsing episodes and/or heavy symptoms. Finally, identifying warning signs or predictors of poor outcomes would allow for earlier intervention that would ultimately lead to lower overall exposure to OCS and other rescue medications. Using terminology such as "asthma at risk" [1] would be easier to adopt by the general population and could lead to improved adherence, as it might improve understanding of the need for a maintenance treatment even in the absence of symptoms, as is the case in management of dyslipidemia. It may also help physicians to screen and to identify early modifiable and non-modifiable factors more accurately. Beyond behavioral (poor adherence, poor understanding, toxicomania, smoking, etc.) and environmental/occupational issues (non-avoidance of known allergens, pollution and smokes, high viral burden, etc.), biomarkers such as blood eosinophils and FeNO may have a place in patients with identified risk factors (poor symptom control, low lung function, nonadherence, reliever overuse, previous intubation/critical asthma attack, selected comorbidities, environmental exposures) [42]. Beyond biomarkers, evidence of small airway involvement, T2 comorbidities among which nasal polyposis ranks first [43], genetic inheritance and epigenetic predispositions [44] are potentially promising predictors useful for identifying whether the asthma patient in front of you is "at risk" and deserving a significant intervention.

21.4 CONCLUSION

Asthma can kill. Still. Mostly through ignorance or inappropriate behaviors. Changing paradigms and communication in all healthcare sectors have the potential to reverse undesirable trajectories. Whereas most of the unmet needs are potentially addressable today, new drugs and new therapeutic schemes in managing exacerbations and life-threatening episodes are still required.

REFERENCES

1. Global Strategy for Asthma Management and Prevention, Global Initiative for Asthma (GINA). Date last updated: April 2019. Available from: http://www.ginasthma.org. [Internet]. Available from: http://www.ginasthma.org.
2. Bourdin A, Bjermer L, Brightling C, Brusselle GG, Chanez P, Chung KF, Custovic A, Diamant Z, Diver S, Djukanovic R, Hamerlijnck D, Horváth I, Johnston SL, Kanniess F, Papadopoulos N, Papi A, Russell RJ, Ryan D, Samitas K, Tonia T, Zervas E, Gaga M. ERS/EAACI statement on severe exacerbations in asthma in adults: facts, priorities and key research questions. *Eur. Respir. J.* 2019; 54.
3. Healthcare Quality Improvement Partnership, Royal College of Physicians of London. Why asthma still kills: The national review of asthma deaths (NRAD). Confidential enquiry report May 2014 Confidential enquiry report May. 2014.
4. Blakey J, Chung LP, McDonald VM, Ruane L, Gornall J, Barton C, Bosnic-Anticevich S, Harrington J, Hew M, Holland AE, Hopkins T, Jayaram L, Reddel H, Upham JW, Gibson PG, Bardin P. Oral corticosteroids stewardship for asthma in adults and adolescents: A position paper from the thoracic society of Australia and New Zealand. *Respirol. Carlton Vic.* 2021; 26: 1112–1130.
5. Bourdin A, Charriot J, Boissin C, Ahmed E, Suehs C, De Sevin A, Volpato M, Pahus L, Gras D, Vachier I, Halimi L, Hamerlijnck D, Chanez P. Will the asthma revolution fostered by biologics also benefit adult ICU patients? *Allergy*. 2021 Aug;76(8): 2395–2406. doi: 10.1111/all.14688. Epub 2020 Dec 26. PMID: 33283296.
6. James AL, Elliot JG, Abramson MJ, Walters EH. Time to death, airway wall inflammation and remodelling in fatal asthma. *Eur. Respir. J.* 2005; 26: 429–434.
7. McGeachie MJ, Yates KP, Zhou X, Guo F, Sternberg AL, Van Natta ML, Wise RA, Szefler SJ, Sharma S, Kho AT, Cho MH, Croteau-Chonka DC, Castaldi PJ, Jain G, Sanyal A, Zhan Y, Lajoie BR, Dekker J, Stamatoyannopoulos J, Covar RA, Zeiger RS, Adkinson NF, Williams PV, Kelly HW, Grasemann H, Vonk JM, Koppelman GH, Postma DS, Raby BA, Houston I, et al. Patterns of growth and decline in lung function in persistent childhood asthma. *N. Engl. J. Med.* 2016; 374: 1842–1852.
8. Bisgaard H, Jensen SM, Bønnelykke K. Interaction between asthma and lung function growth in early life. *Am. J. Respir. Crit. Care Med.* 2012; 185: 1183–1189.
9. Diver S, Khalfaoui L, Emson C, Wenzel SE, Menzies-Gow A, Wechsler ME, Johnston J, Molfino N, Parnes JR, Megally A, Colice G, Brightling CE, CASCADE study investigators. Effect of tezepelumab on airway inflammatory cells, remodelling, and hyperresponsiveness in patients with moderate-to-severe uncontrolled asthma (CASCADE): a double-blind, randomised, placebo-controlled, phase 2 trial. *Lancet Respir. Med.* 2021; 9: 1299–1312.
10. Sverrild A, Andreasen AH, Westergaard CG, von Bülow A, Udesen PB, Thomsen SF, Allin KH, Backer V, Porsbjerg C. Airway hyperresponsiveness to inhaled mannitol identifies a cluster of noneosinophilic asthma patients with high symptom burden. *J. Allergy Clin. Immunol. Pract.* 2021; 9: 4029–4036.e2.
11. Sont JK, Willems LN, Bel EH, van Krieken JH, Vandenbroucke JP, Sterk PJ. Clinical control and histopathologic outcome of asthma when using airway hyperresponsiveness as an additional guide to long-term treatment. The AMPUL study group. *Am. J. Respir. Crit. Care Med.* 1999; 159: 1043–1051.
12. Young RE, Jones M-K, Hines EA, Li R, Luo Y, Shi W, Verheyden JM, Sun X. Smooth muscle differentiation is essential for airway size, tracheal cartilage segmentation, but dispensable for epithelial branching. *Dev. Cell* 2020; 53: 73–85.e5.
13. Woodruff PG, Dolganov GM, Ferrando RE, Donnelly S, Hays SR, Solberg OD, Carter R, Wong HH, Cadbury PS, Fahy JV. Hyperplasia of smooth muscle in mild to moderate asthma without changes in cell size or gene expression. *Am. J. Respir. Crit. Care Med.* 2004; 169: 1001–1006.
14. Venegas JG, Winkler T, Musch G, Vidal Melo MF, Layfield D, Tgavalekos N, Fischman AJ, Callahan RJ, Bellani G, Harris RS. Self-organized patchiness in asthma as a prelude to catastrophic shifts. *Nature* 2005; 434: 777–782.
15. Harris RS, Winkler T, Tgavalekos N, Musch G, Melo MFV, Schroeder T, Chang Y, Venegas JG. Regional pulmonary perfusion, inflation, and ventilation defects in bronchoconstricted patients with asthma. *Am. J. Respir. Crit. Care Med.* 2006; 174: 245–253.
16. Bonta PI, d'Hooghe J, Sterk PJ, Bel EH, Annema JT. Reduction of airway smooth muscle mass after bronchial thermoplasty: are we there yet? *Am. J. Respir. Crit. Care Med.* 2015; 191: 1207–1208.
17. Pretolani M, Dombret M-C, Thabut G, Knap D, Hamidi F, Debray M-P, Taille C, Chanez P, Aubier M. Reduction of airway smooth muscle mass by bronchial thermoplasty in patients with severe asthma. *Am. J. Respir. Crit. Care Med.* 2014; 190: 1452–1454.
18. André-Grégoire G, Dilasser F, Chesné J, Braza F, Magnan A, Loirand G, Sauzeau V. Targeting of Rac1 prevents bronchoconstriction and airway hyperresponsiveness. *J. Allergy Clin. Immunol.* 2018; 142: 824–833.e3.
19. Girodet P-O, Dournes G, Thumerel M, Begueret H, Dos Santos P, Ozier A, Dupin I, Trian T, Montaudon M, Laurent F, Marthan R, Berger P. Calcium channel blocker reduces airway remodeling in severe asthma. A proof-of-concept study. *Am. J. Respir. Crit. Care Med.* 2015; 191: 876–883.
20. Chan R, Lipworth B. Efficacy of biologic therapy on airway hyperresponsiveness in asthma. *Ann. Allergy. Asthma. Immunol.* 2023; 131: 37–41.

21. Brightling CE, Bradding P, Symon FA, Holgate ST, Wardlaw AJ, Pavord ID. Mast-cell infiltration of airway smooth muscle in asthma. *N. Engl. J. Med.* 2002; 346: 1699–1705.
22. Grainge CL, Lau LCK, Ward JA, Dulay V, Lahiff G, Wilson S, Holgate S, Davies DE, Howarth PH. Effect of bronchoconstriction on airway remodeling in asthma. *N. Engl. J. Med.* 2011; 364: 2006–2015.
23. Balzar S, Wenzel SE, Chu HW. Transbronchial biopsy as a tool to evaluate small airways in asthma. *Eur. Respir. J.* 2002; 20: 254–259
24. Carroll N, Elliot J, Morton A, James A. The structure of large and small airways in nonfatal and fatal asthma. *Am. Rev. Respir. Dis.* 1993; 147: 405–410.
25. Mauad T, Silva LFF, Santos MA, Grinberg L, Bernardi FDC, Martins MA, Saldiva PHN, Dolhnikoff M. Abnormal alveolar attachments with decreased elastic fiber content in distal lung in fatal asthma. *Am. J. Respir. Crit. Care Med.* 2004; 170: 857–862.
26. Ruckwardt TJ, Morabito KM, Phung E, Crank MC, Costner PJ, Holman LA, Chang LA, Hickman SP, Berkowitz NM, Gordon IJ, Yamshchikov GV, Gaudinski MR, Lin B, Bailer R, Chen M, Ortega-Villa AM, Nguyen T, Kumar A, Schwartz RM, Kueltzo LA, Stein JA, Carlton K, Gall JG, Nason MC, Mascola JR, Chen G, Graham BS, VRC 317 study team. Safety, tolerability, and immunogenicity of the respiratory syncytial virus prefusion F subunit vaccine DS-Cav1: a phase 1, randomised, open-label, dose-escalation clinical trial. *Lancet Respir. Med.* 2021; 9: 1111–1120.
27. Bartlett NW, Walton RP, Edwards MR, Aniscenko J, Caramori G, Zhu J, Glanville N, Choy KJ, Jourdan P, Burnet J, Tuthill TJ, Pedrick MS, Hurle MJ, Plumpton C, Sharp NA, Bussell JN, Swallow DM, Schwarze J, Guy B, Almond JW, Jeffery PK, Lloyd CM, Papi A, Killington RA, Rowlands DJ, Blair ED, Clarke NJ, Johnston SL. Mouse models of rhinovirus-induced disease and exacerbation of allergic airway inflammation. *Nat. Med.* 2008; 14: 199–204.
28. Contoli M, Message SD, Laza-Stanca V, Edwards MR, Wark PAB, Bartlett NW, Kebadze T, Mallia P, Stanciu LA, Parker HL, Slater L, Lewis-Antes A, Kon OM, Holgate ST, Davies DE, Kotenko SV, Papi A, Johnston SL. Role of deficient type III interferon-lambda production in asthma exacerbations. *Nat. Med.* 2006; 12: 1023–1026.
29. Corne JM, Marshall C, Smith S, Schreiber J, Sanderson G, Holgate ST, Johnston SL. Frequency, severity, and duration of rhinovirus infections in asthmatic and non-asthmatic individuals: a longitudinal cohort study. *Lancet Lond. Engl.* 2002; 359: 831–834.
30. Fraenkel DJ, Bardin PG, Sanderson G, Lampe F, Johnston SL, Holgate ST. Lower airways inflammation during rhinovirus colds in normal and in asthmatic subjects. *Am. J. Respir. Crit. Care Med.* 1995; 151: 879–886.
31. Bønnelykke K, Sleiman P, Nielsen K, Kreiner-Møller E, Mercader JM, Belgrave D, den Dekker HT, Husby A, Sevelsted A, Faura-Tellez G, Mortensen LJ, Paternoster L, Flaaten R, Mølgaard A, Smart DE, Thomsen PF, Rasmussen MA, Bonàs-Guarch S, Holst C, Nohr EA, Yadav R, March ME, Blicher T, Lackie PM, Jaddoe VWV, Simpson A, Holloway JW, Duijts L, Custovic A, Davies DE, et al. A genome-wide association study identifies CDHR3 as a susceptibility locus for early childhood asthma with severe exacerbations. *Nat. Genet.* 2014; 46: 51–55.
32. Djukanović R, Harrison T, Johnston SL, Gabbay F, Wark P, Thomson NC, Niven R, Singh D, Reddel HK, Davies DE, Marsden R, Boxall C, Dudley S, Plagnol V, Holgate ST, Monk P, INTERCIA Study Group. The effect of inhaled IFN-β on worsening of asthma symptoms caused by viral infections. A randomized trial. *Am. J. Respir. Crit. Care Med.* 2014; 190: 145–154.
33. Carroll NG, Mutavdzic S, James AL. Increased mast cells and neutrophils in submucosal mucous glands and mucus plugging in patients with asthma. *Thorax* 2002; 57: 677–682.
34. Extracorporeal membrane oxygenation (ECMO) and beyond in near fatal asthma: a comprehensive review—PubMed [Internet]. [cited 2024 Mar 4]. Available from: https://pubmed.ncbi.nlm.nih.gov/37245648/.
35. Persson EK, Verstraete K, Heyndrickx I, Gevaert E, Aegerter H, Percier J-M, Deswarte K, Verschueren KHG, Dansercoer A, Gras D, Chanez P, Bachert C, Gonçalves A, Van Gorp H, De Haard H, Blanchetot C, Saunders M, Hammad H, Savvides SN, Lambrecht BN. Protein crystallization promotes type 2 immunity and is reversible by antibody treatment. *Science* 2019; 364.
36. Fahy JV, Dickey BF. Airway mucus function and dysfunction. *N. Engl. J. Med.* 2010; 363: 2233–2247.
37. Schuijs MJ, Willart MA, Vergote K, Gras D, Deswarte K, Ege MJ, Madeira FB, Beyaert R, van Loo G, Bracher F, von Mutius E, Chanez P, Lambrecht BN, Hammad H. Farm dust and endotoxin protect against allergy through A20 induction in lung epithelial cells. *Science* 2015; 349: 1106–1110.
38. Bourdin A, Molinari N, Vachier I, Pahus L, Suehs C, Chanez P. Mortality: a neglected outcome in OCS-treated severe asthma. *Eur. Respir. J.* England; 2017; 50.
39. Price DB, Trudo F, Voorham J, Xu X, Kerkhof M, Ling Zhi Jie J, Tran TN. Adverse outcomes from initiation of systemic corticosteroids for asthma: long-term observational study. *J. Asthma Allergy* 2018; 11: 193–204.
40. Bleecker ER, Menzies-Gow AN, Price DB, Bourdin A, Sweet S, Martin AL, Alacqua M, Tran TN. Systematic literature review of systemic corticosteroid use for asthma management. *Am. J. Respir. Crit. Care Med.* 2020; 201: 276–293.
41. Bloechliger M, Reinau D, Spoendlin J, Chang S-C, Kuhlbusch K, Heaney LG, Jick SS, Meier CR. Adverse events profile of oral corticosteroids among asthma patients in the UK: cohort study with a nested case-control analysis. *Respir. Res.* 2018; 19: 75.
42. Couillard S, Laugerud A, Jabeen M, Ramakrishnan S, Melhorn J, Hinks T, Pavord I. Derivation of a prototype asthma attack risk scale centred on blood eosinophils and exhaled nitric oxide. *Thorax* 2022; 77: 199–202.
43. FitzGerald JM, Bleecker ER, Menzies-Gow A, Zangrilli JG, Hirsch I, Metcalfe P, Newbold P, Goldman M. Predictors of enhanced response with benralizumab for patients with severe asthma: pooled analysis of the SIROCCO and CALIMA studies. *Lancet Respir. Med.* 2018; 6: 51–64.
44. Meyers DA, Bleecker ER, Holloway JW, Holgate ST. Asthma genetics and personalised medicine. *Lancet Respir. Med.* 2014; 2: 405–415.

22 Learning from Asthma Deaths to Prevent Attacks

Mark L. Levy

CASE PRESENTATION

A tragic case history (true story, published with permission from her mother).

Tamara Mills died of asthma, a totally treatable disease, just before her 14th birthday. She had 47 asthma attacks during the last 4.5 years of her life, including 21 hospital admissions, 24 Emergency Department/Accident and Emergency Department (ED/A&E) attendances, and 19 consultations with her general practitioner (GP) for asthma attacks. One of these attacks involved a near-fatal event where she deteriorated dramatically after being in hospital for 36 hours. The specialist paediatrician and an anaesthetist managed to save her life on that occasion; however, her chronic management remained unchanged following that episode, which occurred five months before she died. She reattended either at her doctor's office or the ED on 20 occasions shortly after being treated for attacks without follow-up or referral to an asthma specialist. Tamara's asthma was uncontrolled despite prescription for high-dose inhaled corticosteroids (ICSs) in combination with a long-acting bronchodilator (LABA) and excess as-needed short-acting beta-2 agonist bronchodilators (SABAs). She adhered strictly to her medication, and her mum was extremely diligent in seeking medical assistance every time her asthma flared up. Her attacks were usually treated with high-dose bronchodilators, often initiated by her mom, as instructed before going to hospital, and short courses of oral corticosteroids (OCS) for fixed duration of three to five days on most occasions without amendments to her chronic treatment or a post-attack review of her chronic asthma in most of these attacks. Her last two attacks, before her final, fatal one were treated in a major teaching hospital ED, and on neither occasion was she seen by a senior doctor. In the second of these attacks, she was discharged to her grandfather's ground-floor apartment "because she was 'too breathless to climb the stairs to her parents apartment"—according to the junior doctor's discharge letter to her family doctor. Tamara died at home from a severe acute asthma attack at home two days later.

Comment on the Case

Despite requiring high-dose controller treatment, 50 prescriptions for a SABA inhaler during the previous year, numerous hospital admissions, and a near-fatal asthma attack four months before she died from acute asthma, Tamara was never referred to a severe asthma specialist by the hospital or general practice clinicians and was never considered for an escalation of her therapy. Her attacks were treated as if she had repeated episodes of an acute illness; no one addressed her asthma as a chronic disease (1). One of the most important issues related to Tamara's care was that her attacks were treated with fixed duration courses of oral corticosteroids of three to five days without formal follow-up post-attack reviews, which would have alerted clinicians to the fact that her asthma was not being controlled despite very high doses of inhaled corticosteroids. In fact, the only occasion she was prescribed a 14-day post-attack course of oral corticosteroids was when she was discharged form hospital following the life-threatening attack—this was the only time a paediatrician with an interest in asthma saw her—and even that was fortuitous because that hospital doctor came on duty the morning after she was treated. No formal referral was made to this doctor in the four previous admissions at that same hospital during the year, and furthermore Tamara's usual paediatrician declined this doctor's offer to take over the care. Another major problem identified in Tamara's care was that the general practice records did not explicitly detail and code each of her attacks as "acute asthma attacks" in her records. Had this been done, the clear fact that her asthma was severely uncontrolled would have been obvious to anyone Tamara consulted, and she may have been referred to a specialist with a different outcome.

Sadly, this pattern of events where modifiable risk factors for asthma deaths were missed or where there was a failure to take appropriate action, occurs repeatedly in the United Kingdom (2–6). Modifiable risk factors that were missed include excess SABA inhaler prescriptions, insufficient doses or prescriptions of controller medication,

DOI: 10.1201/9781003287209-27

and failure to refer to a specialist paediatrician who may have been able to escalate her treatment by prescribing a biologic anti-asthma drug, and when her final attack before her death was treated, she was discharged from the emergency department without an assessment by a senior specialist doctor.

22.1 INTRODUCTION

Worldwide about 300 million people have asthma, and there are over 250,000 deaths ascribed to this disease every year. This chapter is focussed on clinical experience, research, and inquest findings in the United Kingdom (UK) where there are high numbers of asthma deaths and many published examples of clinical management of patients who have died from acute asthma. While the focus is on experience in the UK, this chapter should assist primary healthcare professionals in primary care (by general practitioners and trained asthma nurses), as well as secondary care and emergency departments in reducing asthma attacks and the incidence of severe and fatal episodes of acute asthma. Sadly, the findings and lessons learned repeatedly in the UK over the last six decades have still not been implemented nationally, with the result that most of the 1000–1400 annually reported UK asthma deaths continue to be potentially preventable. Studies in the UK consistently demonstrate potentially modifiable risk factors in patients themselves or their health professionals, that could have prevented many of these deaths (1, 3–11). The modifiable risk factors for poor asthma control and deaths have been updated annually in the Global Initiative for Asthma (GINA) strategy document, shown in Figure 22.1 (section B (12)) and also in the UK British Thoracic Society/Scottish Intercollegiate Guidelines Network (BTS/SIGN) guidelines. (see Table 14 [13].) Factors related to UK asthma management and deaths are summarised, and findings and recommendations provide practical recommendations for their implementation, which are also relevant worldwide.

22.2 LESSONS FROM CONFIDENTIAL INQUIRIES AND ASTHMA DEATH REVIEWS

A number of themes emerge from the confidential inquiries on asthma death. This chapter is focussed on issues related to asthma assessment during and after acute attacks, the underlying chronic disease, chronic and acute management, patient education, and safeguarding issues related to children and young people with asthma.

22.3 ASSESSMENT

Failure to assess asthma control routinely and to assess the severity of asthma exacerbations are modifiable risk factors that have been recognised for over 60 years (7, 8, 14). In the British Thoracic Association's (now British Thoracic Society) confidential inquiry into 92 asthma deaths in 1979, the authors concluded that a possible explanation for the perception that many of the 92 cases they studied were precipitous or sudden occurrences was that patients, clinicians, and families had underestimated the underlying severity of asthma in these people (9). In fact, only about 20% of deaths are sudden where it was not possible to proactively predict and take action to prevent asthma deaths (15, 16). Where attacks occur suddenly, of course there may not be enough time to do a detailed assessment of the severity of the attack in time to prevent future deaths; however, in most cases, asthma attacks are not initiated suddenly (17) (18) (19) and the mechanism in these cases is unclear. However, in most asthma deaths, warning signs develop gradually. For example, Tattersfield et al., in their 12-month study of 425 severe attacks, demonstrated that a gradual fall in peak expiratory flow (PEF) developed over a number of days, followed by rapid decline with increasing symptoms before attacks occurred a week later (20).

Lack of patient education accounts for many deaths where patients fail to identify warning signs or to act accordingly to prevent attacks from developing or worsening. This occurs in many cases where patients have not been adequately taught how to assess severity of asthma attacks and when to seek medical assistance (2, 21).

Failure by healthcare professionals to include or take note of objective measurements is another potentially modifiable risk factor related to asthma deaths. For example, in the case of Tamara as described, her forced expiratory volume in 1 second (FEV_1) was only 40% predicted when she was transferred from one hospital to another during her final fatal attack, and the ED doctor either failed to note or act on this before she was discharged home (1). Another example from the ongoing confidential enquiry by Harrison et al. (16) found that PEF monitoring was inadequate in 38% in 1988–2001, and, while this dropped to 17% in 2001–2003, this level is still relatively high in people who subsequently died from asthma.

Sturdy et al. (22), in their large case-control study, noted that among those who died from asthma there were fewer general practice contacts in the previous year and fewer PEF recordings in the three months preceding their index attacks.

In the UK, general practitioners (GPs) are incentivised financially to perform annual reviews of people with asthma. While this is a good idea to ensure all patients have an assessment at least once a year, it is difficult to justify this as the only review they get. Asthma is a chronic, ongoing disease that flares up from time to time, and therefore if an assessment is performed when the person is well controlled, objective measurements will not be abnormal, and the doctor may be falsely reassured that their asthma

A. Recent asthma symptom control (but also ask the patient/caregiver about the whole period since last review*)

In the past 4 weeks, has the patient had:		**Well controlled**	**Partly controlled**	**Uncontrolled**
• Daytime asthma symptoms more than twice/week?	Yes☐ No☐	None of these	1–2 of these	3–4 of these
• Any night waking due to asthma?	Yes☐ No☐			
• SABA† reliever for symptoms more than twice/week?	Yes☐ No☐			
• Any activity limitation due to asthma?	Yes☐ No☐			

B. Risk factors for poor asthma outcomes

Assess risk factors at diagnosis and periodically, including after an exacerbation.

Measure FEV_1 at start of treatment, after 3–6 months of ICS-containing treatment to record the patient's personal best lung function, then periodically for ongoing risk assessment.

i. Risk factors for exacerbations

Uncontrolled asthma symptoms: Having uncontrolled symptoms is an important risk factor for exacerbations.

Factors that increase the risk of exacerbations even if the patient has few asthma symptoms:‡

SABA over-use: High SABA use (≥3 x 200-dose canisters/year associated with increased risk of exacerbations, increased mortality particularly if ≥1 canister per month)

Inadequate ICS: not prescribed ICS, poor adherence, or incorrect inhaler technique

Other medical conditions: Obesity, chronic rhinosinusitis, GERD, confirmed food allergy, pregnancy

Exposures: Smoking, e-cigarettes, allergen exposure if sensitized, air pollution

Psychosocial: Major psychological or socioeconomic problems

Lung function: Low FEV_1 (especially <60% predicted), high bronchodilator responsiveness

Type 2 inflammatory markers: Raised blood eosinophils, high FeNO (see biomarker overview)

Exacerbation history: Ever intubated or in intensive care unit for asthma, ≥1 severe exacerbation in last year

ii. Risk factors for developing persistent airflow limitation

History: Preterm birth, low birth weight and greater infant weight gain, frequent productive cough

Medications: Lack of ICS treatment in patient with history of severe exacerbation

Exposures: Tobacco smoke, noxious chemicals, occupational or domestic exposures

Investigation findings: Low initial FEV_1, sputum or blood eosinophilia

iii. Risk factors for medication side-effects

Systemic: Frequent OCS, long-term, high-dose and/or potent ICS, P450 inhibitors§

Local: High-dose or potent ICS, poor inhaler technique

FIGURE 22.1 Global Initiative for Asthma (GINA) Assessment of asthma control in adults, adolescents, and children aged 6–11 years. (© www.ginasthma.com, reproduced with permission.) (The reference citations refer to those in the online Strategy Document at www.ginasthma.com/reports)

is well controlled. In the author's view, it is more efficient and logical to do an asthma review after treating every single asthma attack. The purpose of this post-attack review is first to ascertain whether the attack has resolved or if further treatment is needed and also to identify any modifiable risk factors that need to be addressed to optimise treatment. A flow chart summarising the process followed in a post-asthma-attack review is shown in Figure 22.2. Follow-up and assessment of patients after an acute attack are recommended by national and international guidelines, and yet failure to do this has been noted as a problem in repeated UK coronial inquests on preventable asthma deaths (1, 3, 4, 6).

22.4 CHRONIC MANAGEMENT

Following the early asthma death confidential inquiries (9, 15) and an international task force meeting (23)

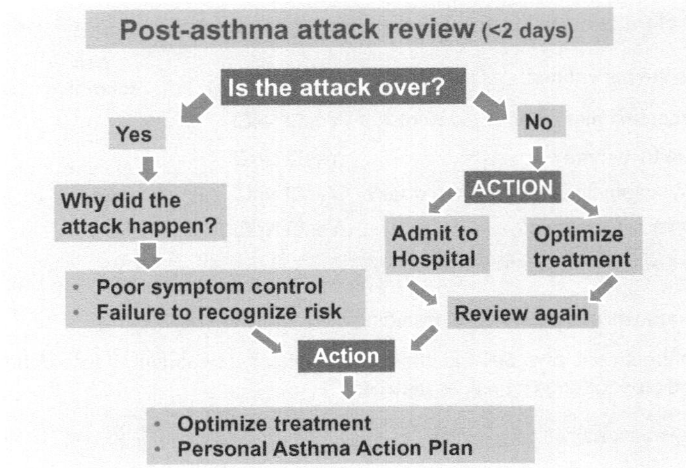

FIGURE 22.2 Post-attack reviews. Flow chart summarising an asthma post-attack review ideally performed a few days after treatment of the attack. (Reproduced with permission from the author's website at https://bigcatdoc.com/2023/01/03/end-asthma-attacks-post-attack-review/.)

convened to discuss lessons learned from these studies, both national and international guidelines and strategy documents were published from the early 1990s onwards. Despite these developments, implementation of asthma guidelines by primary and secondary care health professionals remains a major challenge and varies considerably. Inadequate prescribing of preventer medication, particularly inhaled corticosteroids, as well as underuse of systemic corticosteroids in acute attacks, has been a common observation in confidential inquiries, as well as in case-control studies of severe asthma attacks. The association between excess use of short-acting beta-2 adrenergic agonists (SABAs) and increased risk of asthma death has been identified in a number of studies, one of the earliest being in 1994 (24), and emphasised in the 2019 call from GINA to replace as-needed SABA with a combination inhaler with ICS-formoterol (12). Yet excessive reliance on SABAs by both patients and health professionals persists. In addition, studies demonstrate that health professionals under-prescribe inhaled corticosteroids for prevention (2) and systemic corticosteroids for acute asthma, and fail to implement routine management and follow-up (9, 16, 25, 26). Surprisingly, incorrect drug treatment was noted in one study where nearly 40% of the 20 children who died from asthma attacks were prescribed long-acting beta-agonists (LABAs) alone as monotherapy without concurrent inhaled corticosteroids (11). In the NRAD, 29 of the 185 confirmed deaths due to asthma occurred in people prescribed LABAs alone without inhaled corticosteroids; correspondence from secondary and primary care colleagues made it clear that these people were being inappropriately treated as if they had chronic obstructive pulmonary disease (COPD). These people had asthma, many with fixed airflow obstruction due to severe asthma (2). One paediatric study found that 18 out of 35 (51%) children under 16 who died from asthma had been chronically undertreated (25), while another reported inadequate assessment or therapy of asthma in 68% of 51 people under 20 years who died from asthma (26).

Organisation of care provision has been implicated in poor outcomes for people with asthma. Delayed access to care is associated with asthma deaths. For example, case-control study comparing near-fatal and fatal cases due to asthma concluded there was a delay in access to acute treatment in 28% of the 80 fatalities studied (27). In addition, other studies provide evidence of undue delays in receiving treatment for fatal attacks of asthma (22, 27). In the author's view, a major factor contributing to recurrent asthma attacks and deaths is that asthma is often managed as if it's an acute illness. Asthma is clearly a chronic illness prone to flare-ups or attacks, yet the attacks are treated without systematic follow-up or determining modifiable risk factors, which, if dealt with, could prevent future attacks (2–6). See Figure 22.2 for a suggested process for performing post-attack reviews and Figure 22.1 from the GINA Strategy for details of modifiable risk factors.

Lack of education of healthcare professionals and inappropriate delegation of asthma care to untrained individuals (2, 28) (6) results in failure to recognise poor prognostic risk factors of dying from asthma, with subsequent failure to take appropriate action to gain and maintain control of the disease has often been noted in studies on asthma deaths (1–6).

22.5 PATIENT EDUCATION

While a number of studies report cases of nonadherence to medical advice by patients, a number also report delays in seeking help during fatal attacks (2, 9, 29). This is possibly due to poor adherence to treatment advice but is more likely to be related to a lack of educational provision by health professionals or under-use of personal asthma action plans by patients. In the East of England's ongoing enquiry into asthma deaths, less than half of the 50 subjects had been adequately educated in asthma (21). The National Review of Asthma Deaths (NRAD) (2) found that 45% of those who died either did not seek or get emergency assistance in their final, fatal attack. This was not surprising, however, because over 75% of those who died did not have a record of having received a personal asthma self-management plan, despite many who had repeated asthma attacks treated in hospitals and in the community (2). While clinicians are very busy, asthma attacks should be seen as opportunities to prevent future attacks, which would reduce their future workload by proactively identifying modifiable risk factors as part of the management of acute attacks. These include excess SABA prescribing, insufficient ICS prescribing, lack of provision of patient education, and personal asthma self-management plans (see Figure 22.1).

22.6 ACUTE ASTHMA MANAGEMENT

An asthma attack is a signal that something serious has happened and action is needed to identify and deal with modifiable risk factors. With asthma attacks themselves being one of the main predictors for future attacks, these episodes are probably the most important opportunities for changes in treatment of individuals as well as to make systemic changes in provision of care.

While there is appropriate emphasis on accurate diagnosis of asthma, it is also important that there is early recognition and diagnosis of uncontrolled episodes of asthma, along with assessment of the severity and progress of these exacerbations. General practitioners and emergency department doctors manage a large variety of conditions in patients presenting for care, and it can be sometimes very challenging to identify those developing an asthma exacerbation. While the management of acute asthma exacerbations is detailed elsewhere in this book, the key challenge for the health professional in primary care or ED is to diagnose an asthma attack or exacerbation in a very busy care setting, the key being to differentiate minor from major ailments. Therefore, maintaining a high index of suspicion for an impending asthma attack in any patient presenting with respiratory symptoms, regardless of whether or not they had been previously diagnosed with asthma, is essential. While the symptoms may be sudden and associated with overt wheezing, an asthma exacerbation in many patients may be insidious without obvious clues preceding an impending attack. For example, a child who presents with a history from the mother of severe wheezing and coughing during the night may look perfectly well with a clear chest examination. However, the deceptively normal findings may simply be due to the effect of a high-dose bronchodilator or oral corticosteroids administered during the night if the mother has followed an asthma action plan previously provided. It would be a mistake to discharge such a child home without appropriate advice or management, preferably by someone trained in asthma care. Similarly, it would be a mistake not to recognise risk factors, for example, to take seriously a patient's history of using an excessive amount of short-acting bronchodilator prior to their consultation for respiratory symptoms. Primary care physicians as well as those working in an ED department, therefore, need to be very familiar with the natural history and management of asthma exacerbations to prevent the development of severe attacks. Clues to developing asthma attacks in these settings need to be detected through a very careful history including a history of more frequent use of or reduced effectiveness of reliever drugs; ongoing night-time waking due to respiratory symptoms; ongoing respiratory symptoms following a virus infection or allergic trigger; and increased variability of lung function (peak flow or spirometry) measurements. In those patients with allergic rhinitis, increased symptoms on exposure to indoor or outdoor allergic and nonallergic triggers could herald an asthma exacerbation. Furthermore, an exacerbation could be precipitated on exposure to a variety of environmental triggers in poorly controlled asthma. Therefore, someone with poorly controlled asthma consulting with respiratory symptoms should be assessed and treated fairly rigorously according to published guidance and evidence. Depending on their reported triggers, consideration should be given for a consultation with an allergist.

The severity of the attack can be determined using clinical experience, published guidance (12) (30), and validated tools for assessing severity (31). These assessments are based on history, examination, oxygen saturation, and vital signs. It is helpful to have a reference copy of these tables and tools in each consulting room. However, in some cases, none of these features of severity may be present on examination, so clinicians need to be vigilant in their assessment of patients attending with a history suggestive of uncontrolled asthma. Establishing asthma attack severity helps determine whether it is necessary to transfer the patient to secondary care. Clearly someone with an acute severe or life-threatening attack should be transferred to an appropriate facility as soon as possible. In other cases, a system for ongoing assessment during treatment is helpful in order to facilitate decisions on management as the situation progresses and also on decisions regarding discharge home. A validated tool such as the Canadian Pediatric Respiratory Assessment Measure (PRAM) should be used in ED to utilise objective evidence to support clinical decisions. In addition, accurate clinical records detailing timing of vital signs, lung function, vital signs, levels of consciousness and confusion, oxygen saturation, and oxygen flow rates could be helpful in guiding nursing and medical staff on when to escalate care in inpatients being treated for acute asthma exacerbations. Unfortunately, many of the early warning score charts used for assessing acute paediatric and adult inpatients do not include lung function. For example, the systems used in the UK are the national paediatric and adult early warning systems (PEWS and NEWS2) scores (https://www.england.nhs.uk/publication/national-pews-observation-and-escalation-charts/ and https://www.rcplondon.ac.uk/projects/outputs/national-early-warning-score-news-2).

Ideally, asthma-specific charts and scoring systems should be used for inpatients being treated for acute attacks. In the case of Tamara, she was an inpatient for 36 hours before she went into respiratory failure—without anyone systematically recording her gradual deterioration over the time period. The PEWS chart was used for monitoring her, which does not allow nurses to specify frequency of high-dose SABA administration or lung function measurements. Similarly, primary care clinicians could use a template to record timed measurements (pulse, respiratory rate, oximetry, PEF, levels of exhaustion, etc.) and treatment interventions. This information should be included when referring patients to hospital for treatment of acute exacerbations, if that decision is taken. This could be beneficial for patients because many general practitioners have had the experience where patients with acute asthma attacks referred to hospital are discharged home after a short time span because hospital colleagues assume the attack is over, but the acute drugs administered by the GP are still exhibiting an effect. In those patients not admitted to hospital following emergency treatment with high-dose SABA, in addition to a home supply of oral corticosteroids, what is needed is optimisation of treatment and checking inhaler technique, providing a peak flow meter and diary to enable the patient or parent to monitor progress until the episode has resolved. This could benefit a primary care clinician in deciding whether to escalate care in those seeking further advice if the exacerbation is not resolving. Additionally, in this way an informed decision can be made as to when it may be safe to discontinue oral corticosteroids.

Lack of objective assessment before, during, and after treatment of acute asthma is a major factor that contributes to preventable asthma death. In addition, failure to understand and interpret these objective measurements when they are preformed is a further factor. For example, failure to recognise that high normal arterial carbon dioxide levels are a signal of impending respiratory failure (2) or that a raised respiratory rate is a danger signal (3) or that reassurance by the absence of signs of severe attacks, such as audible wheeze or borderline oximetry, are false (32, 33).

Undertreatment of acute asthma attacks, especially the failure to use systemic corticosteroids, initiating inhaled corticosteroids has been a recurrent theme underlying the conclusions of asthma death studies (6, 9, 15, 16, 23). Either these drugs are not used at all or they are not used in adequate doses for a long enough time; fixed duration, short courses of three to five days following attacks, instead of continuing until the attacks were over (13), was usual in one sad preventable childhood asthma death (1).

Most asthma attacks and deaths are preventable. Clinicians and healthcare managers could put an end to these preventable events by implementing recommendations and lessons learned from published literature on asthma attacks and deaths.

Asthma is often treated as if it is an acute illness, where attacks are managed without dealing with the underlying chronic disease. In three childhood asthma deaths where the author was the coroner's expert witness for the inquests, the children had 7, 48, and 47 asthma attacks respectively during their final year (3), 10 years before (4), and 4.5 years (1) respectively before they died from the disease. Many people are sent home after hospital and primary care treatment for an attack, without any change in their chronic management or an assessment by someone trained in asthma care (34). Unsurprisingly, many of these people re-attend subsequently with new attacks. The logical solution is firstly for asthma attacks to be recognised by clinicians as an indication that something serious has gone wrong with the chronic asthma management. Secondly, their duty is to implement systems for ensuring after-treatment of the attack in order to identify modifiable risk factors and deal with these by optimising the person's care and also by implementing changes in the system of care to prevent future attacks. Every patient should be seen by an appropriately trained clinician, ideally before discharge from hospital or ED and within a few days after an asthma exacerbation for a post-attack review. The need for a post-attack review applies to all exacerbations whether they occur in a primary or secondary care setting, or even where patients have self-treated an attack according to a previously agreed self-management action plan. This is often not done, as evidenced by the numerous studies on near-fatal attacks and in confidential inquiries on asthma deaths where the individuals had suffered a previous attack. The post-attack review has two functions: first, to establish whether the attack is over or additional treatment or readmission to hospital is required. Secondly, modifiable risk factors must be identified in order to optimise the person's care to prevent future attacks. (See Figure 22.1[b].) Actually asking the patient or parent what their PEF readings are and reviewing a PEF chart with them help to reinforce the use of objective measurements to identify future attacks. Questions to consider asking at this review include: When did the symptoms start? How bad were they? Was there any response to self-treatment? Did the person have and follow an action plan? Did they try and get an appointment to see the doctor or asthma nurse? What happened? Were they seen in an ED or urgent care centre? (Listen to an explanation by the author of a system for performing a post-attack review at https://www.pcrs-uk.org/resource/current/demand-webinar-keeping-people-asthma-safe.)

Optimisation of care could include replacing the use of SABA for relief with one of the anti-inflammatory, two-in-one inhalers containing inhaled corticosteroid and formoterol, a quick-acting, long-acting bronchodilator (35–37).

In addition, this post-attack review is an opportunity to add or amend the person's self-management plan (see Figure 22.2). So this review is an opportunity not only to monitor the person's progress towards satisfactory recovery of the attack and to optimise treatment but also to identify and act on barriers to adherence and other modifiable risk factors.

Essentially, by conducting a thorough review after initial treatment of attacks, both the health professional and the patient can learn how to prevent future attacks from this experience.

22.7 SYSTEM FOR ASSESSING PATIENTS AND PROVISION OF ASTHMA CARE

In addition to performing a post-asthma attack review, primary care (and acute) services could set up a system for routinely assessing all patients cared for by the service, who have had an asthma attack with the aim of eradicating preventable attacks in the practice. By way of illustration, for primary care, the author's seven-step plan (see Table 22.1) could both improve individual care and also reduce future attacks through changes in the system of care. This is based on a study in 29 general practices in North London, UK, where paediatric hospital admissions were reduced by 16% in the year following the intervention (38). The seven-step plan starts with accurate recording in the medical record that an asthma attack has occurred. This could be based on correspondence from secondary care following an admission, an ED attendance for acute asthma, or treatment with high-dose SABA and/or a short course of oral (systemic) corticosteroids. Then someone is allocated the patient's records with the purpose of extracting details of modifiable risk factors preceding the attack. These factors include excess SABA prescriptions, insufficient inhaled corticosteroids, poor inhaler technique, and previous attacks (see Figure 22.1). This is then followed by a meeting attended by all front-line staff, including receptionists and clinician assistants, with subsequent optimisation of the patient's care as well as implementing any changes in the provision of care by the primary care service. This exemplar could be used as a basis for proactively implementing change in secondary care or ED services.

22.8 INAPPROPRIATE DELEGATION OF ASTHMA CARE

An asthma review is not simply a tick box exercise. While performing a review is not complicated, a considerable level of knowledge and experience is required by the person doing the review. The processes involved in the review are summarised in the GINA cycle in Figure 22.3. So delegation of any or all of these tasks, assessments, adjustments, or reviews should only be done if the doctor is sure the person has the necessary training and competence to perform the task(s).

Inappropriate delegation of asthma care to untrained individuals is a major factor implicated in preventable asthma deaths. Although the nature of general practice varies from country to country, there are a number of similarities in their working practices. Most general practitioners deal with hundreds of different medical conditions presented by their patients, and most have very limited time for each consultation. As a result, only the acute presenting symptom or problem is managed at the time rather than dealing with any underlying chronic cause. Also, depending on the systems in place, if there is time, some preventative action is included, for example to offer vaccinations or routine investigations. Some general practices offer specialist services for some chronic diseases such as asthma. In the UK, it has become commonplace, and even incentivised financially, for primary care/general practice services to employ non-medically trained staff who are delegated to provide some services. So asthma care, as well as other chronic disease care, may be delegated to inadequately trained individuals (physician assistants, nurse assistants, general nurses, healthcare assistants). Sadly, risk factors for poor asthma outcome are often not recognised or dealt with by these untrained individuals, sometimes with tragic

TABLE 22.1
7-Step Plan for Reducing Asthma Attacks in Primary Care (could be adapted for other settings)

1. Agree on a regular meeting to discuss at-risk patients (ideally chaired by someone with some asthma expertise).
2. Establish a system to record and accurately code all asthma attacks in each patient (i.e. following admission or ED/A&E treatment for an attack, or administration of emergency high-dose SABA, or prescription for a short course of oral corticosteroids for an attack).
3. Allocate a clinician to urgently assess the records of each one of those who had an attack using a pro forma designed for this purpose.
4. Identify modifiable risk factors.
5. Agree, in a meeting, to address problems identified in the patient's record that can be dealt with.
6. Refer those with possible severe asthma to an asthma specialist.
7. Agree who will review the patient to optimise care, and who will implement any changes identified in the system for providing care in the primary care centre.

ED/A&E: Emergency Department/Accident and Emergency Department, SABA: short-acting beta$_2$-bronchodilator
Source: Author's website: https://bigcatdoc.com/2024/01/10/2024-identify-that-an-asthma-attack-is-a-red-flag/

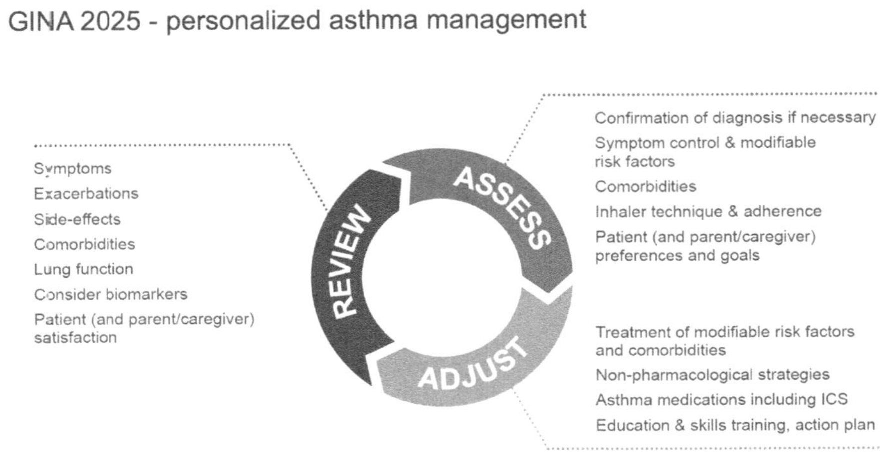

FIGURE 22.3 Asthma assessment, adjustment, review cycle for personalised care. (© www.ginasthma.com, reproduced with permission.)

consequences (6). So there is an urgent need to institute systems for ensuring appropriate training and supervision for these individuals. However, these non-medically trained individuals are not a substitute for a fully trained doctor or asthma-trained nurse who would be able to perform a systematic detailed asthma assessment, which includes confirmation of the diagnosis, identification of and dealing with risk factors, educating the patient, adjusting medication, and then reviewing the patient after an appropriate time period to ascertain whether the interventions have been successful or if referral to a specialist is needed.

22.9 OPPORTUNITIES FOR INTERVENTION

A number of issues have been identified in research and individual patient factors that, had they been dealt with, could have prevented asthma attacks and deaths. Accepting that frontline clinicians have an extremely difficult task, with limited time, to deal with all sorts of medical and social problems, health professionals in primary care and the ED need to try to move away from an approach that deals only with the patient's presenting symptoms at the time. By identifying patients at risk, in a dynamic ongoing manner, patients' well-being can be improved and doctors' workload can be reduced through reduction of unscheduled care for acute crises in future.

The one major barrier to reducing asthma attacks is a failure to recognise that asthma is a chronic, not an acute disease. Therefore, recognising that an attack/exacerbation, is a clear signal that something has gone wrong with the chronic management of the underlying chronic disease and that it is essential to optimise the chronic care to prevent future attacks and deaths.

The advent of computerised record systems in medical care has been extremely positive in some respects, but, as is often the case, the value of the system depends entirely on the quality of information entered by the human operator. Medical record entries are often in the form of short, coded items, often using unrecognisable abbreviations, without much information describing any critical thinking underlying the rationale for clinical decisions. In essence, many primary care computerised record systems are simply used as a system for prescribing and a repository for sometimes very brief records. The power of using the data dynamically and interactively has not yet been systematically harnessed in routine clinical practice. A key lesson from the UK NRAD and subsequent inquests is the failure to code asthma attacks clearly in computerised (and written) records so that alerts can be generated, and clinicians could, in subsequent consultations, be reminded to do a detailed chronic asthma assessment.

Prescribing has certainly been made safer with computerisation, with alerts on past allergies and potential drug interactions, and through maintenance of a clear, legible record of prescriptions issued. These prescribing records have been used for years by funders, researchers, and advisers to management, although there is little evidence in the literature that these records are integrated automatically with risk factors for poor asthma control in primary care and used dynamically in assessing risk and identifying patients in need of optimisation of care. With modern computer systems it should be possible for software to flag certain issues during the consultation. For example, when a patient with asthma consults, an alarm flag could alert the practitioner to the number of beta-2 agonist bronchodilator and ICS prescriptions issued and the number of attacks in the last year. More than three SABAs a year is associated with increased unscheduled care for attacks (39–41). In the absence of a computer system, a manual record could be organised to provide the same sort of information. For example, a page in the record could be dedicated to each repeat drug prescribed, perhaps a page for each SABA, and one for each inhaled corticosteroid prescribed, numbered and dated so a quick glance will reveal those under- or overusing their drugs. These types of systems could alert the clinician, at the time the patient consults, that further intervention may be needed. Suissa and colleagues (42) noted many years ago that a pattern of increased use of beta-2 agonist inhalers was associated with an increased risk of having a life-threatening asthma attack, yet a high proportion of those who died in the last few decades from asthma had been prescribed excess SABAs (2, 16). Ideally, there should be systems for integrating pharmacy records—for example, on dispensing or actual "pick-up rates" by patients collecting medication with those in primary care. Therefore, by implementing systems for recognising this pattern, general practitioners and pharmacists are uniquely placed to identify people in need of an urgent asthma evaluation. Another example from general practice is that many patients in the UK are able to obtain refill prescriptions without seeing a doctor or nurse. A quick perusal of the prescribing history by the doctor, before signing one of these refills, could help identify those who are receiving an excess of SABAs or too few controller medications. These patients could be instructed to make an office appointment when coming to pick up their prescription. Furthermore, in keeping with prescribing advice, those taking LABAs as monotherapy without inhaled corticosteroids could also be identified and told to make an office appointment immediately.

Post-asthma-attack reviews have been discussed, and in the author's view, these are more important than routine "annual" asthma reviews. The main reason being that asthma is a disease that fluctuates from day to day, and a review performed on a day when the disease is well controlled will often reveal no information regarding the person's overall asthma control. The biggest problem is that many clinicians seem to believe or have been taught that a validated "current" symptom questionnaire is sufficient for assessing control. This is why the Global Initiative for Asthma (GINA, www.ginasthma.org/reports) has defined asthma control in two domains: symptom control and future risk (see Figure 22.1). These tests are very useful if they indicate poor current symptom control and, clearly, immediate action is needed by the clinician administering the test. The validated questionnaires often used for assessing symptom control, e.g. the Asthma Control Test (ACT) and the Asthma Control Questionnaire (ACQ), only provide valid information on the previous month and week respectively. Bateman et al. (43) demonstrated a sixfold increased risk of future asthma exacerbations in people with poorly controlled asthma using the GINA Control Tool (part A, Figure 22.1). Wei et al. showed that both partly and poorly controlled patients (using the ACT) were at risk of having future asthma exacerbations as well as unplanned and emergency visits (44). Therefore, it seems sensible to assess asthma symptom control at every opportunity in the primary care setting. However, if the symptom test is normal on the day of testing, this may be very misleading. So while these questionnaires are useful, if abnormal, they do not provide the full picture of asthma control. That's why future risk (Figure 22.1B) is included in the second GINA domain for assessing asthma control. For example, someone who has a perfect ACT or ACQ score on the day of assessment and who had an asthma attack a few months before is clearly uncontrolled! So it is pretty unhelpful for a patient if the clinician relies only on a once-a-year pre-planned asthma assessment to decide whether their asthma is well controlled or not. The GINA Strategy document (www.ginasthma.org/reports) was the first to focus on assessment of asthma control and risks, with the aim of achieving and maintaining control to prevent asthma attacks.

There is also some confusion between the terms "control" and "severity" when classifying asthma patients, which may result in inconsistent care provided for those with this disease, including their current need for treatment and frequency of routine office visit follow-ups. Essentially, chronic severity of asthma relates to the amount of chronic ongoing treatment required to achieve symptom control, whereas acute severity is determined by the history of response to SABAs, the presence of symptoms, signs, and physiological indices. Difficult-to-treat asthma is where someone is prescribed asthma medication, sometimes high doses, and despite this remains poorly controlled. The key question here is whether the person is collecting and correctly taking their medication, and this needs to be dealt with if poor adherence to medical advice is an issue.

Having determined that a person's asthma is poorly controlled, it is clearly incumbent upon the clinician to then ascertain the possible reason(s) for this and to take appropriate action to gain control. This would include an assessment of adherence to medication and inhaler technique. As described previously, the former can be straightforward to establish in primary care by simply counting the number of prescriptions issued for SABAs and preventer medication. Of course, this is incomplete, as it's also important to establish whether the prescriptions have been dispensed and are being taken as prescribed. Information on asthma control can be derived from prescription data (prescription of more than three SABA inhalers a year indicates possible poor control), and the proportion of prescribed inhaled corticosteroid prescriptions collected acts as a surrogate measure for both the clinician's and the patient's adherence to asthma guidelines. Clearly, patients using excess, regular SABAs should be prescribed a preventer medication (12). Similarly, someone who has had prescriptions for short courses of systemic corticosteroids is possibly at risk for further exacerbations. Of course, while this will establish the number of prescriptions issued, it will not determine whether the medication has been dispensed by a pharmacist or has actually been taken by the person.

The principles of asthma reviews have been well described in international and national guidelines and should include confirmation of the diagnosis, assessment of asthma control, identification of risk factors particular to that patient, checking of adherence, inhaler technique, optimisation of medication, and provision or updating of a personal asthma action plan. All of this could be dealt with during a post-attack review and if necessary, could be coded as an "annual review" in the records for the purpose of meeting requirements for payment, such as in the UK.

One of the major criticisms of primary care management of asthma relates to delay and accuracy of diagnosis. One of the functions of an asthma review includes confirmation of the diagnosis, and that is one of the reasons for ensuring that asthma care and reviews are performed by trained individuals. Furthermore, because many people are prescribed inhaled medication, without a clear diagnosis, a post-attack review for anyone treated with high-dose SABA or oral corticosteroids is an opportunity to confirm and record whether the person has asthma.

Some have suggested setting up asthma "at-risk registers" in primary care. The justification for this would be to prioritise those patients at risk for severe asthma and to reduce workload. This would result in a list of patients that should be more closely monitored and more aggressively treated in the outpatient setting. However, this argument is flawed particularly since asthma control is a dynamic process, and therefore a classification of an asthma sufferer as "at risk" is valid only on the day of assessment. Since asthma control status may change from day to day, it is possible for someone to be well controlled one day and admitted to an intensive care unit for an acute severe attack on another. Therefore, unless there is a dynamic system for updating patients' risk status, it may be very dangerous to rely on a fixed at-risk register. This is another strong argument for performing a detailed post-attack review every time someone has an attack/exacerbation. Having said this, it is really important to identify those who may have severe asthma; these people should indeed be on a register and require referral to an asthma specialist, both to confirm the diagnosis and to decide whether more specialised treatment, such as biologic anti-asthma treatment, is advised.

Patients unable to use their inhalers (particularly pressurised metered-dose inhalers) should be either taught to do so or prescribed a spacer or an alternative device. There is mounting evidence that asthma control is adversely affected by poor inhaler technique, and therefore it is vital to ensure that patients can take their medication properly.

22.10 CONCLUSION

Lessons learned from the circumstances surrounding the tragic avoidable deaths due directly or indirectly to poorly controlled asthma provide an extremely rich source of educational and research information to guide health professionals as well as patients and their families through proper asthma management. Case reviews, medical audit, and participation in confidential inquiries following an acute attack or asthma death provide a method for learning from our patients and improving asthma care overall.

REFERENCES

1. Carney T. Regulation 28 statement in the matter of tamara mills (Deceased). 2015 [Available from: https://www.judiciary.gov.uk/wp-content/uploads/2016/01/Mills-2015–0416.pdf].
2. Royal Coll Physicians London. National review of asthma deaths (NRAD) London 2014 [Available from: https://www.rcplondon.ac.uk/projects/outputs/why-asthma-still-kills].
3. Radcliffe S. Regulation 28 statement in the matter of Michael Uriely (Deceased) 2017 [Available from: https://www.judiciary.gov.uk/wp-content/uploads/2017/03/Uriely-2017–0069_Redacted.pdf].
4. Radcliffe S. Regulation 28 Statement in the matter of Sophie Holman (Deceased) 2019 [Available from: https://www.judiciary.uk/wp-content/uploads/2019/05/Sophie-Holman-2019–0035_Redacted.pdf].
5. Persaud N. Senior Coroner East London. REGULATION 28: report to prevent future deaths 2020 [Available from: https://www.judiciary.uk/wp-content/uploads/2021/01/Kalila-Griffiths-2020–0299_Redacted.pdf].
6. Hayes S, AC, for the coroner area of Essex. Regulation 28 report to prevent further deaths 2023 [Available from: https://www.judiciary.uk/prevention-of-future-death-reports/william-gray-prevention-of-future-deaths-report/].
7. MacDonald JB, MacDonald ET, Seaton A, Williams DA. Asthma deaths in Cardiff 1963 to 1974: 53 deaths in hospital. *Br Med J.* 1976;2(6038):721–3.
8. MacDonald JB, Seaton A, Williams DA. Asthma deaths in Cardiff 1963–1974: 90 deaths outside hospital. *Br Med J.* 1976;1(6024):1493–5.
9. Hills A, Sommer AR, Adelstein AM. Death from asthma in two regions of England. *Br Med J.* 1982;285(6350):1251–5.
10. Johnson AJ, Nunn AJ, Somner AR, Stableforth DE, Stewart CJ. Circumstances of death from asthma. *Br Med J.* 1984;288(6434):1870–2.
11. Anagnostou K, Harrison B, Iles R, Nasser S. Risk factors for childhood asthma deaths from the UK Eastern Region Confidential Enquiry 2001–2006. *Prim Care Respir J.* 2012;21(1):71–7.
12. Global Initiative for Asthma (GINA). The global strategy for asthma management and prevention. 2023 [Available from: http://www.ginasthma.org].
13. Scottish Intercollegiate Guideline Network (SIGN), the British Thoracic Society (BTS). British guideline on the management of asthma 2019 [Available from: https://www.sign.ac.uk/media/1048/sign158.pdf].
14. Cochrane GM, Clark TJH. A survey of asthma mortality in patients between ages 35 and 64 in the Greater London hospitals in 1971. *Thorax.* 1975;30(3):300–5.
15. Fraser PM, Speizer FE, Waters SDM, Doll R, Mann NM. The circumstances preceding death from asthma in young people in 1968 to 1969. *Br J Dis Chest.* 1971;65(2):71–84.
16. Harrison B, Stephenson P, Mohan G, Nasser S. An ongoing confidential enquiry into asthma deaths in the Eastern Region of the UK, 2001–2003. *Prim Care Respir J.* 2005;14(6):303–13.
17. Elliot JG, Abramson MJ, Drummer OH, Walters EH, James AL. Time to death and mast cell degranulation in fatal asthma. *Respirology.* 2009;14(6):808–13.
18. Rodrigo GJ, Rodrigo C. Rapid-onset asthma attack: a prospective cohort study about characteristics and response to emergency department treatment. *Chest.* 2000;118(6):1547–52.
19. Carroll N, Carello S, Cooke C, James A. Airway structure and inflammatory cells in fatal attacks of asthma. *Eur Respir J.* 1996;9(4):709–15.
20. Tattersfield AE, Postma DS, Barnes PJ, Svensson K, Bauer CA, O'Byrne PM, Löfdahl CG, Pauwels RA, Ullman A. Exacerbations of asthma: a descriptive study of 425 severe exacerbations. The FACET international study group. *Am J Respir Crit Care Med.* 1999;160(2):594–9.
21. Mohan G, Harrison BDW, Badminton RM, Mildenhall S, Wareham NJ. A confidential enquiry into deaths caused by

asthma in an English health region: implications for general practice. *Br J Gen Pract*. 1996;46(410):529–32.
22. Sturdy PM, Butland BK, Anderson HR, Ayres JG, Bland JM, Harrison BDW, Peckitt C, Victor CR. Deaths certified as asthma and use of medical services: a national case-control study. *Thorax*. 2005;60(11):909–15.
23. Proceedings of the Asthma Mortality Task Force. November 13–16, 1986, Bethesda, Maryland. *J Allergy Clin Immunol*. 1987;80(3 Pt 2):361–514.
24. Suissa S, Blais L, Ernst P. Patterns of increasing beta-2-agonist use and the risk of fatal or near-fatal asthma. *Eur Respir J*. 1994;7(9):1602–9.
25. Fletcher HJ, Ibrahim SA, Speight N. Survey of asthma deaths in the Northern region, 1970–85 [see comments]. *Arch Dis Child*. 1990;65(2):163–7.
26. Robertson CF, Rubinfeld AR, Bowes G. Pediatric asthma deaths in Victoria: the mild are at risk. *Pediatr Pulmonol*. 1992;13(2):95–100.
27. Campbell DA, McLennan G, Coates JR, Frith PA, Gluyas PA, Latimer KM, Luke CG, Martin AJ, Roder DM, Ruffin RE, Yellowlees PM. A comparison of asthma deaths and near-fatal asthma attacks in South Australia. *Eur Respir J*. 1994;7(3):490–7.
28. Levy ML. The national review of asthma deaths: what did we learn and what needs to change? *Breathe*. 2015;11(1):15–24.
29. Bucknall CE, Slack R, Godley CC, Mackay TW, Wright SC. Scottish confidential inquiry into asthma deaths (SCIAD), 1994–6. *Thorax*. 1999;54(11):978–84.
30. Todd GRG, Acerini CL, Ross-Russell R, Zahra S, Warner JT, McCance D. Survey of adrenal crisis associated with inhaled corticosteroids in the United Kingdom. *Arch Dis Child*. 2002;87(6):457–61.
31. Arnold DH, Gebretsadik T, Hartert TV. Spirometry and PRAM severity score changes during pediatric acute asthma exacerbation treatment in a pediatric emergency department. *J Asthma*. 2013;50(2):204–8.
32. Noviski N, Cohen L, Springer C, Bar-Yishay E, Avital A, Godfrey S. Bronchial provocation determined by breath sounds compared with lung function. *Arch Dis Child*. 1991;66(8):952–5.
33. McFadden ER, Jr., Kiser R, DeGroot WJ. Acute bronchial asthma. Relations between clinical and physiologic manifestations. *N Engl J Med*. 1973;288(5):221–5.
34. Bucknall CE, Moran F, Stevenson RD. A retrospective survey of asthma management in hospital. *Scottish Med J*. 1988;33(5):328–30.
35. Levy ML, Beasley R, Bostock B, Capstick TG, Crooks MG, Fleming L, Freeman D, Marsh V, Rupani H, Whittamore A, Barnes PJ, Bush A. A simple and effective evidence-based approach to asthma management: ICS-formoterol reliever therapy. *Br J Gen Pract*. 2024;74(739):86–9.
36. Warraich S, Bush A, Levy ML, Fleming L. Regular (up to 10 puffs 4-hourly) inhaled salbutamol should be prescribed at discharge after an asthma attack: myth or maxim? *Breathe (Sheff)*. 2023;19(3):230054.
37. Levy ML, Bateman ED, Allan K, et al. Global access and patient safety in the transition to environmentally friendly respiratory inhalers: the global initiative for asthma perspective. *Lancet*. 2023;402(10406):1012–16. https://doi.org/10.1016/S0140-6736(23)01358-2
38. Levy ML, Ward A, Nelson S. Management of children and young people (CYP) with asthma: a clinical audit report. *NPJ Prim Care Respir Med*. 2018;28(1):[16 p.]. https://doi.org/10.1038/s41533-018-0087-5.
39. Quint JK, Arnetorp S, Kocks JWH, Kupczyk M, Nuevo J, Plaza V, Cabrera C, Raherison-Semjen C, Walker B, Penz E, Gilbert I, Lugogo NL, van der Valk RJP, Fong A, Qian C, Fabry-Vendrand C, Touboul C, Brzostek D, Maslova E, Surmont F, Goike H, Gandhi H, Korevaar JC, Tkacz J, Johnston K, Peres da Costa K, van Dijk L, Vervloet M, Pollack M, Hernandez P, Boarino S, Noorduyn SG, Beekman-Hendricks W, Weesie YM. Short-acting beta-2-agonist exposure and severe asthma exacerbations: SABINA findings from Europe and North America. *J Allergy Clin Immunol Pract*. 2022;10(9):2297–309.e10.
40. Nwaru BI, Ekström M, Hasvold P, Wiklund F, Telg G, Janson C. Overuse of short-acting β-2-agonists in asthma is associated with increased risk of exacerbation and mortality: A nationwide cohort study of the global SABINA programme. *Eur Respir J*. 2020. https://doi.org/10.1183/13993003.01872-2019.
41. Bloom CI, Cabrera C, Arnetorp S, Coulton K, Nan C, van der Valk RJP, Quint JK. Asthma-related health outcomes associated with short-acting β2-agonist inhaler use: an observational UK study as part of the SABINA global program. *Adv Ther*. 2020;2020/07/27:1–13. https://doi.org/10.1007/s12325-020-01444-5.
42. Suissa S, Ernst P, Boivin JF, Horwitz RI, Habbick B, Cockroft D, Blais L, McNutt M, Buist AS, Spitzer WO. A cohort analysis of excess mortality in asthma and the use of inhaled beta-agonists. *Am J Respir Crit Care Med*. 1994;149(3 Pt 1):604–10.
43. Bateman ED, Reddel HK, Eriksson G, Peterson S, Ostlund O, Sears MR, Jenkins C, Humbert M, Buhl R, Harrison TW, Quirce S, O'Byrne PM. Overall asthma control: The relationship between current control and future risk. *J Allergy Clin Immunol*. 2010;125(3):600–8.e6.
44. Wei H, Zhou T, Wang L, Zhang H, Fu J, Ji Y, Wang G. Current asthma control predicts future risk of asthma exacerbation: A 12-month prospective cohort study. *Chinese Med J*. 2012;125(17):2986–93.

Section VI

Asthma and Special Populations

23 Occupational Asthma

Joshua S. Bernstein and Jonathan A. Bernstein

CASE PRESENTATION

A 49-year-old male worker for a chemical manufacturing company presents with increased shortness of breath, chest tightness, and wheezing, which began approximately seven months after starting his job. His symptoms begin within one hour after arriving at work and persist throughout his shift. Initially the symptoms resolved after leaving the workplace, but over time they persisted at home, causing him to wake up two to three times a night. His symptoms improve when the plant is closed for holidays and when he is on vacation, but they resume immediately after returning to work. He has no history of asthma but has some spring and fall seasonal upper respiratory symptoms consisting of sneezing, nasal congestion, and rhinorrhea. Other than some mild hypertension and hypercholesterolemia controlled with diet, he is healthy. His work process involves operating a forklift in a warehouse where finished powdered chemicals in 1-ton plastic bales are stored. He wears no personal protective equipment such as a respirator. His physical exam reveals some mild inspiratory wheezing but is otherwise normal. His peak expiratory flow (PEF) is 350, which is decreased for his age and height (normal for 72-inch male: 632 L/min). Spirometry reveals an FEV_1 of 2.4 L (60% predicted), which improves to 4 L (100% predicted) after bronchodilators. Exhaled nitric oxide level is 72 ppb (normal <20 ppb). The worker is provided with a PEF meter and diary and asked to record PEF every two hours while in the workplace and every three to four hours at home while awake. He is given an albuterol inhaler to use as needed for chest tightness and wheezing. He also is asked to obtain material safety data sheets (MSDSs) for review.

During his return visit two weeks later, he is still very symptomatic. His PEF is 30% lower at work than at home. MSDSs reveal he is exposed to trimellitic anhydride (TMA), phthalic anhydride (PA), and maleic anhydride (MA) powders. Blood is obtained for specific IgE and IgG to TMA, PA, and MA from a commercial laboratory. He is started on an inhaled corticosteroid and instructed not to go into the warehouse. After discussion with the company safety supervisor, the worker is able to be placed in an area of the plant where there is no chemical exposure. A return visit four weeks later reveals that the worker is symptomatically much improved and that his PEF has increased to 560 L/min; his FEV_1 has improved to 3.7 L, and his exhaled nitric oxide has decreased to 20 ppb. Results of his blood testing reveal increased specific IgE and IgG to TMA only. The worker is instructed to continue to avoid exposure to TMA and continue his inhaled corticosteroid as prescribed. A return visit eight weeks later reveals he is completely asymptomatic and his FEV_1 has increased to 4 L.

Diagnosis: TMA-induced occupational asthma.

23.1 INTRODUCTION

Occupational asthma (OA) is defined as "a disease characterized by variable airflow limitation and/or hyperresponsiveness and/or inflammation due to causes and conditions attributable to a particular occupational environment and not to stimuli encountered outside the workplace"[1]. OA classically is characterized by a latency period during which time workers are exposed to either a high-molecular-weight (HMW) or low-molecular-weight (LMW) agent for a varying amount of time before becoming sensitized and subsequently developing asthma symptoms [2, 3]. HMW agents include plant or animal proteins larger than 1000 kD, which include natural rubber latex, enzymes, or laboratory animal allergens [3]. LMW agents include chemicals smaller than 1000 kD that require conjugation with an endogenous protein (i.e. human serum albumin) to form a complete antigen capable of eliciting a specific immune response; they include isocyanates, acid anhydrides, and metallic salts [3]. However, it is now well recognized that OA can occur in the absence of a latency period after a large exposure to an irritating or toxic material, resulting in airway hyperresponsiveness (AHR) and asthma within 24 hours, referred to as reactive airways dysfunction syndrome (RADS) or irritant-induced asthma [4]. The term *work-exacerbated asthma* has been recommended for patients with pre-existing asthma that later develop worsening of asthma due to exposures in the workplace [5].

23.2 EPIDEMIOLOGY

Throughout history, physicians have increasingly recognized the relationship between asthma and a variety of occupations. A description of breathing problems related

DOI: 10.1201/9781003287209-29

to a worker's trade, which would be considered OA in modern times, was first provided by Hippocrates (460–370 BCE) in reference to metalworkers, tailors, horsemen, farmhands, and fishers [1]. The increasing prevalence of respiratory allergies in the 20th century coinciding with increases in traffic-related air pollutants, such as diesel exhaust particles, secondhand tobacco smoke exposures, use of formaldehyde-releasing resins in building materials, and the use of phthalates in consumer products, has further exacerbated occupational susceptibilities [6].

The incidence of OA per year varies among countries, ranging from 10 to 114 cases per million per year. Differences in incidence are mainly due to methodological differences in calculating incidence and the types of occupations and employment opportunities in each country [7].

The Sentinel Event Notification System for Occupational Risks (SENSOR) was first developed in several US states in the 1980s to encourage reporting of OA cases by physicians and to put them in contact with public health agencies responsible for investigating high-risk workplaces [8]. This program was successful at increasing awareness among physicians about OA, but underreporting of cases has been a continuous problem [8]. Other countries have developed voluntary reporting registries to identify the ongoing incidence and prevalence of OA with varying degrees of success [9–13]. The evaluation of asthma cases being considered for workers' compensation or disability benefits has been another source of estimated incidence rates of OA.

Between 15% and 54% of all adult asthma is attributable to exposures at work, affecting up to 11 million adults [14]. More than 300 agents in the workplace have now been associated with causing OA [15]. Cross-sectional studies have provided prevalence data for a number of agents known to cause OA. Prevalence of OA varies widely between occupations. Studies have found the prevalence of OA for laboratory animal workers to be approximately 20%, for western red cedar-induced OA approximately 5%, for baker's asthma 7–9%, for isocyanate-induced OA 5–21%, platinum-exposed workers 20–50%, and enzyme-exposed workers to be as high as 60% [7, 16–18]. The prevalence of OA within a specific occupation depends on environmental conditions within the plant, exposure levels, durations of exposure, and the effectiveness of procedures implemented in the workplace to reduce worker exposure [7]. There is also an evolving understanding of the socioeconomic and racial disparities contributing to occupational respiratory disease, since financial status, healthcare access, and exposure to hazardous substances leads to medical inequities [14].

Using cross-sectional studies to determine OA prevalence can result in an underestimation due to the "healthy worker effect," which refers to the occurrence of symptomatic workers leaving the workplace without documenting the work relatedness of their illness, leading to what appears to be a healthier workforce [19]. To obtain more accurate prevalence data information about the causes, risk factors, and natural course of OA, surveillance programs for some high-risk manufacturing industries have been established in developed countries, including the United Kingdom, United States, and Finland. The Surveillance of Work-Related and Occupational Respiratory Disease (SWORD) program established in the United Kingdom involves voluntary reporting of occupational illnesses from a variety of industries by pulmonologists and occupational medicine physicians [20]. This program has been very useful for generating prevalence data due to the excellent response rate from participating physicians. The SWORD database has found that OA is the most frequently reported occupational respiratory illness and that isocyanates are the most common specific cause of OA [20]. As mentioned, the SENSOR program established in the United States has not been as successful in obtaining useful epidemiologic data due to a poor response rate from participating physicians [8]. In contrast, the Finnish program has been successful over a relatively short period in estimating the country's yearly incidence of OA and hypersensitivity pneumonitis [11].

23.3 IMMUNOPATHOGENESIS

The pathogenic features of OA are similar to those observed in non-OA patients. In general, lung biopsies of patients with OA demonstrate increased numbers of inflammatory cells with a predominance of eosinophils and lymphocytes, increased intercellular spaces between epithelial cells, and thickening of the reticular basement membrane due to deposition of types I, III, and V collagen [21]. It has been demonstrated that the degree of reticular basement membrane thickening differs between different forms of OA. For example, workers with RADS have been demonstrated to have basement membrane thickening as great as 30–40 μm compared with workers with diisocyanate-induced OA (6–15 μm) and normal subjects (3–8 μm) [22]. Similar bioactive mediators and pro-inflammatory cytokines occur in OA and non-OA [21]. Interestingly, agents including natural rubber latex, mushroom spores, acrylates, and epoxy resins can cause work-related lower respiratory symptoms that manifest as eosinophilic bronchitis, characterized as a chronic cough with sputum eosinophilia, in the absence of bronchial AHR [23]. Although less common, OA can manifest as neutrophilic inflammation with some LMW agents [24]. For non-OA, the presence of neutrophils is believed to be a marker of severity, but their role in different causes of OA is still unclear [25]. Patients with OA and non-OA can exhibit similar inflammatory/physiologic phases of asthma [26]. However, different causes of OA characteristically exhibit different airway responses. For example, whereas an early airway response (EAR) is more characteristic of HMW agents, the late airway response (LAR) and dual airway response (DAR) are more commonly observed in workers with isocyanate-induced OA [26]. It is possible to miss a diagnosis of isocyanate-induced OA, as workers who exhibit a LAR may not manifest clinical symptoms until leaving the workplace [26].

23.4 MECHANISMS

Occupational asthma is a heterogeneous disease with T-helper type 2 (Th2), non-Th2, and mixed inflammation. Frequently used biomarkers to differentiate endotypes are similar to common asthma and include eosinophils, neutrophils, total or specific IgE, fractional exhaled nitric oxide (FeNO), and microRNA profiles [27]. HMW and LMW agents known to cause OA involve Th2 pro-inflammatory cytokines characteristic of IgE-mediated allergic asthma [21]. Enzymes are a good example of HMW agents, whereas acid anhydrides are a good example of LMW agents known to cause OA through an IgE-mediated mechanism. Although HMW agents classically induce Th2 inflammation, it has been demonstrated that HMW can also initiate non-Th2 and mixed immune responses, driven by environmental factors such as endotoxins and/or host-related factors such as genetics and airway microbiome [27]. Microbiome dysbiosis specifically is an area of ongoing research as a predisposition for development of occupational lung disease [28].

In contrast to HMW agents, most LMW chemicals (plicatic acid and diisocyanates) cause OA through as of yet unknown non-IgE-mediated mechanisms. Several mechanisms have been proposed for different clinical presentations associated with a number of causative agents [21]. For acid anhydrides, specific IgE, cytotoxic, immune complex, and cell-mediated immune responses have all been reported (Table 23.1) [29, 30]. The mechanism(s) for irritant-induced asthma or RADS caused by a single high exposure or chronic low exposure to a chemical (i.e. anhydrous ammonia) also remains elusive [4]. It is speculated that chronic inflammatory changes occur in these workers as a result of toxic injury to bronchial epithelial cells leading to loss of epithelial-derived relaxing factors combined with neurogenic inflammation and release of bioactive mediators and pro-inflammatory cytokines by nonspecific activation of mast cells [4]. A number of OA animal models have been developed in an attempt to better elucidate the role of innate and adaptive immune responses in causing a variety of IgE- and non-IgE-mediated induced OA [31–33].

It is also worth acknowledging outdoor and indoor air pollution exposures as an underlying risk factor for compromised airway health. Classical outdoor air pollutants include particulate matter (PM), ozone (O_3), nitrogen oxides

TABLE 23.1
Trimellitic Acid Anhydride Clinical Syndromes

Characteristics	Rhinitis/ Asthma	Late Asthma	Late Respiratory Systemic Syndrome (LRSS) akaTMAFlu	Pulmonary Disease-Anemia	Irritant-Induced Asthma
Latency period	Yes	Yes	Yes	Yes	No
Onset of symptoms after work exposure	Immediate (30–60 min)	4–12 hours	4–12 hours	Progressive with further work exposure	Variable depending on exposure
Clinical symptoms	Cough, wheeze, chest tightness, shortness of breath, rhinorrhea, nasal congestion, sneezing, postnasal drainage	Coughing, sneezing, tightness in chest wheezing due to constriction of airways, sneezing, itching of nose	Resembles hypersensitivity pneumonitis, Coughing. wheezing and dyspnea often accompanied by malaise, chills, fever, muscle and joint pains	Hemoptysis, dyspnea. pulmonary infiltrates, restrictive lung disease, and anemia, as well as the same symptoms as LRSS	Cough, chest tightness, wheezing, shortness of breath and upper airway and eye irritation, lacrimation, sneezing, and nasal discharge
Specific IgE	+	±	–	–	–
Specific IgG	+	±	+	±	–
Gell–Coombs classification	IgE mediated	Type I (late-phase asthmatic response)	Type III (immune-complex-mediated hypersensitivity)	Type II (antibody-dependent cytotoxic hypersensitivity); type III (immune-complex-mediated hypersensitivity)	–

Source: Zeiss, C.R., Mitchell, J.H. Van Peenen, P.F. Kavich, D. Collirn, M.J. Crammer. L. et al. A clinical and immunologic study of employees in a facility manufacturing trimellitic anhydride. *Allergy Proc.* 13, 193–198. 1992; Zeiss, C.R., Patterson, R. Pruzansky, J.J. Miller, M.M. Rosenberg, M. Levitz, D. Trimellitic anhydride-induced airway syndromes: Clinical and immunologic studies. *Allergy Clin. Immunol.* 60, 96–103. 1977.

(NO_x), sulfur dioxide (SO_2) and carbon monoxide (CO) [34]. $PM_{2.5}$ refers to particles with an aerodynamic diameter ≤2.5 μm. Short-term exposure is known to exacerbate asthma and COPD and, with long-term exposure, lead to decreased lung function and lung cancer [34]. Indoor air pollution encompasses the infiltration of not only outdoor air pollution into the indoor space but also unique indoor sources such as particulate matter from combustion processes (cooking, heating, candles, incense, tobacco), dust, cleaning products, personal care products, and chemicals generating volatile organic compounds (VOCs) [35]. Additionally, the use of cleaning and disinfecting products both at work and at home has increased since the COVID-19 pandemic, increasing exposure to surfactants, acids/bases, carcinogens such as chloroform, and endocrine-disrupting chemicals such as cyclosiloxanes, phthalates, and synthetic fragrances [36].

23.5 GENETICS

Genetic associations in workers with OA have been reported. For example, workers who develop acid anhydride OA express the class II HLA molecule DQB1*501 [37]. Interestingly, this genetic marker may be protective against developing OA secondary to isocyanates or plicatic acid [38, 39]. In laboratory animal handlers, the HLADRB1*07 phenotype was more commonly expressed in workers sensitized to rat lipocalin allergens [40]. Glutathione-S transferase (GST) polymorphisms, associated with reduction in oxidative stress, have been reported to protect isocyanate-exposed workers from developing asthma in a way similar to what has been observed with non-OA-induced by ozone and diesel exhaust particulate exposures [41]. Subsequently, GST, microsomal epoxide hydrolase, and manganese superoxide dismutase have been demonstrated to be associated with diisocyanate OA [42]. More recently, polymorphisms of a-catenin gene (CTNNA3), a key protein of the adherence junctional complex on epithelial cells important for cell adherence, have been found to be associated with diisocyanate OA [43]. In addition, previous studies have found that N-acetyltransferase genotypes, specifically the slow acetylator genotype, increased the risk of isocyanate-exposed workers for developing OA almost eightfold [44]. Over the last several years, IL-4R gene polymorphisms have been found to be associated with isocyanate-induced OA, and, more recently, linkages with IL4RA, CD14, and IL-13 have been reported [45, 46].

There are also possible epigenetic effects from occupational exposures. A recent meta-analysis indicated that parental occupational exposure to allergens and irritants was associated with an increased risk of childhood asthma and wheezing [47]. The risk of asthma development in offspring was greatly affected by maternal occupational exposure, potentially alluding to an increased incidence of *de novo* mutations and epigenetic changes as environmental toxins accumulate in reproductive cells [47].

23.6 DIAGNOSIS

23.6.1 History

The criteria for diagnosis of OA proposed by the American College of Chest Physicians are summarized in Table 23.2 [48]. To successfully diagnose OA, the physician must be familiar with known causative HMW and LMW agents, which are continuously increasing each year. A comprehensive review of old and new causes of OA has recently been published [15].

The classic presentation of a worker with OA consists of symptoms that begin while at work and resolve or improve either shortly after leaving the workplace at night, during weekends, or while on vacation [49]. However, a worker with OA may not improve away from the workplace because of chronic airway inflammation with or without fixed obstruction of the airways as a result of persistent workplace exposure to an agent for months or years after the initial onset of symptoms [49]. In addition, patients with RADS typically do not improve away from work [4]. Therefore, the diagnosis of OA should not be overlooked because of the apparent lack of correlation of symptoms with workplace exposure.

Omission or an inadequate history pertaining to the workplace can often delay the diagnosis of OA for months or years. Figure 23.1 is an algorithmic approach for the evaluation and diagnosis of OA [50]. Structured occupational

TABLE 23.2
Criteria for Defining OA Proposed by the American College of Chest Physicians

A. Diagnosis of asthma
B. Onset of symptoms after entering the workplace
C. Association between symptoms of asthma and work
D. One or more of the following criteria:
1. Workplace exposure to an agent or process known to give rise to OA
2. Significant work-related changes in FEV, or PEF rate
3. Significant work-related changes in nonspecific airway responsiveness
4. Positive response to specific inhalation challenge tests with an agent to which the patient is exposed at work
5. Onset of asthma with a clear association with a symptomatic exposure to an irritant agent in the workplace RADS

Requirements
OA:
Surveillance case definition: A + B+C + D1 or D2 or D3 or D4 or D5
Medical case definition: A + B + C + D2 or D3 or D4 or D5 Likely OA: A + B + C + D1
Work-aggravated asthma: A + C (i.e. the subject was symptomatic or required medication before and had an increase in symptoms or medication requirement after entering a new occupational exposure setting)

Source: Tarlo. S.M., Balmes, J., Balkissoon, R., Beach, J. Beckett, W., Bernstein, D., et al. Diagnosis and management of work-related asthma: American College Of Chest Physicians consensus statement. *Chest*. 134. IS-4IS, 2008.

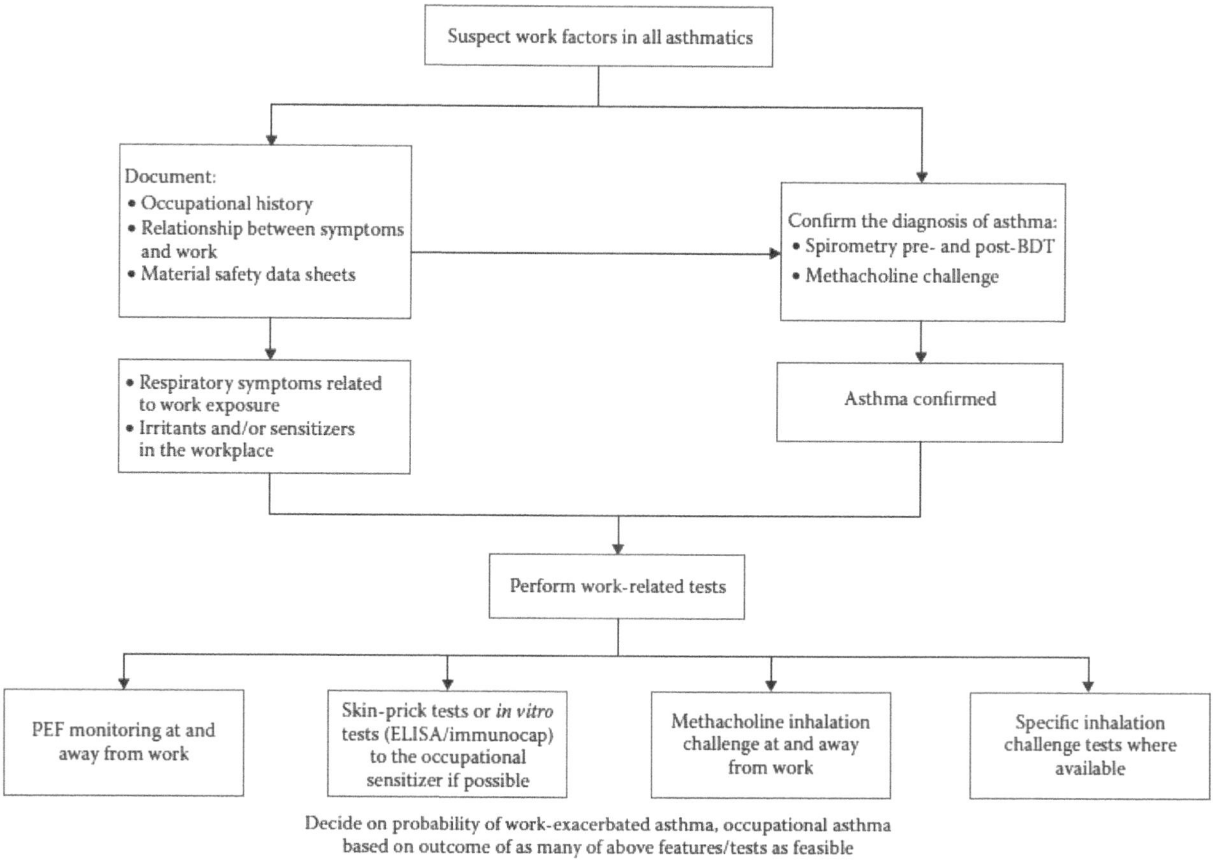

FIGURE 23.1 An algorithmic approach for the evaluation and diagnosis of occupational asthma.

questionnaires have been developed as tools for determining the probability of OA [48]. The basic components of a structured occupational questionnaire include an employment history and medical history (Table 23.3) [48]. The employment history should ascertain the following information: the worker's past and present employment history; their work process, including all jobs that could be related to specific exposures; work processes in adjacent areas; work-shift hours; previous jobs where the worker may have been exposed to similar or identical agents; relationship of symptoms experienced before, during, or after work to a specific exposure in the workplace; duration of symptoms after leaving the workplace; improvement of symptoms on weekends or vacations; associated upper respiratory and dermatologic symptoms; systemic symptoms such as fever, chills, and temperature; smoking history; pre-existing allergy/asthma history; previous chemical spill exposure; and potential risk factors for OA [48]. Although occupational questionnaires are helpful in ascertaining invaluable information that determines the likelihood of workplace-related asthma, history alone is sensitive but not specific and therefore cannot be relied upon to make a definitive diagnosis of OA without confirmatory objective testing.

Material safety data sheets (MSDSs) are an essential component of the occupational history [51]. They provide invaluable information regarding generic chemical names and specific constituents of raw materials being used in the workplace. They also provide standard information about threshold limit values (TLV) and permissible exposure levels (PEL) of potentially toxic and/or sensitizing agents [51]. When available, assistance from industrial hygienists or safety officers familiar with the workplace and the worker's exposure history should be sought. On occasion, these documents have proprietary agents not specifically listed that could cause OA. Therefore, it may be necessary for the clinician to contact the company to obtain additional exposure information [51].

23.6.2 Occupational Specific Exposures

To properly diagnose and treat OA, it is important to recognize some common occupational exposures (see Table 23.4). Following is a general overview, although this is by no means an exhaustive list.

Isocyanates are commonly used in the automotive industry, footwear, construction, foundries, tanneries, the electronics industry, the production of molded parts, printing, and painting maintenance [52]. The most frequently used isocyanates in industry are TDI, HDI, MDI, and less commonly NDI and IDPI. Isocyanates are generally introduced in the air via aerosols [52]. Interestingly, the incidence rate of isocyanate-induced occupational asthma in

TABLE 23.3
Key Elements of the Occupational History in the Evaluation of OA

I. Demographic Information
  A. Identification and address
  B. Personal data including sex, race, and age
  C. Educational background with quantitation of the number of school years completed
II. Employment History
  A. Current department and job description including dates begun, interrupted, and ended
  B. List all other work processes and substances used in the employee's work environment. A schematic diagram of the workplace is helpful to identify indirect exposure to substances emanating from adjacent workstations.
  C. List prior jobs at current workplace with description of job, duration, and identification of material used.
  D. Work history describing employment preceding current workplace. Job descriptions and exposure history must be included.
III. Symptoms
  A. Categories:
    1. Chest tightness, wheezing, cough, shortness of breath
    2. Nasal rhinorrhea, sneezing, lacrimalion, ocular itching
    3. Systemic symptoms such as fever, arthralgias, and myalgias
  B. Duration should be quantitated.
  C. Duration of employment at current job prior to onset of symptoms
  D. Identify temporal pattern of symptoms in relationship to work.
    1. Immediate onset beginning at work with resolution soon after coming home
    2. Delayed onset beginning 4–12 hours after starting work or after coming home
    3. Immediate onset followed by recovery with symptoms recurring 4–12 hours after initial exposure to suspect agent at work
  E. Improvement away from work
IV. Identify potential risk factors.
  A. Obtain a smoking history along with current smoking status and quantitate number of pack-years
  B. Asthmatic symptoms preceding current work exposure
  C. Atopic status
    1. Identify consistent history of seasonal nasal or ocular symptoms.
    2. Family history of atopic disease
    3. Confirmation by epicutaneous testing to a panel of common aeroallergens
  D. History of accidental exposures to substances such as heated fumes or chemical spills

Source: Tarlo, S.M., Balmes, J., Balkissoon, R., Beach, J., Beckett, W., Bernstein, D. et al. *Chest.*, 134. 1S–41S. 2008.

TABLE 23.4
Common Associations for Occupational Asthma by Industry

Industry	Low Molecular Weight Agent
Carpenters, woodworkers	Monoterpenes, resin acids (plicatic acid in western red cedar wood dust)
Automotive industry, painters, insulators, roofers	Isocyanates (TDI, MDI, HDI)
Cosmetologists, dental hygienists, plastic manufacturers	Acrylates, epoxy
Metal/chemical workers, welders, mining and refinery industry	Metals (platinum salts, potassium dichromate)
Cosmetologists, hairdressers, fabric dyers	Dyes and bleaches (persulfate, carmine, henna)
Manufacturers of paint, plastics, and epoxy	Anhydrides (phthalic, trimellitic)
Chemists, cleaners, plastics manufacturers	Amines
Hospital workers, laboratories	Formaldehyde, glutaraldehyde
Firefighters, emergency workers, military veterans	Pollutants (PM, CO, PAH, benzene, SO_2, NO_x)
Cannabis factory workers	Bioaerosols
	High molecular weight agent
Food industry, bakers	Flours (wheat, rye, buckwheat, barley)
Lab workers, vets	Animal proteins (domestic and laboratory)
Bakers, pharmaceutical workers	Enzymes (amylase, lipase, pectinase, subtilisins)
Seafood handlers	Crab/lobster

the US has fallen from 5% before 1980 to 0.9% in 2017, possibly alluding to either reduced use of isocyanate-containing products or more effective implementations of preventive measures from labor laws [52, 53].

Among food industry workers, common exposures are from HMW aerosolized, IgE-mediated exposures. Specific irritants include cereals and flours (wheat, rye, buckwheat, barley), animals (farms, laboratory, and seafood), latex, and enzymes (amylase, subtilisins, maxatase, pancreatin, bromelain) [54, 55]. These risks are further exacerbated by poor ventilation systems and lack of training on safety and health [55].

Wood dust production is the result of machines or tools used in wood-cutting and processing, which generate unwanted by-products during the work process. Airborne wood dust exposure is one of the most common occupational hazards in the wood industry and affects workers in construction, furniture, builders' carpentry, joinery, sawmilling, and forestry [56]. Dust generated from wood processing is a heterogeneous mixture of inorganic and organic particles comprising wood fragments, microorganisms, endotoxins, mycotoxins, and allergens, as well as other LMW chemical compounds that can cause adverse respiratory health effects. Monoterpenes and resin acids (e.g. abietic and pimaric acids in pine, plicatic acid in western red cedar) have been shown to have sensitizing and irritative properties [56].

Hairdressers have increased risk of developing sensitization against *p*-phenylenediamine, ammonium persulfate, and glyceryl thioglycolate. Of these exposures, persulfate salts are most likely to induce respiratory sensitization [57].

Exposure to platinum and its salts occur in the mining and (primary and secondary) refinery industries and in downstream industries (jewelry, dentistry, pharmaceutical, electrical, and chemical industries). In the secondary refining industry, precious metals are reclaimed from scrap material. The most widespread use of platinum at present is used as a catalyst, in particular in the automobile and petrochemical industry [58]. Although platinum salt exposures are a less common occupational exposure, the risk for exposed workers to develop platinum salt respiratory allergy is relatively high with a cumulative risk higher than 50% over a period within five years of exposure [58].

Wildfire smoke poses unique risks to firefighters and other emergency workers, with dangerous exposures to high levels of pollutants including particulate matter (PM), carbon monoxide (CO), polycyclic aromatic hydrocarbons (PAHs), benzene, sulphur dioxide (SO_2), and nitrogen oxides (NOx) [59]. Wildfire research studies have consistently reported decreased lung function, increased airway dysfunction and inflammation, increased respiratory symptoms, and increased risk for asthma incidence [59].

Millions of military veterans have been exposed to burn pit smoke during combat deployment over the past three decades. Toxic compounds contributing to respiratory disease include dioxins, polyaromatic hydrocarbons (PAHs), particulate matter (PM), among others [60]. The Veterans Administration established the Airborne Hazards and Open Burn Pit Registry in 2014. However, specific causality of airway disease from burn pits has been difficult to prove, and ongoing research is required [60].

Lastly, with the ongoing legalization of cannabis across the United States, more insight has been shed on the occupational hazards of bioaerosols generated in indoor cannabis cultivation and manufacturing facilities [61]. Preliminary studies demonstrate a significant fraction of airborne particles in cannabis facilities comprise fungal spores, bacteria, and plant material, which may also contain hazardous microbial metabolites and allergens. These bioaerosols may pose pathogenic, allergenic, toxigenic, and pro-inflammatory risks to workers [61].

23.6.3 Differential Diagnosis

Diagnosis of OA can be incorrectly made in individuals with pre-existing asthma due to nonworkplace allergens. In these cases, symptoms are aggravated by exposure to irritants, physical factors (e.g. cold air), or common indoor allergens (e.g. dust mites) in the workplace [48]. However, it should be emphasized that pre-existing asthma does not preclude the development of OA. In these cases, workers may be experiencing work-exacerbated asthma or asthma due to a new workplace allergen or chemical exposure. At times, OA must also be distinguished from other diseases, such as vocal cord dysfunction, chronic obstructive lung disease, pneumoconiosis, bronchiolitis obliterans, and endotoxin-induced asthma-like syndromes such as grain fever or byssinosis [48]. These disorders are differentiated from OA by history, chest radiograph, chest computerized tomography (CT) scan, lung volumes with diffusion capacity, and, if necessary, open lung biopsy. Chest radiographs and diffusing capacity of lung for carbon monoxide (DLCO) are normal in workers with OA [48].

23.6.4 Immunologic Assessment

Immunologic mechanisms have been confirmed for many causes of OA. Therefore, it is important to investigate whether specific immune responses to suspected agents with allergenic potential are involved. Although identification of an immunologic response to a specific agent helps phenotype different forms of OA, it is usually not diagnostic. Such a response may only reflect exposure and the immunogenic nature of the inciting agent [48]. Cutaneous sensitization to an offending agent indicates a high risk for OA but lacks the specificity needed to diagnose OA. Several types of immune responses are associated with HMW and LMW agents that cause OA. Type I IgE-mediated immune responses have been identified for the majority of HMW proteins derived from a variety of plant and animal sources known to cause OA. IgE-mediated immune responses have also been identified as the underlying mechanism for several LMW chemical agents, such as acid anhydrides and platinum salts. Although type II cytotoxic, type III immune-complex, and type IV cell-mediated immune responses have been linked to certain causes of OA, measures of specific IgE are usually the simplest and most readily available tests for diagnosing OA [48].

HMW antigens are considered complete allergens because they do not require structural modification to elicit a specific immune response. *In vivo* skin testing and *in vitro* immunoassays have been used to identify sensitized individuals to these specific allergens. Examples of HMW allergens include proteins from animal dander, insect scales, food products, and enzymes used in the food manufacturing and pharmaceutical industries. LMW chemical agents in most instances require structural modification to act as complete antigens. Exceptions to this rule are platinum salts and sulfonchloramide (chloramide T). To investigate specific immune responses of these chemicals, typically they are coupled to a carrier molecule such as an autologous human protein (e.g. human serum albumin [HSA]). The chemical hapten protein conjugate forms new antigenic determinants, which can induce an IgE-mediated response [48].

Skin test or *in vitro* reagents used in the diagnosis of OA must be characterized and standardized as well as possible. Standardization should include identification of the allergen source, the extraction procedure, and its biochemical composition. Proper characterization should include total protein content, molecular weight range of proteins, isoelectric points of each protein, and identification of immunologic and allergenic components. The latter can be determined by a variety of techniques, such as enzyme-linked immunosorbent assay (ELISA), western blotting, leukocyte histamine release assays, and end-point skin test titration techniques [48]. A limitation of skin or serologic testing to HMW and LMW agents is the lack of standardized skin test reagents and immunoassays. Studies comparing IgE serum-specific assays with skin prick testing have found fairly good correlations for some LMW agents like TMA [62]. Similarly, specific IgE assays and skin test reagents for natural rubber latex and cat and dog allergens have been found to have high positive and negative predictive values for occupational sensitization [48].

Measurement of specific IgG antibodies by ELISA is often performed as part of immunosurveillance programs in industries where workers are exposed to agents known to cause OA. The significance of elevated specific IgG antibodies to a workplace allergen is less clear, but for some agents such as isocyanates and acid anhydrides there is evidence to suggest it could represent a biologic marker of exposure [62, 63].

The proper interpretation of an immunologic test used in the diagnosis of OA requires validation against an accepted benchmark, such as the specific bronchoprovocation test (SBPT). In addition, proper standardization of an immunoassay always requires the use of well-established positive and negative control sera [48]. Other *in vitro* assays that have been proposed as biomarkers for OA include monocyte chemoattractant protein-1 (MCP-1), lymphocyte proliferation, and leukocyte histamine release, which have been used primarily as research tools in the investigation of workers with OA induced by various agents [48, 64]. Skin test responses and *in vitro* specific antibody responses may decline within months or years after removal from exposure to the causative agent, which may limit their clinical utility in the evaluation of workers remotely exposed to an incriminated agent. Table 23.5 summarizes a representative number of HMW and LMW causes of OA and immunologic tests used for diagnosis [15, 48].

TABLE 23.5
Etiologic Agents (HMW and LMW OA) and Reported Immunologic Tests

Agent	In Vitro	In Vivo
Azodicarbonamide	Prick tests with 0.1%, 1%, and 5% azodicarbonamide	Not done
Baby's breath	Intradermal titration testing	RASR/histamine release
Bacillus subullis enzymes	Prick tests with 0.05, 0.5, 5, and 10 mg/mL	RASR/radial immunodiffusion
Buckwheat flour	Prick tests with 10 mg/mL	Reverse enzyme immunoassay/histamine
Carmine dye	Skin test with Coccus cactus	RAST or ELISA to dyes
Castor bean	Prick tests with 1:100 extract	Not done
Chloramine T, halazone	Scratch test at 10^{-3} dilution	Not done
Chromate	Prick tests at 10, 5, 1, and 0.1 mg/mL $Cr_2(SO_4)_3$	RAST or ELISA to HSA-chromium sulfate
Cobalt	Patch tests	RAST or ELISA to HSA-cobalt sulfate
Coffee bean	Intradermal titration to coffee bean extract	RAST or ELISA to coffee bean extract
Diazonium tetrafluroborate (DIFB)	Not done	RAST or ELISA to HSA-DTFB
Dimethylethanolamine	Prick tests to dimethylethanolamine undiluted at 1:10, 1:100, and 1:1000	Not done
Douglas fir tussock moth	Cutaneous tests with 1:25 extract	Histamine release
Dyes, textiles	Prick or scratch tests to dyes At 10 mg/mL in 50% glycerine	ELISA to HSA dye
Egg proteins	Prick tests with 1:10 w/v egg yolk, whole egg; prick tests to 10 mg/ml egg white fractions	RAST or ELISA to egg proteins
Ethylenediamine	Intracutaneous test to 1:100 ethylenediamine	Not done
Furan binder	Not done	RAST or ELISA to catalyst, sans, and furfuryl alcohol
Garlic	Prick tests titrations beginning at 10^{-3} garlic extract	PTRIA for IgE against garlic extract
Grain dust, grain dust mite	Prick tests intracutaneous tests with grain dust, grain dust mite	Not done
Grain weevil	Skin test to weevil extract	Not done
Gum acacia	Skin test with gum acaia	Not done
Guar gum	Prick tests with 1 mg/mL guar gum	RAST or ELISA with guar gum
Hexamethylene-diisocyanate (HDI)	Prick test to HSA-HDI	ELISA to HSA-HDI
Hexahydrophthalic anhydride (HHPA)	Not done	RAST or ELISA to HSA-HHPA
Hog trypsin	Skin test to trypsin	Histamine release
Laboratory animals	Skin test with serum and urine extracts from animals	ELISA
Latex	Prick test using low ammonia latex solution	Not done

HMW = High Molecular Weight; LMW = Low Molecular Weight; OA = Occupational Asthma

(Continued)

TABLE 23.5 (*Continued*)
Etiologic Agents (HMW and LMW OA) and Reported Immunologic Tests

Agent	In Vitro	In Vivo
Locusts	Prick test with locust extract at 0.1, 1, and 10 mg/mL	ELISA
Mealworm	Prick test titration beginning at 1:20 w/v *Tenebrio molitor* (TM) extract	RAST or ELISA to TM extract
Diphenol methane duusocyanate (MDI)	Prick test with 5 mg/mL HSA-MDI; intradermal test with 1 and 10 mg/mL	ELISA to HSA-MDI
Mushroom	Prick test with mushroom extract	Not done
Nickel	Prick test with $NiSO_4$ at 100, 10, 5, 1, and 0.1 mg/mL	RAST or ELISA to TM $NiSO_4$
Papain	Skin test with papain at 1.25–20 mg/mL	RAST or ELISA to papain
Pancreatic extract	Prick test with 1:1000 extract	Not done
Penicillin	Prick test with ampicillin at 10^{-3}–10^{-2} mol/L, benzyl penicillin	Not done
Penicillamine	Prick test with penicillamine Major and minor penicillin	Not done
Phthalic anhydride (PA) and tetrachlorophthalic anhydride (TCPA)	Prick test intradermal test to HSA-PA and HSA-TCPA	ELISA; PTRIA to HSA-PA only
Platinum	Prick test with complex platinum salts from 10^{-3} to 10^{-11} g/mL	RAST or ELISA to $(NH_4)_2PtCl_2$, RAST to HSA-platinum and histamine release
Poultry mites	Skin test with 1:10 w/v northern fowl mite (NFM)	RAST or ELISA to NFM
Protease bromelain	Prick test with bromelain at 10 mg/mL	RAST or ELISA to bromelain
Redwood	Prick test with redwood sawdust extract	Not done
Spiramycin	Prick test with 10 and 100 mg/mL spiramycin	Not done
Tobacco	Skin tests with green tobacco extract 10 mg/mL	RAST or ELISA with green tobacco extract
Toluene diisocyanate (TDI)	Prick test to 5 mg/mL HSA-TDI	RAST and ELISA to HSA-TDI, histamine release
Trimellitic anhydride (TMA)	Prick test to 3.4 mg/mL HSA-TDI and TMA in acetone	PTRIA with HSA-TMA
Western red cedar (WRC)	Prick test with 25 mg/mL WRC extract; intracutaneous testing with 2.5 mg/mL WRC	Not done
Wheat flour	Prick test with 10% w/v extract	RAST or ELISA to wheat flour and wheat flour components

Source: Quirce, S., Bernstein, J.A., *Immunol Allergy Clin. North Am*, 31, 677–698, 2011.

23.6.5 Physiologic Assessment

Many approaches have been used in measuring lung function in workers suspected of OA. It is recommended that lung function be monitored in the workplace during a known exposure to a suspected causative agent. However, this is not always logistically possible. Personnel experienced in proper performance of pulmonary function testing may not be readily available to conduct serial testing of lung function, and employers may not be cooperative. Spirometry should include the forced expiratory volume in 1 second (FEV_1), forced vital capacity (FVC), and the maximum mid-expiratory flow rate (FEF25–75) [48]. Assessment of cross-shift lung function (i.e. pre- and post-shift FEV_1) has been used to correlate asthma symptoms to workplace exposure, but this approach lacks sensitivity for confirming OA [48]. Multiple assessments of PEF at work (4–5 times per day) often capture enough data to diagnose or exclude OA [48]. Furthermore, cross-shift changes in a worker's lung function have been found to be directly proportional to their level of exposure to the sensitizing agent. Serial measurements of PEF, when performed properly, correlate moderately well with results of the SBPT used in the diagnosis of OA [48]. Serial PEF measurements should be interpreted with caution due to patient noncompliance and the potential for falsification of measurements. Using computerized peak flow meters that record effort associated with each measurement, reproducibility, and the exact time of the reading may circumvent these problems [48]. Although not diagnostic, nonspecific bronchial hyperresponsiveness (NSBH) testing with agonists such as methacholine, histamine, and mannitol is essential for confirming the presence or absence of AHR, a central feature of asthma. Subjects with a positive methacholine test and evidence of specific

IgE to a HMW are more likely to exhibit a positive SBPT to that agent. Negative tests of NSBH are most useful in excluding a current diagnosis of OA in a currently symptomatic exposed worker [48].

The SBPT is considered the gold standard for diagnosis of OA. This test should only be administered in specially equipped centers under the supervision of physicians experienced in conducting this procedure [48]. Specific provocation testing is very time-consuming and expensive to perform and therefore not readily available. However, if performed properly, the SBPT can be performed with minimal risk. Several airway response patterns may be elicited that are characteristic for workers presenting with OA [48]. An isolated EAR is characterized by the immediate onset of asthma symptoms after exposure to an agent that is more commonly associated with IgE-mediated OA. An isolated LAR, which occurs for 4–12 hours after exposure to the challenge agent, is more characteristic of nonimmunologic OA induced by LMW chemical agents [48]. Finally, workers with OA may exhibit a DAR characterized by an EAR followed by a recovery period and then an LAR. Multiple physiologic patterns have been observed in OA caused by chemicals. For example, workers with diisocyanate-induced OA present 30–50% of the time with DARs, 40% of the time with an isolated LAR, and <10% of the time with an isolated EAR [26, 48].

Asthma occurring in the workplace in the absence of a latency period is characteristic of RADS, also referred to as irritant-induced OA [4]. RADS typically occurs after one or more repetitive large inhalational exposure to a toxic chemical agent such as ammonia gas, acidic fumes, smoke, or spray paints [4]. RADS must be differentiated from the irritant symptoms that occur in patients with pre-existing asthma. Irritant symptoms disappear promptly after cessation of exposure and are not associated with prolonged bronchoconstriction or bronchial hyperresponsiveness characteristic of RADS [4]. Workers with RADS typically do not manifest airway response patterns seen with OA induced by HMW and LMW agents.

TABLE 23.6
Screening Survey for Occupational Respiratory Disorders

Survey for work-related respiratory symptoms[12]

(1) Do you experience cough, shortness of breath, or chest tightness that is worse when you are at work?
(2) Do you experience nasal symptoms and/or eye symptoms that are worse when at work?
(3) Do your asthma or nasal symptoms get better during times away from work such as on the weekends or vacations or other extended times you are away from work?
(4) Were there any changes to your job or the work process before your chest symptoms began?
(5) Was there an unusual exposure or event on the job that occurred within 24 hours before your chest symptoms began?

If you answered yes to any of these questions, alert the physician about your work-related symptoms.

Source: Bernstein DI, Pacheco K, Lemiere C. *J Allergy Clin Immunol Pract.* 2024;12(8):1951–1958.

23.7 CLINICAL ASSESSMENT OF A PATIENT WITH OCCUPATIONAL ASTHMA

As in the case summary presented in this chapter, the first step for assessing a suspected case of OA is to obtain a careful physician-administered history (see Table 23.6) [48, 50]. This can be greatly enhanced by using a validated occupational questionnaire to capture the necessary clinical and exposure information and to help validate information obtained by the physician-administered history [48, 65].

Workers with OA may present with dyspnea, chest tightness, wheezing, and cough in or outside the workplace. Upper airway symptoms such as rhinorrhea, nasal congestion, and ocular pruritus preceding the onset of asthmatic symptoms are especially characteristic of IgE-mediated sensitization to HMW agents [66]. Symptoms may begin after immediately starting a work shift (within 1–2 hours) or several hours after starting work. Review of MSDSs is often very helpful for identifying agents known to cause OA [51]. If the history is positive for OA, a test of NSBH (i.e. methacholine or histamine provocation) should be performed. A negative methacholine test (PC20 >10 mg/mL) excludes AHR and is a good negative predictor for asthma. A positive methacholine test indicates the presence of AHR suggestive of asthma but is nonspecific and does not confirm a diagnosis of OA. In this case, assessment of lung function performed at and away from the workplace to demonstrate AHR around the suspected agent is very useful for supporting a diagnosis of OA [50]. When possible, a workplace challenge, which consists of supervised measurements of lung function (i.e. FEV_1) in the actual work site before and during work shifts for at least one week of work exposure, should be conducted. Improvement of symptoms and lung function after removal from the workplace with subsequent deterioration after reintroduction into the workplace further supports a diagnosis of OA, except in the case of RADS [50]. If a workplace challenge cannot be performed, PEF monitoring should be conducted over 2–3 weeks at work [50]. The worker should measure and record his or her PEF every two hours at work and every 3–4 hours while awake at home or at least four times a day. Work exposure, symptoms, and medication usage should be recorded in a diary during this time. Diurnal variability of >20% at work as compared with normal variability at home is consistent with OA [48, 50].

The gold standard for the diagnosis of OA is the SBPT [48, 50]. If a specific substance in the workplace is suspected of causing OA and the workplace challenge is equivocal, an SBPT may be necessary [48, 50]. The PC20 ascertained by methacholine or histamine testing may be helpful for estimating the initial dose of an occupational agent prior to the specific inhalation challenge test. An SBPT should not be performed in workers with severe cardiac or pulmonary disease (FEV_1 <60%) [48, 50]. Specific inhalation challenge tests have also been used to document causation of OA by new substances in index cases and for medical/legal purposes in proving or excluding a worker's eligibility for workers' compensation. Although specific challenge tests confirm a diagnosis of OA if positive, negative tests do not always exclude the diagnosis in workers who have been removed from the workplace for a period of time, during which bronchial AHR to the suspected agent may have resolved. It is therefore important to perform an SBPT either before or shortly after removing the worker from his or her workplace. Other potential problems with specific inhalation challenge testing are poor standardization of methods used among different centers and inability to reproduce workplace exposure conditions in the laboratory including temperature, atmospheric pressure, and concentration [48, 50]. As with any specific inhalation challenge, false positive and false negative tests can occur, and therefore results must be interpreted with caution [50]. In addition to lung function assessment, it is important to identify the worker's allergic status by skin testing to common seasonal and perennial aeroallergens, especially for workers exposed to HMW agents. Skin prick testing to the suspected causative agent and/or specific IgE *in vitro* assays can also be performed when appropriate [48, 50].

23.8 TREATMENT

Once the diagnosis of OA has been confirmed, the treatment of choice is to remove the worker from further exposure [50]. Studies evaluating the clinical course of workers after removal from the workplace have found that persistence of their asthma was correlated with the duration of exposure and symptoms prior to diagnosis. Individuals with OA caused by diisocyanates or western red cedar wood dust had a better prognosis if they were diagnosed early, had relatively well-preserved lung function, and less AHR compared with symptomatic workers who remained in the workplace for longer periods of time and had greater deterioration of lung function, leading to chronic persistent asthma requiring increased medication use even after being removed from exposure. Use of respirators and other personal protective equipment (PPE) should be enforced for workers exposed to known causes of OA such as enzymes, isocyanates, and acid anhydrides. However, once OA has been established, use of PPE does not always prevent or reduce exposure or prevent clinical deterioration [67]. Some studies have suggested that certain types of respirators such as airstream helmets may offer adequate protection for the worker from the offending agent; however, they are generally not considered adequate substitutes for absolute avoidance measures [68]. Pharmacologic treatment of acute or chronic OA is similar to that of non-OA, which involves inhaled corticosteroids, with or without long-acting beta-2 adrenergic agonists, leukotriene-modifying agents, xanthine oxidase inhibitors like theophylline, and, for severe asthma exacerbations, oral corticosteroids [67, 68]. Medications can be used in various combinations depending on the severity of the worker's symptoms. Immunotherapy is rarely indicated to treat occupational respiratory allergies but may play a role in the treatment of some forms of OA caused by HMW protein allergens such as laboratory animal proteins [68, 69]. The use of biologics is understudied in occupational asthma; however, there have been some data to suggest a beneficial role of omalizumab in workers with OA with continued exposure to the causal agent [69].

23.9 PREVENTION AND IMMUNOSURVEILLANCE

The primary categories of prevention include reducing exposure to known occupational inciting agents, identifying susceptible workers and removing them from exposure, and administering workplace controls to reduce the number of workers exposed and the duration of their exposure.

It is important to educate at-risk atopic individuals about avoidance of occupations where the likelihood for developing OA is increased (e.g. laboratory handlers) [48, 50, 67, 68]. Effective prevention of OA requires cooperation between management and workers in the implementation of good industrial measures aimed at preventing exposure to agents known to cause OA. Every attempt should be made to minimize a worker's exposure to a potentially problematic agent(s) through the institution of strict handling procedures. Workers should be continually educated about the importance of adhering to those procedures to avoid inadvertent exposures such as chemical spills [48, 50, 67, 68]. Pre-screening of already hired workers for atopy should be considered before assigning employees to jobs where they would have inhalational exposure to sensitizing proteins (e.g. latex, laboratory animals, and enzyme proteins). Comprehensive immunosurveillance programs for detecting and monitoring workers at increased risk for exposure to known inducers of OA have been successfully implemented in industries that utilize enzymes and acid anhydrides in their manufacturing processes [48].

REFERENCES

1. Tarlo, S., O. Vandenplas, D. Bernstein, Jean-Luc Malo, *Asthma in the Workplace*, 5th ed. CRC Press; 2021.
2. Bernstein, D.I., *Allergic reactions to workplace allergens*. JAMA, 1997. **278**(22): p. 1907–13.
3. Malo, J.L. and O. Vandenplas, *Definitions and classification of work-related asthma*. Immunol Allergy Clin North Am, 2011. **31**(4): p. 645–62, v.
4. Brooks, S.M. and I.L. Bernstein, *Irritant-induced airway disorders*. Immunol Allergy Clin North Am, 2011. **31**(4): p. 747–68, vi.
5. Szema, A.M., *Work-exacerbated asthma*. Clin Chest Med, 2012. **33**(4): p. 617–24.
6. Shusterman, D., *History of pollutant adjuvants in respiratory allergy*. Front Allergy, 2024. **5**: p. 1374771.

7. Smith, A.M., *The epidemiology of work-related asthma.* Immunol Allergy Clin North Am, 2011. **31**(4): p. 663–75, v.
8. Reilly, M.J., et al., *Surveillance for occupational asthma-Michigan and New Jersey, 1988–1992.* MMWR CDC Surveill Summ, 1994. **43**(1): p. 9–17.
9. Bonneterre, V., et al., *Programmed health surveillance and detection of emerging diseases in occupational health: contribution of the French national occupational disease surveillance and prevention network (RNV3P).* Occup Environ Med, 2010. **67**(3): p. 178–86.
10. Latza, U. and X. Baur, *Occupational obstructive airway diseases in Germany: Frequency and causes in an international comparison.* Am J Ind Med, 2005. **48**(2): p. 144–52.
11. Oksa, P., *Occupational asthma in Finland.* Duodecim, 2011. **127**(20): p. 2225–30.
12. Popin, E., et al., *The incidence of occupational asthma in Alsace from 2001 to 2002. Results of intensification of the ONAP project in Alsace (2001–2002). Regional specificities.* Rev Mal Respir, 2008. **25**(7): p. 806–13.
13. To, T., et al., *Feasibility of a provincial voluntary reporting system for work-related asthma in Ontario.* Can Respir J, 2011. **18**(5): p. 275–7.
14. Gandhi, S.A., et al., *Occupational contributions to respiratory health disparities.* Clin Chest Med, 2023. **44**(3): p. 635–49.
15. Quirce, S. and J.A. Bernstein, *Old and new causes of occupational asthma.* Immunol Allergy Clin North Am, 2011. **31**(4): p. 677–98, v.
16. Bakerly, N.D., et al., *Fifteen-year trends in occupational asthma: data from the Shield surveillance scheme.* Occup Med (Lond), 2008. **58**(3): p. 169–74.
17. Bush, R.K. and G.M. Stave, *Laboratory animal allergy: an update.* ILAR J, 2003. **44**(1): p. 28–51.
18. Hur, G.Y., et al., *Prevalence of work-related symptoms and serum-specific antibodies to wheat flour in exposed workers in the bakery industry.* Respir Med, 2008. **102**(4): p. 548–55.
19. Le Moual, N., et al., *The healthy worker effect in asthma: work may cause asthma, but asthma may also influence work.* Am J Respir Crit Care Med, 2008. **177**(1): p. 4–10.
20. Meyer, J.D., et al., *SWORD '99: surveillance of work-related and occupational respiratory disease in the UK.* Occup Med (Lond), 2001. **51**(3): p. 204–8.
21. Lummus, Z.L., A.V. Wisnewski, and D.I. Bernstein, *Pathogenesis and disease mechanisms of occupational asthma.* Immunol Allergy Clin North Am, 2011. **31**(4): p. 699–716, vi.
22. Gautrin, D., et al., *Is reactive airways dysfunction syndrome a variant of occupational asthma?* J Allergy Clin Immunol, 1994. **93**(1 Pt 1): p. 12–22.
23. Quirce, S., *Eosinophilic bronchitis in the workplace.* Curr Opin Allergy Clin Immunol, 2004. **4**(2): p. 87–91.
24. Lemiere, C., et al., *Airway inflammation and functional changes after exposure to different concentrations of isocyanates.* J Allergy Clin Immunol, 2002. **110**(4): p. 641–6.
25. Douwes, J., et al., *Non-eosinophilic asthma: importance and possible mechanisms.* Thorax, 2002. **57**(7): p. 643–8.
26. Bernstein, J.A., *Overview of diisocyanate occupational asthma.* Toxicology, 1996. **111**(1–3): p. 181–9.
27. Mason, P., M. Biasioli, and F. Liviero, *Endotypes of occupational asthma.* Curr Opin Allergy Clin Immunol, 2024. **24**(2): p. 58–63.
28. Peer, A. and D.R. Samuelson, *The role of the microbiome in allergy, asthma, and occupational lung disease.* Curr Allergy Asthma Rep, 2024. **24**(8): p. 415–23.
29. Zeiss, C.R., et al., *A clinical and immunologic study of employees in a facility manufacturing trimellitic anhydride.* Allergy Proc, 1992. **13**(4): p. 193–8.
30. Zeiss, C.R., et al., *Trimellitic anhydride-induced airway syndromes: clinical and immunologic studies.* J Allergy Clin Immunol, 1977. **60**(2): p. 96–103.
31. Ban, M., et al., *Simultaneous analysis of the local and systemic immune responses in mice to study the occupational asthma mechanisms induced by chromium and platinum.* Toxicology, 2010. **277**(1–3): p. 29–37.
32. Regal, J.F., *Immunologic effector mechanisms in animal models of occupational asthma.* J Immunotoxicol, 2004. **1**(1): p. 25–37.
33. Ward, M.D. and M.K. Selgrade, *Animal models for protein respiratory sensitizers.* Methods, 2007. **41**(1): p. 80–90.
34. Yatera, K. and C. Nishida, *Contemporary concise review 2023: environmental and occupational lung diseases.* Respirology, 2024. **29**(7): p. 574–87.
35. Radbel, J., et al., *Indoor air pollution and airway health.* J Allergy Clin Immunol, 2024. **154**(4): p. 835–46.
36. Salonen, H., et al., *Cleaning products: their chemistry, effects on indoor air quality, and implications for human health.* Environ Int, 2024. **190**: p. 108836.
37. Taylor, A.N., *Role of human leukocyte antigen phenotype and exposure in development of occupational asthma.* Curr Opin Allergy Clin Immunol, 2001. **1**(2): p. 157–61.
38. Jones, M.G., et al., *Association of HLA-DQ5 and HLA-DR1 with sensitization to organic acid anhydrides.* Clin Exp Allergy, 2004. **34**(5): p. 812–6.
39. Mapp, C.E., et al., *Association between HLA genes and susceptibility to toluene diisocyanate-induced asthma.* Clin Exp Allergy, 2000. **30**(5): p. 651–6.
40. Jeal, H., et al., *HLA associations with occupational sensitization to rat lipocalin allergens: a model for other animal allergies?* J Allergy Clin Immunol, 2003. **111**(4): p. 795–9.
41. Mapp, C.E., et al., *Glutathione S-transferase GSTP1 is a susceptibility gene for occupational asthma induced by isocyanates.* J Allergy Clin Immunol, 2002. **109**(5): p. 867–72.
42. Yucesoy, B., et al., *Genetic variants in antioxidant genes are associated with diisocyanate-induced asthma.* Toxicol Sci, 2012. **129**(1): p. 166–73.
43. Bernstein, D.I., et al., *CTNNA3 (alpha-catenin) gene variants are associated with diisocyanate asthma: a replication study in a Caucasian worker population.* Toxicol Sci, 2013. **131**(1): p. 242–6.
44. Wikman, H., et al., *N-Acetyltransferase genotypes as modifiers of diisocyanate exposure-associated asthma risk.* Pharmacogenetics, 2002. **12**(3): p. 227–33.
45. Bernstein, D.I., *Genetics of occupational asthma.* Curr Opin Allergy Clin Immunol, 2011. **11**(2): p. 86–9.
46. Bernstein, D.I., et al., *Diisocyanate asthma and gene-environment interactions with IL4RA, CD-14, and IL-13 genes.* Ann Allergy Asthma Immunol, 2006. **97**(6): p. 800–6.
47. Ren, X., et al., *Association between parental occupational exposure and the risk of asthma in offspring: A meta-analysis and systematic review.* Medicine (Baltimore), 2023. **102**(48): p. e36345.
48. Tarlo, S.M., et al., *Diagnosis and management of work-related asthma: American College of Chest Physicians Consensus Statement.* Chest, 2008. **134**(3 Suppl): p. 1S–41S.
49. Nicholson, P.J., et al., *Concise guidance: diagnosis, management and prevention of occupational asthma.* Clin Med (Lond), 2012. **12**(2): p. 156–9.

50. Tarlo, S.M., G.M. Liss, and P.D. Blanc, *How to diagnose and treat work-related asthma: key messages for clinical practice from the American college of chest physicians consensus statement.* Pol Arch Med Wewn, 2009. **119**(10): p. 660–6.
51. Bernstein, J.A., *Material safety data sheets: are they reliable in identifying human hazards?* J Allergy Clin Immunol, 2002. **110**(1): p. 35–8.
52. Coureau, E., et al., *Is isocyanate exposure and occupational asthma still a major occupational health concern? Systematic literature review.* Int J Environ Res Public Health, 2021. **18**(24).
53. Collins, J.J., et al., *Incidence of occupational asthma and exposure to toluene diisocyanate in the United States toluene diisocyanate production industry.* J Occup Environ Med, 2017. **59** (Suppl 12): p. S22–S27.
54. Jeebhay, M.F., et al., *Food processing and occupational respiratory allergy- An EAACI position paper.* Allergy, 2019. **74**(10): p. 1852–71.
55. Md Zamri, A.S.S., et al., *Factors associated with occupational asthma among food industry workers: A systematic review.* PLOS ONE, 2023. **18**(6): p. e0287040.
56. Baatjies, R., P. Chamba, and M.F. Jeebhay, *Wood dust and asthma.* Curr Opin Allergy Clin Immunol, 2023. **23**(2): p. 76–84.
57. Uter, W., et al., *Diagnostics and prevention of occupational allergy in hairdressers.* Curr Allergy Asthma Rep, 2023. **23**(5): p. 267–75.
58. Heederik, D. and F. van Rooy, *Update on occupational allergy, including asthma, to soluble platinum salts.* Curr Opin Allergy Clin Immunol, 2024. **24**(2): p. 69–72.
59. Wah, W., et al., *Systematic review of impacts of occupational exposure to wildfire smoke on respiratory function, symptoms, measures and diseases.* Int J Hyg Environ Health, 2025. **263**: p. 114463.
60. Wang, X., T.A. Doherty, and C. James, *Military burn pit exposure and airway disease: Implications for our Veteran population.* Ann Allergy Asthma Immunol, 2023. **131**(6): p. 720–25.
61. Eidem, T., T. Nordgren, and M. Hernandez, *Bioaerosol exposures and respiratory diseases in cannabis workers.* Curr Allergy Asthma Rep, 2024. **24**(7): p. 395–406.
62. Bernstein, J.A., et al., *Is trimellitic anhydride skin testing a sufficient screening tool for selectively identifying TMA-exposed workers with TMA-specific serum IgE antibodies?* J Occup Environ Med, 2011. **53**(10): p. 1122–7.
63. Pronk, A., et al., *Respiratory symptoms, sensitization, and exposure response relationships in spray painters exposed to isocyanates.* Am J Respir Crit Care Med, 2007. **176**(11): p. 1090–7.
64. Lummus, Z.L., et al., *Diisocyanate antigen-enhanced production of monocyte chemoattractant protein-1, IL-8, and tumor necrosis factor-alpha by peripheral mononuclear cells of workers with occupational asthma.* J Allergy Clin Immunol, 1998. **102**(2): p. 265–74.
65. Bernstein, D.I., K. Pacheco, and C. Lemiere, *How allergists can perform an occupational history in every patient.* J Allergy Clin Immunol Pract, 2024. **12**(8): p. 1951–58.
66. Sublett, J.W. and D.I. Bernstein, *Occupational rhinitis.* Immunol Allergy Clin North Am, 2011. **31**(4): p. 787–96, vii.
67. Fishwick, D., et al., *Standards of care for occupational asthma: an update.* Thorax, 2012. **67**(3): p. 278–80.
68. Peden, D.B. and R.K. Bush, *Advances in environmental and occupational respiratory disease in 2010.* J Allergy Clin Immunol, 2011. **127**(3): p. 696–700.
69. Smith, A.M. and J. Sastre, *The role of immunotherapy and biologic treatments in occupational allergic disease.* J Allergy Clin Immunol Pract, 2020. **8**(10): p. 3322–30.

24 Pregnancy and Asthma

Arzu Yorgancioglu

CASE REPRESENTATION

A 28-year-old woman 30 weeks pregnant was admitted to the emergency department for an asthma exacerbation. She had a history of asthma for 10 years. She had not been taking any maintainance asthma treatment since she became pregnant as she was previously well-controlled by means of medications with no daytime or nocturnal symptoms. One week prior to her admission, she started to experience increased chest tightness and wheezing, which quickly progressed to exertional shortness of breath with coughing. In the emergency room, she was tachypneic, with a BP 152/91 and audible wheezing. A blood gas revealed a pH of 7.35, $PaCO_2$ 42 mmHg, PaO2 75 mmHg. Her breathing was labored, and she appeared to be in moderate distress. She was started on O2 2 L nasal canula, given nebulized beta-2 agonist bronchodilator treatments × 3 in the first 60 minutes, and a dose of IV methylprednisolone 60 mg. She was also dosed with IV magnesium sulfate 2 grams over 20 minutes due to the severity of her asthma exacerbation. Her breathing started to improve, she became less short of breath with normal oxygenation, and she was no longer in respiratory distress. Her blood pressure decreased to 125/78. After 23-hour observation, she was discharged home on a tapering course of oral corticosteroids, inhaled budesonide/formoterol 160/4.5 ug two puffs twice a day to be used as maintenance and as a rescue inhaler, and scheduled to see her primary care doctor that week for further evaluation and management.

24.1 INTRODUCTION

The most common respiratory system disease during pregnancy is asthma with a rate of 4–8% (1,2). While the physiological changes that occur during pregnancy, including changes in hormones and a growing uterus, do not cause problems in a healthy pregnancy, they cause significant issues for an asthma patient during pregnancy (1–3).

Pregnancy and asthma mutually affect each other. According to classical information, asthma worsens during pregnancy in about one-third of pregnant women with asthma, while disease severity decreases in one-third, and no changes are seen in one-third. However, recent studies questioning these estimates indicate that asthma gets more severe in less than one-third of patients, indicating that asthma worsening has decreased over the past decades (4). In general, it appears that asthma worsens during pregnancy in more severe patients with a lower Asthma Control Test (ACT) score and who require higher doses of inhaled corticosteroids (ICSs) (4).

The most severe asthma exacerbations are observed between the 24th and 36th weeks of gestation, whereas symptoms decrease in the last four weeks, with 90% of women having no problems during delivery (1,2,5,6). In 11–18% of asthma pregnancies, 18% have been reported to experience at least one emergency admission, and of these 62% were hospitalized (6,7).

Worsening asthma can also be expected in severe or uncontrolled asthmatics during pregnancy, which may differ within the same individual during different pregnancies (1,2,5–7).

Maintaining asthma control during pregnancy is most important for the health of both mother and baby. Therefore, close follow-up during pregnancy with appropriate medication adjustments, measures, and objective assessments with spirometry based on patient-reported outcomes is necessary.

Hypoxia that develops in a pregnant woman with uncontrolled asthma is an ominous situation that can have significant consequences for the mother and her child (1–3).

In the mother, hyperemesis can cause maternal complications such as hypertension, miscarriage, preeclampsia, gestational diabetes, antepartum or postpartum vaginal bleeding, placenta previa, and cesarean delivery birth complications. In a cohort of 220,000 pregnancies, the risk of gestational diabetes was found to be 11%, and in the same study, it was shown that the risk of pulmonary embolism increased (0.06%/0.12%) compared to non-asthmatic pregnancies (8). Viral respiratory tract infections are also more common in asthmatic pregnancies than in non-pregnant women (71%/46%) [Question: any type of tumor] (8). Women who are midwives are at risk of influenza and H1N1, and therefore routine flu vaccination is recommended for these individuals, especially for pregnant women they are caring for in the second and third trimesters (3,7).

Pregnant women with severe asthma can lead to many fetal complications, such as intrauterine growth retardation, premature birth, low birth weight, increased perinatal mortality, and neonatal hypoxia (3,8).

The risk of prematurity and low birth weight (LBW) infants was found to be much higher in women with severe

DOI: 10.1201/9781003287209-30

asthma. Although the true cause of these complications cannot be fully elucidated, hypoxia is considered the most important factor. Partial pressure of oxygen (PO_2) in umbilical veins is lower than in placental venous ducts, so maternal hypoxemia will cause insufficient oxygen supply to the fetus, affect intrauterine growth, and cause a low birth weight (3). If asthma is under control, the risk of this complication is considered negligible (5,7).

Smoking during pregnancy increases the risk of prematurity, low birth weight (LBW), dysdiadochokinesia (DDK), and respiratory disorders. Exposure to cigarettes during gestation or infancy is associated with the development of asthma in the baby (1,2,5–7).

24.2 DIAGNOSIS

The algorithm for diagnosing asthma while pregnant in people who have not previously been diagnosed is not very different from non-pregnant women. However, allergen skin tests or methacholine or other provocation tests are not recommended (3,9).

"Pregnancy dyspnea," which is important for differential diagnosis, is often present at rest and can be seen in 70% of pregnant women. This is a progesterone-related event and is distinguished from asthma by the absence of airway obstruction, coughing, and wheezing (3).

Gastroesophageal reflux (GERD), postnasal drip, laryngeal dysfunction, hyperventilation, pulmonary edema, and pulmonary embolism should also be considered in the differential diagnosis (9).

24.3 FOLLOW-UP AND MANAGEMENT (3,4,6–8)

During pregnancy, people with asthma tend to use less medication, physicians tend to prescribe less medication, and the compliance is lower than in non-pregnant asthma patients (3). People who have been provided with accurate information about their asthma have low anxiety levels and a good perception of asthma control, have reduced probability of attacks (OR = 0.92), less risk for premature babies (OR = 0.84), and risk of cesarean delivery (OR = 0.84) (3).

24.3.1 Education

Asthma education should ideally be provided for all women of reproductive age with asthma before pregnancy. Education should include possible changes that may occur in the woman's body during pregnancy, how asthma may affect the baby, and how to avoid these adverse consequences. In addition, information should be provided on the correct use of inhalers, a written personal asthma action plan detailing how to recognize and deal with uncontrolled asthma, and how to obtain medical assistance if needed. Information about asthma drugs that are safe to use during pregnancy should be provided. In contrast, a detailed explanation should be provided of the harm imposed by poor asthma control if these medications are not used correctly.

24.3.2 Follow-Up

It is recommended that pregnant asthma patients should be followed more closely with shorter intermittent monthly follow-up visits. Monitoring should use standardized patient-reported outcome instruments such as the Asthma Control Test (ACT), Global Initiative for Asthma (GINA) Symptom Score, or the Asthma Control Questionnaire (ACQ). Monitoring should include spirometry or peak expiratory flow rates (PEFR).

Fetal monitoring should be monitored after 32 weeks.

24.3.3 Triggers

For atopic pregnant women, all sensitizing agents should be avoided when possible, including household pets, dust mites, cockroaches, indoor mold, and indoor air pollutants such as chemical volatile organic compounds (perfumes, fragrances, detergents, aerosols), sources of ozone (e.g. electrical appliances and filtration devices), and nitrogen dioxide (e.g. outdoor drive-by traffic, indoor tobacco exposure, wood-burning fireplaces, and kerosene-fueled heaters without ventilation).

Indoor smoking should be strictly prohibited. Active smoking increases day and night symptoms and causes fetal growth impairment resulting in low birth weight (LBW) in the baby. In addition, passive smoke exposure can contribute to the development of asthma in the child (RR = 1.34, 95% CI: 1.01–1.76). In addition, asthmatic pregnant women who smoke and develop influenza infections are at significantly increased risk of severe asthma exacerbations requiring intensive care (RR = 2.77, 95% CI: 1.19–6.45) (3). Nicotine replacement therapy as a smoking cessation method during pregnancy has been associated with a high risk for LBW and premature birth. Varenicline and bupropion, which are smoking cessation medication aids, are rated as category C (7).

24.3.4 Comorbidities

Comorbidities frequently associated with asthma such as allergic rhinitis, gastroesophageal reflux disease, depression/anxiety, and obesity should be properly managed to improve asthma control in pregnant asthmatics. Proton-pump inhibitors (PPIs) for GERD except omeprazole are category B, and all H2-receptor blockers are category B. Of the H1-antihistamines, cetirizine, loratadine, and levocetirizine, fexofenadine, desloratadine, and azelastine are category C. All intranasal ICSs except budesonide are C. Intranasal triamcinolone and epinephrine are category D (7).

Obesity in pregnancy can cause metabolic syndrome, behavioral disorders, and worsening asthma (8). More asthma exacerbations (OR = 1.3), cesarean delivery (OR =

1.6), gestational hypertension/preeclampsia (OR = 1.7), and gestational diabetes (OR = 4.2) are seen in obese asthmatics.

24.4 PHARMACOLOGICAL TREATMENT

24.4.1 Asthma Medications

Possible side effects due to drugs used in the treatment of asthma can be easily ignored as well as complications caused by asthma that is not under control. Therefore, asthma treatment should not be changed during pregnancy (1–5).

The drugs and safety categories that can be used in pregnant asthmatics are summarized in Table 24.1 (1,2,7).

After 2015, the US Food and Drug Administration (FDA) replaced the letter system, which ranged from category A (no risk in human studies) to category X (evidence of fetal abnormalities in animals or humans) to a pregnancy, and the lactation labeling rule, which included an overview of known safety for use of a drug during pregnancy, lactation, and for males and females of reproductive potential. This system replaced the letter system, as some clinicians and patients were misinterpreting this system for grading risk rather than a categorization for available safety data. As there is insufficient data for pregnancy risk for fewer than 9 out of 10 medications, this system emphasizes weighing risks of side effects of a medication on a fetus against the potential benefits it may have. Because there is heterogeneity between risks and benefits for each individual, the decision to use medication during pregnancy should be individualized using shared decision-making between the patient and the physician. For the purpose of this discussion, we will include the letter system while discussing what is known about the medications risk on the fetus during pregnancy (10).

TABLE 24.1
Asthma Medications and Safety Categories Used in Pregnancy Prior to 2015 (1,2)

Medications	FDA Security Category (7)
Short-Acting Beta$_2$-Agonists	
Salbutamol	C
Terbutaline	C
Albuterol	C
Long-Acting Beta$_2$-Agonists	
Formoterol	C
Salmeterol	C
Inhaled Corticosteroids	
Beclamethasone	C
Budesonide	B
Fluticasone	C
Mometasone	C
Triamcinolone	C
Ciclesonide	C
Flunisolide	C
Systemic Corticosteroids	C
Inhaled Corticosteroid-Long-Acting Beta$_2$-Agonist Combination	
Salmeterol/fluticasone	C
Leukotriene Receptor Antagonists	
Montelukast	B
Zafirlukast	B
Theophylline	C
Anti IgE (Omalizumab)	B

24.5 USE OF ASTHMA DRUGS DURING PREGNANCY

Table 24.2 summarizes the stepwise management of asthma during pregnancy.

24.5.1 Short-Acting Beta-2 Agonists (SABA)

Sufficient data is available on usage and reliability. Terbutaline is the first option.

In 190 systematic reviews and 156 case-control studies on the use of SABA in pregnancy, there was no increase in the risk of congenital malformation, premature birth, or preeclampsia observed (3). An interesting observation is that, while a decrease in fertility is observed in asthmatic patients who use SABA alone, this has not been observed for use of inhaled corticosteroids (ICS) alone or in combination with LABA. These findings support the utility of asthma control with ICS. Therefore, women with asthma planning pregnancy should be encouraged to use these controller drugs (11–14).

24.5.2 Long-Acting Beta-2 Agonists (LABA)

Although limited data is available, salmeterol is considered safe to use during pregnancy based on its safety profile and long-term prescribing results. Patients who are taking salmeterol or formoterol should continue taking it, but it should not be initiated during the first trimester if possible. In addition, LABAs should always be used in conjunction with ICS (1–3).

24.5.3 Inhaled Corticosteroids (ICSs)

Inhaled corticosteroids are the recommended first-line treatment to control asthma and prevent exacerbations in pregnant asthmatic patients. No relationship between the use of ICS and fetal complications has been demonstrated. Regular use of ICS during pregnancy has been shown to reduce the frequency of exacerbations and hospital admissions (11). As a general principle, ICSs should be used at the lowest dose needed to control the asthma. The ICS budesonide is the preferred ICS during pregnancy, as it has been found to have the best safety profile. However, no data suggests that any ICS is unsafe to use during pregnancy (3,9). However, there are studies that demonstrate some safety concerns for use of high-dose ICSs (9).

24.5.4 Fixed Combination Inhalers

There are insufficient studies assessing the efficacy and safety of ICS in pregnancy, and until more information is available, it is recommended to use ICS as monotherapy or in combination (low-dose budesonide + formoterol) to maintain asthma control (8).

24.5.5 Systemic Corticosteroids

There is sufficient evidence demonstrating that use of ICS is not teratogenic. Most studies have not shown a significant relationship between use in the first trimester and cleft palate. Although prenatal complications are more common in patients who require oral systemic corticosteroids for their asthma during pregnancy, it is unclear whether this complication is related to the drug's effect or to the severity of asthma.

When there is an indication for systemic corticosteroids in pregnant women with severe asthma, it is advisable not to avoid their use, as these are at high risk both from asthma morbidity and their comorbid complications. Prednisone, prednisolone, and methylprednisolone pass through the placenta in very low concentration, whereas dexamethasone and betamethasone pass through in higher concentration, and therefore these formulations should be avoided if possible. Typically, a dose of prednisone of at least 40 mg should be prescribed daily for 5–14 days (1,2,8).

24.5.6 Leukotriene Receptor Antagonists (LTRAs)

The results of animal studies with LTRAs have demonstrated that they are safe, but there is insufficient evidence in humans. Continuation is recommended in cases where these agents were the only suitable option for asthma control in a patient prior to pregnancy (1,8).

24.5.7 Theophylline

Studies have shown that theophylline preparations can be used orally or via IV, provided they are maintained in the therapeutic range, which has been recommended to be between 10 and 15 υg/ml, but others have suggested 8–13 υg/ml to safeguard against unforeseen drug–drug interactions. Furthermore, this lower therapeutic level may be sufficient, as protein binding decreases during pregnancy and free drug levels will increase. However, nausea and reflux-enhancing side effects should be considered when prescribing (1,8). Theophylline is no longer readily available for prescription in the United States.

24.5.8 Omalizumab

Omalizumab, which is considered by the FDA to be category B, can be used during pregnancy if it was started before pregnancy; however, initiation is not recommended during pregnancy (6). If allergic rhinitis is also present, intranasal corticosteroids should be added, and leukotriene receptor antagonists (LTRAs) can also be added, if necessary, as can second-generation antihistamines such as loratadine or cetirizine.

In the omalizumab pregnancy registry data (Xolair Pregnancy Registry [EXPECT]) study, no major congenital malformations, evidence of prematurity, or an increase in LBW have been observed. However, due to the low risk of anaphylaxis, omalizumab should not be initiated during pregnancy but can be continued if started before pregnancy (8).

A review of 25 non-randomized studies (two cohort studies and 23 case reports/series) involving biologics for atopic diseases during pregnancy reported 313 exposures to biologics prior to, at conception, or during pregnancy of which 311 were maternal exposures and two were paternal exposures. This review suggests that women who inadvertently become pregnant while taking biologics can be assured that continuing these therapies does not impose an increased health risk to themselves or their children. It should be emphasized that among the 313 pregnancies reviewed, 298 describe the outcomes after omalizumab exposure, whereas among the remaining 15 pregnancies, 11 were exposed to dupilumab, 3 to mepolizumab, and 1 to benralizumab. There was no included published human pregnancy data regarding reslizumab, tezepelumab, or tralokinumab. Therefore, there is currently insufficient data for most biologic medications to make a firm conclusion about drug-associated risks in pregnancy. We should also keep in mind that biologics are more commonly used in patients with severe disease activity, which might also adversely influence pregnancy outcomes, which can potentially confound safety data recommendations, especially if data from pregnant women on biologics is not compared to pregnant women with a similar degree of asthma severity not treated with biologics. Finally, many reports lacked information on maternal age, disease activity, birth weights, comorbidities, or concomitant medications (11,12).

24.5.9 Medications That Should Never Be Used During Pregnancy

Brompheniramine, epinephrine, adrenaline (except for anaphylaxis), alpha-adrenergic drugs, decongestants, tetracycline, sulfonamide, ciprofloxacin, and iodine therapy should not be used during pregnancy. For pregnant women on allergen immunotherapy, the dose should be held at the last dose before pregnancy until birth. However, allergen immunotherapy should not be administered during pregnancy (2).

24.5.10 Attack Treatment

A recent cohort study of 103,976 asthma pregnancies reported an increase in hospitalizations but a decrease in routine physician visits, which suggests these patients receive less preventive treatment and more acute emergency treatment. This emphasizes the importance of controller

TABLE 24.2
Stepwise Treatment for Asthma Management During Pregnancy (1,3,7,13)

Step 1: SABA as needed; if more than two uses of a SABA per week, then advance to Step 2. For mild intermittent asthma patients with normal FEV_1 and eNO could also consider as-needed low-dose budesonide in combination with albuterol or formoterol as needed.

Step 2: Low-dose ICS (budesonide 360 mg (2×1) (180–600 mcg; equivalent fluticasone HFA 88–264 mcg) An ICS + LABA, ICS + LTRA or ICS + theophylline can also be used according to the guidelines.

Step 3: Medium-dose ICS (budesonide > 600–1200 mcg; equivalent fluticasone HFA 264–440 mcg)

Step 4: Medium-dose ICS (budesonide > 600–1200 mcg-; equivalent fluticasone HFA 264–440 mcg) + LABA

Step 5: High-dose ICS + LABA (budesonide > 1200 mcg; equivalent-dose fluticasone HFA > 440–800 mcg) + LABA

Step 6: Step 5 + oral corticosteroids

therapy in this vulnerable population to prevent hospitalization (15).

Asthma exacerbations, which often occur with viral infections and inadequate controller therapy in conjunction with outpatient monitoring, increase the risk of LBW in the baby. However, maintenance and acute treatment for pregnant asthma patients is no different from non-pregnant women with asthma. Medication dose changes should be made throughout pregnancy to maintain control (1–5).

Radiography is not routinely recommended during pregnancy but may be used in an emergency such as to diagnose a uterine tear. If venous thromboembolism is suspected, lower extremity dopplers or ventilation/perfusion scintigraphy can be performed, but CT angiography should be avoided due to radiation risk.

To prevent fetal hypoxia, rapid intervention to keep the mother's pO_2 above 70 mmHg and oxygen saturation above 95% is essential using nebulized short-acting beta-2 agonists, oxygen, and systemic corticosteroids (2,3).

Hospitalization is indicated if low oxygen levels persist, the peak expiratory flow rate (PEFR) drops below 70%, and there is evidence of fetal distress, mental changes exhibited by the mother, and an increase in pCO_2 if response to treatment is delayed. If hypoxemia is severe, or if there is evidence of preeclampsia or laryngeal edema, the patient should be admitted to an intensive care unit (3). Adrenaline should not be used, as it may disrupt utero-placental perfusion. The risk of using a helium-oxygen mixture (heliox) is small, but its actual risk in pregnant women is not well documented, nor is the use of magnesium therapy (8).

24.6 DELIVERY

Due to the production of endogenous glucocorticoids, symptoms due to asthma during childbirth are very rare. In 90% of patients, SABA alone may be sufficient to prevent symptoms during delivery. In pregnant women with mild to moderate asthma that is well controlled, treatment during delivery is similar to treatment of pregnant women without asthma. In general, asthma is not considered an indication for a cesarean section. An increase in the frequency of postpartum asthma attacks for women undergoing cesarean sections has been reported, which may reflect the fact that cesarean section is performed more frequently for women with severe asthma.

In women requiring anesthesia, epidural or spinal anesthesia is preferred over general to minimize respiratory complications.

All asthma medications used during pregnancy should be continued during childbirth. In those women using pre-delivery prednisolone above a dose of 7.5 mg/day for more than two weeks, systemic corticosteroids should be administered during delivery. If needed, prostaglandins and oxytocin are considered safe to be used for induction (1,2).

24.7 POSTPARTUM PERIOD

No harmful effects of asthma drugs used during breastfeeding have been demonstrated in babies. Regardless of the asthma medications required postpartum, mothers should be encouraged to breastfeed due to the known health benefits of human breastmilk for the baby (1,2).

24.8 CONCLUSION

Pregnancy is a normal physiological event that should be allowed to follow its natural course as much as possible in women with asthma. Common mistakes made in asthma management during pregnancy are related to underestimation of asthma severity, overreliance on rescue medication, underuse of ICS controller medication and overuse of systemic corticosteroids, failure to provide patients with a personal written asthma action plan, and failure to refer these patients to an asthma specialist when appropriate. Patient education using shared decision-making principles about the hazards of active or passive smoke exposure during pregnancy, the importance of getting an influenza vaccination before or during pregnancy, and the importance of treatment adherence and drug safety during pregnancy will ensure a healthy outcome for the mother and child (1,9).

REFERENCES

1. Global Initiative for Asthma Global Strategy for Asthma Management and Prevention, Revised ed., 2023. Available from www.ginasthma.org. Accessed 2/September/2025.
2. Turkish Thoracic Society National asthma diagnosis and treatment guide *Turkish Thoracic Journal* 2022: Supp 1; 15.
3. Kelly W, Massoumi A, Lazarus A Asthma in pregnancy: Physiology, diagnosis, and management *Postgraduate Medicine* 2015; 127(4):349–358.
4. Grosso A, Locatelli F, Gini E et al The course of asthma during pregnancy in a recent, multicase–control study on

respiratory health *Allergy, Asthma & Clinical Immunology* 2018; 14:16.

5. Available from https://www.brit-thoracic.org.uk/document-library/ clinical-information/asthma/btssign-guideline-on-the-management- of-asthma/. Accessed 2/September/2025.
6. Asthma Management Handbook, The National Asthma Council Australia Revised and updated 2006.
7. National Asthma Education and Prevention Program *Session 4. Expert panel report III: Guidelines for the diagnosis and management of asthma* Bethesda, MD: National Heart, Lung, and Blood Institute; 2007; NIH publication no. 08–4051.
8. Bonham C, Patterson KC, Strek ME Asthma outcomes and management during pregnancy *Chest* 2018; 153(2):515–527.
9. Alqalyoobi S, Zeki AA, Louie S Asthma control during pregnancy: avoiding frequent pitfalls *Consultant* 2017; 57(11):662–665.
10. Jin J Safety of medications used during pregnancy *JAMA*. 2022;328(5):486. doi:10.1001/jama.2022.8974
11. Gemicioğlu B, Yalçin AD, Havlucu Y, Karakaya G, Özdemir L, Keren M, et al. Country-based 357report: the safety of omalizumab treatment in pregnant patients with asthma *Turkish Journal of Medical Sciences* 2021; 51(5):2516–2523.
12. Shankuntulla F, Chiarella SE Safety of biologics for atopic diseases during pregnancy *The Journal of Allergy and Clinical Immunology: In Practice* 2022 August 17; 10:3149–3155. S2213–2198(22)00817–0. https://doi.org/10.1016/j.jaip.2022.08.013.
13. Dombrowski MP, Schatz M ACOG committee on practice bulletins-obstetrics. ACOG practice bulletin: clinical management guidelines for obstetrician-gynecologists number 90, February 2008: asthma in pregnancy. *Obstetrics & Gynecology* 2008; 111:457–464.
14. Grzeskowiak LE, Smithers LG, Grieger JA, Bianco-Miotto T, Leemaqz SY, Clifton VL, Poston L, McCowan LM, Kenny LC, Myers J, Walker JJ, Norman RJ, Dekker GA, Roberts CT Asthma treatment impacts time to pregnancy: evidence from the international SCOPE study. *European Respiratory Journal* 2018 February 14; 51(2):1702035.
15. To T, Feldman LY, Zhu J et al Asthma health services utilization before, during and after pregnancy: a population-based cohort study *European Respiratory Journal* 2018; 51.

25 Anxiety and Depression and Asthma

Alison C. McLeish

CASE PRESENTATION

KB was a 42-year-old White male with a history of progressive worsening of lower respiratory symptoms consisting of shortness of breath, chest tightness, wheezing, and cough. These symptoms developed gradually and resulted in four hospitalizations in the past six years. He reported that his symptoms were triggered by exercise, cold air, viral infections, dust, smoke, cleaning agents, and weather changes. He had been corticosteroid dependent for over five years with a minimal effective prednisone dose of 20 mg/day. He had no history of allergies or asthma as a child but did have a family history of asthma. He was diagnosed with nasal polyps 10 years ago and underwent sinus surgery for a polypectomy. After the surgery, however, he continued to experience nasal congestion, anosmia, and postnasal drainage. Previously, he worked as a diesel machinist but was forced to quit work and apply for disability due to the fumes. He was married with two children and was the primary homecare provider, as his wife traveled extensively for work.

At presentation, KB appeared very calm but was hesitant to volunteer information beyond answering specific questions he was asked. His past medical history was remarkable for acid reflux and weight gain from the prednisone. He denied a history of anxiety or depression. Allergy testing to seasonal and perennial aeroallergens was negative. His FEV_1 was 41%, which improved by 20% after administration of a bronchodilator, and no environmental factors at home were identified as triggering his symptoms. Extensive asthma education was provided, and KB demonstrated good compliance with medications and office visits. However, repeated attempts to taper him off prednisone were unsuccessful, despite using other disease-modifying agents.

Further questioning to determine why the patient was unable to taper prednisone revealed that he was experiencing high levels of anxiety about recent financial and marital problems. He had recently moved out of the family home, and he and his wife were seeing a marriage counsellor in an attempt to resolve their problems. KB also acknowledged that the physical limitations of his disease and inability to financially support his family contributed to his increased anxiety. As he was not receptive to treatment with anxiolytic medication, it was recommended that he see a psychologist for cognitive behaviour therapy to treat his anxiety. This therapy helped him identify and change maladaptive thoughts and behaviours that contributed to his anxiety. As his symptoms decreased, KB began to exercise more and lose weight, and ended up moving back home with his wife and children. With continued therapy, he has been able to taper his daily prednisone dose to 7.5 mg/day while his asthma and nasal polyps have remained well controlled.

25.1 INTRODUCTION

It has long been appreciated that co-occurring psychological symptoms and disorders are common among asthma patients. Indeed, epidemiological work indicates that individuals with asthma are nearly 1.7 times more likely than those without to have a lifetime history of any mental disorder.[1] Moreover, the presence of co-occurring psychopathology is related to greater difficulties in achieving and maintaining asthma control as well as more frequent asthma-related emergency department visits.[2]

The purpose of the current chapter is to examine the association between asthma and anxiety and depressive symptoms and disorders, as they are the most common classes of psychological disorders.[3] The chapter will begin with a description of anxiety and depressive symptoms and disorders as well as a clarification of appropriate terminology. Next, the prevalence of anxiety and mood disorders among individuals with asthma will be reviewed. Then the effect of anxiety and depression on asthma-related outcomes will be examined, followed by an examination of psychological interventions to address comorbid asthma and panic disorder. Next, a potential mechanism that contributes to the asthma–anxiety association, anxiety sensitivity (fear of one's own anxiety symptoms), will be examined. Lastly, limitations of the current literature and directions for future research will be discussed.

25.2 DEPRESSION AND ANXIETY OVERVIEW

Approximately 45% of the US population will experience one or more psychiatric disorders at some point in their lifetime.[3] Of these disorders, mood and anxiety disorders are the most common, with lifetime prevalence rates of

DOI: 10.1201/9781003287209-31

21% and 25%, respectively.[3] Aside from a high prevalence rate, mood and anxiety disorders generally maintain a chronic, fluctuating course, resulting in substantial impairment across the life span. In addition, anxiety and mood disorders place a large burden on the financial and social resources of society. For example, it is estimated that major depressive disorder alone results in approximately $236 billion in direct and indirect costs in the United States each year.[4]

25.3 MOOD DISORDERS

Mood disorders, also called affective disorders, represent a category of mental health problems in which the primary underlying problem is an individual's persistent emotional state or mood. Three primary mood disorders are relevant to the current literature review: major depressive disorder (MDD), persistent depressive disorder (PDD), and bipolar disorder. The lifetime prevalence rate of any mood disorder is 20.8%, with MDD being the most common (16.6%), followed by bipolar disorder (3.9%), and PDD (2.5%).[5] Mood disorders affect individuals of all ages, but they typically manifest in the mid-twenties and are more common in women than men.[6]

MDD is what is often thought of by the term "depression" and is characterized by the presence of one or more major depressive episodes that cause significant distress and impairment. A major depressive episode is a period of two or more weeks of a depressed or irritable mood and/or markedly diminished interest or pleasure in all or almost all activities. These primary symptoms are accompanied by a combination of the following additional symptoms: significant changes in weight or sleep patterns, fatigue, psychomotor agitation or retardation, feelings of worthlessness, difficulty concentrating, and suicidal ideation.[6] PDD is characterized by a chronic, depressed mood that occurs for most of the day, for more days than not, for at least two years. Bipolar disorder, in its most classic form, can be thought of as alternating periods of major depressive and manic episodes or unusual shifts in mood, energy, activity levels, and the ability to carry out everyday tasks. A manic episode is a period of abnormally elevated or irritable mood that lasts for at least one week and is accompanied by symptoms of inflated self-esteem, decreased need for sleep, pressured speech, racing thoughts, and increased activity.[6]

25.4 ANXIETY DISORDERS

Anxiety is a future-oriented, negative mood state that results in feelings of helplessness due to a perceived inability to control or predict events. Anxiety consists of symptoms across physiological (e.g. sympathetic nervous system activation), cognitive (e.g. hypervigilance, worry), and behavioural domains (e.g. avoidance, exaggerated startle response). While anxiety is a normal response to stressful events or the anticipation of such events, anxiety becomes abnormal when it is pervasive, persistent, and accompanied by excessive avoidance and clinically significant impairment. The most common anxiety disorder is specific phobia with a lifetime prevalence rate of 15.6%, followed by social phobia (10.7%), generalized anxiety disorder (GAD; 4.3%), separation anxiety disorder (5.2%), panic disorder (3.8%), and agoraphobia (2.5%).[7] Until the publication of the 5th edition of the *Diagnostic and Statistical Manual of Mental Disorders* (*DSM-5*), obsessive-compulsive disorder (OCD), and posttraumatic stress disorder (PTSD) were also considered to be part of the anxiety disorders category. Given this historical precedent and their similarity to anxiety disorders, they will be included in the discussion of anxiety disorders as well.

A specific phobia is an extreme or irrational fear of a specific object or situation (e.g. heights, snakes, flying).[6] Social phobia is a marked or persistent fear of social or performance situations involving unfamiliar people or scrutiny by others. Generalized anxiety disorder is typically what is thought of by the term "anxiety" and consists of periods of intense worry that are excessive, pervasive, and uncontrollable. Separation anxiety disorder is a disorder of childhood only that is characterized by developmentally inappropriate and excessive anxiety regarding separation from home or from those to whom the individual is attached. Panic disorder consists of recurrent or unexpected panic attacks (discrete periods of fear in which physical symptoms develop abruptly and peak within 10 minutes) as well as worry about future panic attacks and avoidance of situations that might produce panic attacks. Agoraphobia consists of anxiety about being in a place or situation where escape might be difficult or help might not be available in the event of developing panic-like or other incapacitating or embarrassing symptoms. OCD consists of intrusive and recurring thoughts (obsessions) that often result in repetitive behaviours or rituals that are repeated excessively to reduce anxiety (compulsions). PTSD consists of intrusive symptoms (e.g. flashbacks), avoidance, changes in cognitions or mood, and physiological arousal following exposure to a traumatic event.[6]

25.5 TERMINOLOGY

In the literature reviewed in the remainder of the chapter, mental health terms are not always used consistently. Thus there is a need to clarify terms that will be used throughout the chapter. The terms "anxiety" and "depression" will be used to refer to global levels of anxiety and depression *symptoms*, which can include clinical levels of anxiety and depression (i.e. *disorders*) but also subclinical and nonclinical levels. When referring to clinical levels of anxiety and depression, the terms "anxiety disorders" and "mood disorders" will be used, or the specific anxiety or mood disorder will be identified. Although not an officially recognized category of disorders, the term "depressive disorders" is often used to indicate mood disorders that only include depression (e.g. MDD, PDD) and not mania (e.g. bipolar disorder) by many researchers. This term will be utilized in this manner throughout the chapter as well.

25.6 CO-OCCURRENCE OF ASTHMA AND ANXIETY AND MOOD DISORDERS

In addition to being common in the general population, anxiety and mood disorders are even more common among individuals with asthma. The presence of asthma has been linked with anxiety and mood disorders across developmental periods, across clinical and nonclinical samples, and using a variety of methodologies (e.g. longitudinal, cross-sectional, epidemiological).

25.7 CHILDREN

Epidemiological data indicate that children with asthma, compared to those without, are more likely to have any anxiety disorder (OR = 1.6), specific phobia (OR = 1.70), separation anxiety (OR = 1.82), and GAD (OR = 1.89), while children with a chronic illness other than asthma are more likely to meet criteria for any depressive disorder.[8] Similarly, in a nonclinical sample, adolescents with asthma, compared with those without, were nearly twice as likely to have an anxiety or depressive disorder.[9] Factors associated with the presence of comorbid anxiety or depressive disorders included female gender, more recent asthma diagnosis, living in a single-parent household, greater externalizing behaviours, and greater functional impairment.[9] Adolescents with asthma are also more likely than those without to report suicidal ideation and suicide attempts and are twice as likely to die by suicide.[10,11] In terms of temporality, longitudinal work has found that an asthma diagnosis at age five was associated with greater risk of affective (OR = 1.5) and anxiety (OR = 1.64) problems in later childhood and adolescence.[12] Similarly, adolescents with asthma have been shown to have a higher risk of developing MDD and bipolar disorder later in life.[13] Recent research also indicates a potential shared genetic contribution to MDD and childhood asthma, though only a small proportion of asthma risk could be attributed to a higher genetic liability for MDD.[14]

25.8 ADULTS

Findings from studies among adults generally mirror what is found in children and adolescents. On average, the prevalence rate of any anxiety disorder among adults with asthma is 24%, which is approximately twice the rate found in the general population.[15] The most common co-occurring anxiety diagnoses among adults with asthma are panic disorder (12%), agoraphobia (12%), and GAD (9%).[16] Prevalence rates for these disorders are significantly higher than those found among individuals without asthma, while rates of specific phobia, social phobia, and PTSD are similar to, or lower than, rates among individuals without asthma.[16] Adults with asthma are also more likely to have greater depression symptom severity,[17] and the incidence of asthma among adults with MDD is higher than among those without.[18] Similar to what is found in adolescents with asthma, the risk for suicidal ideation and suicide attempts among adults with asthma is significantly higher than among those without asthma.[19–21]

The association between asthma and anxiety and depression appears to be bidirectional. Asthma has been found to be associated with a twofold increased risk of later anxiety disorder and vice versa.[22] Similarly, a diagnosis of MDD, bipolar disorder, panic disorder, GAD, specific phobia, and PTSD prior to age 21 was associated with adult-onset asthma (i.e. after age 21).[23, 24] In terms of differential associations based on asthma severity, current non-severe asthma has been found to be associated with a nearly 2.5 times greater likelihood of having any mood disorder, and current severe asthma has been associated with increased risk for any anxiety disorder (OR = 2.65), specific phobia (OR = 4.78), and panic disorder (OR = 4.61).[25] In this same study, a lifetime history of severe asthma was associated with an increased risk for any anxiety disorder, panic disorder, specific phobia, social phobia, GAD, and bipolar disorder, while a lifetime history of non-severe asthma was associated with increased odds of any anxiety disorder.

25.9 ASTHMA AND PANIC PSYCHOPATHOLOGY

Although extant research has clearly documented an association between asthma and both depressive and anxiety disorders, there is evidence for a relatively specific association between asthma and panic psychopathology (i.e. panic attacks, panic disorder, and agoraphobia). Indeed, rates of panic attacks and panic disorder are consistently higher among individuals with asthma compared with the general population.[25, 26] Moreover, there appears to be a dose–response relationship, such that, with every additional panic symptom, the likelihood of asthma increases.[26, 27] A recent 20-year longitudinal study found a significant bidirectional relationship between the two; asthma was a significant predictor of future panic disorder (OR = 4.5), and panic disorder predicted later asthma activity (OR = 6.3).[27]

25.10 IMPACT OF CO-OCCURRING ANXIETY AND DEPRESSION

25.10.1 Asthma Severity

Due to the high rates of co-occurrence between asthma and both anxiety and depression, researchers have begun to examine the effects of these comorbid mental health conditions on asthma severity, including asthma symptoms and pulmonary function. Among youth, the presence of one or more anxiety or depressive disorders has been found to be associated with greater asthma symptoms, with a linear increase in asthma symptoms as severity of anxiety and depressive disorders increases.[28] Similarly, adults with asthma and comorbid depression have been shown to have greater asthma severity,[29] and those with comorbid anxiety or depression are more likely to have had an asthma attack in the past 30 days.[30]

In terms of pulmonary function, one study found that the presence of depression but not anxiety was associated with decreased FEV_1 and FEV_1/FVC values, independent of asthma severity.[31] The nonsignificant findings for anxiety, however, may be due to the small sample size in this study ($n = 38$). Hayatbakhsh et al. also found that a current or lifetime diagnosis of MDD but not GAD, panic disorder, or PTSD, was predictive of slightly lower FEV_1 and FEV25–75, but only among males.[32] However, other studies in both adults and children have found no differences between those with and without a mood or anxiety disorder in terms of objective measures of lung function.[33–35]

There are a few studies examining associations between anxiety and depression and asthma-related death, with conflicting results. In one historical cohort and nested case-control study, there was an increased mortality rate among asthma patients with comorbid depression (OR = 1.87);[36] however, the authors caution that the cause of this association has yet to be examined. On the other hand, other work has found similar or even lower mortality rates among asthma patients reporting depression or anxiety symptoms.[37, 38] There are, however, a number of methodological limitations to many of the studies in this area; thus further research is needed before any definitive conclusions about the impact of depression or anxiety on asthma-related death can be made.

25.10.2 Asthma Control

The results for asthma control, on the other hand, are more consistent. The majority of studies in this domain have found that anxiety and depression (both symptoms and disorders) are associated with poorer asthma control, with a specific association for panic disorder.[33, 39–41] Compared with individuals with asthma without comorbid psychiatric disorders, individuals with comorbid anxiety and depressive disorders report greater bronchodilator use, more nocturnal waking, and worse symptoms in the morning, shortness of breath, and wheezing, despite no differences in measures of lung function.[40] Further, individuals with a lifetime history of an anxiety disorder were nearly twice as likely to have used an inhaler more than 30 times in the past 30 days compared with those without such a history.[30]

There is some question as to whether the effects of depression on asthma are stronger or more severe than the effects of anxiety. Although the body of literature is small, a few studies have found that only those with depressive but not anxiety disorders reported poorer asthma control.[33, 42] However, there are also studies that have found that both anxiety and depression are independent predictors of asthma control.[39] Similar contradictory findings can be seen when looking at the interaction of anxiety and depression. Lavoie and colleagues found no significant increase in risk for poorer asthma control associated with the presence of both anxiety and depressive disorders.[33] However, another study found that only a combination of anxiety and depression was a significant predictor of poor asthma control.[43]

25.10.3 Symptom Perception

One potential explanation for the association between anxiety and depression and poor asthma control is that these conditions affect symptom perception, a key component in asthma management. Previous research indicates that anxiety and depression are associated with greater frequency of self-reported hyperventilation and airway obstruction symptoms.[44] However, it is unclear whether individuals with comorbid asthma and anxiety or depression perceive, report, or recall their asthma symptoms differently, or whether they are truly experiencing more symptoms. One study examined symptom perception in childhood asthma and found that, after controlling for pulmonary function, trait anxiety was associated with heightened symptom perception at baseline but not during a methacholine challenge.[45] Such findings lend support to the idea that individuals with high anxiety tend to pay more attention to (i.e. overperceive) ambiguous (i.e. mild) symptoms but are able to accurately perceive symptoms of changes in bronchoconstriction. However, patients with comorbid asthma and panic disorder have been found to report greater levels of dyspnoea, compared with those with asthma only, when experiencing the same reduction of lung function during a histamine challenge.[46]

25.10.4 Quality of Life

Given these reports of poorer asthma control, it is not surprising that anxiety and depression are associated with poorer asthma-related and overall quality of life as well as increased functional limitations.[29, 33, 35, 40, 47–50] For example, it is estimated that comorbid depressive symptoms reduce quality of life by 43%.[35] Indeed, individuals with asthma and a lifetime diagnosis of an anxiety or depressive disorder are more likely to report frequent physical distress, mental distress, and activity limitations as well as fair/poor general health, greater life dissatisfaction, and lack of social support.[30] The findings are less clear when trying to discern the unique effects of symptoms of depression and anxiety on quality of life. Some studies have found that when controlling for the effects of anxiety, depression is no longer a significant predictor of quality of life.[43] On the other hand, in a study of patients with poorly controlled asthma, when controlling for the effects of anxiety, only depression was found to be a significant predictor of poorer quality of life.[44] The substantial overlap between depression and anxiety symptoms may partly explain these inconsistent findings. Similar inconsistencies have been found when trying to determine whether the presence of both anxiety and depression is worse than either alone. One study found an additive negative effect of having depression in addition to anxiety in terms of quality of life;[43] however, no such additive effect was found in a study of patients with poorly controlled asthma.[44]

25.10.5 Healthcare Use

Depression and anxiety have also been associated with greater asthma-related healthcare use. Higher levels of anxiety and depression among both children and adults with asthma have been associated with higher rates of emergency department visits, more frequent routine and unscheduled medical visits and overnight hospitalizations, greater use of short-acting beta-agonists, and more frequent need for oral corticosteroid treatment.[29, 30, 39, 51, 52] Indeed, independent of objective pulmonary functioning, individuals with anxiety tend to overuse short-acting beta-agonist medication, receive more intensive corticosteroid regimens, and have longer and more frequent hospitalizations.[34, 53–55] However, Lavoie and colleagues did not find any differences between adults with and without a mood or anxiety disorder in terms of number of emergency department visits or hospitalizations in the past year.[33] Thus it is possible that the impact of comorbid anxiety and depression accumulates over time and may not be seen in the short term. Comorbid asthma and panic disorder seem to be particularly problematic. These patients are over six times as likely to visit their primary care provider and report greater use of short-acting beta-agonists compared with those with asthma only.[47, 56]

At least two studies have found that depression but not anxiety is associated with greater healthcare use. In one, depression but not anxiety was found to be associated with more frequent unscheduled doctor's visits.[44] Another found that depression was associated with more hospital visits and greater number of days on oral corticosteroids in the past year, even after controlling for anxiety.[48] While the majority of studies have focused on asthma-related healthcare use, at least one study found that the increase in healthcare costs among individuals with asthma and comorbid anxiety and depression was related to treatment of the mental health condition and not to asthma.[50]

25.11 INTERVENTIONS FOR CO-OCCURRING ANXIETY AND DEPRESSION

With the high rates of depression and anxiety found among individuals with asthma and the resulting increases in morbidity and functional impairment, there is a clear need for interventions to treat these comorbid problems. Thus it is surprising that, despite the existence of well-validated and highly efficacious cognitive behavioural treatments for anxiety and depressive disorders, there has been little attempt to apply cognitive behavioural principles to develop efficacious treatments for asthma patients with comorbid anxiety or depression. Cognitive behavioural therapy (CBT) in this context would focus on understanding and changing dysfunctional behaviours and beliefs about bodily symptoms and the asthma diagnosis itself (e.g. perceived burden associated with asthma management).

Due to their high rates of co-occurrence, the majority of work in this area has focused on developing interventions to treat comorbid asthma and panic disorder. To date, there have been two different CBT interventions developed to treat comorbid asthma and panic disorder that combined CBT for panic disorder with asthma education.[57, 58] The CBT portion of the treatment programmes consisted of (1) psychoeducation regarding the nature of anxiety and panic; (2) cognitive therapy techniques to modify cognitive misappraisals that contribute to and maintain panic symptoms; (3) training on diaphragmatic breathing to reduce physical symptoms that may elicit panic attacks; and (4) interoceptive exposure exercises designed to reduce fear of the bodily sensations associated with anxiety and panic attack symptoms. Both interventions successfully reduced anxiety and asthma symptoms and improved quality of life.[57, 58]

Two additional CBT interventions have been developed for comorbid anxiety and depression and asthma. The first is an eight-week, group-based CBT intervention for adults with severe asthma and clinical levels of either anxiety or depression symptoms.[59] Although no large-scale randomized clinical trial of the intervention has been conducted to determine efficacy, the feasibility trial indicated that participants found the intervention to be helpful, but attrition rates were relatively high.[59] The second CBT intervention, Creating Opportunities for Personal Empowerment (COPE) for Asthma, was developed for children between the ages of 8 and 12 with comorbid anxiety and asthma to be delivered in schools.[60] The seven-week programme was feasible to implement in small groups during the school day, acceptable to participants, and resulted in reductions in separation and social anxiety and improvements in quality of life. However, there were no changes in depression symptoms or asthma control.[60]

There has been one examination of a CBT-based prevention programme to treat individuals with asthma and high levels of anxiety and asthma-related panic fear, which would place these individuals at higher risk for developing a comorbid anxiety disorder.[61] As with the previous two studies, this intervention combined education about asthma and anxiety, CBT, and asthma self-management. Results indicated that the intervention resulted in a significant reduction of asthma-related panic fear but not general anxiety by the end of treatment, and this reduction was maintained at the six-month follow-up. There were also significant improvements in asthma-related quality of life and depression at the end of treatment, but these gains were not maintained at the six-month follow-up. Overall, these interventions appear to be successful in reducing anxiety symptoms but are less consistently effective in improving asthma outcomes.

25.12 ANXIETY SENSITIVITY: A POTENTIAL PSYCHOLOGICAL MECHANISM

Research has clearly documented substantial negative health effects as well as personal and economic costs associated with co-occurring asthma and depression and/or anxiety, particularly for co-occurring panic disorder. However, little is known about the etiology of these associations and what factors may serve to maintain them. Efforts to understand these underlying mechanisms would not only fill an important gap within the empirical literature but would also provide specific targets for intervention efforts that could improve asthma control and ultimately reduce healthcare costs. One way in which to accomplish this task is to identify malleable psychological risk factors for not only mood and anxiety symptoms and disorders but also for poor asthma control. Given the particularly strong relationship between asthma and panic disorder, we focus here on one panic-related risk factor that has been receiving increased research attention in terms of its association with asthma, namely anxiety sensitivity.

Anxiety sensitivity is a modifiable cognitive predisposition defined as the fear of anxiety or arousal symptoms that is theoretically and empirically distinct from the tendency to experience negative affect.[62] Anxiety sensitivity acts as an amplifier to stress and encompasses three lower-order dimensions—physical, cognitive, and social concerns—that load onto a single higher-order factor.[63] It exacerbates the experience of somatic and emotional sensations, leading to increased distress and desire to escape/avoid. Essentially, individuals high in anxiety sensitivity misinterpret and overreact to stress and anxiety symptoms. In line with this theory, anxiety sensitivity is concurrently and prospectively associated with an increased risk of anxiety symptoms and with the onset of certain anxiety disorders, most notably panic disorder and PTSD.[64, 65]

A cognitive behavioural model may help explain how anxiety sensitivity impacts asthma. Individuals with asthma tend to be fearful of pulmonary-based and other bodily sensations and may react with greater levels of anxiety or related negative affect when confronted with such stressors. Since anxiety sensitivity results in the amplification of negative emotional experiences, an individual with asthma who is high in anxiety sensitivity would perceive bodily sensations associated with autonomic arousal as a sign of imminent harm, resulting in greater distress about these physical sensations and an increased tendency to catastrophize about them, resulting in avoidance of situations that may elicit such sensations. As a result, this asthma patient with high anxiety sensitivity would likely experience elevated levels of anxiety and be at risk for developing panic disorder as well as increased asthma symptoms and exacerbations. In support of this theory, individuals with asthma who are high in anxiety sensitivity have demonstrated greater physical and affective reactivity to asthma-like sensations.[66]

A growing body of research has demonstrated further associations between anxiety sensitivity and asthma outcomes. For example, anxiety sensitivity has been shown to significantly predict panic in response to symptoms of asthma independently of asthma severity.[67] Other work has found that patients with atopic asthma have higher levels of anxiety sensitivity than those with non-atopic asthma.[68] In terms of asthma-related outcomes, anxiety sensitivity, particularly the physical concerns facet, has been found to significantly predict poorer asthma control and asthma-related quality of life as well as increased risk for ED visits.[41, 69, 70] These findings suggest that individuals with asthma who are fearful of physiological arousal are a particularly "at risk" population for poor asthma control and that there may be utility in reducing anxiety sensitivity levels to improve asthma control. To date, there has been one intervention developed to reduce anxiety sensitivity in adults with asthma and nonclinical levels of anxiety using high-intensity interval training.[71] Results of this six-week intervention indicate that it successfully improved anxiety sensitivity but not FEV_1.

25.13 SUMMARY

Overall, extant research indicates a significant association between asthma and depression and anxiety in terms of both global symptoms and specific disorders, most notably panic disorder. The presence of co-occurring anxiety and depression negatively impacts asthma, particularly in terms of asthma control, quality of life, and healthcare usage. Although the findings are not consistent, co-occurring anxiety and depression do appear to be associated with greater asthma severity in terms of more severe and frequent symptoms, more frequent hospitalizations, and greater medication use. However, the majority of studies also found that there was no effect of co-occurring anxiety and depression on objective measures of lung function. Indeed, it appears as if one of the primary ways in which anxiety, in particular, exerts its influence on asthma is through increased symptom perception, particularly for ambiguous symptoms. Such over-perception of symptoms is problematic, as individuals with asthma rely on their subjective experience of asthma symptoms to guide the management of their asthma and physicians tend to rely more heavily on patients' subjective reports of asthma symptoms than on objective assessments of lung function to inform treatment decisions (e.g. medication class or dosage).[72] As a result, co-occurring anxiety and depression appear to result in poorer asthma outcomes in the absence of actual physical causes. Thus interventions to treat anxiety and depression are needed to reduce this over-perception. Although there are psychological treatments for comorbid asthma and panic disorder, they have been relatively less effective in improving asthma outcomes compared to anxiety outcomes. Moreover, little attention has been given to developing preventive interventions for asthma patients that would target risk factors for developing comorbid anxiety or mood disorders. One potential target that has been identified is anxiety sensitivity. Using exposure-based techniques to reduce anxiety sensitivity has shown some initial promise in asthma patients;[71] however, more work is needed to determine how to improve efficacy for asthma outcomes.

25.14 LIMITATIONS AND FUTURE DIRECTIONS

Although a great deal of research attention has been paid to co-occurring asthma and depression and anxiety, a number of directions for research in this area remain relatively unexplored. Much of this research has focused on documenting this co-occurrence and its effects, and less research attention has been paid to developing and testing theoretical models to explain the etiology and maintenance of this co-occurrence. Such a theory would not only guide research but also provide a framework for understanding how data from various studies fit together. Furthermore, it is difficult to draw definitive conclusions about the associations between anxiety and depression and asthma based on the numerous discrepancies found in extant research. These discrepancies are due, in part, to the types of samples used (e.g. community vs. clinical) but also to what specifically is being examined (e.g. anxiety or depression or both) and how variables are defined. In terms of anxiety and depression, both have been looked at as symptoms as well as clinical disorders. No studies, to our knowledge, have examined the differential effects on asthma outcomes of subclinical levels of anxiety and depression symptoms compared with actual clinical anxiety and depressive disorders. Such work would provide important information about which levels of anxiety and depression are particularly problematic and what specific effects these differing levels have on asthma. Further, it may be useful to clarify the definition of the constructs used as well as the method of their assessment to increase consistency across studies.

Along these same lines, researchers often combine a wide range of anxiety or mood disorders into one group, rather than examining each disorder individually. This strategy is understandable, as relatively large sample sizes are needed to have sufficient representation of each disorder. However, it is then difficult to ascertain associations between specific anxiety or mood disorders and asthma. Moreover, studies looking at classes of disorders do not necessarily include all disorders within a certain class. That is, when researchers examine anxiety disorders, they typically do not include every anxiety disorder. Thus even the conclusions about anxiety disorders as a class can be somewhat misleading since they do not cover all anxiety disorders. Similarly, researchers have focused primarily on the depression end of the spectrum of mood disorders, and little research has been done on the effects of disorders involving mania (e.g. bipolar disorder). This lack of attention is unfortunate, as at least one study found that bipolar disorder is associated with lifetime severe asthma.[25]

More research is needed to examine the differential effects of depression and anxiety on asthma. Several studies attempted to determine whether anxiety or depression, or both, exerted a stronger negative effect on asthma, with conflicting results.[33, 39, 42–44] There is substantial symptom overlap between anxiety and depression, and most self-report measures of depression and anxiety do not take this overlap into consideration. The tripartite model is one attempt to differentiate between anxiety and depression. This model posits that negative affectivity serves as a general distress factor, lack of positive affect is specific to depression, and autonomic arousal is specific to anxiety.[73] Measures based on this conceptualization (e.g. inventory of depression and anxiety symptoms) contain scales that assess symptoms specific to anxiety and specific to depression.[73] Use of such measures in future research may help clarify the differential effects of depression and anxiety. In addition, there is a need to more clearly differentiate between subjective and objective measures of asthma outcomes. Research has shown that asthma patients with co-occurring anxiety, in particular, tend to perceive more symptoms than would be expected based on objective measures of lung function.[46] Unfortunately, various measures of asthma control and asthma severity are largely based on patients' subjective reports of symptoms. Thus it is unclear to what extent anxiety and depression exert a negative influence on asthma outcome measures as the effects of depression and anxiety on symptom perception could confound significant findings.

The majority of studies have compared individuals with asthma to those without; however, anxiety and depression are commonly found among most chronic medical conditions. Thus it is important to understand how much of the link between anxiety and depression and asthma is specific to asthma, rather than related to having a chronic medical condition in general. Future research would also benefit from examining the role of so-called third variables in the co-occurrence of anxiety and depression and asthma. For example, there appear to be certain differential effects based on age[23] and gender[32] that need further examination. Moreover, recent research examining the role of anxiety-related risk factors (e.g. anxiety sensitivity) in this association highlights the importance of examining malleable psychological risk factors as well. Lastly, this body of literature would benefit from greater use of laboratory-based studies. Such studies could examine "online" responding to symptoms of depression and anxiety among individuals with asthma. For example, laboratory-based emotion elicitation procedures could be used to examine how experiencing anxiety or depression symptoms impact physiological responding, perceptions of asthma control, and medication use. This information would not only inform theoretical models of co-occurring asthma and anxiety and depression but also facilitate the examination of the individual and interactive effects of depression and anxiety. Ultimately, such knowledge could be used to develop targeted interventions for individuals with co-occurring asthma and depression or anxiety that would improve asthma management and reduce asthma-related healthcare costs.

REFERENCES

1. Goodwin et al., *Journal of Psychosomatic Research* (2010). https://doi.org/10.1016/j.jpsychores.2009.06.005
2. Pilipenko et al., *Psychology, Health, and Medicine* (2016). https://doi.org/10.1080/13548506.2015.1131995

3. Alvarez et al., *Social Psychiatry and Psychiatric Epidemiology* (2019). https://doi.org/10.1007/s00127-018-1644-5
4. Greenberg et al., *Pharmacoeconomics* (2021). https://doi.org/10.1007/s40273-021-01019-4
5. Kessler et al., *Archives of General Psychiatry* (2005). https://doi.org/10.1001/archpsyc.62.6.593
6. American Psychiatric Association. (2013). *Diagnostic and statistical manual of mental disorders* (5th ed.). https://doi.org/10.1176/appi.books.9780890425596
7. Kessler et al., *International Journal of Methods in Psychiatric Research* (2012). https://doi.org/10.1002%2Fmpr.1359
8. Ortega et al., *Journal of Nervous and Mental Disease* (2002). https://doi.org/10.1097/00005053-200205000-00001
9. Katon et al., *Journal of Adolescent Health* (2007). https://doi.org/10.1016/j.jadohealth.2007.05.023
10. Kyung et al., *Journal of Asthma* (2021). https://doi.org/10.1080/02770903.2020.1847930
11. Kuo et al., *American Journal of Psychiatry* (2010). https://doi.org/10.1176/appi.ajp.2010.09101455
12. Goodwin et al., *Psychological Medicine* (2013). https://doi.org/10.1017/S0033291712001754
13. Chen et al., *Journal of Psychiatric Research* (2014). https://doi.org/10.1016/j.jpsychires.2013.10.015
14. Liu et al., *Brian, Behavior, and Immunology* (2020). https://doi.org/10.1016%2Fj.bbi.2020.07.030
15. Ye et al., *Psychological Medicine* (2021). https://doi.org/10.1017/S0033291720005097
16. Weiser, *Journal of Clinical Psychology in Medical Settings* (2007). https://doi.org/10.1007/s10880-007-9087-2
17. Akula et al., *Journal of Asthma* (2018). https://doi.org/10.1080/02770903.2017.1418885
18. Shen et al., *Epidemiology and Psychiatric Services* (2017). https://doi.org/10.1017/S2045796016000664
19. Goodwin et al., *American Journal of Public Health* (2005). https://doi.org/10.2105%2FAJPH.2003.019109
20. Goodwin et al., *Journal of Psychiatric Research* (2012). https://doi.org/10.1016/j.jpsychires.2012.04.024
21. Chung et al., *Annals of General Psychiatry* (2016). https://doi.org/10.1186/s12991-016-0122-2
22. Lee et al., *Journal of Affective Disorders* (2016). https://doi.org/10.1016/j.jad.2015.09.040
23. Patten et al., *General Hospital Psychiatry* (2008). https://doi.org/10.1016/j.genhosppsych.2008.05.001
24. Alonso et al., *Journal of Psychiatric Research* (2014). https://doi.org/10.1016/j.jpsychires.2014.09.007
25. Goodwin et al., *Archives of General Psychiatry* (2003). https://doi.org/10.1001/archpsyc.60.11.1125
26. Goodwin et al., *Journal of Asthma* (2003). https://doi.org/10.1081/jas-120017984
27. Hasler et al., *American Journal of Respiratory and Critical Care Medicine* (2005). https://doi.org/10.1164/rccm.200412-1669oc
28. Richardson et al., *Pediatrics* (2006). https://doi.org/10.1542/peds.2006-0249
29. Eisner et al., *Annals of Allergy, Asthma, and Immunology* (2005). https://doi.org/10.1016/s1081-1206(10)61135-0
30. Strine et al., *Journal of Asthma* (2008). https://doi.org/10.1080/02770900701840238
31. Krommydas et al., *Respiratory Medicine* (2004). https://doi.org/10.1016/j.rmed.2003.09.018
32. Hayatbakhsh et al., *Journal of Asthma* (2010). https://doi.org/10.3109/02770903.2010.489141
33. Lavoie et al., *Chest* (2006). https://doi.org/10.1378/chest.130.4.1039
34. Feldman et al., *Journal of Pediatric Psychology* (2013). https://doi.org/10.1093/jpepsy/jst052
35. Mangold et al., *Journal of Asthma* (2018). https://doi.org/10.1080/02770903.2017.1350968
36. Walters et al., *PLOS ONE* (2011). https://doi.org/10.1371/journal.pone.0020750
37. Kolbe et al., *Thorax* (2002). https://doi.org/10.1136/thorax.57.4.317
38. Sturdy et al., *Thorax* (2002). https://doi.org/10.1136/thorax.57.12.1034
39. Di Marco et al., *Respiratory Medicine* (2010). https://doi.org/j.rmed.2009.08.005
40. Lavoie et al., *Respiratory Medicine* (2005). https://doi.org/10.1016/j.rmed.2005.03.003
41. Favreau et al., *Psychosomatic Medicine* (2014). https://doi.org/10.1097/PSY.0000000000000032
42. Trzcinska et al., *Medical Science Monitor* (2012). https://doi.org/10.12659%2FMSM.882524
43. Urrutia et al., *Journal of Asthma* (2012). https://doi.org/10.3109/02770903.2011.654022
44. Deshmukh et al., *Respirology* (2008). https://doi.org/10.1111/j.1440-1843.2008.01310.x
45. Chen et al., *Health Psychology* (2006). https://doi.org/10.1037/0278-6133.25.3.389
46. Van Peski-Oosterbaan et al., *Behaviour Research and Therapy* (1996). https://doi.org/10.1016/0005-7967(95)00080-1
47. Feldman et al., *Journal of Asthma* (2005). https://doi.org/10.1081/jas-200054633
48. Kullowatz et al., *Respiratory Medicine* (2007). https://doi.org/10.1016/j.rmed.2006.06.002
49. Mancuso et al., *Journal of General Internal Medicine* (2000). https://doi.org/10.1046/j.1525-1497.2000.07006.x
50. McCauley et al., *General Hospital Psychiatry* (2007). https://doi.org/10.1016/j.genhosppsych.2007.02.003
51. Bardach et al., *Pediatrics* (2019). https://doi.org/10.1542/peds.2019-0856
52. Ahmedani et al., *Psychosomatic Medicine* (2013). https://doi.org/10.1097/PSY.0b013e3182864ee3
53. Dahlem et al., *Journal of Allergy and Clinical Immunology* (1977). https://doi.org/10.1016/0091-6749(77)90108-7
54. Dirks et al., *Psychosomatic Medicine* (1978). https://doi.org/10.1097/00006842-197802000-00003
55. Dirks et al., *Journal of Asthma Research* (1977). https://doi.org/10.3109/02770907709098953
56. Feldman et al., *Journal of Anxiety Disorders* (2009). https://doi.org/10.1016%2Fj.janxdis.2008.06.005
57. Ross et al., *Clinical Nursing Research* (2005). https://doi.org/10.1177/1054773804273863
58. Lehrer et al., *Journal of Anxiety Disorders* (2008). https://doi.org/10.1016%2Fj.janxdis.2007.07.001
59. Yorke et al., *Journal of Asthma* (2017). https://doi.org/10.1080/02770903.2016.1229335
60. McGovern et al., *School Psychology* (2019). https://doi.org/10.1037/spq0000310
61. Parry et al., *Respiratory Medicine* (2012). https://doi.org/10.1016/j.rmed.2012.02.006
62. McNally, *Biological Psychiatry* (2002). https://doi.org/10.1016/s0006-3223(02)01475-0
63. Taylor et al., *Psychological Assessment* (2007). https://doi.org/10.1037/1040-3590.19.2.176
64. Schmidt et al., *Journal of Abnormal Psychology* (1997). https://doi.org/10.1037//0021-843x.106.3.355
65. Feldner et al., *Depression and Anxiety* (2008). https://doi.org/10.1002/da.20281

66. McLeish et al., *Behavior Modification* (2016). https://doi.org/10.1177/0145445515607047
67. Carr et al., *Health Psychology* (1995). https://doi.org/10.1037//0278-6133.14.5.421
68. Barone et al., *Journal of Behavioral Medicine* (2008). https://doi.org/10.1007/s10865-008-9164-5
69. McLeish et al., *Journal of Health Psychology* (2011). https://doi.org/10.1177/1359105310382584
70. Avallone et al., *Journal of Asthma* (2012). https://doi.org/10.3109/02770903.2011.641048
71. O'Neill et al., *Journal of Physical Activity & Health* (2020). https://doi.org/10.1123/jpah.2019-0521
72. Apter et al., *Journal of Allergy and Clinical Immunology* (1997). https://doi.org/10.1016/s0091-6749(97)70020-4
73. Watson et al., *Psychological Assessment* (2007). https://doi.org/10.1037/1040-3590.19.3.253

Section VII

Approach to Asthma Worldwide and in the Primary Care Setting

26 Managing Asthma and Allergy *The Need for a Countrywide Approach to Integrating Care*

Luane Marques de Mello and Álvaro Augusto Cruz

CASE

A 29-year-old man showed up at a public primary healthcare unit (PCU), requesting an appointment because he had asthma and the device he used was no longer working. His family recently moved to the area, and he wanted to be followed up by the PCU because he couldn't afford private care. He reported that where he previously lived, there was no PCU, which is why he never had regular follow-up care for his asthma. During the consultation, the patient reported asthma symptoms since childhood, but the diagnosis was only confirmed at age 18. He used the emergency room (ER) as his primary source of care when he became symptomatic but was only medicated with a short-acting beta-2 agonist bronchodilator (SABA) aerosol to relieve symptoms. On occasion, he received a prescription for oral corticosteroids upon discharge. He was never referred to an allergy specialist for allergy testing but, at the time of his diagnosis, had a normal chest X-ray and spirometry. He had no previous asthma hospitalizations but had several 23-hour visits to the ER, where he was treated and observed until stable for discharge. His only medication was albuterol to relieve symptoms as needed, which he used one to two times a month. However, he had noticed progressive worsening of asthma symptoms over the last year, requiring more SABA use, which helped to relieve symptoms for a few hours. Approximately two weeks before his current visit, coughing and wheezing symptoms started to worsen, requiring albuterol two times a day or more. He was unable to carry out daily activities and was waking up at night due to shortness of breath, coughing, and wheezing at least twice a week, He was also unable to participate in regular leisure activities such as playing football (soccer) with his friends during this time.

On physical examination, the patient was anxious but in good condition overall. He was afebrile, slightly tachypneic (RR = 28 bpm) with a HR = 96 bpm and BP 128/89 mmHg. Auscultation revealed diffuse wheezing but no difficulty speaking or signs of respiratory fatigue. His peak flow was 30% lower relative to the predicted values based on his height, gender, and age. He reported using two puffs of albuterol less than two hours before.

At the conclusion of the patient's evaluation, the general practitioner confirmed a clinical diagnosis of poorly controlled asthma, pending objective confirmation by spirometry pre- and post-bronchodilators. The patient was prescribed a course of oral corticosteroids for seven days and instructed on the proper use of his albuterol inhaler as a rescue medication, while prescribing a medium-dose generic inhaled corticosteroid as controller therapy. The patient was also provided with a rescue plan in case of worsening symptoms or an asthma exacerbation. The patient was referred for allergy testing as well as spirometry and a follow-up appointment was scheduled. The physician emphasized to the patient the importance of adhering to treatment and follow-up recommendations.

26.1 ABOUT THE CASE

That is a typical case of a public healthcare system user and the approach taken by the physician in Brazil. He had never received treatment for asthma because there was no PCU in the neighborhood where he previously lived, which had very low primary healthcare coverage for patients who could not afford to pay for their own healthcare. Therefore, due to impaired access to outpatient care, he overutilized the ER, which is much more costly. Furthermore, he was never referred to a primary care physician or a specialist for outpatient management, which perpetuated his fragmented care. Once he relocated to an area that had better PCU coverage, he was able to have his respiratory complaints better evaluated, leading to an appropriate asthma management plan based on GINA guidelines that incorporated the daily use of a controller therapy, an assessment for allergies, and ongoing outpatient follow-up to ensure asthma control was maintained.

Most importantly, GINA guidelines emphasize the importance of adapting management and therapeutic recommendations to local realities, especially regarding access to medication for underserved or economically stressed populations (1), which in this case was what the treating

DOI: 10.1201/9781003287209-33

physician implemented. In the Brazilian public health system, other branded inhaled corticosteroids (ICS) alone or in combination with a long-acting β2-agonist are available only to patients who are followed by a specialist.

In addition, this patient was referred to the Allergy and Pulmonology specialty center to obtain further diagnostic testing, as some specialized care is unavailable for PHC providers in Brazil, which is a hierarchical medical care system that can impact the integration of medical care.

At the end of his appointment, the patient received a written plan with instructions in case of exacerbations. He also was given an appointment for follow-up with the PCU for his asthma and other healthcare needs to ensure continuity of care.

This individual case report unfortunately represents the reality for thousands of asthma and allergy patients in Brazil who have a delayed diagnosis and fragmented care due to poor access to a healthcare clinic even though the country's national healthcare policy guarantees comprehensive and universal healthcare wherever you live.

26.2 STRUCTURING COMPREHENSIVE HEALTHCARE IN BRAZIL

For many years, access to Brazilian public healthcare services was restricted to individuals with a formal employment relationship. For the remaining population, medical assistance is obtained through direct payment for private healthcare services or is free healthcare through charitable institutions (2).

The Unified Health System (SUS) in 1989 was created to provide healthcare and rehabilitation services that promoted health and prevented disease for the entire population regardless of economic or social status. The underlying premise was to meet the needs of everyone's health needs according to the principles of universality and equity of care (3).

Over the last few decades, the morbidity and mortality profile of the Brazilian population has improved correspondingly to improved living conditions and the quality of healthcare delivery in association with the effects of an accelerated demographic transition to areas where healthcare is more accessible. Consequently, the overpopulation of certain regions has led to increased needs for controlling and reducing infectious diseases, preventing malnutrition, and addressing reproductive health issues. In addition, there is an increase in chronic diseases and their risk factors including active and passive smoke exposure, obesity, poor eating habits, sedentary lifestyle, and stress, which further increase the complexity of patients' healthcare needs (4).

The Primary Health Care (PHC) approach was selected as the country's overall healthcare model and, more specifically, the Family Health Strategy was chosen for administering healthcare through the PHC in the public health system (5).

To ensure the principles of adequate regional distribution of integrated healthcare, it was necessary to reorganize the components of the health system according to the Health Care Networks (HCN) model. Thus health professionals and patients interact through a broad network of services where the PHC functions to ensure there is coordination of care and appropriate longitudinal follow-up (6).

26.3 INTEGRATED ASTHMA CARE

Presently, Brazil does not have any national policy specifically targeting asthma. Other allergic diseases, such as anaphylaxis, drug and food allergy, urticaria, and angioedema, also have no national policy for management. Thus there is still an unmet need to recognize these common conditions and provide resources that can educate caregivers on how to reduce their associated morbidity and, in the case of anaphylaxis, potential death.

In recent years we have witnessed a significant increase in the prevalence of allergic diseases around the world, generating a significant socioeconomic impact and impairment in quality of life. About 25% of the population in industrialized countries has some form of allergic disease such as allergic rhinitis, asthma, atopic dermatitis, chronic rhinosinusitis, allergic conjunctivitis, or food allergy. These conditions have been reported to affect more people in low- and medium-income countries, such as Brazil, where the repercussions are even worse due to the general scarcity of resources (7). Whereas hospitalizations and mortality rates are decreasing in some countries of the world, data from a recent study showed rising levels of poor symptom control (12.3%) and treatment adherence (32%) in Brazilian asthma patients (8).

However, even though there are insufficient resources in Brazil, asthma, among all allergic diseases, has been receiving some attention from the public authorities due to its higher morbidity and mortality. Recently, the Clinical Protocol and Therapeutic Guidelines (CPTG) for asthma were approved to provide improved access to healthcare and medications for asthma. This document is expected to serve as a guide for Health Care Networks and more specifically the asthma referral centers (9).

Two legal frameworks were pivotal for getting asthma care and treatment included into the public health system. The first was the National Medicines Policy by the Ministry of Health, which provides free access to some asthma medications, i.e. the ICS beclomethasone and the SABA fenoterol and salbutamol. This plan especially favors patients with milder asthma conditions, who, despite having less intense symptoms, have frequent exacerbations requiring hospitalizations as often as patients with severe asthma (10). This milder group, which feels well in between or has a poor sense of dyspnea, receives the most benefits from being monitored in the PHC system (11).

The second milestone was the ministerial decree that determined the creation of therapeutic guidelines and clinical protocols for severe asthma, making available drugs such as budesonide, formoterol, fluticasone, and salmeterol, thus favoring the specialized treatment of patients with severe asthma (12).

In recent years, a national plan aimed at the group of chronic diseases (13), recently updated for the next eight years (Plan of DANT 2022–2030), began to define strategic actions aimed at the prevalent chronic disease conditions in the country. The plan includes cardiovascular diseases, cancer, diabetes mellitus, and chronic respiratory diseases, which consists of asthma as well as COPD, chronic cough, obstructive sleep apnea, dyspnea, and pulmonary nodules (14).

However, this agenda was instituted only recently, and there still is no priority for asthma. Over the years, the prevalence of chronic diseases, including allergic diseases and asthma, continues to rise without a corresponding "call to action" response from the public healthcare sector.

A Brazilian Consensus on Education in Asthma was published 25 years ago, resulting from the dedicated work of pulmonology, allergy, and pediatric societies frustrated with the inertia of public authorities. The Consensus advocated programs to educate patients and recommended self-management skills while encouraging family involvement in asthma management, with oversight by qualified professionals to improve disease management, and to modify asthma morbidity and mortality risk factors considering cultural and social beliefs and economic capabilities (15).

Several programs emerged in response to the Consensus. Due to the efforts of specialty societies, the National Asthma Control Plan (NACP) was created to clarify care for patients with asthma by guaranteeing access to comprehensive care and continuous free-of-charge medication (16).

Although the NACP was not implemented as expected, it served as a reference for individual programs and other initiatives throughout the country to offer specialized and high-quality asthma care (17) (Table 26.1).

Over the years, some initiatives were discontinued while others were strengthened and consolidated. Among the successful initiatives for asthma, the two programs that succeeded in offering qualified asthma care and modifying

TABLE 26.1
Successful Asthma Experiences in Brazil

Asthma Programs in Brazil

Program	Year	Place	Goals	Financing
The Wheezing Child Program	1996	Belo Horizonte (MG)	Team training Education on asthma Systematize care Guarantee access to free-of-charge medicines	Federal University of Minas Gerais (UFMG) Public funding: Use of the public facilities network at the municipal and state levels of health; National Medicines Plan–SUS
Comprehensive Care Program for Asthmatic Children (PROAICA)	1996	Fortaleza (CE)	Train and qualify the assistance on asthma Education on asthma Scientific research	Public funding: Use of the public facilities network at the municipal and state levels of health; National Medicines Plan–SUS
Asthma Patient Assistance Program (PAPA)	1996	São Luís (MA)	Create asthma referral centers Education on asthma Professional qualification	Hospital of the Federal University of Maranhão
Program–Respiratory Infections and Allergies	2000	Curitiba (PR)	Organize care flows Free-of-charge medicines Professional qualification Reduce morbidity and mortality	Municipal public facility network Clinical hospital of the Federal University of Paraná (UFPR) and Pequeno Príncipe Children's Hospital
Back to Home & Asthma	2001	Porto Alegre (RS)	Offer training and continuing health education Guidelines and flow charts for diagnosis and treatment Reduction in hospitalizations for asthma	Public funding: Use of the public facilities network at the municipal and state levels of health National Medicines Plan–SUS
Asthmatic Patient Care Program of the Federal District	2001	Brasília DF)	Education on asthma Access to free-of-charge medicines Professional training	Public funding: Use of the public facilities network at the municipal and state levels of health National Medicines Plan—SUS
Program–Breathe London	2002	Londrina (PR)	Permanent Education active search Timely diagnosis and treatments Access to free-of-charge medicines Comprehensive care	Public funding: Use of the public facilities network at the municipal and state levels of health National Medicines Plan—SUS

(*Continued*)

TABLE 26.1 (*Continued*)
Successful Asthma Experiences in Brazil

Asthma Programs in Brazil

Program	Year	Place	Goals	Financing
Asthma Control Program in Bahia (ProAR)	2003	Salvador and Feira de Santana (BA)	Integrated care Free-of-charge medicines Create referral centers for severe asthma Health education Professional qualification	Foundation for Research Support of the State of Bahia (FAPESB) Public funding: use of the public facilities network at the municipal and state levels of health National Medicines Plan—SUS
Asthma Control Program (CATAVENTO)	2003	Goiânia (GO)	Permanent education Search patients actively Free-of-charge medicines Qualified healthcare Know and improve local epidemiological indicators	Public funding: Use of the public facilities network at the municipal and state levels of health National Medicines Plan—SUS
Asthma Control Program (Respira Niterói)	2003	Niterói (RJ)	Diagnosis and treatment Integrated care Public manager awareness Improve local epidemiological indicators	Public funding: Use of the public facilities network at the municipal and state levels of health National Medicines Plan—SUS
Care plan for patients with asthma and rhinitis in the city of Rio de Janeiro (RespiraRio)	2004	Rio de Janeiro (RJ)	Reduce morbidity and mortality Professional training Permanent education Create asthma centers to ensure access to medicines and diagnostic tests Improve the information system	Public funding: Use of the public facilities network at the municipal and state levels of health National Medicines Plan—SUS
CreAs Program–Rhinitis and Asthma Control at Santa Casa de Misericórdia	2006	Vitória (ES)	Create reference asthma centers Health permanent education Search and control the comorbidities	Public funding: Hospital of the Santa Casa de Misericórdia School of Medicine (EMESCAM)

Source: Adapted from Cerci Neto A, org. Asma em Saúde Pública (2006).

asthma-related morbidity and mortality indicators in their regions of operation were The Wheezing Child Program and Asthma Control Program in Bahia (ProAR).

The Wheezing Child program was developed to respond to a problem identified in the city of Belo Horizonte through a study conducted in 1994 and 1995. The results showed that 90% of the children and adolescents with asthma evaluated attended the ER 1–2 times a month because of asthma symptoms, that 64% had been previously hospitalized for asthma, and that 71% required readmission. The study also showed that the approach to patient care was limited to treating only asthma exacerbations either in the outpatient setting or as a hospital inpatient. The economic cost of care was increasing in large part due to treating patients with reliever SABA medications as opposed to using controller medications (ICS or ICS+ LABA) that are known to improve clinical disease by reducing airway inflammation (18).

The program was made possible through a technical cooperation contract between the Federal University of Minas Gerais (UFMG) and the Health Department of the Municipality of Belo Horizonte, using the available capacity and resources of the public health network.

The program began in 1996 to offer training to the health team and education for asthma and their families, reorganize assistance to children with asthma in the public health system at all levels of care, and provide medications to treat exacerbations and control the disease.

The training of professionals from PCU who participated in the in-service training program was essential for changing the care provided to patients from a treatment focused on acute care to one emphasizing long-term anti-inflammatory preventive care (19).

Based on the 1995 Global Initiative for Asthma (GINA) document, this training was primarily recommended for pediatricians, general practitioners, nurses, and pharmacists.

Two referral centers for specialized care in pediatric pulmonology were created. The children initially assisted were patients <5 years of age, as they were the most vulnerable risk for hospitalization, according to clinical study data. Children over five years of age and adolescents were initially seen in asthma referral centers and then followed up in primary care units.

The health education actions involved the health team, patients, and family members, all important stakeholders in the management of asthma (20).

The patient's relationship to a primary care unit was essential for continuing educational activities that addressed important topics such as adherence, environmental control including allergen avoidance measures, encouragement of physical activities, and recognition of early warning signs of worsening asthma that can lead to exacerbations.

As a result of this program, the use of ICSs increased, and the sensitivity of the team to the patient's medical and social needs improved, which had an overall favorable impact on disease control. There was a significant increase in prescriptions for ICSs, use of aerosolized bronchodilators with a spacer, and a 79% reduction in hospitalization rates several years after the program's implementation (21).

Ten years after the program's implementation, the authors have reported the positive impact on local morbidity indicators, the improvement in quality of life, the quality of care provided to patients, and the generation of new scientific knowledge (22). However, their report highlights some of the challenges encountered over the launch of this program including low adherence (50–60%) affecting asthma control of many children; issues pertaining to the willingness and interest between the healthcare managers in the public sector and the university to cooperate so that implementation of the program was successful; and the increased coverage of healthcare by primary care throughout the country, which, although providing increased access, depends on professionals with less experience and knowledge for diagnosis and management of asthma and offers poor access to more potent ICS by primary care to treat more complex severe cases (22).

Another successful example is the Asthma Control Program in Bahia (ProAR), which positively impacted the outcomes of patients with severe asthma and reduced morbidity disease indicators in Salvador and Feira de Santana, Bahia.

ProAR is a multi-institutional program of teaching, research, and specialized assistance based on the NACP, coordinated by the Federal University of Bahia, funded by the Fundação de Amparo à Pesquisa do Estado da Bahia (FAPESB), and operated with the support and collaboration of the public sectors.

The program, which has been operating since 2003, was implemented as a referral center for severe asthma patients from primary care in the City of Salvador, Feria de Santana, and the region in the State of Bahia. The initiative arose from the need for developing an adequate approach for specialized monitoring of patients with the most severe forms of asthma, most of whom did not have access to long-term controller anti-inflammatory treatment (23, 24).

The main goals of the program were to provide comprehensive care to asthma patients in the public health system, offer free asthma medication, structure referral outpatient clinics for severe cases, and train primary care teams to care for patients with mild and moderate forms of the disease.

In the first years of the program, four reference centers in Salvador and one in Feira de Santana were established, expanding access to specialized asthma care, and positive results began to emerge. With ProAR, it was possible to observe a reduction in 85% of urgent care and 90% of hospitalizations, 86% lower school and work absenteeism, and 67% reduced need for oral corticosteroid use by the affected population (25).

The direct and indirect costs of the disease for families were reduced by 50% in the time spent on commuting, 59% in time spent in waiting rooms because of asthma, and 80% in school absenteeism. At the same time, there was an increase of 10% in the average family income and a reduction in treatment costs by 86.3%, generating an average annual increase in family income of 50% concerning the income before the program. Asthma medications were the costliest budget items for asthma patients, which was reduced after the program from 37.5% to 4.5% of the total cost to families related to asthma management (26).

Regarding public health, essential reductions in costs with hospitalizations, ICUs, and emergency visits were also identified, despite an increase in expenses with inhaled medications, healthcare visits, and consultations (27).

The ProAR experiences supported several studies, generating specific knowledge of important relevance. One of these studies compared demographic, clinical, and pulmonary function characteristics between two cohorts of adults with severe asthma. The Brazilian ProAR cohort and a European cohort formed from a consortium of academic institutions, the pharmaceutical industry, and patient organizations (U-BIOPRED) and controls mild/moderate asthma from Brazil and 11 European countries. The results showed that, despite some differences, phenotypic similarities endorse asthma as a nosological entity, which allows studies to be conducted between groups from different regions in order to seek answers to important questions that explain the phenotypic variability of asthma and treatment responses (28).

Other studies conducted with the ProAR cohort of severe asthma showed that asthma patients have a 53% greater likelihood of having depression, possibly due to the decreased quality of life impacted by symptoms that can be disabling, especially for severe asthma patients who are more prone to exacerbations. In this study, the authors further proposed that asthma can constitute a negative adverse life event causing suffering as well as physical and mental stress. Psychological stress could lead to increased pro-inflammatory markers that could underlie the relationship between asthma and depression (29).

26.4 FINAL CONSIDERATIONS

Brazil has not yet implemented national public policies specifically aimed to address allergic diseases and asthma. However, immeasurable advances and benefits obtained to date result from the various local experiences that changed the lives of thousands of patients in low- and medium-income countries by reducing local morbidity indicators, which influenced others to reproduce and adapt the models, thus extending favorable outcomes to a larger sector of the population.

Problems with under-diagnosed asthma, as reported in the illustrative case presented in this chapter, are also common in many other countries, such as those published recently from observations in Vietnam (30). These evolving healthcare systems, like Brazil, are slowly recognizing the importance of extending healthcare symptom resources to include asthma education and management programs. Brazil is but one example of a low- to medium-income country where asthma, initially considered a low-priority disease by the public health system, became associated with a high morbidity and economic burden to the healthcare system. However, with effective healthcare initiatives, slow but steady progress is being made that is making a significant impact on asthma outcomes. It is important that asthma experts continue international advocacy efforts with a focus on low- and medium-income country healthcare systems to promote asthma educational resources and guidelines that can improve asthma outcomes globally.

REFERENCES

1. Reddel HK et al. *Am J Respir Crit Care Med* (2022). PMID: 34658302 https://doi.org/10.1164/rccm.202109-2205PP
2. Souza RR. O Sistema Público de Saúde Brasileiro (2002). Available at: https://bvsms.saude.gov.br/bvs/publicacoes/sistema_saude.pdf
3. Mendes EV. *Estudos avançados* (2013). https://doi.org/10.1590/S0103-40142013000200003
4. Malta DC et al. *Popul Health Metr* (2020). https://doi.org/10.1186/s12963-020-00224-1
5. Pan American Health Organization. World Health Organization. 44th Directing Council. 55th Session of the Regional Committee (2003). Available at: https://iris.paho.org/bitstream/handle/10665.2/238/cd44-r6-e.pdf?sequence =1&é permitido=y
6. Mendes EV. *As redes de atenção à saúde*. Brasília: Organização Pan-Americana da Saúde (2011). Available at: https://bvsms.saude.gov.br/bvs/publicacoes/redes_de_atencao_saude.pdf
7. Meghji J et al. *Lancet* (2021). PMID: 33631128 https://doi.org/10.1016/S0140-6736(21)00458-X
8. Cançado JED et al. *J Asthma* (2019). PMID: 29595345 https://doi.org/10.1080/02770903.2018.1445267
9. Portaria Conjunta N° 14, de 24 de agosto de 2021. Available at: https://www.gov.br/conitec/pt-br/midias/protocolos/20210830_pcdt_asma_pt14.pdf
10. Ponte EV et al., *Pediatr Pulmonol* (2021). PMID: 34932729 https://doi.org/10.1002/ppul.25363.
11. Technical Institutional Reports: National medicines policy. *Health Policy Dept Rev Saúde Pública* (2000). https://doi.org/10.1590/S0034-89102000000200018
12. PORTARIA N° 1.318, DE 23 DE JULHO DE 2002. Available at: https://abcd.org.br/wp-content/uploads/2014/02/doc_portaria_1318.pdf
13. [Strategic Action Plan to Tackle Noncommunicable Diseases (NCD) in Brazil 2011–2022] (Plano de DCNT 2011–2022). Available at: https://bvsms.saude.gov.br/bvs/publicacoes/plano_acoes_enfrent_dcnt_2011.pdf
14. [Strategic Actions Plan for Takle Chronic Diseases and Noncommunicable Diseases in Brazil 2021–2030] (Plano de DANT 2022–2030). Available at: http://bvsms.saude.gov.br/bvs/publicacoes/plano_enfrentamento_doencas_cronicas_agravos_2021_2030.pdf
15. Sociedade Brasileira de Pneumologia e Tisiologia. *J Pneumol* (1996) Available at: https://storage.googleapis.com/bkpsbpt/programas_congressos_cursos/sup01_96.pdf
16. Silva LC et al. *J Pneumol* (2002). Available at: https://www.scielo.br/j/jpneu/a/b9DYhFFFQZ7YLyczW6NSZNq/?format=pdf&lang=pt
17. Cerci Neto A et al. *J Bras Pneumol* (2008). PMID: 18345454 https://doi.org/10.1590/s1806-37132008000200007
18. Lasmar LMLB et al. *Rev. méd. Minas Gerais* (2000). Available at: http://bases.bireme.br/cgi-bin/wxislind.exe/iah/online/?IsisScript=iah/iah.xis&src =google&base=ADOLEC&lang=p&nextAction=lnk&exprSearch=613721&indexSearch=ID
19. Camargos PAM et al. *Protocolo de asma brônquica e curso teórico-prático de abordagem da asma na infância e adolescência e aplicações da terapia inalatória*. UFMG, 2000.
20. Camargos PAM et al. In search of comprehensive care for asthma patients in Brazil.In: Cruz AA. Asma, *um grande desafio* (2004). São Paulo, Ateneu, P343–57.
21. Fontes MJ et al. *J Pediatr* (2011). https://doi.org/10.2223/JPED.2129
22. Lasmar LM et al. In: Cerci Neto A, *org. Asma em Saúde Pública* (2006). São Paulo: Manole, P93–102.
23. Ponte EV et al. *Revista Baiana de Saúde Pública* (2004). Available at: http://www.luzimarteixeira.com.br/wp-content/uploads/2009/11/doencas-ocupacionais-em-professores1.pdf
24. Brandao HV et al. *Gazeta Médica da Bahia* (2008). Available at: http://www.gmbahia.ufba.br/index.php/gmbahia/article/viewFile/751/734
25. Ponte EV et al. *J Bras Pneumol* (2007). https://doi.org/10.1590/S1806-37132007000100006
26. Franco RA et al. *BMC Public Health* (2007). https://doi.org/10.1186/1471-2458-7-82
27. Souza-Machado C et al. *Gazeta Médica da Bahia* (2008). Available at: https://gmbahia.ufba.br/index.php/gmbahia/article/viewFile/750/733
28. Cruz AA et al. *Respir Med* (2020). PMID: 31790928 https://doi.org/10.1016/j.rmed.2019.105817
29. Vázquez VS et al. *J Thorac Dis* (2021). PMID: 34795954 https://doi.org/10.21037/jtd-20-3197
30. Huang WC et al. *ERJ Open Res* (2021). PMID: 33681343 https://doi.org/10.1183/23120541.00572-2020

27 Primary Care Setting and Integrating Care Across Primary/Secondary Care Interface

Alan G. Kaplan and Barbara P. Yawn

CASE PRESENTATION

Cases

Mary and John are 12-year-old twins whose asthma was diagnosed at ages 10 and 6 years, respectively. Both were diagnosed with persistent asthma, and both began therapy with moderate-dose inhaled corticosteroid (ICS). After this, the courses of their diseases differed.

John is an athlete whose asthma was adequately controlled until about two years ago. Now he consistently has problems during soccer and basketball practice. In addition, he awakes several nights a month. While his spirometry is within normal limits, he continues to remain poorly controlled. Over the past two years, he has progressed from his moderate-dose ICS to a high-dose combination of ICS and long-acting beta-adrenoceptor agonist (LABA) but continues to use his short-acting beta-2 adrenoceptor agonist (SABA) almost daily with limited results. He is waking up two to three nights a month coughing and had to sit out the last soccer practice. His family physician has assessed potential allergens with in vitro assays with positive results for grasses and trees. John does not appear to have seasonal symptoms, but with the constant problems, seasonal assessment is difficult. His family physician recognizes that John is not in control and wonders if it is time to consider stepping up to therapy with a biologic and arranges a referral to a local allergist. The physician recognizes that there are a number of different biologics and has ordered a CBC for the eosinophil count as well as a total IgE level. These are both biomarkers that may allow the specialist to choose the appropriate biologic for John. A FENO (fractionated exhaled nitric oxide) measurement (which is a surrogate marker for eosinophilic inflammation) may also be available to the specialist to give yet another biomarker for the decision.

On the other hand, Mary's asthma had been well controlled with moderate-dose ICS and remains controlled most of the time. However, in the spring and fall for the past two years, Mary has had severe exacerbations even requiring hospitalization this March. After the hospitalization, Mary finished a 10-day course of oral steroids, and her asthma has been under good control on moderate-dose ICS plus LABA combination inhaler for May, June, and July. The fall allergy season is approaching, and Mary, her parents, and her family physician are concerned that they do not know about all of Mary's allergies nor how to prevent another severe exacerbation. In addition, Mary and her family report they do not see the need for medications to be continued year-round and plan to stop the medications between the fall and spring allergy seasons. Her family physician wants a better assessment of Mary's allergic triggers and thinks the allergist can address this and support recommendations for year-round asthma therapy. So she arranges for her to see the allergist on the same day as her brother.

THE ALLERGIST'S OFFICE

John's visit reveals a common but often unrecognized problem. John's inhaler technique is very poor for both his dry powder inhaler and his metered-dose inhaler. Thinking back, it becomes clear that John's problems began when he started using his medications in his room rather than with parental supervision. Since then, his inhaler technique has apparently deteriorated, although he is very motivated to take his medication, as he wants to excel in soccer. With an appropriate technique over the next four weeks, John's asthma is again well-controlled on moderate-dose ICS and pre-exercise use of SABA without needing to step up to combination therapy or a biologic treatment. The allergist returned John to the care of his family physician with an updated asthma action plan and a suggestion to the family physician to assess inhaler technique at each visit, providing links to online inhaler technique videos the family medicine office staff can use to help teach and review inhaler technique. There are many resources for this

DOI: 10.1201/9781003287209-34

including lung association websites, YouTube, and medical organizations such as the one at https://www.fpagc.com/tools-resources.

Mary's visit included a detailed allergy history and targeted allergy skin testing. The allergist recommended consideration of allergy desensitization as the first choice, as her asthma is currently under good control between allergy seasons but with severe asthma flares and disabling seasonal allergic rhinoconjunctivitis. They discussed biologics being a possible future consideration if seasonal exacerbations requiring oral corticosteroids continued despite desensitization therapy and the use of seasonal intranasal corticosteroids. The allergist provided a detailed consultation summary to the family and Mary's family physician. All agreed that Mary's asthma care would be a collaboration between her family physician with continued follow-up by the allergist.

Comment

John's consultation may well have been able to be avoided if the primary care physician had a systematic approach to not only assessing control but also assessing the common causes of asthma being out of control. This list should include affirming the diagnosis, medication adherence, observing and ensuring proper inhaler technique, treating comorbidities, and possibly assessing phenotypic differences. Many tools are available to assist in this review. For example, the SIMPLES tool, created by the IPCRG (International Primary Care Respiratory Group).[1]

Mary's frequent exacerbations and hospitalization were an indication for the detailed review of triggers and possible consultation; this is recommended in virtually all current asthma guidelines to provide options that are seldom available in primary care for diagnosis, monitoring, and treatment (e.g. fractionated exhaled nitric oxide or FENO, detailed allergy assessments, and considerations for further step-up therapies including biologics).

27.1 INTRODUCTION

Asthma is one of the most common chronic conditions for both adults and children. Rates vary by country and are consistently high in the most high-income countries: 14–15% in the United Kingdom, New Zealand, Canada, Australia, and Ireland and 11% in the United States. Low- and middle-income countries report wider variations: 13% in Peru, 12% in Costa Rica, 8% in Africa, and only 2% in China; however, many cases are likely to be unreported or undiagnosed. Rates in schoolchildren are higher than those in adults.[2,3,4] The decline in rates from childhood to adults may be due to more careful assessment and diagnostic tool availability in adults; asthma-like symptoms common in children, which may not be asthma; and asthma remission during transition into adulthood. The estimated percentage of those with asthma who have mild asthma varies widely but is usually more than 50% of all patients with asthma.[5,6,7] As asthma is common, usually of mild to moderate severity and amenable to well-known treatments, it is not surprising that the vast majority of people with asthma and asthma exacerbations are cared for by primary care physicians.

Yet data from many countries demonstrate the vast opportunities to improve asthma care and patient outcomes.[8] Specialist care can potentially improve asthma management. For example, in the United States, people whose asthma management includes an asthma specialist have better outcomes then when cared for only in primary care. Whether this is due entirely to the additional training and expertise of the allergist or to the allergists' care system or both is not clear.[9] Based on information from management of other chronic conditions, improving the primary care systems is very likely to improve asthma outcomes,[10] as it has improved outcomes for people with diabetes.[11,12] Many aspects of asthma specialists' care systems can be adapted and transferred to primary care sites, as demonstrated in many asthma management quality-improvement (QI) programs. Not all attempts at improvement have been successful, but some specific tasks appear to be universally helpful. The next section of this chapter will address asthma care in primary care practices. Many of the issues discussed are addressed in greater depth in other chapters in this book. When possible, reference is made to other chapters to guide you to tools and information that can facilitate implementation of suggestions in this chapter.

27.2 ASTHMA GUIDELINES IN PRACTICE

Several national and international guidelines have been produced to direct asthma management—Global Initiative for Asthma (GINA), Scottish Intercollegiate Guidelines Network (SIGN), National Heart, Lung, and Blood Institute (NHLBI), International Primary Care Respiratory Group (IPCRG), Dutch GP guidelines, and Canadian and Australian guidelines (see Chapter 5, this volume). Unfortunately, few of the guidelines can be transferred directly to daily practice activities.[13,14,15,16] For example, asthma control tools have been developed to facilitate assessment of asthma response to therapy and the adequacy of asthma management. These tools were developed in response to identified gaps in practice, specifically the failure of most medical encounter notes to include the information required to quantify control based on asthma signs and symptoms or the most common reasons for inadequate control (see GINA Table 2-2b in: A summary guide for Asthma management and prevention in adults, adolescents and children aged 6–11 years. Available at: https://ginasthma.org/wp-content/uploads/2024/12/GINA-Summary-Guide-2024-WEB-WMS.pdf). The control tools are used to calculate a score that suggests the patient's asthma is "in control," "poorly controlled," or somewhere in between at the time of testing; for example, Asthma Control Test (ACT),[17] Asthma Therapy Assessment Questionnaire (ATTAQ), Asthma Control Questionnaire (ACQ),[18] and Asthma APGAR.[19] The ACT and ACQ both have separate tools for children,[20] while the Asthma APGAR is designed to be used by parents of very young children, adolescents, and adults. Using any of these tools ensures that the right questions are asked to assess control, after which the physician or other clinician needs to determine the next steps. Only the Asthma APGAR also addresses issues such as triggers, adherence with links to a next steps algorithm.

All the asthma guidelines suggest management steps in response to asthma control problems. For example, in the 2021 Canadian Asthma guidelines,[21] an often-ignored box (see Figure 27.1) to the top left corner of the steps of therapy says, "assess control, risk of exacerbation, lung function, adherence, triggers, inhaler techniques and comorbidities before stepping it up." A similar box appears in the NHLBI 2007 and updated 2021 guidelines.

The British Thoracic Society guidelines[23] also specifically state, "Before initiating a new drug therapy practitioners should check compliance with existing therapies, inhaler technique, and eliminate trigger factors." Despite these statements, in most primary patient care settings, poor control results in an increase in medication without further assessment of why the current therapy is not effective. Common causes of poor or inadequate control include lack of adherence to current management program, inability to afford medications, poor inhaler technique, and triggers that are unrecognized or not avoided and undertreated comorbidities.

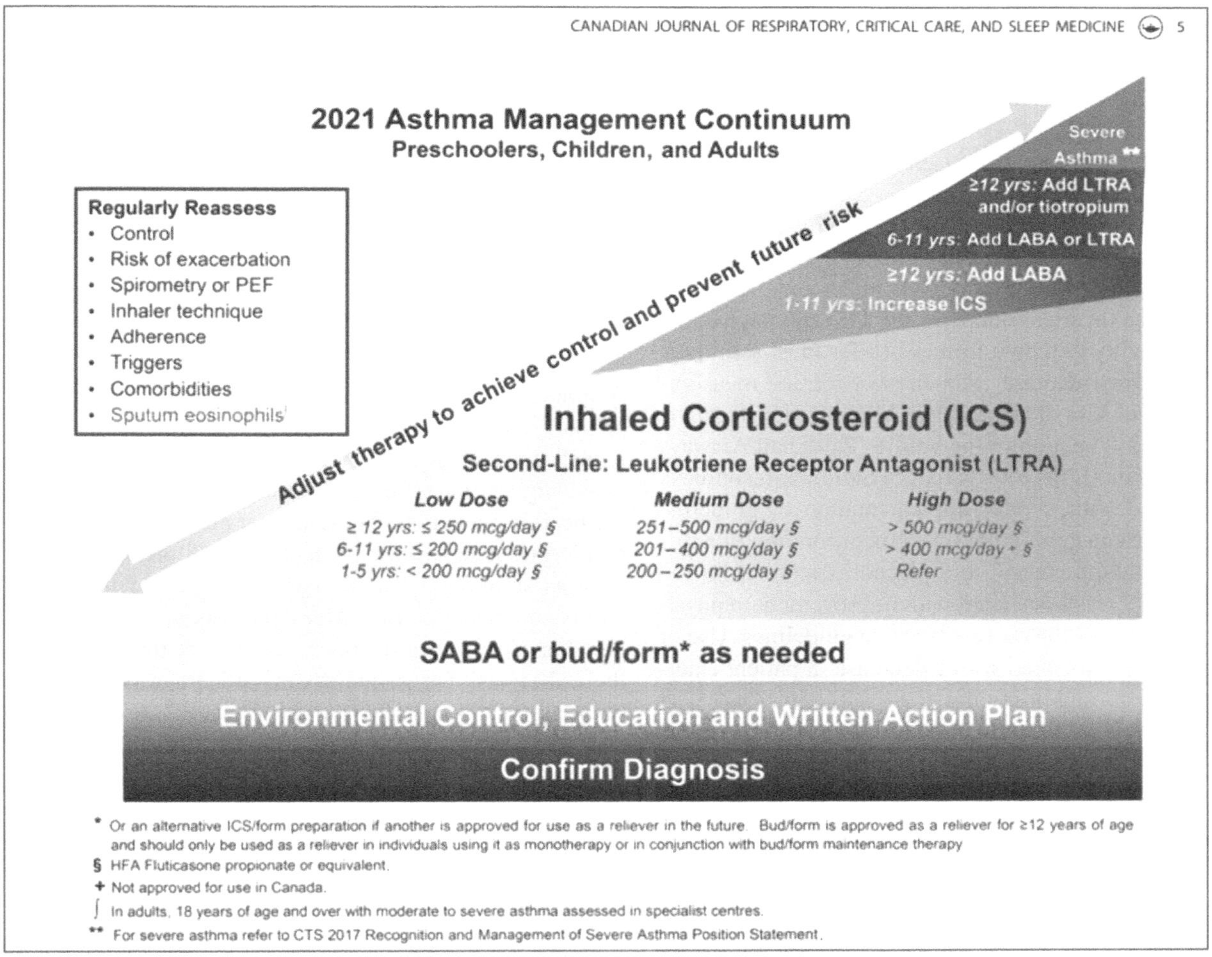

FIGURE 27.1 Extract from the 2021 Canadian Asthma Guidelines. (© 2021 Canadian Thoracic Society, reprinted by permission of Taylor & Francis Ltd, http://www.tandfonline.com on behalf of © 2023 Canadian Thoracic Society.[22])

27.3 ASSESSING ASTHMA CONTROL

Clinicians require an approach to the uncontrolled asthma patient. Tools such as the ACT, the ATTAQ, the Asthma APGAR Score, and the ACQ have proven to be valid and reliable at quantifying asthma control, some in many languages. But as noted, most national and primary care asthma guidelines require more than a simple control score to guide asthma care, such as the additional questions and linked care algorithm of the Asthma APGAR tool. When available, the use of exhaled nitric oxide (FeNO) may also be helpful but can be expensive. While usually considered a test to identify out-of-control asthma, it may also be used to demonstrate to patients the impact of actually using their medications. In busy primary care practices where physicians address multiple conditions in any single visit, having a system and tools that quickly assess control that also guide the next steps may improve outcomes to a greater degree than a simple assessment of control status.

Physicians and other clinicians cite time constraints, discomfort in "confronting" patients about adherence, and limited knowledge of inhaler techniques as reasons to skip these steps and move forward with step-ups of therapy.[24] Failing to assess the common causes of poor or inadequate asthma control can result in a perception of a person having "difficult to control asthma" with resultant over-medication.[25] Stepping up may not result in improved outcomes if basics of care such as actually taking the medication (adherence) or having it reach the lungs (inhaler technique) are missed.

Unfortunately, while this makes sense in theory, only limited data are available on the impact of incorporation of these tools into routine practice. Implementation often depends on healthcare systems. In the UK, the payment is based on a quality outcome framework for most asthmatic patients and does increase frequency of routine measurements of control. Use of the Asthma APGAR, which can be found in the tools section of the Family Physician Airways Group of Canada (https://www.fpagc.com/tools-resources), was associated with greater implementation of guideline concordant asthma care in the US.[26] Incorporation of a different novel asthma control tool placed as a stamp in the patients' chart[27] was associated with improvement in physicians' knowledge of the current practice guidelines. Use of both tools were associated with a decrease in patient emergency room visits and hospitalizations.

27.4 ASSESSING INHALER TECHNIQUE

If inhaled medication does not reach the lungs, it will not work. Critical errors in inhaler technique are ones wherein no medication will reach the lung, such as failure to take off a device's cap or loading it improperly. Less obvious errors can include not coordinating inhalation and device triggering or even exhaling into the device. Accurate inhaler technique is essential to asthma control, even when adherence is otherwise perfect. Ensuring good inhaler technique can become an issue on several levels. First, healthcare professionals (HCP) including physicians, nurses, nursing assistants, pharmacists, and even respiratory therapists may not know all the proper techniques,[28] especially with the availability of multiple different inhalers. In observational studies, neither the HCP nor the patient demonstrated adequate inhaler technique more than half the time. When the health professional has a poor grasp of inhaler technique, who is competent to teach the patient?[29] The use of inhaler videos in the office can overcome this gap (see Chapter 15, this volume), Secondly, whose responsibility is it to teach this? Often it gets assumed that the next HCP such as the pharmacist will ensure this is done, but it does not actually happen. Even when well-taught, over time, technique can deteriorate and, if not corrected, will result in poor delivery of the medication into the lungs. Clinicians often prescribe medications in two or more different types of devices to a patient, which can cause confusion and errors. As a rule, a pressurized metered-dose inhaler (pMDI) needs to be inhaled with slow, deep inhalations to prevent medication impacting the back of the throat, while a dry powder inhaler needs to be inhaled forcefully for the medication to reach the lungs. The pMDI pushes the medication in, but the patient has to pull in the dry powder. Use of a valved holding chamber with a pMDI can minimize upper airway side effects and improve lung deposition.[30] Therefore, it is imperative that we all must take responsibility for ensuring proper inhaler technique by teaching and observing regularly. In some countries additional support is available from asthma educators including trained asthma nurses and pharmacists in the UK and certified asthma educators in Canada and the United States.

27.5 IDENTIFICATION OF AND EDUCATION ABOUT ASTHMA TRIGGERS

Asthma trigger assessment is an essential part of every primary care evaluation of asthma.[31] Even if the patient is well controlled, identifying and confirming methods to avoid triggers may prevent future exacerbations or allow a medication reduction. These triggers can be broken down to allergic, such as animals, plants, and foods, and irritants such as smoking tobacco or cannabis, wood fire smoke, and occupational causes. Many patients are aware of triggers but have just never been asked what they believe are their allergies. The primary care office can be the site of blood tests (IgE specific testing) to investigate allergens or even perform skin testing that is then linked with confirmatory history of problems on exposure. In other countries or regions, in-depth allergy assessment and initiation of immunotherapy is best considered part of shared care with an allergist (see Chapter 10). Shared care will be the focus of the later part of this chapter.

27.6 COMORBID CONDITIONS

Often overlooked but an important part of asthma and allergy evaluation is assessment for allergic rhinitis. Allergic rhinitis can be a substantial barrier to good asthma control.

Evidence shows that treating the nose helps the lung, and treating the lung helps the nose. *Allergic Rhinitis and Its Impact on Asthma* (ARIA) provides guidelines for allergic rhinitis in asthma.[32] Unfortunately, few practical tools have been developed to translate these guidelines into everyday practice. However, a few simple questions may begin this process, and many patients are aware of allergies and have been treating their allergic rhinitis using over-the-counter drugs and nasal sprays, which they may forget to report to you (see Chapter 8).

Other comorbidities[33] that can worsen asthma control and/or response to current therapies include GERD (gastro-esophageal reflux) and obesity.[34] GERD is often treated successfully in primary care and can improve asthma control. Some conditions may mimic[35] asthma including COPD, upper airway conditions like vocal cord dysfunction (VCD), and aspergillosis. Upper airway obstruction can often be diagnosed by reviewing the inspiratory loop on spirometry.

27.7 ASSESSING ADHERENCE

Adherence is a known barrier to management of all chronic diseases, and asthma is no exception.[36] A non-confrontational approach is preferable, and comments about medication adherence should be prefaced with comments such as, "Many people find it difficult to take all of their medications all of the time. During the past two weeks, how many days have you been able to take your medications?" Finding unexpectedly elevated fractional exhaled nitric oxide (FeNO) measurements can lead to a suspicion of adherence issues, as it is quite sensitive to use of ICS in most patients with non-severe asthma. Nonadherence is generally be divided between intentional and non-intentional.

27.7.1 Unintentional Nonadherence

Unintentional nonadherence includes forgetting medications or taking them incorrectly, for example, or poor inhaler technique. Reminders, medication placement near the site of a common activity, use of phone applications ("apps") or simplifying a complex therapy regimen can improve unintentional nonadherence. Knowing that failure to take the medication is unintentional saves the primary care office personnel the time that might be spent trying to convince the patient that they need the medication and allows them to move directly to problem solving with the patient.

27.7.2 Intentional Nonadherence

Intentional nonadherence may vary from inability to afford the medications to fear of side effects, concerns about medication dependency, failure to accept the diagnosis for multiple reasons including stigma, and failure to accept the chronic nature of asthma and need for daily therapy. One of the most common types of nonadherence is discontinuing medications when control is good—because symptoms are in abeyance. Intentional nonadherence will be more time-consuming to address. Motivational interviewing to establish patient goals and then align treatment with their goals can help improve adherence. For some solutions to intentional nonadherence, collaboration with others such as a social worker to identify financial resources or an asthma educator or pharmacist to help affirm the risk and benefit of asthma medication usage can be helpful and reduce time burden on office staff.

27.8 ASSESSING LUNG FUNCTION

The diagnosis of asthma[37] is based on a history of characteristic symptom patterns and evidence of variable expiratory airflow limitation obtained with bronchodilator reversibility testing with spirometry. If spirometry is normal, a bronchial provocation test, wide variability during peak flow monitoring, or wide variation in FEV_1 from visit to visit, or a 200 ml or 12% increase in FEV_1 after a trial of ICS treatment can confirm the diagnosis. It is important to try to confirm the diagnosis of asthma before starting daily maintenance or controller treatment to avoid inappropriate treatment or missing other important diagnoses.[38] Diagnosis is often more difficult later after therapy is started.

Ideally, by most guidelines, spirometry is recommended for the confirmation of reversible airflow obstruction and therefore a diagnosis of suspected asthma in adults and children over ages 5–7 years. Good-quality spirometry with reliable interpretation is an important tool for primary care practices[39,40,41] and should be available for assessment of asthma diagnosis,[42,43,44] especially in those with less clear clinical assessment for asthma, when trying to differentiate COPD from asthma and for patients whose asthma is difficult to control or requires multiple therapies. The data to support the use of spirometry for monitoring asthma care are less sound. The SIGN guidelines suggest spirometry for monitoring difficult to control asthma and for people with occupational exposures in order to assess possible reversible lung function when exposed and disease progression. Yearly spirometry in stable asthma has not been shown to improve outcomes.

When spirometry is available on site, problems may arise related to the quality of tests performed and the accuracy of the interpretation of the results.[45] Sharing spirometry care with a respiratory therapist, a respiratory nurse specialist, another primary care physician with expertise in performing quality assured spirometry, or a specialist in this field may improve both the quality of the tests performed and the interpretation and use of the results for clinical practice. In fact, working together to make high-quality-assured spirometry available to primary care patients may be a first simple step to implementing shared care as part of ensuring that we systemize care to ensure the best outcomes (Table 27.1).

Many primary care practices do not have onsite or easily accessible spirometry testing. Peak flow monitoring can be done at home or in the office and has been suggested for monitoring some people with asthma, especially poor symptom perceivers,[46] but is less sensitive in confirming an asthma diagnosis. It can also be an adjunct for diagnosis in

TABLE 27.1
Systematizing Primary Care for Asthma

- Ensure or confirm an accurate asthma diagnosis.
- Consider supplementing asthma visits with routine telephone reviews.
- People and families with asthma require asthma and device education with regular reviews based in primary care.
- When available, enhance care and education with an asthma educator or respiratory nurse.
- The review should incorporate a written action plan.
- Maintain and use a register of people with asthma to support regular care.
- Use structured and standardized reviews of asthma to ensure all aspects are covered.
- Audit and feedback to clinicians and office staff should link guideline recommendations to the management of individual patients.

TABLE 27.2
Reasons for Referral for Additional Asthma Care

- Level of asthma problems (control and medication adverse effects)
- Recurrent or high risk of exacerbations, especially an asthma hospitalization
- Excessive use of systemic corticosteroids (greater than one course per year or any long-term use)
- Age of the person with asthma with special attention paid to the very young
- Inability of the primary care team to help the patient/family obtain and maintain adequate asthma control
- Number and type of trained asthma staff and expertise available in the local office
- Local availability and accessibility of other needed asthma support HCPs
- Primary care physician comfort and expertise in caring for people with asthma
- Financial and/or social issues

occupational asthma with improvement in peak flow during times away from exposures.

Some patients require more care or more intensive care than is feasible in the primary care office. While guidelines often define when patients with asthma should be referred for specialty care, that decision is best made by the physician and the patient and family. Some primary care teams are quite comfortable caring for patients with moderate to moderately severe asthma and do so. Other primary care teams have trouble caring for even mild or intermittent asthma, usually due to the lack of an asthma care system.

27.9 PRIMARY CARE TEAMS

Developing primary care teams and delegating responsibilities to appropriately trained individuals, rather than relying on physicians alone, is a major advance when developing care systems. Teams can help alleviate system deficiencies and facilitate implementation of the medical home concept.[47] In several countries that have national health systems, other groups of HCPs like asthma nurses have been developed to provide or supplement asthma care for those with stable asthma as well as with severe or difficult to control asthma. Some practice nurses are trained to provide routine asthma care and support the primary care physicians' practices.[48] Some sites define "specialty respiratory nurses" who see complicated patients and help monitor their asthma. Certified respiratory educators in Canada are required to pass examinations by the Canadian Network for Asthma Care and can be helpful in multiple facets of asthma care, where they are available. The final level of referral remains the specialist physician—an allergist or a respirologist/pulmonologist. All of these levels and layers should work together to provide shared care with clearly established roles and goals to improve long-term asthma care. Shared care can assure that the patient has access to the specialty services they need while retaining the whole-person care that all children and adults require, including care for other acute or chronic conditions and preventive services. This is also the basic premise of the medical home and family medicine.

27.10 SPECIALIST REFERRAL

The timing for referral of a person with asthma to additional services will vary based on many factors (Table 27.2). While guidelines have suggested benchmarks for referral, each guideline is a little different and not easily translated to a global set of recommendations. The primary care physician/team and the patient/family are the final arbiters of this decision. A request for additional care and support from either group should result in discussion of the referral, including what is desired from the referral and whether and how asthma care will also continue at the primary care site.

The Global Initiative for Asthma has clearly listed those people who are at increased future risk of exacerbations.[49] Although patients with poor symptom control are more likely to have exacerbations, patients with few or no symptoms can still have severe or even fatal exacerbations, usually from external triggers such as viral respiratory infections. Factors that increase a patient's future risk of exacerbations, even if they have few symptoms, include having had one or more exacerbations in the previous year, overuse of SABA (e.g. >2 canisters of short-acting beta-2 agonist per year,[50] inadequate ICS use (undertreatment, poor adherence, incorrect inhaler technique), some comorbidities (including obesity, chronic rhinosinusitis, gastroesophageal reflux, confirmed food allergy), a low forced expiratory volume in 1 second (FEV_1), a high blood eosinophil count or other markers of type 2 inflammation, and major psychological or socioeconomic problems.

Asthma exacerbations are important events to assess and attempt to prevent. They reduce a patient's quality of life,[51] may cause further loss of lung function,[52] may lead to the fixed airway obstruction[53] as seen in COPD, and increase the risk of mortality.[54] In addition, exacerbations almost always necessitate the use of systemic steroids, which have well-known deleterious side effects including psychiatric effects, risk of osteoporosis and fracture, diabetes, glaucoma, cataracts, and atypical infections.[55]

27.10.1 Communication in Shared Care

Communication is the biggest issue in implementing successful shared care. Before communicating, the primary care physician or team must consider three things: (1) Why is a referral being made? (2) To whom should communication be made? (3) What information should be shared with the referral, and what information do you want back following the referral? The purpose of the communication is to prevent some of the potential adverse outcomes of shared care, such as fragmented care; patient/family confusion due to multiple and differing healthcare messages; and patient and HCP uncertainty of the role(s) of each of the individuals involved in the patient's care. Inadequate communication can lead to failure to address the whole person and potential comorbidities in the context of developing asthma management plans. Each of these concerns can be addressed briefly in the referral communication. For example, in your referral letter or even on the asthma action plan, list the prescriptions that were issued in the previous 12 months and list the terms that you and the patient use to talk about asthma, reactive airway disease, recurrent wheezing, and so on. Be sure to include terms the primary care team uses to identify medications like inhalers, puffers, or rescue therapy in addition to outlining current and past medications prescribed and why changes were made. Share the asthma action plan to show specific instructions for patients like the use of rescue medications or acute medications, e.g. short-acting bronchodilators; controller, maintenance, or anti-inflammatory medications, e.g. ICSs; and combination medications or leukotriene modifiers. In addition, the referrer should detail medications prescribed or taken over the counter for comorbidities, such as allergic rhinitis including intranasal steroids or antihistamines. Therapies should also be outlined for any comorbidity such as depression, anxiety, and GERD, as well as noting the possibility of coexisting asthma and COPD so these can be considered in the consultant's care and recommendations and are not re-evaluated with the tests you have already completed.

The other times when communication needs to be maximized are the post-ER visit and post-hospital admission. These are both considered severe exacerbations by GINA and will likely have necessitated a course of systemic steroids, with their intrinsic risks. Communication would be effective if it included barriers to control established at the visit, such as lack of adherence, trigger management, and inhaler technique. Management in hospital followed by treatment given on discharge will be important for the primary care clinician to reinforce continued care and management. Hopefully, some suggestions for management can help prevent further exacerbations but also the recommended follow-up time suggested in primary care and other information about secondary care or an educational initiative would be important to know.

27.10.2 Referral Template Letters

Referral template letters have been created by many different organizations. While none have an evidence base behind them, they highlight the need for the transfer of appropriate information. The International Primary Care Respiratory Group has a resource available on their website, which is reproduced here (see Table 27.3). In this resource you see the emphasis on reviewing the clinical factors involved prior to referral. Issues like why the referral is being made now, how the diagnosis was made, the level of control, current and past treatments and their results, adherence, device technique, comorbidities, triggers, phenotypes, and social factors should be included. It is very important to state what follow-up you as the referrer anticipates, i.e. desired repeat specialty assessments and by whom and when should follow-up be done. Care for people with more severe illness or medication complications or those needing biologic treatments are more

TABLE 27.3
Suggested Content for Inclusion in a Referral Letter to a Specialist

- Reason for referral today/current concern (for example: poor control despite optimal treatment, to confirm diagnosis of asthma, for management suggestions; what is concerning or bothering the patient regarding their asthma)
- The criteria on which the original diagnosis was made if available (for example: symptoms; demonstration of reversibility, with PEF or spirometry)
- Duration of asthma
- Any measures of current control (including symptom scores, evidence of variable airflow dysfunction)
- Risk factors for poor outcome: (including exacerbations in the last year, poor inhaler technique, steroid use, hospitalization, need for mechanical ventilation, life-threatening asthma episodes)
- Current treatments and prescriptions issued in last 12 months (including: generic name, brand name, dosage, inhaler type)
- Inhaler technique checked by observing
- Adherence with asthma therapy checked against prescribing record
- How the patient understands their condition and its treatment
- Impact on quality of life
- Any concomitant rhinitis, eczema, or anaphylaxis. If so, how this is treated
- Smoking history; (including: pack-years; quit attempts; motivation to quit)
- Exposure to pollution
- Other factors in a patient's life (such as depression, psychological factors, etc.) that may affect asthma management, which the difficult-to-manage asthma service could offer support better than primary care

Source: Modified with permission from the International Primary Care Respiratory Group (IPCRG).[56]

likely to continue under regular specialists' care. If you are using an electronic medical record, this could all be put in an electronic template to make the process faster and more efficient. Creation of an effective referral letter can be shared by the primary care HCP and asthma educators or asthma nurses if they are part of the care team.

Patients may get referred from an emergency or urgent care setting usually if they are a frequent visitor, recognized as a high-risk patient, or do not have a home for primary care medical care. In these cases, it may be more difficult but equally important to ensure that the patient will have follow-up care after the consultation.

In all situations, people with asthma should have their healthcare anchored in a setting that not only provides and coordinates care of asthma but also helps integrate asthma care into the care for the whole person. It is preferrable if the primary care setting is viewed as a medical home, which is now a concept around the world.

27.11 SHARING CARE WITH OTHERS BEYOND SPECIALIZED SERVICES

Involvement of family can reinforce messages, assess adherence and attitudes, and be the clinicians' eyes in the home. Empowerment of families[57] has been shown to improve control in children and adolescents[58] with asthma. For children, shared care will go beyond the patient, family, practice team, respiratory nurses, and specialists. Children spend a good portion of their day in school and often experience asthma problems during school. Adults commonly work outside the home and many preschoolers with asthma attend day care. Therefore, care will need to be shared with the school, work, or day care staff. In schools and in some workplaces, nurses are on-site all or part of each day. Many school and worksite nurses have limited asthma care knowledge or experience.[59] They require clear and thorough guidance in the assessment and treatment of asthma problems. This guidance is often provided in an asthma action plan that can be provided to both the person (family) with asthma and their school, day care, or work site.

Sharing care with schools has been expanded beyond care of those with identified asthma to include identifying those with asthma who remain unrecognized and undiagnosed.[60,61] In less developed countries, the International Study of Asthma and Allergies in Childhood (ISAAC) was successful in identifying those with potential asthma. Unfortunately, providing the required follow-up evaluation and care was often beyond the ability and resources of the county's healthcare system.[62] In both Canada and the United States, school-based asthma screening has not been found to be successful in identifying new cases; however, it was able to identify and help intervene in children whose asthma was out of control. Therefore, working with schools may facilitate the broad-based care anchored in the community that is likely to be most effective in improving asthma control, especially in children.

27.12 SUMMARY

Primary care HCP continue to have many opportunities to improve asthma diagnosis and its chronic continuing management and to reduce emergency and hospital-based utilization for asthma. This requires a willingness and ability to share care within the office team and with patients and their families, as well as to extend the shared management to include appropriate others from school, work, or day care personnel and to respiratory nurses/educators or asthma specialists. Asthma management is a team exercise, whenever teams can be mobilized. Teams are more likely to succeed when they include the patient and family and have an integrated management plan with a designated role for each member, from diagnosis to control measurements, management of causes of lack of control, and referral when appropriate with systems in place to ensure effective communication to reassess the process of care provision and patient outcomes so adjustments can be made when necessary.

REFERENCES

1. https://www.ipcrg.org/desktophelpers/desktop-helper-no-2-difficult-to-manage-asthma
2. Braman SS. The global burden of asthma. *Chest* 2006; 130:4s–12s.
3. Mannino DM, Homa DM, Pertowski CA, Ashizawa A, Nixon LL, Johnson CA, Ball LB, Jack E, Kang DS. Surveillance for asthma: United States, 1960–1995. *MMWR Morb Mortal Wkly Rep* 1998;47(SS-1):1–28.
4. WHO (World Health Organization). *Bronchial asthma.* Fact sheet no. 206. WHO, Geneva, www.who.int/mediacentre/factsheets/fs206/en. (Accessed 23 October 2011).
5. Bandiola C, Badiella L, Plaza V, Prieto L, Molina J, Villa JR, Cimas E. Women, patients with severe asthma and patients attended by primary care physicians are at higher risk of suffering from poorly controlled asthma. *Prim Care Respir J* 2009; 18:294–299.
6. Shah S, Sawyer S, Mellis CM, et al. Improving paediatric asthma outcomes in primary health care: A randomised trial. *Med J Aust* 2011;195:405–409.
7. Barton C, Proudfoot J, Amoroso C, et al. Management of asthma in Australian general practice: care is still not in line with clinical practice guidelines. *Prim Care Respir J* 2009;18(2):100–105.
8. Dharmage SC, Perret JL, Custovic A. Epidemiology of asthma in children and adults. *Front Pediatr.* 2019 Jun 18;7:246. https://doi.org/10.3389/fped.2019.00246. PMID: 31275909; PMCID: PMC6591438.
9. Vollmer WM, O'Hollaren M, Ettinger KM, et al. Specialty difference in the management of asthma: a cross-sectional assessment of allergists' patients and generalists' patients in a large HMO. *Arch Intern Med* 1997;137:1201–1208.
10. Yawn BP. The role of the primary care physician in helping adolescent and adult patient improve asthma control. *Mayo Clin Proc* 2011;86:894–902.
11. Grimshaw JM, Shirran L, Thomas R, et al. Changing provider behavior: An overview of systematic reviews of interventions. *Med Care* 2001;39:112–145.
12. Haynes RB, Ackloo E, Sahota N, et al. Interventions for enhancing medication adherence. *Cochrane Database Syst Rev* 2009;3:CD00011.

13. Burgers JS, Grol RP, Zaat JO, et al. Characteristics of effective clinical guidelines for general practice. *Br J Gen Pract* 2003;53:15–19.
14. Weinberger M. Seventeen years of asthma guidelines: Why hasn't the outcome improved for children? *J Pediatr* 2009;154:786–788.
15. Cabana MD, Rand CS, Powe NR, et al. Why don't physicians follow clinical practice guidelines. A framework for improvement. *JAMA* 1999;282:1458–1465.
16. Yawn BP, van der Molen T, Humbert M. Asthma management: Are GINA guidelines appropriate for daily clinical practice? *Prim Care Respir J* 2005;14(6):294–302.
17. Nathan RA, Sorkness CA, Kosinski M, et al. Development of the asthma control test: a survey for assessing asthma control. *J Allergy Clin Immunol* 2004;113(1):59–65.
18. Juniper EF, Bousquet J, Abetz L, Bateman ED. Identifying 'well-controlled' and 'not well-controlled' asthma using the Asthma Control Questionnaire. *Respir Med* 2006;100(4):616–621.
19. Yawn BP, Bertram S, Wollan P. Introduction of Asthma APGAR tools improve asthma management in primary care practices. *J Asthma Allergy* 2008;1:1–10.
20. Liu AH, Zeiger R, Sorkness C, et al. Development and cross-sectional validation of childhood asthma control test. *J Allergy Clin Immunol* 2007;119(4):817–825.
21. Yang CL, Hicks EA, Mitchell P, Reisman J, Podgers D, Hayward KM, Waite M, Ramsey CD. 2021 Canadian Thoracic Society Guideline—A focused update on the management of very mild and mild asthma. *Can J Respir Crit Care Sleep Med.* 2021;5(4):205–245. doi:10.1080/24745332.2021.1877043
22. Yang CL, Hicks EA, Mitchell P, Reisman J, Podgers D, Hayward KM, Waite M, Ramsey CD. 2021 Canadian Thoracic Society Guideline—A focused update on the management of very mild and mild asthma. *Can J Respir Crit Care Sleep Med.* 2021;5(4):205–245. doi:10.1080/24745332.2021.1877043
23. British Thoracic Society. *British guideline on the management of asthma: quick reference guide.* British Thoracic Society, 2011. http://www.sign.ac.uk/pdf/qrg101.pdf.
24. Bender B. Physician-patient communication as a tool that can change adherence. *Ann Allergy Asthma Immunol* 2009;103(1):1–2.
25. Hancox RJ, Le Souef PN, Anderson GP, Reddel HK, Change AB, Beasley R. Asthma: time to confront some inconvenient truths. *Respirology* 2010;15:194–201.
26. Yawn BP, Rank MA, Cabana MD, Wollan PC, Juhn YJ. Adherence to asthma guidelines in children, tweens, and adults in primary care settings: a practice-based network assessment. *Mayo Clin Proc.* 2016;91(4):411–421. https://doi.org/10.1016/j.mayocp.2016.01.010
27. Renzi PM, Ghezzo H, Goulet S, Dorval E, Thivierge RL. Paper stamp checklist tool enhances asthma guidelines knowledge and implementation by primary care physicians. *Can Respir J.* 2006 May–Jun;13(4):193–7. https://doi.org/10.1155/2006/825281. Erratum in: *Can Respir J.* 2006 Jul–Aug;13(5):279. PMID: 16779463; PMCID: PMC2683278.
28. Guidry GG, Roche N. Incorrect use of metered-dose inhalers by medical personnel. *Chest* 1992;101:31–33.
29. Fink JB, Rubin BK. Problems with inhaler use: A call for improved clinician and patient education. *Respir Care* 2005;50:1360–1374.
30. McIvor RA, Devlin HM, Kaplan A. Optimizing the delivery of inhaled medication for respiratory patients: the role of valved holding chambers. *Can Respir J.* 2018 Apr 4;2018:5076259. https://doi.org/10.1155/2018/5076259. PMID: 29849831; PMCID: PMC5904796.
31. Rank MA, Wollan P, Li JT, Yawn BP. Trigger recognition and management in poorly controlled asthmatics. *Allergy Asthma Proc* 2010;31(6):99–105.
32. Bousquet J, Schünemann HJ, Zuberbier T, et al. Development and implementation of guidelines in allergic rhinitis: An ARIA-GA2LEN paper. *Allergy* 2010;65(10):1212–21.
33. Haughney J, Price D, Kaplan A, Chrystyn H, Horne R, May N, Moffat M, Versnel J, Shanahan ER, Hillyer EV, Tunsäter A, Bjermer L. Achieving asthma control in practice: understanding the reasons for poor control. *Respir Med.* 2008 Dec;102(12):1681–93. https://doi.org/10.1016/j.rmed.2008.08.003. Epub 2008 Sep 23. PMID: 18815019.
34. Kaplan A, Kim J. Asthma exacerbations and glucagon-like peptide-1 receptor agonists: a review of the current evidence. *Pulm Ther.* Oct 17, 2022. https://doi.org/10.1007/s41030-022-00203-x
35. Helen K Reddel, Common conditions that mimic asthma. *Med J Aust* 2022; 216 (7): 337–340. || https://doi.org/10.5694/mja2.51467
36. Williams LK, Pladevall M, Hi H, et al. Relationship between adherence to inhaled corticosteroids and poor outcomes among adults with asthma. *J Allergy Clin Immunol* 2004;114:1288–1293.
37. Reddel HK, Bacharier LB, Bateman ED, Brightling CE, Brusselle GG, Buhl R, Cruz AA, Duijts L, Drazen JM, FitzGerald JM, et al. Global initiative for asthma strategy 2021: executive summary and rationale for key changes. *Eur Respir J.* 2022;59(1):2102730. https://doi.org/10.1183/13993003.02730-2021
38. Aaron SD, Vandemheen KL, FitzGerald JM, Ainslie M, Gupta S, Lemière C, Field SK, McIvor RA, Hernandez P, Mayers I, Mulpuru S, Alvarez GG, Pakhale S, Mallick R, Boulet LP; Canadian respiratory research network. Reevaluation of diagnosis in adults with physician-diagnosed asthma. *JAMA.* 2017 Jan 17;317(3):269–279. https://doi.org/10.1001/jama.2016.19627. PMID: 28114551.
39. Dombkowski KJ, Hassan F, Wasilevich EA, Clark SJ. Spirometry use among pediatric primary care physicians. *Pediatrics* 2010;126(4):682–687.
40. Poels PJ, Schermer TR, Thoonen BP, Jacobs JE, Akkermans RP, de Vries Robbe PF, Quanjer PH, Bottema BJ, van Weel C. Spirometry expert support in family practice: a cluster-randomised trial. *Prim Care Respir J* 2009;18(3):189–197.
41. Gillette C, Loughlin CE, Sleath BL, Williams DM, Davis SD. Quality of pulmonary function testing in 3 large primary care pediatric clinics in rural North Carolina. *N C Med J* 2011;72(2):105–110.
42. Holton C, Crockett A, Nelson M, Ryan P, Wood-Baker R, Stocks N, Briggs N, Beilby J. Does spirometry training in general practice improve quality and outcomes of asthma care? *Int J Qual Health Care* 2011;23(5):545–553.
43. Kaplan A, Stanbrook M. Must family physicians use spirometry in managing asthma patients? YES. *Can Fam Physician.* 2010;56(2):126–128.
44. Rebuttal: Must family physicians use spirometry in managing asthma patients? *Alan Kaplan, Matthew Stanbrook Canadian Family Physician* 2010 Feb;56(2):e4.
45. Yawn BP, Enright PL, Lemanske RF, Israel E, Pace W, Wollan P, Boushey H. Spirometry can be done in family physicians' offices and alters clinical decisions in management of asthma and COPD. *Chest* 2007;132(4):1162–1168.

46. Brusasco V. Usefulness of peak expiratory flow measurements: is it just a matter of instrument accuracy? *Thorax* 2003;58:375–376.
47. O'Dell ML. What is a patient-centered medical home? *Mo Med.* 2016 Jul–Aug;113(4):301–304. PMID: 30228482; PMCID: PMC6139911.
48. Lindberg M, Ahlner J, Ekstrom T. Asthma nurse practice improves outcomes and reduces costs in primary health care. *Scand J Caring Sci* 2002;16:73–78.
49. Global Strategy for Asthma Management and Prevention. Available at: https://ginasthma.org/reports/
50. Nwaru BI, Ekström M, Hasvold P, Wiklund F, Telg G, Janson C. Overuse of short-acting β(2)-agonists in asthma is associated with increased risk of exacerbation and mortality: a nationwide cohort study of the global SABINA programme. *Eur Respir J.* 2020;55(4).
51. Briggs, A., Nasser, S., Hammerby, E. et al. The impact of moderate and severe asthma exacerbations on quality of life: a post hoc analysis of randomised controlled trial data. *J Patient Rep Outcomes* 2021;5:6. https://doi.org/10.1186/s41687-020-00274-x
52. Soremekun S, Heaney LG, Skinner D, et al. Asthma exacerbations are associated with a decline in lung function: a longitudinal population-based study. *Thorax*, August 3, 2022. https://doi.org/10.1136/thorax-2021-217032
53. Asamoah-Boaheng M, Farrell J, Bonsu KO, Oyet A, Midodzi WK. Association between medication adherence and risk of COPD in adult asthma patients: a retrospective cohort study in Canada. *Clin Epidemiol* 2022;14:1241–1254. https://doi.org/10.2147/CLEP.S370623
54. Tupper OD, Ulrik CS. Long-term predictors of severe exacerbations and mortality in a cohort of well-characterised adults with asthma. *Respir Res.* 2021;22:269. https://doi.org/10.1186/s12931-021-01864-z
55. Bleecker ER, Al-Ahmad M, Bjermer L, Caminati M, Canonica GW, Kaplan A, Papadopoulos NG, Roche N, Ryan D, Tohda Y, Yáñez A, Price D. Systemic corticosteroids in asthma: A call to action from world allergy organization and respiratory effectiveness group. *World Allergy Organ J.* 2022;15(12):100726. https://doi.org/10.1016/j.waojou.2022.100726.
56. https://www.ipcrg.org/resources/search-resources/referral-letter-for-difficult-to-manage-asthma-outside-uk
57. Kashaninia Z, et al. Effect of family empowerment on asthma control in school-age children. *Tanaffos* 2018;17:47–52.
58. Rhee H, Belyea MJ, Brasch J. Family support and asthma outcomes in adolescents: barriers to adherence as a mediator. *J Adolesc Health.* 2010 Nov;47(5):472–478. https://doi.org/10.1016/j.jadohealth.2010.03.009. Epub 2010 May 14. PMID: 20970082; PMCID: PMC2963868.
59. Wilson KD, Moonie S, Sterling DA, Gillespie KN, Kurz RS. Examining the consulting physician model to enhance the school nurse role of children with asthma. *J Sch Health* 2009;79(1):1–7.
60. Yawn BP. Asthma screening, case identification and treatment in school-based programs. *Curr Opin Pulm Med* 2006;12(1):23–27.
61. Moricca ML, Grasska MA, BMarthaler M, Morphew T, Wiesmuller PC, Galant SP. School asthma screening and case management: Attendance and learning outcomes. *J Sch Nurs* 2013;29(2):104–112.
62. Ellwood P, Asher MI, Beasley R, Clayton TO, Stewart AW. ISAAC Steering Committee. The international study of asthma and allergies in childhood (ISAAC): Phase three rationale and methods. *Int J Tuberc Lung Dis* 2005;9(1):10–16.

Index

Note: Page numbers in *italics* indicate a figure and page numbers in **bold** indicate a table on the corresponding page.

Q

R

S

T